Cannabis in Medicine

Kenneth Finn

Editor

Cannabis in Medicine

An Evidence-Based Approach

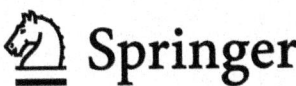 Springer

Editor
Kenneth Finn
Springs Rehabilitation PC
Colorado Springs, CO
USA

ISBN 978-3-030-45967-3   ISBN 978-3-030-45968-0   (eBook)
https://doi.org/10.1007/978-3-030-45968-0

This Springer imprint is published by the registered company Springer Nature Switzerland AG
The registered company address is: Gewerbestrasse 11, 6330 Cham, Switzerland

Equo ne credite, Teucri. Quidquid id est,
timeo Danaos et dona ferentes
    – Publius Vergilius Maro, 19 B.C.

Medicus necesse est dicere quod possit ex
antecedentibus, quia praesens et futura
dicamus - haec medium est, et in intuitu
obiecti specialem duo de morbo, scilicet
facere bonum non est non nocere
    – Hippocrates, Of the Epidemics, 400 B.C.

Dedicated to those who have been affected
or have lost loved ones to any substance of
abuse and addiction, including marijuana,
and to the memory of Peggy Mann, and other
pioneers, not afraid to speak the truth.

Foreword

Losing Ground: The Rise of Cannabis Culture

Addressing the Wider Implications of Increasing Marijuana Use

Why Our Knowledge of the Risks in Cannabis Exposure Has Increased

As ongoing science enhances our understanding of the health risks of cannabis/ marijuana exposure, two dimensions of the problem have been revealed. First, the range of health concerns has grown. Second, our confidence has grown that the risk lies in the impact of cannabis exposure itself, as an independent variable, rather than in a constellation of potential confounders.

To be sure, genetic propensity and co-morbidity issues affect the risk of cannabis exposure, placing some populations at higher risk than others, but the exposure to cannabis has a clear effect on the course of the propensity and/or the expression of the co-morbidity over and above the simple fact of a predisposition.

More broadly, of the known health concerns that were visible in research over the past 20 years (to pick an arbitrary period), it is reasonable to argue that few have been allayed or disconfirmed, while the majority of concerns have been not only confirmed but, in several instances, rendered even more worrisome, fraught, and widespread in terms of populations affected and the severity of the effects.

Results are surely still contested, but in general cautions are increasingly becoming questions more of the persistence and depth of the effects, rather than rejection of the validity of strong correlations between cannabis exposure and increased risk of negative effects.

Studies increasingly support some attributional role to the elements of cannabis themselves as producing risk and, in some instances, even strengthen suspicions of a more direct or even causal role from cannabis exposure, particularly when prolonged. This generalization seems to hold especially regarding susceptibility to psychotic episodes and other emotional or cognitive adverse outcomes.

A major reason for the growing confidence in findings of negative health effects has been a series of changes affecting both the cannabis drug itself as currently marketed, as well as the power and subtlety of the research methods brought to bear on our understanding of the effects.

Simply put, the science has changed, growing more robust, as the drug and exposure to it has changed, the result being a more urgent sense of individual as well as population damage.

Specifically, the science informing our portrait of cannabis consequences has become more refined and more grounded in neurophysiology, as better techniques utilizing brain scans or animal models increasingly show what appear to be profound changes in brain physiology and function under certain circumstances of exposure.

In addition, wider and more careful evaluation of the consequences of *in utero* and perinatal exposure (as well as the potential impact of exposure of infants through maternal use and lactation) are all informing our understanding of the basis for epidemiological and behaviorally based evidence long seen with regards to the consequences of cannabis exposure.

That is, widespread population findings are now being provided with enhanced biologically based cognitive and neurophysiological reinforcement that the impact of cannabis consumption produces elevated behavioral and mental performance risks.

The drug as consumed likewise has changed from as recently as 20 years ago, not only with respect to average potency on the market (rising from roughly 3% THC to a national average of no less than 15% THC for smoked marijuana plant material), but further with respect to the relative market share of high potency product. Potency is not only rising as an average, but the proportions available in the commercial market are also shifting upwards towards higher potency smoked cannabis, such as found with sinsemilla, averaging nearly 20% potency, becoming the market standard.

Today, with respect to the "industrialized" ultra-high potency product accelerated by commercialization (still reportedly replete with heavy metal and fungal contaminates), we find available potencies routinely ranging from 20% THC to upwards of 40% as found in smoked joints filled with plant product, now supplemented by new products presenting concentrates of nearly pure THC (reported at 60–90% potency) capturing high-end commercial market share.

One corollary of these changes in potency is that longitudinal studies of youth, begun several years in the past, are therefore based on THC exposure at relatively low potencies, and as such their findings may not be reliably projected onto the impact that today's initiates may experience over their lifetime, given the far stronger doses that constitute their initiation experience.

That is, the marijuana of the past has been supplanted by a drug with qualitatively different characteristics and potential impact, with changes even found in shifting ratios of the cannabinoids presented (smaller percentages of CBD, for instance, diminished in favor of concentrated THC). Moreover, while there is evidence of some positive or at least ameliorative effect from CBD exposure, there are concerns that greater doses of CBD may produce biphasic responses. This potential is only now being explored. Nevertheless, much of the modern commercial product has been deliberately selected for THC concentration at the expense of other cannabinoids, such as CBD.

Moreover, early blandishments from cannabis activists that such changes in the product, showing increasing potency of THC, were not "real" but were a function of measurement artifacts, or second if the changes were "real" that they need not signal greater ingestion of THC because users might titrate their dosages, or even arguments that stronger doses at higher potencies would not necessarily present greater risks of intoxication and potential dependency profiles, have all been shown to be illusory reassurances.

Instead, we have learned that users, especially naïve users, do not show a profile of careful titration, but instead seem to be getting dramatically more intoxicated, for longer periods than heretofore, coupled with growing evidence [1] that higher potency exposure is indeed correlated with increased risk of dependency or the onset of Cannabis Use Disorder (CUD).

Further, the modes of consumption of cannabis (principally THC) have changed, largely as a function of commercialization, generating not only new products but also new forms of their being consumed, such as in the form of edibles or drinks, or concentrated forms of the drug consumed no longer as smoked leaves but rather as forms of "shatter" or purified THC extraction products, often "vaporized" rather than smoked, or orally ingested.

One potential effect of such novel products is that our surveys of self-reported usage, especially by youth, are rendered less reliable as a measure of cannabis prevalence, since survey questionnaires built around models of smoked leaf consumption struggle to capture the proportions of consumption represented by the new modes of ingestion.

Increasingly, for instance, we learn that "edibles" [2] may now represent as much as half of new youth consumption, according to sales data from state dispensaries [3], while questions concerning "vaporizing" over and beyond "smoking" are only now being incorporated into standard youth surveys.

That is, the overall reliability of our measures of use is declining, and changes in the relative trajectory of youth use, in particular, are becoming less certain because of survey discontinuities (in particular, changes to the NSDUH survey methodology leading to a discontinuity with years prior to 2001).

The changes to the drug itself, and our means of detecting its effects, are intersecting with yet additional changes in the patterns of consumption, particularly by youth at developmentally susceptible periods. The window of susceptibility for developmental impact ranges from early adolescent exposure (not uncommonly at ages 12–15) up through early adulthood, at ages 18–25, when brain development still presents a vulnerability.

It should trouble us, for instance, that the age group showing the greatest increase in cannabis prevalence rates is the young adult population ages 18–25, as found in national surveys. Though subjects are in early adulthood, in terms of brain development they are still at a vulnerable period for negative cannabis effects to become long-standing adult problems.

Further, many of this age group live in a college or university setting, where nearly half of the student population is still legally underage for legal commercial purchase, comingling there with the young adults who are not only the heaviest users but are "legal" commercial product consumers. Do colleges present a particular domain of underage access to high-potency commercial cannabis acquired from peers?

Not only are more youth now exposed to cannabis markets as a function of state legalization and the rise of commercial markets, but the patterns of use are increasingly intensifying, in the sense that the frequency of use in youth populations is moving towards daily or near-daily exposure.

For instance, data from the largest national survey of drug use (discussed in detail below) show that the percentage of users of marijuana within the past year who used "more than 300 days" during the past year has risen steeply, from 12.2% of the total in 2002 to 19.8% of Past Year users in 2017, the most recent data available.

Hence, not only are more people using cannabis today than before, but they are using the drug more frequently, and at considerably higher potencies than before.

That is, a larger share of youth and young adult users, in particular, is gravitating towards a profile of use that presents the greatest developmental threat: frequent, repeated exposure at a developmentally sensitive period, an exposure that moreover is sustained for multiple years. The risk of developing Cannabis Use Disorder (CUD), for instance, becomes more pronounced with every year of use; according to recent research, for each succeeding year of exposure after initiation, the percentage of users experiencing CUD increases [4] steadily, rising to more than 20% of users at the fourth year of use beyond initiation.

As we have noted, longitudinal studies of the impact of early exposure traced over time into adulthood are worrisome enough, without taking into account that the THC potency routinely encountered at first exposure was likely a fraction of what an early adolescent is presented with today. This fact leads to the realization that the true developmental impact of early exposure, traced into maturity, is likely to understate the current potential impact, as the career of users initiating with high-potency THC products and then progressing to daily use at an early age has not yet been seen in current longitudinal studies.

In 1992, only 9% of Past Month cannabis users reported being heavy users (25 or more days per month). By 2014, that figure had risen to 40%. Recent analyses of dispensary users show that those "daily/near-daily" users consume about three times as much per day of use as less-frequent smokers and are estimated [5] to account for more than 80% of cannabis sales. Under the impact of high-potency THC consumption, tolerance progresses rapidly, and in order to sustain sufficient intoxication, dosages offered at unprecedented levels are now a routine share of all cannabis sales, and are escalating.

Hence, the damage that we observe today is best understood as a retrospective grasp of the consequences of cannabis exposure from a period when, in relative terms, the drug was less dangerous, while the impact of adolescent exposure today has as yet to be manifested, and is likely far worse than we have yet to witness. The future may yet reveal a greater risk for early, frequent, high-potency use than we have anticipated.

These changing factors taken together will likely produce an enhanced understanding of the "disease burden" of greater cannabis prevalence following from "legal" commercialization, and resultant normalized attitudes towards ingestion in the wider society, and the likely correlative impact of heavy cannabis use on the use of other substances of abuse.

That "burden" may considerably exceed our current estimates, and even require us to rethink our sense of the "ranking" of drug threats, with vastly greater cannabis prevalence elevating substantially whatever impact is found at the individual level.

That is, this current experiment with cannabis, underway nationwide, is leading us towards a future of unanticipated consequences, a future already established in the patterns of use "seeded" in the population but as yet unmanifested.

To be sure, studies of cannabis risk are largely "correlational" or show "associations" with relative risk, and are not clear demonstrations of cannabis "causality," a rarity in any epidemiological undertaking.

Nevertheless, the correlations are compelling, especially when there is found a robust relative risk signal, a demonstration of a dose-response relationship between the exposure and the impact, and plausible biological pathways or mechanisms for the exposure to be linked to the effect, such as found in studies of brain development and in animal models.

Moreover, critics of the notion that cannabis exposure is causally linked to negative effects often fail to recognize that the "correlation" arguments constitute not just single dimensions of damaging effects, limited to one domain of biological consequences, but rather present a striking and wide-ranging "constellation" of studies and effects across a wide horizon of biological domains. What we increasingly see in research reports is a convergence of findings regarding cannabis risk that are mutually reinforcing.

That is, the dangers of exposure are found not only in brain physiology and function, ranging across a variety of functions and performances including cognition, memory, emotion, motivation, and potential psychological pathologies, but are further compounded by multiple behavioral studies and outcomes, involving school performance, lifetime achievement, susceptibility to social pathologies and disorders, and troubling propensities, such as suicide [6] risk.

In general, the literature shows not only multiple negative effects on large proportions of regular cannabis users, but we learn that for some specialized populations, such as those with mental or genetic predispositions or histories of pathologies or co-morbidities, cannabis exposure can be elevated beyond the risky to the level of the catastrophic, involving psychotic breaks and dissociations.

An added perversity is that many advocates, as well as those promoting greater commercial access and use of the drug, encourage exposure for populations already known to be at risk, such as sufferers of Post Traumatic Stress Disorder (PTSD), pregnant or nursing women, those with compromised immune systems, or those already at risk from substance use disorders, such as dependent opioid users.

That is, populations at high risk of developing cannabis abuse disorders and suffering disproportionately the consequences are being, perversely, targeted with messages to use cannabis as a putative protection or relief from their condition, either through so-called "medical marijuana" programs found in multiple states or through commercial, "recreational" market advertising and promotion. There are even direct targeted inducements [7] for pregnant women to consume marijuana to ease their afflictions, or unproven efforts to provide cannabis as an alternative to medications available for opioid use disorder, or even as a pain management regime thought to be superior to opioids.

In summary, each of these factors, when taken together, renders what dangers we thought were likely risks, as seen in the current literature, as being in fact likely understatements of the real risk now presented to the generation now affected, those coming of age in the era of a normalized, widespread, and aggressive market promoting drug exposure.

Limitations to Our Knowledge: Inadequate Measures, No Real Baseline

Before turning to current data showing the extent of cannabis use, it is important to stress the dismaying limitations on our knowledge. In some measure because drug use has been an illicit activity, our grasp of the true scope of prevalence, as well as accurate trajectories of change, has been deficient, perhaps presenting more uncertainty than found for any other large-scale medical challenge.

There are three major surveys providing information on use at the national level. The National Survey on Drug Use and Health (NSDUH), run under the auspices of the federal Department of Health and Human Services, is performed annually on a sample population of roughly 70,000 persons, with summed state-level data being reported every 2 years. The scope of coverage is taken to represent all Americans aged 12 and older living in households.

In addition, there are two surveys directed specifically at the youth/young adult population. Monitoring the Future (MTF) is conducted, under a grant from the National Institute on Drug Abuse (NIDA) to the University of Michigan, in select high schools (with a separate college age population segment), reporting on 8th, 10th, and 12th grade drug use. MTF routinely samples, on an annual basis, approximately 44,000 youth. The 12th grade data extend back to 1975, while the addition of 8th and 10th grade data begins since 1991.

The third is the Youth Risk Behavioral Survey (YRBS), overseen at the state level by the Centers for Disease Control (CDC). This survey is biennial, and questions a wide array of health-risk behaviors, only some of which behaviors include a substance use component. Prevalence rates are affected by the setting of the survey instrument, with school-based responses commonly exceeding those reported from households. Limitations on the YRBS as a national-level survey, (such as low response rates, incomplete state coverage, and even under-coverage within states – the Colorado YRBS version has not had participation from the largest school district since 1995) render it less useful for our purposes.

None of the three surveys is an ideal surveillance instrument for a variety of reasons, the most prominent deficiency being that they all rely on self-reports of behavior, with the reports not subject to any objective evidence of actual exposure.

Moreover, the coverage of the sample populations presents an inherent limitation, given that either residence in stable households or current school attendance are necessary preconditions in order to be captured in the survey response. Hence, we may be systematically missing the very population most at risk for heavy substance use, since they may have suffered attrition from the sample population, being found neither in stable households nor enrolled in school.

While it is possible to supplement the findings of these surveys by reference to data such as drug-related arrests, incarcerations, treatment admissions, and hospital emergency department episodes, efforts to capture these data at the national level are inadequate, and poorly funded.

In fact, several sources of supplemental federal data on populations most at risk, such as the nationwide data-collections known as the Drug Abuse Warning Network (DAWN), which was focused on emergency department admissions (and/or mortality data), or the Arrestee Drug Abuse Monitoring (ADAM) program, focused on law enforcement intake populations, are currently unfunded at the national level, their operation suspended under the Obama administration.

Finally, though we can review the most recent survey reports (restricted in this discussion to the most reliable instruments, the NSDUH and the MTF), it remains a surprising fact that analysts at the federal level face considerable uncertainty establishing either the volume of illicit substances produced domestically or globally (Supply), and have even less reliable information on the volume of such substances consumed, or the market value of the products (Demand).

It follows that authorities trying to implement national drug control strategies that integrate "supply reduction programs" with "demand reduction programs" are faced with the reality that measurements of both supply and demand are woefully uncertain.

The challenge is particularly acute when it comes to cannabis production and consumption, since the metrics may rely on metric tons of organic material, while the most consequential variable should be the quantity of intoxicant actually consumed. Obviously, a marijuana plant with average THC potency of 3% available for market consumption is simply not comparable to a concentrated chemical product sold at 70% THC. Hence, the true metrics of actual THC consumption are exceedingly uncertain.

Current Measurements of Marijuana Use Showing the Comparative Scope of the Problem

Deficiencies aside, we can nevertheless observe relative changes over time in the self-reported data, even acknowledging that important populations with heavy use are likely not being measured at all.

American society has been plagued by various forms of substances of abuse throughout its history. But until the later half of the twentieth Century they did not include widespread consumption of cannabis, particularly by youth.

Before chronicling the most recent findings regarding cannabis use in the USA, as reflected in the 2018 National Survey on Drug Use and Health (NSDUH), it is worth a momentary reflection on the contemporary status of alcohol consumption as reflected by the same measuring instrument.

Surely some of the disease burden of a substance like alcohol is a function of its legal status for adults, producing prevalence rates of routine use that are multiples greater than the rates of use of cannabis, prior to legalization. If the impact of commercial legalization produces for cannabis prevalence rates in emerging generations that approach those of alcohol use, not only will cannabis use itself register as a more grave public health problem than it has been, its use somewhat truncated by legal risk, but the resultant impact of the concomitant use of alcohol and cannabis as dual public health threats could well exceed the damage of either of the substances taken alone.

That is, the future may present us with an intensifying "additive" model of substance misuse, as emerging and increasing cannabis patterns of use intersect with already prevalent alcohol use, there being little support for the hopeful speculation that cannabis use might supplant, rather than complement, concurrent alcohol consumption. Needless to say, measures of their interactive effects are as yet poorly developed.

A second reason to view contemporary alcohol consumption is that it might prefigure the potential scale of future cannabis consumption, after legalization and normalization of cannabis use becomes the context in which future generations acquire their norms of substance misuse.

Alcohol is more widely used, to be sure. But at least some of the disparity in prevalence is a function of the heretofore inhibitory effect on cannabis use deriving from the fact of societal prohibition, backed by legal sanction. Once those legal sanctions are removed, at least for adults 21 and older, we might be seeing in alcohol use the potential scale to which cannabis use might well grow, once promoted, fully commercialized, and normalized for a generation or more.

Accordingly, for the use of alcohol, in 2017, according to the NSDUH survey, there were in the population 12 and older 140.6 million current (Past Month) alcohol users, 66.6 million of which were "binge drinkers," 16.7 million of which were "heavy drinkers" during the Past Month, while 7.4 million drinkers were "under-aged."

While by no means inevitable, we see at least a plausible model for the scale of nationwide cannabis use following full legalization, a figure approaching fully half of the American population 12 and older routinely consuming an additional addictive substance.

Moreover, it would be a substance, cannabis, that has its greatest negative impact relatively early in life, compared to the worst negative health effects of alcohol, most commonly manifested later in life after years of abuse. In this regard one may further note recent research arguing that cannabis exposure is even more damaging [8] to adolescent brain development than is alcohol exposure.

To grasp the scale of illicit drug use, and its steep recent rise, we should look to what NSDUH terms Past Month (or "Current") use for the set substances identified as constituting use of "Any Illicit" drug (which category is inclusive of marijuana use).

Retrospectively, for 2015, shortly after early state-level commercial legalization of marijuana, NSDUH reported that during the course of that year, Past Month use of "Any Illicit" drug in the population 12 and older stood at 27.1 million Americans.

Scarcely a year later, however, the 2016 figures show a rise to 28.6 million users, an increase of 1.5 million additional drug users. This increase of Past Month users was nearly 6% in a single year.

The main reason for the overall "Any Illicit" increase can be found in the increased use of marijuana, which rose between 2015 and 2016 from 22.2 million Past Month marijuana users to 24 million users, an increase of 1.8 million users. The increase was just over 8%.

Since those data came out, NSDUH has advanced one more year to 2017 data (the survey results are released in September of the succeeding year, so the 2018 NSDUH report contains the 2017 data).

First, the new figures for "Any Illicit" drug use: In 2017, 30.5 million Americans 12 and older (that's about 1 in 9 Americans) were Past Month users of "Any Illicit" drug. That rise once again represents a slightly greater than 6% increase in a single year over 2016's 28.6 million users. That is, in two short years we have witnessed an increase in regular illicit drug use of 12%.

More specifically, focused just on marijuana, the 24 million Past Month users from 2016 has now risen to 26 million users in 2017. Again, for marijuana use, for the second consecutive year, the rise is just over 8% in a single year – yielding slightly greater than a 16% rise in what could arguably be seen as the first 2 years of the period post commercialization.

Marijuana use far outstrips the self-reported use of any other "illicit" substance.

The second-ranked "illicit" drug used is found in the misuse of prescription analgesics, with 3.2 million Current or Past Month misusers.

From there, the numbers drop even further, with the third-ranked drug, cocaine, having no more than 2.2 million Past Month users, while both methamphetamine and heroin both report fewer than 1 million Past Month users.

The contrast with marijuana use, the first-ranked illicit drug by far, is striking. While still lower than current use of alcohol, currently, the estimated 26 million Americans 12 and older reporting regular marijuana use in 2017 far exceeds any other substance use problem (leaving aside the issue of tobacco). The 26 million persons corresponds to 9.6% of the population 12 and older, and as we have seen, the figure is increasing by 8% with each passing year.

Where, then, is the population limit? What happens to our calculation of the relative "disease burden" of marijuana compared to alcohol when the number of users moves towards parity? Bear in mind that we are just now discovering the impact of legalization, which is still recent and partial across the states.

Moreover, the NSDUH survey allows the breakdown [9] of the population 12 and older into age groups, those 12–17, those 18–25, and those 26 and older. In addition to Past Month use, they also inquire as to Past Year use and Lifetime use.

Past Year use shows an enormous segment of the American population engaged in regular drug use. For Americans 12 and older, for 2017, there were 51.7 million Past Year users of any illicit drug. Of these, there were 40.9 million Past Year users of marijuana, or 15% of the population 12 and older. (By way of contrast, for the second and third leading illicit drugs, 6.6% misused psychotherapeutic drugs and 2.2% used cocaine.)

The increase since 2008, when there were 25 million Past Year marijuana users, is a stunning 64%. The percentage of users for 2017 exceeds any year, based on data that track back to 2002, before which year the survey was rendered discontinuous because of changes in methodology. The increase is driven most by those aged 18–25 and by those 26 and older. In 2017, among those aged 18–25, Past Year use of marijuana stood at 11.9 million (34.9% of this age group).

Switching categories now to the more regular Past Month users, how are the drug usage patterns distributed? Of adolescents, 12–17 years old (those arguably most at risk for damage), 6.5% were Past Month (Current Users) of marijuana. That figure represents approximately 1.6 million adolescents.

For 18–25 year olds, 22.1% (more than 1 in 5) were Past Month marijuana users. The figure has risen in a statistically significant manner every year since 2012, when it stood at 18.7%. That figure represents about 7.6 million young adults.

For adults 26 and older, the percentage for Past Month marijuana use is 7.9%, nearly double of what it was in 2008 at 4.2%. The current percentage represents about 16.8 million adult Past Month marijuana users.

Summarized 2017 Findings in Brief Tabular Form for Past Month and Past Year Marijuana Use:

- NSDUH 2017 [10] (reported in 2018): among approximately 70,000 people 12 and older surveyed:

- Past Year Marijuana Use ages 12–17: 12.4%
- Past Month Marijuana Use ages 12–17: 6.5%

- Past Year Marijuana Use ages 18 and older: 15.3%
- Past Month Marijuana Use ages 18 and older: 9.9%

- Past Year Marijuana Use ages 18–25: 34.9% (the increase from 2007, which showed 27.5% using, is 27%)
- Past Month Marijuana Use ages 18–25: 22.1% (the increase from 2007, which showed 16.5% using, is 34%)

- Past Year Marijuana Use ages 26 and older: 12.2% (the increase from 2007, which showed 6.8%, is 79%)
- Past Month Marijuana Use ages 26 and older: 7.9% (the increase from 2007, which showed 3.9%, is 102%)

In addition to overall increases in prevalence, we also see the "intensification" of use patterns. For all ages 12 and older, among Past Year users, the percentage of "daily/near daily" marijuana use stands at 19.8%, and at 21.9% for those 18–25.

Among Past Month marijuana users 12 and older, the average number of days used during the past month is 14.5 days, while the percentage of Past Month users consuming marijuana "daily/near daily" is a remarkable 41.7%. (NSDUH [11] table 7.21 B).

For those Past Month users who are aged 12–17, 25.1% were "daily/near daily" users.

For the 22.1% of those aged 18–25 who are Past Month users, the "daily/near daily" percentage stood at 44.3%.

Use of marijuana on a "daily/near daily" basis is the pattern of exposure most likely to produce Marijuana Use Disorder (the term for Cannabis Use Disorder or CUD). For 2017, CUD in the Past Year was reported as 5.2% for the category of 18–25 year olds.

Cannabis Use Disorder (CUD) is rising, in general. Data [12] from the National Epidemiology Survey on Alcohol and Related Conditions (NESARC), comparing successive waves of data between the years 2001–2002 and the years 2012–2013, show that the prevalence of marijuana use more than doubled, which prevalence was accompanied by a large increase in CUD experienced within the past year, largely because of the increase in the number of users.

According to NESARC, nearly 3 in 10 marijuana users experienced CUD. (The rate of CUD among marijuana users, however, did not increase, potentially owing to the fact that the "pool" of new users may have dampened the overall rate of disorder; subsequent NESARC waves, especially given the steeply rising potencies now experienced, may disambiguate the factors behind changes in CUD rates.)

Moreover, based on the same survey data set, additional research [13] has shown that the increase in CUD prevalence was greater in states that had passed "medical marijuana" laws than in states that had not.

Marijuana Use in Sub-populations at High Risk

Even further insight [14] regarding our future threat can be seen in use of marijuana by specialized populations presenting particular risks.

For pregnant women, aged 15–44, 7.1% report using marijuana during the Past Month. This represents an increase since 2015, when it stood at 3.4%, of 108% in two years. On the whole 3.1% of pregnant women report "daily/near daily" marijuana use, up from 1.2% in 2015.

For youth aged 12–17 who are Past Year "daily/near daily" marijuana users, 15.5% report a co-morbidity of past month "heavy alcohol use" while 24.1% report a Major Depressive Episode (MDE).

On the whole 31.8% of Past Year "daily/near daily" marijuana users suffer a co-morbidity of past-year opioid misuse (reported by only 1.6% of non-marijuana users for this co-morbidity).

The corresponding figures for the age group 18–25, by Past Year "daily/near daily" marijuana use, are: 20.7% Heavy Alcohol Use, 17% past year Major Depressive Episode, and 24.1% past year Opioid Use Disorder, respectively, for the co-morbidities reported.

Monitoring the Future School-Based Data

Some additional insights on the scope of youth exposure can be gained from the Monitoring the Future Survey of high-school youth. MTF 2018 [15] is a school-based survey reporting on 44,482 students from 392 public and private schools, examining self-reported substance use amongst 8th, 10th, and 12th graders (as mentioned earlier, the trajectory for 8th and 10th grades begins since 1991, while reports from 12th graders have been gathered since 1975).

For 12th graders, 22% report Current, or Past Month, marijuana use (a rate that exceeds cigarette use, which has fallen to 7.6%; binge drinking, at 13.8%, has been in steady decline since 1998). Past Year marijuana use stands at 36.9%.

Of current enrolled students, 5.8% of 12th graders report daily marijuana use.

In a troubling recent development, 37% of 12th graders report vaping some substance, primarily nicotine, while the 13.1% report vaping marijuana or hash oil. The rise between 2017 (the first year that inquired about vaping) and 2018 for all grades reporting vaping marijuana is significant (for 8th and 10th graders, it is 63%).

For vaping marijuana (only), the rise for 12th graders is from 4.9% in 2017 to 7.5% in 2018, an increase of 53% in a single year.

It may well be that we are failing to capture the full extent of marijuana use prevalence because of the rise of vaping and consumption of comestible forms of the drug are only now being systematically included in the survey instruments.

Additionally, MTF [16] reports that marijuana use among college age students, seen among a cohort that they track beyond high school, has risen steeply. They report that 30-day use of marijuana has increased significantly by 5.1% across the past 5 years, ending in 2018 at 24.1%, an all-time high for the study. In fact, annual and 30-day marijuana use among young adults aged 19–28 are at the highest levels in the 33 years that MTF has been monitoring their use.

Finally, MTF has for years measured subjective norms regarding the acceptability of smoking marijuana, as well as asked concerning student perceptions [17] of risk in using. These two metrics are often seen as harbingers of future prevalence; for instance, when perceptions of risk rise, prevalence rates tend to fall shortly after. Disturbingly, therefore, we learn from the most recent MTF perceptions by high school seniors of harmfulness in regular use of marijuana have fallen from high of 78.6% in 1991 to only 26.7% in 2018, a fact which may well show the triumph of the misleading "medical marijuana" campaign.

Widening Societal Impact of Increased Marijuana Prevalence

It is disturbing to realize that no one knows the full societal impact of these kinds of drug use changes spreading into every sector of the nation. Surely we can expect some societal consequences, not least on educational attainment, on workforce performance, on economic attainment, and even military recruitment, over and above the consequences found in strictly public health or criminal justice dimensions.

A recent (and proprietary) publication from Baron Public Affairs, a risk-assessment firm that provides analysis and guidance to public policy and corporate decision makers, evaluated the possible impact of commercial marijuana in a document entitled "The Unintended Consequences of Marijuana Legalization."

While by no means exhaustive, their research nevertheless identified several areas of societal concern over the emerging levels of marijuana use, which concerns extend beyond just the public health and criminal justice impact.

The Baron report anticipated widespread impact on individual initiative and motivation, affecting the economic prospects not only for the generation of heavy users but for the wider economy. They noted such effects as those who smoked marijuana regularly had lower social class as adults than their parents experienced. They also had greater levels of welfare dependency and higher levels of unemployment.

Given further effects, such as those on family formation and collapsing social capital, Baron anticipated even greater social stratification, income inequality, greater damage to those with fewer economic resources, and greater class conflict.

Baron further anticipated a link to the multi-billion dollar opioid crisis, to which the coming marijuana epidemic will add further addiction and greater need for government services, welfare relief, and public funding, particularly for treatment purposes, to address the consequences of widespread marijuana use.

To these effects they add alarms concerning the available pool of warfighters and the potential erosion of military standards through either drug use waivers or tolerance of on-going use, which could render users compromised as decision-makers and vulnerable as security risks.

Even after the acute effects of intoxication have faded, users may experience reduced [18] cognitive/executive function, long-term, with strongest effect on adolescents.[19]

Finally, with regards to economic impacts, Baron notes that in one rural area, half of all job applicants were reported to have failed their employment drug test, which in a tight labor market is an obstacle to growth. In fact, data [20] from the largest national drug testing business, Quest, show that those who fail an employment drug test stands at its highest level (4.4% in 2018) in 14 years.

We are only at the beginning of the consequences of commercialization. The recent political calculus of both California and Canada to enter commercial marijuana markets has during the last 2 years added a combined population of nearly 77 million persons now living under "legal" marijuana regimes.

No wonder, as Baron concludes, has cannabis investment nearly quadrupled during the year 2018, built on major investments from well-established tobacco, pharmaceutical, and alcohol companies.

The Societal Impact of Expanded Cannabis Extends to the Use of Other Substances Of Abuse

First, we should recognize that trafficking networks for all drugs penetrate expanding marijuana markets. These criminal networks operate with a business model that is polydrug and polyfinance, operating with violence, coercion, and corruption as standard modes of behavior, capitalizing on addiction.

There are multiple ways in which the spread of marijuana prevalence is tied to the continued strengthening [21] of the illicit criminal market not only for marijuana but also for the trafficking in all illicit drugs, including the opioids.

Criminal organizations are polydrug traffickers, and wherever they establish a presence by capitalizing on the expanding commercial prevalence of marijuana, they begin to exploit their access to traffic other substances, thereby feeding [22] not only the opioid crisis (responsible for 47,000 of the overall 70,000 overdose deaths from all drugs in 2017) but further fueling the overdose crisis in cocaine (deaths rising rapidly to over 13,000 in 2017) and methamphetamine (contributing to over 10,000 deaths nationwide in that same year).

To take but one example, in Colorado [23], between 2015 and 2016, after steady rise since 2002, pharmaceutical opioid overdose deaths declined by 6%. But in that same year, overdoses from heroin increased 23% (subsequent data have shown that even the pharmaceutical overdose deaths have rebounded upward). Numerous communities, such as Pueblo, note that rapid expansion of homeless populations following the proliferation of marijuana dispensaries has been accompanied by increased trafficking and use of methamphetamine, illicit opioids, and cocaine, the effects of which can be observed in local emergency rooms.

Moreover, the financial profits accruing to the criminal cartels from marijuana sales serve to fund the full scope of their trafficking activities, supporting their capacity to insulate themselves not only financially but also politically.

To understand the broader relationship between adolescent drug use, including the initiation of marijuana, and the persistence of our current opioid overdose epidemic, we can turn to the work of Dr. Robert DuPont, a psychiatrist who is President of the Institute on Behavior and Health.

DuPont recently authored [24] *"A New Narrative to Understand the Opioid Epidemic,"* noting that for many opioid-addicted individuals, drug use frequently began in early adolescence, particularly with the use of alcohol and marijuana. "Early poly-drug use often sets the stage for later transition from medical to addictive use of opioids that are prescribed for pain. These patients' brains have been primed for the addictive response to opioids."

As DuPont notes, opioid overdose deaths nearly always involve the use of other addictive drugs, such as marijuana, cocaine, methamphetamine, and alcohol. About 95% of current opioid overdose deaths, according to studies of particular populations, involve other drugs, with an average of 2–4 and a maximum of 11 in addition to the opioids.

The standard overdose narrative, DuPont argues, overstates the degree to which physician prescribing of opioid medications is the primary pathway for overdose risk and ignores the significant role of adolescent initiation to drug use in the opioid overdose epidemic, occurring at older ages. While for many opioid addicted people their first use of an opioid was a prescribed opioid from a physician, it is also true that the majority of these individuals first used other drugs before or with their first use of opioids.

Further, only about 4% of people who use prescription opioids non-medically initiate heroin within 5 years of first prescription opioid use. For example, among 4493 individuals treated for opioid addiction whose first exposure to opioids was through a prescription from their physician, notably 94.6% reported prior or coincident use of other psychoactive drugs. Alcohol was used by 92.9%, and marijuana by 87.4%, and excluding these top substances, fully 70.1% reported other prior or coincident drug use.

The clear message is that in order to comprehensively address the current drug abuse crisis and accompanying fatalities, we must address early adolescent exposure to marijuana as a contributing factor.

Multiple accounts now found in the literature clearly show that cannabis use, especially persistent use of high-potency cannabis in adolescence, is a risk [25] factor for the development of subsequent opioid use disorder.

To take but one example, a 2017 study [26] using NESARC data found specifically that cannabis use is linked to prescription opioid disorder: "… cannabis use at wave 1 was associated with increased incident nonmedical prescription opioid use (odds ratio = 5.78) and opioid use disorder (odds ratio = 7.76) at wave 2."

As the Centers for Disease Control succinctly summarized [27] the matter, "People addicted to marijuana are three times more likely to be addicted to heroin." In addition, multiple studies, particularly using animal [28] models, show an effect of brain "priming" and "cross-sensitization" between cannabis exposure and opioid exposure. Overall, we are witnessing increasing validation of a marijuana "gateway" [29] effect on subsequent drug use. Indeed, there is increasing evidence [30] that "early marijuana use by itself, even after control for other covariates, increases [31] significantly the use of other illicit drugs."

Final Thoughts on the Wider Implications of Increased Use

The full scope of the potential negative effects of increased marijuana use, particularly as accelerated by commercial legalization, is now emerging, and the damage affects many domains of national life.

First, we should be concerned over the future impact of a marijuana "gateway" effect, whereby early adolescent exposure increases the risk of subsequent initiation of other addictive substances, and further heightens the risk of multiple drug use disorders in later life.

To the extent that the gateway thesis is validated, we can expect that the surging crisis in the use of drugs such as opioids, cocaine, methamphetamine, and other emerging synthetic drug threats will continue at an epidemic level, as widespread marijuana prevalence serves to feed vulnerable users into polydrug dependency and disorders.

Moreover, it is not just the users of such substances who are placed at risk, we recognize that major criminal enterprises, those that traffic lethal poisons, find in the "legal" marijuana market an open pathway for their operation, thereby enhancing their revenue, and reinforcing their violent and corrupting methods.

But the public health impact is not limited to the effect on users. We should acknowledge that the rise of "medical marijuana" treated as though it were a legitimate medicine approved through clinical trials, scientific rigor, and demonstrations of safety and therapeutic efficacy, shows the consequence of allowing a political process to supplant strict medical trials as the basis for legal acceptance.

As such, the integrity of the drug approval process itself, and the authority of the criteria upon which it is based, has been compromised by resort to illegitimate mechanisms.

Further, there are lessons to be learnt in how both "medical" and commercial marijuana progressed at the state level, in settings such as Colorado. Promises were made by advocates, seeking a political appeal to sway voter approval. Promises were made of enhanced state revenue sufficient to compensate for possible public health or law enforcement costs. Promises were made of more effective means for protecting youth from access to the drug. Promises were made of forcing out criminal activity, with its attendant violence, coercion, and fear. Promises were made of reducing supposed injustices in legal enforcement of anti-drug laws.

In fact, so appealing were the promises that the Obama administration's Department of Justice (DOJ) agreed to reorder federal prosecutorial priorities to enable state legislation to operate. In repeated memos from the DOJ we were told that there would be established certain "Red Lines," which, if crossed, would trigger an intervention on behalf of federal law. The "Red Lines" pertained to such issues as drug access by youth, or evidence of smuggling activities, or other signs of criminal activity.

Yet we cannot forget that those "Red Lines" were repeatedly, even flagrantly, violated in succeeding years, as multiple reports from the Rocky Mountain High Intensity Drug Trafficking Area (HIDTA) [32] joint law enforcement command readily demonstrated. But no federal intervention was triggered. (Further, we now see evidence at the state level that the promised taxation revenue has not been sufficient to cover the greater costs to society of increased prevalence, nor have certain putative benefits manifested, and that black market marijuana, offered more cheaply, has captured major market share.)

Suffice it to say that the promises have not been kept. Yet we now see them repeated at the national level.

So as we pull back the lens for a wider picture, we see not only a public health crisis affecting users and medical institutions, but an emerging criminal justice crisis, as the black market thrives in states that have approved commercial marijuana, and as violence, smuggling, and corruption have all persisted in support of strengthened criminal activity, which now seeks to insulate itself by gaining political [33] power.

As noted, there are now efforts in Congress to alter at the federal level not only the Schedule I status of marijuana but further enable banking and financial legislation that could threaten the integrity of the US financial system, were transnational criminal organizations could exploit the proposed changes to mask or launder illicit proceeds from their entire international operations.

If we pull the lens back even further, we now see the international impact of our failure to uphold federal drug law at the state level. Simply put, the position of the USA as the moral leader in drug control, and the primary protector of the global drug control enterprise, has been compromised.

Our international commitments, such as found in treaty obligations in partnership with the United Nations, have been countermanded. Our allies, themselves fighting transnational criminal organization, feel abandoned, and many are yielding the fight. Even US development objectives, seeking to strengthen not only international economies but human rights and democratic institutions, have been eroded by the threatened emergence of corrupt narco-states among international partner nations who once depended on us for protection.

That is, we can now count the costs of the spreading acceptance of legalized drug use as serving to damage not only public health and criminal justice, but national security as well.

None of these developments make our own borders more secure, nor our own citizens safer nor healthier. In fact, US interests and well-being may be facing a coming debacle of major dimensions through unprecedented drug use and the attending criminal attack on our institutions, financial as well as political.

It should finally trouble us greatly that all of these developments represent self-inflicted wounds, against which many have warned us. We may well find that we done no other than to enable a virtual Trojan Horse in our midst, a development likely to occasion great regret.

David W. Murray, Ph.D.
Senior Fellow, Hudson Institute
Washington, DC, USA

Reference Section

[1] https://www.ncbi.nlm.nih.gov/pubmed/?term=Higher+average+potency+across+the+United+States+is+associated+with+progression+to+first+cannabis+use+disorder+symptom

[2] https://www.nytimes.com/2019/03/25/well/eat/marijuana-edibles-may-pose-special-risks.html

[3] https://www.greenentrepreneur.com/article/324383

[4] https://www.ncbi.nlm.nih.gov/pubmed/30474910

[5] https://slate.com/business/2016/11/america-is-legalizing-marijuana-wrong.html

[6] http://www.biblioteca.cij.gob.mx/Archivos/Materiales_de_consulta/Drogas_de_Abuso/Articulos/cannabisdepresion.pdf

[7] https://www.cpr.org/2018/05/09/study-dispensaries-recommend-marijuana-to-pregnant-women-against-medical-advice/

[8] https://ajp.psychiatryonline.org/doi/10.1176/appi.ajp.2018.18020202

[9] https://www.samhsa.gov/data/sites/default/files/cbhsq-reports/NSDUHDetailedTabs2017/NSDUHDetailedTabs2017.pdf

[10] https://www.samhsa.gov/data/sites/default/files/cbhsq-reports/NSDUHDetailedTabs2017/NSDUHDetailedTabs2017.htm#lotsect7pe

[11] https://www.samhsa.gov/data/sites/default/files/cbhsq-reports/
     NSDUHDetailedTabs2017/NSDUHDetailedTabs2017.pdf
[12] https://www.ncbi.nlm.nih.gov/pmc/articles/PMC5037576/
[13] https://jamanetwork.com/journals/jamapsychiatry/fullarticle/2619522
[14] https://www.samhsa.gov/data/sites/default/files/nsduh-ppt-09-2018.pdf
[15] https://www.drugabuse.gov/related-topics/trends-statistics/infographics/
     monitoring-future-2018-survey-results
[16] http://monitoringthefuture.org/pubs/monographs/mtf-vol2_2018.pdf
[17] http://monitoringthefuture.org/pubs/monographs/mtf-overview2018.pdf
[18] https://ro.uow.edu.au/cgi/viewcontent.cgi?article=3163&context=sspapers
[19] https://www.ncbi.nlm.nih.gov/pubmed/19630709
[20] http://newsroom.questdiagnostics.com/2019-04-11-Workforce-Drug-Testing-
     Positivity-Climbs-to-Highest-Rate-Since-2004-According-to-New-Quest-
     Diagnostics-Analysis
[21] https://www.hudson.org/research/15034-the-false-arguments-
     for-legal-marijuana
[22] https://www.hudson.org/research/15168-return-of-the-cocaine-nemesis
[23] https://www.colorado.gov/pacific/sites/default/files/Opioid%20Use%20
     in%20Colorado%20-%20March%202017.pdf
[24] https://www.dfaf.org/wp-content/uploads/2018/11/Opioid-Narrative-3.pdf
[25] https://www.apa.org/monitor/2015/11/marijuana-brain
[26] https://ajp.psychiatryonline.org/doi/full/10.1176/appi.ajp.2017.17040413
[27] https://www.cdc.gov/vitalsigns/heroin/infographic.html
[28] https://www.nature.com/news/2006/060703/full/news060703-9.html
[29] https://www.hudson.org/research/12980-marijuana-threat-assessment-
     part-two-the-opioid-epidemic-fentanyl-deaths-and-marijuana
[30] https://pdfs.semanticscholar.org/676c/4c18c320654a5d9fc5c5df928cadc
     5e81d18.pdf
[31] https://www.researchgate.net/publication/10946401_Does_Marijuana_
     Use_Cause_the_Use_of_Other_Drugs
[32] https://rmhidta.org/files/D2DF/FINAL-%20Volume%205%20UPDATE%20
     2018.pdf
[33] https://www.chicagotribune.com/news/ct-marijuana-legalize-illinois-politics-
     campaign-funds-20190802-lfzjgrn5vnahdlbabfenuukpmi-story.html

Contents

Contributors

Salahadin Abdi, MD, PhD Department of Pain Medicine, Division of Anesthesia, Critical Care and Pain Medicine, The University of Texas MD Anderson Cancer Center, Houston, TX, USA

Reagan Anderson, MD Dermatology, Rocky Vista University, Colorado Springs, CO, USA

Catherine Murer Antley, MD Vermont Dermatopathology, South Burlington, VT, USA

Arpit Arora, MD Department of Medicine, Division of Hematology-Oncology, Division of Geriatric-Palliative Medicine, Department of Rehabilitation Medicine, New York University School of Medicine, New York, NY, USA

LaTisha L. Bader, PhD Women's Recovery, Denver, CO, USA

Jacquelyn Bainbridge, PharmD University of Colorado Anschutz Medical Campus, Skaggs School of Pharmacy and Pharmaceutical Sciences, Department of Clinical Pharmacy and Neurology, Aurora, CO, USA

Andrew Bauer, MD Boulder Neurosurgical Associates, Boulder, CO, USA

Marcio Sommer Bittencourt, MD, MPH, PhD, FACC Dalboni – DASA, São Paulo, Brazil

Hospital Israelita Albert Einstein & School of Medicine, Faculdade Israelita de Ciência da Saúde Albert Einstein, São Paulo, Brazil

Center for Clinical and Epidemiological Research, University Hospital & Sao Paulo State Cancer Institute, University of Sao Paulo, São Paulo, Brazil

Leeann M. Blaskowsky, MSN, NNP-BC University of Colorado School of Medicine, Department of Pediatrics, Aurora, CO, USA

Allen C. Bowling, MD, PhD NeuroHealth Institute, Englewood, CO, USA

Department of Neurology, University of Colorado, Aurora, CO, USA

Elizabeth Brooks, PhD University of Colorado, Aurora, CO, USA
Whole Health Innovation, Denver, CO, USA

Sigita Burneikiene, MD Boulder Neurosurgical Associates, Boulder, CO, USA
Justin Parker Neurological Institute, Boulder, CO, USA

Maria Demma Cabral, MD Department of Pediatric and Adolescent Medicine, Western Michigan University Homer Stryker M.D. School of Medicine, Kalamazoo, MI, USA

Grace S. Chin, PharmD, MS University of Colorado Anschutz Medical Campus, Skaggs School of Pharmacy and Pharmaceutical Sciences, Department of Clinical Pharmacy and Neurology, Aurora, CO, USA
St. Joseph's Hospital, Denver, CO, USA

Matthew Chung, MD Department of Pain Medicine, Division of Anesthesia, Critical Care and Pain Medicine, The University of Texas MD Anderson Cancer Center, Houston, TX, USA

John Cienki, MD Jackson Memorial Hospital, Miami, FL, USA

Ben Cort Cort Consulting, Longmont, CO, USA

Nazar Dubchak, MS Rocky Vista University, Parker, CO, USA

Robert L. Dupont, MD Institute for Behavior and Health, Inc., Rockville, MD, USA

Monica Dzwonkowski, MS Rocky Vista University, Parker, CO, USA

David G. Evans, Esq General Counsel, Cannabis Industry Victims Educating Litigators (CIVEL), Flemington, NJ, USA

Tyler E. Gaston, MD University of Alabama at Birmingham Epilepsy Center, Department of Neurology, Birmingham, AL, USA

Donald E. Greydanus, MD, DrHC Department of Pediatric and Adolescent Medicine, Western Michigan University Homer Stryker M.D. School of Medicine, Kalamazoo, MI, USA

Doris C. Gundersen, MD Department of Psychiatry, University of Colorado, Colorado Physician Health Program, Boulder, CU, USA

Jean R. Hausheer, MD, FACS Department of Ophthalmology, University of Oklahoma Health Sciences Center, Dean McGee Eye Institute, Lawton, OK, USA

Richard L. Hilderbrand, PhD Toxicology Consulting, Penrose, CO, USA

Sabina Hochroth, MS Rocky Vista University, Parker, CO, USA

Michelle Kem Su Hor, MD Springs Gastroenterology, PLLC Colorado Springs, CO, USA
Rocky Vista University, Parker, CO, USA

Edward Hulten, MD Fort Belvoir Community Hospital, Virginia, USA

Cicily Hummer, MS Rocky Vista University, Parker, CO, USA

Monica C. Jackson, PhD Department of Mathematics and Statistics, American University, Washington, DC, USA

Finny T. John, MD Department of Ophthalmology, University of Oklahoma Health Sciences Center, Dean McGee Eye Institute, Oklahoma City, OK, USA

Brian P. Kaskie, PhD University of Iowa, Department of Health Management & Policy, Iowa City, IA, USA

Esther Kim, BA Department of Radiation Oncology, New York University Langone Health, New York, NY, USA

Arum Kim, MD, FAAPMR Department of Medicine, Division of Hematology-Oncology, Division of Geriatric-Palliative Medicine, Department of Rehabilitation Medicine, New York University School of Medicine, New York, NY, USA

Sean Knight, MS Rocky Vista University, Parker, CO, USA

Tesia Kolodziejczyk, MS Rocky Vista University, Parker, CO, USA

Jesse J. LeBlanc III, BSME Engineering Advisor-Ret., League City, TX, USA

Maureen A. Leehey, MD Department of Neurology, University of Colorado School of Medicine, Aurora, CO, USA

Ying Liu, PhD Department of Neurology, University of Colorado School of Medicine, Aurora, CO, USA

Bertha K. Madras, PhD Department of Psychiatry, Harvard Medical School, Boston, MA, USA

McLean Hospital, Belmont, MA, USA

Judith Margulies, RPh, MEd Pharmacology, Timbre Health, Cambridge, MA, USA

Christopher M. Merrick, MD Pulmonary Associates, PC, Memorial Hospital, Colorado Springs, CO, USA

Christine L. Miller, PhD MillerBio, Baltimore, MD, USA

Derek Moriyama, MD Department of Medicine, Division of Geriatric-Palliative Medicine, New York University School of Medicine, New York, NY, USA

Lorne Muir, MS Rocky Vista University, Parker, CO, USA

E. Lee Nelson, MD Boulder Neurosurgical Associates, Boulder, CO, USA

Robert L. Page II, PharmD, MSPH University of Colorado Anschutz Medical Campus, Skaggs School of Pharmacy and Pharmaceutical Sciences, Department of Clinical Pharmacy, Aurora, CO, USA

Sanjog Pangarkar, MD Greater Los Angeles VA Healthcare Service, Department of Medicine, David Geffen School of Medicine at UCLA, Los Angeles, CA, USA

Bhaktasharan Patel, MD Peak Gastroenterology Associates, Colorado Springs, CO, USA

Uday Patel, MS Rocky Vista University, Parker, CO, USA

Cynthia Philip, MD Cardiology Service, Department of Medicine, Walter Reed National Military Medical Center and Uniformed Services University of Health Sciences, Bethesda, MD, USA

Sharad Rajpal, MD Boulder Neurosurgical Associates, Boulder, CO, USA

Justin Parker Neurological Institute, Boulder, CO, USA

Karen Randall, DO, FAAEM Southern Colorado Emergency Medicine Associates, Pueblo, CO, USA

David C. Rettew, MD Child, Adolescent, and Family Unit, Vermont Department of Mental Health, Psychiatry and Pediatrics, University of Vermont Larner College of Medicine, @Pedipsych, Burlington, VT, USA

Quentin Remley, MS Rocky Vista University, Parker, CO, USA

Erica Kirsten Rapp, MD Department of Psychiatry, University of Colorado School of Medicine, Aurora, CO, USA

Paula Riggs, MD Faculty Affairs, Division of Substance Dependence, Department of Psychiatry, University of Colorado School of Medicine, Aurora, CO, USA

Brad Roberts, MD, FAAEM, FACEP Southern Colorado Emergency Medicine Associates, Pueblo, CO, USA

University of New Mexico, Albuquerque, NM, USA

Kevin Sabet, MSc, PhD Department of Psychiatry, Yale University, New Haven, CT, USA

Fabienne Saint-Preux, MD Department of Rehabilitation Medicine, New York University School of Medicine, New York, NY, USA

Jerzy P. Szaflarski, MD, PhD University of Alabama at Birmingham Epilepsy Center, 312 Civitan International Research Center, Birmingham, AL, USA

Tristan Seawalt, BS Department of Neurology, University of Colorado School of Medicine, Aurora, CO, USA

Rebecca Seifried, DO Cardiology Service, Department of Medicine, Walter Reed National Military Medical Center and Uniformed Services University of Health Sciences, Bethesda, MD, USA

Amanjot Mona Sidhu, MHM, MD, FRCPC McMaster University, Hamilton, ON, Canada

Garrett Smith, MS Rocky Vista University, Parker, CO, USA

Stig Erik Sørheim, Cand. Philol Actis-Norwegian Policy Network on Alcohol and Drugs, Oslo, Norway

Thida Thant, MD Department of Psychiatry, The University of Colorado School of Medicine, Aurora, CO, USA

Alan T. Villavicencio, MD Boulder Neurosurgical Associates, Boulder, CO, USA

Justin Parker Neurological Institute, Boulder, CO, USA

George Sam Wang, MD, FAAP, FAACT Section of Emergency Medicine and Medical Toxicology, Department of Pediatrics, University of Colorado Anschutz Medical Campus, Aurora, CO, USA

Peter R. Wilson, MB, BS, PhD Pain Medicine, Mayo Clinic College of Medicine, Rochester, MN, USA

Edward C. Wood, BS, MBA DUID Victim Voices, Morrison, CO, USA

Aaron Wu, MS Rocky Vista University, Parker, CO, USA

Part I
Basic Science

Chapter 1
The Properties and Use of *Cannabis sativa* Herb and Extracts

Richard L. Hilderbrand

Abbreviations

CBD	Cannabidiol
CBDA	Cannabidiolic acid
CBD-COOH	Cannabidiol carboxylic acid
CCR	Colorado Code of Regulations
CSA	Controlled Substances Act
DEA	U.S. Drug Enforcement Administration
FDA	U.S. Food and Drug Administration
Farm Bill	Agricultural Improvement Act of 2018
NAS	National Academies of Sciences, Engineering, and Medicine
SAMHSA	Substance Abuse Mental Health Services Administration
SAMHDA	Substance Abuse Mental Health Data Archives
THCA	Delta-9-tetrahydrocannabinolic acid
THC	Delta-9-tetrahydrocannabinol
THC-COOH	Delta-9-tetrahydrocannabinol-9-carboxylic acid
11-OH-THC	11-Hydroxy-delta-9-tetrahydrocannabinol
U.K.	United Kingdom
U.S.	United States

R. L. Hilderbrand (✉)
Toxicology Consulting, Penrose, CO, USA

© Springer Nature Switzerland AG 2020
K. Finn (ed.), *Cannabis in Medicine*,
https://doi.org/10.1007/978-3-030-45968-0_1

Background

Cannabis sativa (hemp) is in the family *Cannabaceae* and is cultivated in temperate and tropical regions for its fiber and for the drug (known variously as ganja, marijuana, bhang, pot, etc.) produced by the plant. Discussion persists concerning the classification of *Cannabis* as a genus made up of one species *sativa* or of three species *sativa, indica*, and *ruderalis*. *Cannabis sativa* is used in this writing to represent a single species consisting of three cultivars (i.e., *C. sativa sativa, C. sativa indica*, and *C. sativa ruderalis*). *Cannabis* subspecies are frequently crossbred to produce viable hybrid phenotypes for certain purposes or products, such as industrial hemp (fiber, food, and oil) or psychotropic phytocannabinoids. *Cannabis* is the most widely cultivated drug plant across the world. North America has now become a leading producer of *Cannabis* herb while Morocco is the leading producer of *Cannabis* resin. Despite a decline in 2016, *Cannabis* continues to be the drug seized in the greatest quantities worldwide [1]. *Cannabis* is widely used due primarily to the presence of delta-9-tetrahydrocannabinolic acid (THCA), the precursor to the psychotropic delta-9-tetrahydrocannabinol (THC) (Fig. 1.1). In the same manner, the plant contains cannabidiolic acid (CBDA), a precursor to cannabidiol (CBD). Both THCA and CBDA are converted to the active THC and CBD, primarily by heat, but also partially by storage [2]. Over 100 chemicals of the cannabinoid family have been identified [3].

Although this chapter is not intended to fully present the synthesis and degradation of THC and CBD, the chemistry of the plant and the cannabinoids is summarized to assist in the understanding of the methods of preparation and use of *Cannabis* and the extracted substances. Marijuana and cannabis are used interchangeably in this chapter. In contrast to claims of many advocates of legalization that research on marijuana has been greatly restricted, the volume and breadth of scientific literature are so vast that attempts to summarize must only target limited and specific topics. As a result, this writing is to inform the reader as to the reasons for the methods of preparation and the manner of use of both THC and CBD by examining the characteristics of the plant and the chemical behavior of the two phytocannabinoids of primary interest. Cannabis product chemotypes are described (e.g., THC-dominant, CBD-dominant, balanced, or "hybrid" with relatively equal concentrations of THC and CBD), along with product formulations (e.g., edibles, concentrates) and methods of administration (e.g., smoked, vaporized, ingested orally).

The U.S. Drug Enforcement Administration (DEA) includes marijuana and THC in Schedule I of the Controlled Substances Act (CSA) and denied a petition to consider rescheduling marijuana in 2016 [4]. The decision was based on a five-element test of current criteria to establish medical use of a substance and found that marijuana did not meet the elements needed. The Ninth Circuit Court has upheld the

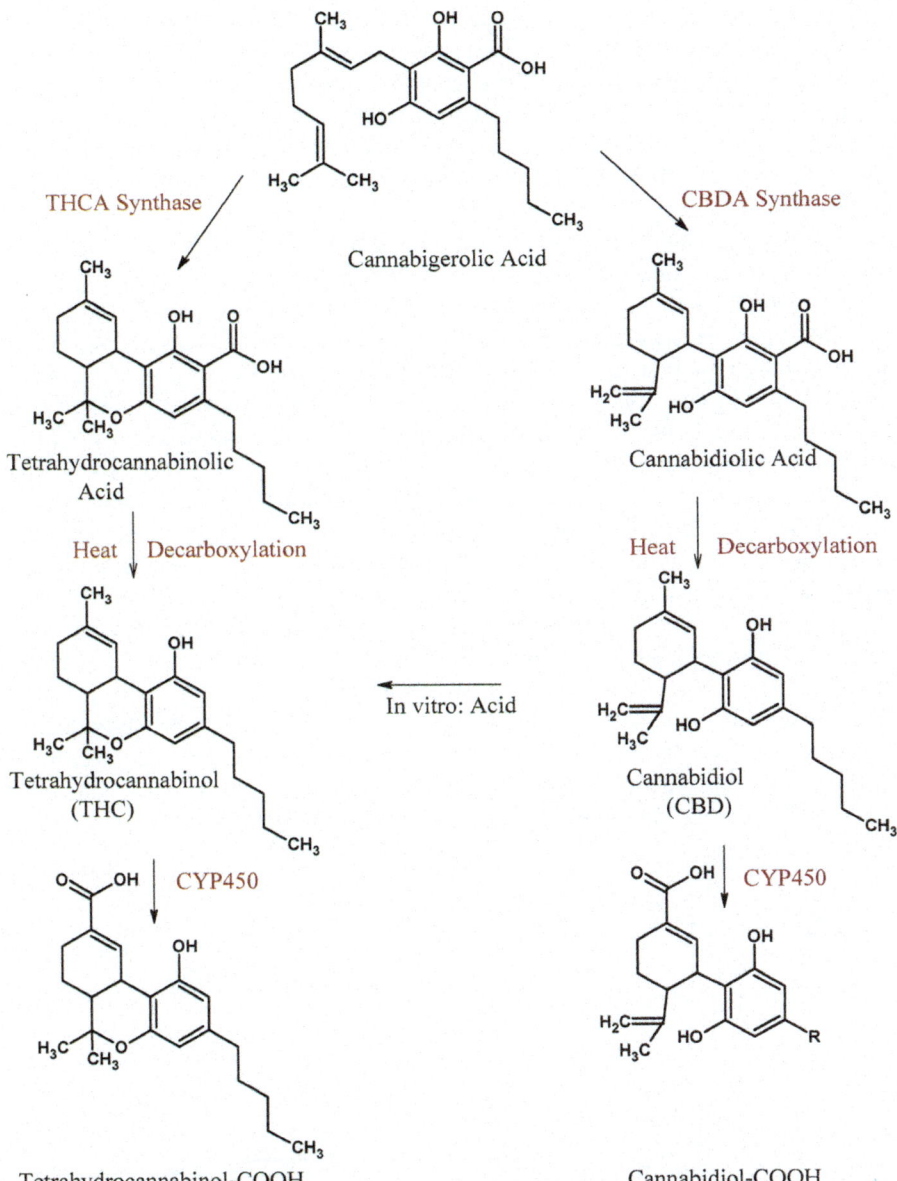

Fig. 1.1 Representative biosynthetic pathways in cannabis to produce THCA and CBDA followed by conversion to THC and CBD by storage and heat. The THC and CBD are each metabolized in vivo to many different cannabinoids

action taken by the DEA [5]. Effective January 13, 2017, the DEA created a new CSA code number (7350) for marijuana extracts [6]. The Agricultural Improvement Act of 2018 (Farm Bill) removed hemp from the controlled substances and removed "…tetrahydrocannabinols in hemp (as defined under section 297A of the Agricultural Marketing Act of 1946)" from Schedule I of the CSA. Hemp is defined as cannabis containing less than 0.3% THC by dry weight measured following decarboxylation of the THCA [7].

A global estimate, produced for the first time by United Nations Office on Drug Control and based on available data from 130 countries, suggests that in 2016 13.8 million young people (mostly students) aged 15–16 years used cannabis at least once in the previous 12 months. That number represents about 5.6% of the population in that age range. The global annual use of cannabis in the 15–16 year old group was slightly higher than among the general population aged 15–64 years (3.9% in 2016) [1]. In 2018 in the U.S. an estimated 15.9% (43.5 million) of persons aged 12 or older used marijuana in the past year. An average of 8400 Americans aged 12 or older tried marijuana for the first time each day in 2018. This is an increase of 100 users per day from the 2017 report. This increase in marijuana use among ages 12 or older reflects increases in marijuana use primarily among adults aged 26 or older (Fig. 1.2) [8]. Table 1.1 shows prevalence of use of marijuana in the last 30 days among individuals 12 years and older in the 10 states with the highest and the 10 states with the lowest prevalence of use in 2016–17 [9].

CBD was first obtained in a pure form in 1940 [10]. THC was subsequently identified by Merchoulam in 1964 and has been investigated thoroughly over many years [11]. Marijuana and industrial hemp are different varieties of the same plant species *C. sativa*. Marijuana typically contains greater than 3% THC on a

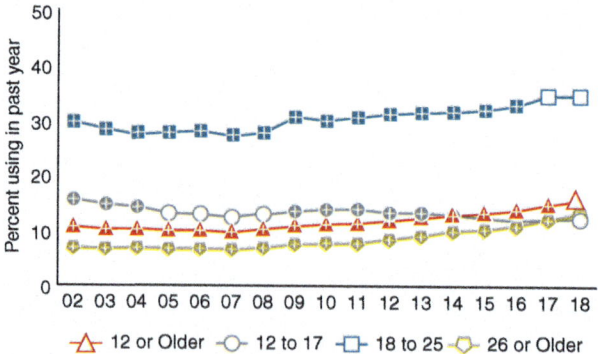

Fig. 1.2 Past year use of marijuana among people aged 12 or older, by age group: Percentages 2002–2018. In 2018, 12.5% (3.1 million) of adolescents aged 12–17, 1 in 3 young adults aged 18–25 (34.8%), and 13.3% of adults aged 26 or older were current users of marijuana. (Ref: Figure 12. Available from: https://www.samhsa.gov/data/report/2018-nsduh-annual-national-report.) + mark shows difference between this estimate and the 2018 estimate is statistically significant at the 0.05 level

Table 1.1 Use of marijuana in the last 30 days among individuals 12 years and older in the 10 states with the highest and 10 states with the lowest prevalence of use in 2016–17

Top 10	%	Low 10	%
Oregon	19.93	Virginia	6.96
Vermont	18.64	Oklahoma	6.90
Wash. DC	17.17	Georgia	6.74
Colorado	16.43	South Carolina	6.66
Alaska	15.81	Iowa	6.65
Maine	15.81	Kansas	6.62
Rhode Island	15.75	North Dakota	6.44
Washington	15.30	Alabama	6.37
Massachusetts	13.38	Utah	6.25
Montana	13.01	Texas	5.98

The current use of marijuana is classified as use in the last 30 days. The states with the highest prevalence of use have the lowest perception of harm from marijuana and states with the lowest prevalence of use have the highest perception of harm

dry-weight basis, while industrial hemp is being defined as cannabis having a THC concentration less than 0.3% THC [12]; however, the two varieties are indistinguishable by appearance. The industrial hemp variety results from the absence or limited activity of THCA-synthase, the enzyme in the plant responsible for production of THCA [13]. DeMeijer et al. [14], in a study of 97 cannabis strains, concluded there was no way to distinguish between marijuana and hemp varieties without chemical analysis [15]. More recently, the varieties of cannabis may be differentiated by gene analysis of THCA-synthase [16].

The growing plant releases a volatile substance with a skunk-like odor that may emanate for hundreds of yards from large commercial grow areas. This odor is in contrast to the more pleasing aroma of the plant in flowering stage. Many growers now spray odor masking agents into the air as the air is exhausted from the grow house. The end result is that anyone breathing the exhausted air is inhaling the volatiles produced by the plant as well as the masking agent; the impact of chronic exposure to the exhausted air on persons with respiratory illness is not known and seems to not be a concern to policy makers. Cannabis contains many cannabinoids and terpenes such as limonene, myrcene, α-pinene, linalool, and β-caryophyllene. Of the many volatiles identified, myrcene appears to predominate [17]. The volatile oils released by fresh and air-dried buds have been evaluated as a means to identify the source of confiscated marijuana, however with limited success. Neither the precursors nor THC and CBD are volatile and so are not released to the atmosphere during the growing phase or in the aroma of the flowering stage.

The THC concentration varies widely in different parts of the plant [18]. The primary production of THCA is in trichomes that develop on various parts of cannabis – primarily the leaves and buds of the female plant – and secrete the phytocannabinoids in resin from the trichomes (Fig. 1.3). Cannabis is being cloned by the use of cuttings [19] to obtain high concentrations of THC (Fig. 1.4), with THC being

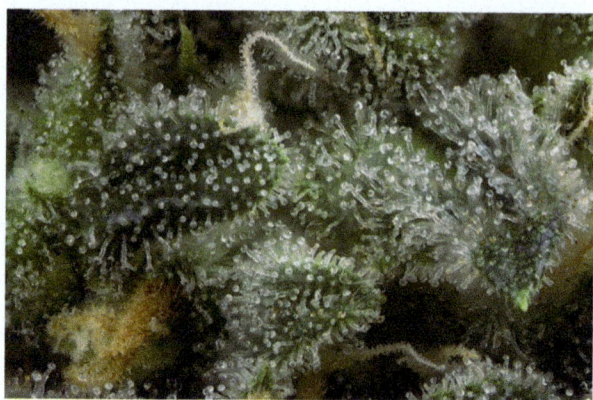

Fig. 1.3 Trichomes are epidural appendages covering the leaves of cannabis. This photo shows two types of trichomes – hair like and glandular with a resin head. Secretory cells at the base of the resin head of the glandular trichomes secrete the phytocannabinoids. The resin head is attached to the leaf by a stalk. Cannabis can be identified by the types of trichomes present and the attachment to the plant [18]. (Photo used by extended license #143447216 from Adobe Stock)

Fig. 1.4 Average THC concentrations in cannabis materials seized by DEA: 1980–2017. The figure shows the concentrations of THC in marijuana plant materials and sinsemilla, the flowering tops of female plants. (Data combined from [21–23])

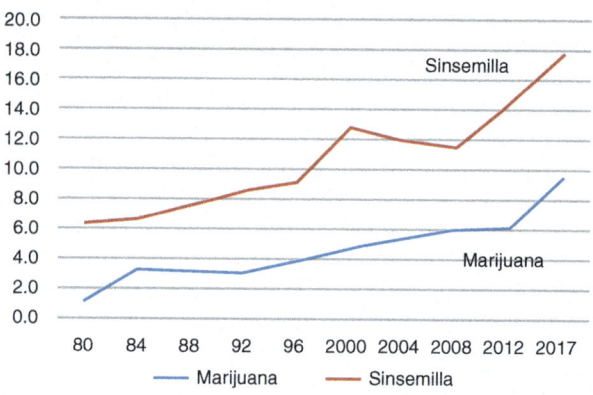

reported as well over 20% of the dry weight of the plant material [18]. The conditions responsible for the high concentrations of THC vary; however, selection of THC-dominant strains along with growth promoters, lighting, and growth conditions contribute to the increasing concentrations. The average THC potency of flower product in Colorado is reported to be 19.6% [20]. THC concentrations in materials seized by DEA have increased remarkably since 1980 [21]. The results of analysis are somewhat inconsistent and difficult to interpret, although ElSohly provides an excellent description of the actual material analyzed and the methods used [22]. In addition, while the THC concentrations in the materials tested have increased, the CBD concentrations fluctuate and have decreased [23]. The full impact of the high THC concentrations on users is not known at this time, since experienced users may attempt to titrate the THC; however, novice users may encounter adverse reactions.

THC

Initial changes to acceptance of marijuana included medicalization (marijuana recommended by a physician for a medical condition) followed by legalization (laws or policies which make the possession and use of marijuana legal under state law). In states with full legalization, the result has been full commercialization of all forms of marijuana with little control over the products or use of the THC. For example, the *Colorado Code of Regulations (CCR) Medical Marijuana Rules*, 1 CCR 212-1 establishes the regulatory framework for medical marijuana and states "Medical Marijuana-Infused Product" means a product infused with Medical Marijuana that is intended for use or consumption other than by smoking, including but not limited to edible products, ointments, and tinctures. Such products *shall not be considered a food or drug for purposes of the "Colorado Food and Drug Act"* [24]. Thus, a marijuana extract that is widely advertised and distributed as a "medicine" and is frequently included as an infusion in a food product is exempt from Colorado food and drug rules.

The high THC content achieved in the plant has resulted in an ease of preparation of extracts containing THC in highly concentrated forms. The THCA and CBDA are lipophilic, and extracts of plant material can be prepared using many lipophilic type solvents, e.g., critical point carbon dioxide, butane, or various alcohols. Butane was favored initially but has been widely replaced as extraction processes performed without appropriate knowledge, and equipment may produce an explosive air:solvent mixture as the butane flashes off the extracted phytocannabinoids. Many house fires and explosions resulted from the evaporating butane being ignited by an electrical spark. The extracted material when dry may appear like an amber glass and is called shatter. If water or other materials are included either intentionally or accidently, or if THCA precipitates, the material may be waxy or butter-like. The THC content is high in all preparations; however, the appearance of the various preparations is quite different. An extract prepared in hemp, coconut, or other oil may be called 710 (reversed OIL). The extractions are not specific to THC and CBD, and as a result the extracts may contain both THC and CBD and a variety of cannabinoids and other substances such as terpenes, heavy metals, pesticides, and plant oils. Contamination is a concern and includes fungi, molds, heavy metals, growth promoters, and substances added for marketing [25]. If leaf and bud material is allowed to dry, the resinous parts may detach and may be collected as a concentrated THC material, known as kief, to be added back to leaves for smoking or other uses. Hashish (Hash) is a cannabis product composed of compressed or partially purified preparations of resin. Sinsemilla is the flower from a female plant that has not been pollinated, and increases in THC concentration of the flower are responsible for much of the increase in THC potency measured in marijuana.

Methods of Use

The psychotropic THC is now consumed in many different ways. In addition, a person may be exposed to THC without knowingly using THC containing materials. Some examples of use or exposure are as follows:

- Oral ingestion of raw plant material: Ingestion of unheated plant material produces little effect since very little active THC is available and the absorption of any available THC is subject to first-pass metabolism [26].
- Smoking: Traditional use of marijuana plant is to smoke joints, blunts, spliffs, or pipes. The joints and blunts contain only marijuana and vary by the paper used and the rolling procedures. The spliffs are a mixture of marijuana and tobacco and blend the effects on the user of the two substances. Countries other than the U.S. may describe preparations in different terms. Various types of pipes are used where the marijuana is placed in the bowl and a flame applied followed by inhalation of combustion products. Smoking produces active drug that goes directly to the lungs and by-passes first-pass metabolism. The user inhales the many combustion products in addition to the THC. A significant percentage of the marijuana is lost by pyrolysis and by side stream smoke. A study of marijuana smoke testing cytotoxicity, mutagenicity, and ability to induce chromosomal damage found that marijuana smoke is more cytotoxic and mutagenic than the corresponding method of smoking tobacco [27]. California completed a comprehensive review in 2009 and concluded there is evidence for the carcinogenicity of marijuana smoke [28].
- Vaping: Vaping is the process of converting a THC-containing material to vapor and activating the THC or CBD without the combustion process. Many procedures are used for vaping but most provide a temperature of 360–375°F. Vape pens are now available with adjustable temperatures so the same pen can be used for a variety of preparations of THC (wax, budder, oil) or other drugs. Without full combustion, the vape pens produce limited smoke or odor.
- Dabbing: A small piece or portion of extracted THC material is a "dab." Figure 1.5 shows a "rig" used for dabbing – a recent method of ingestion of highly concentrated THC [29]. The short cylindrical glass cup to the right is called the "nail." The nail is heated with a torch for 30 seconds or so and the "dab" of THC (wax, shatter, budder, etc.) is added while the nail is hot. The small glass cap is then placed on the top of the nail and the dabber can inhale the vapor through the mouthpiece at the upper left. The user must adjust time, temperature, and air flow so that the dab produces a grayish vapor to be inhaled but does not destroy all the THC in the dab. Dabbing uses a product of up to 80% THC and gives an immediate hit to the user. The rigs come in many sizes and designs and may be used for consuming flower product, as well.
- Sublingual (tinctures and oils): This method requires that the THCA be decarboxylated to THC by heat prior to placing in an oil or tincture (alcohol base). The desired dose of THC or CBD is placed under the tongue and held for a time until the material is absorbed.
- Edibles (oral): Edible products containing active THC have increased in popularity. The products available vary widely from gummy candies, truffles, and the more traditional cookies, brownies, and sauces (Fig. 1.6). The edibles are generally baked or cooked to activate the drugs. The consumption of edibles produces a delayed effect, and the phytocannabinoids are subject to first-pass metabolism

Fig. 1.5 A water pipe rig used for dabbing and identified as a "dab rig" or oil rig and designed specifically for the use of waxes, oils, honey, budder, or shatter (dabs). The user must learn to adjust THC material, times, temperature, and air flow to achieve their desired effect. Dabbing does allow titration of the dose although the THC concentration in the materials used is very high and may approach 80% THC. (Photo used by extended license #142300664 from Adobe Stock)

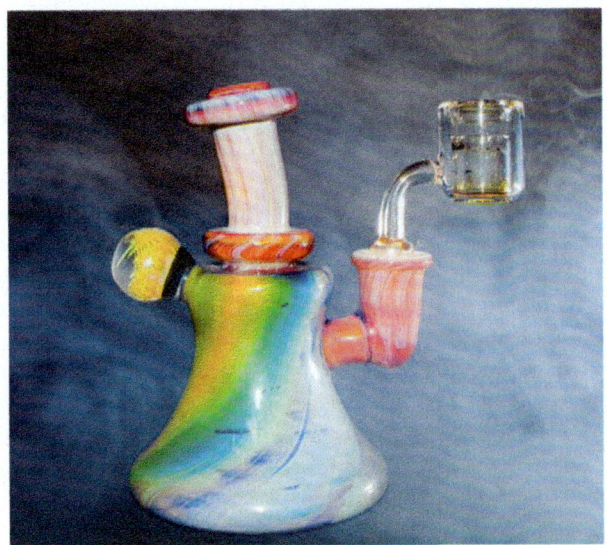

Fig. 1.6 Edible products containing marijuana come in many forms. Representative examples are shown and include cookies, truffles, gummy drops, and brownies. In addition are body creams and lotions

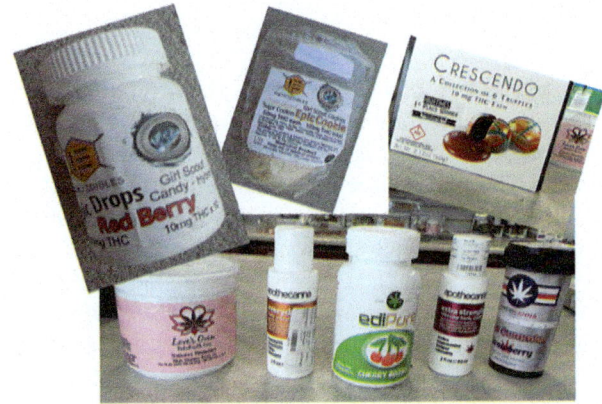

in the liver. The difficulty with edibles is that the delayed effect makes titration of the dose very difficult and easily produces overdose conditions.

- Sidestream smoke: The combustion products emanating from smoked marijuana that are not inhaled by the user contain THC and CBD and may be inhaled by persons in the vicinity of the user. Sidestream marijuana smoke has been found to contain polycyclic aromatic hydrocarbons at a higher concentration than found in the mainstream smoke [30].
- Rectal: Use of suppositories or insertion of extracts of liquid extracts reduces first-pass metabolism and essentially doubles bioavailability over oral ingestion [31].

- Secondhand smoke: Secondhand smoke is exhaled following use of combusted or vaporized marijuana and contains THC that is not absorbed by the inhalation process. Cone et al. [32] have thoroughly investigated the inhalation of second-hand smoke, although the THC concentrations in materials smoked in the studies were not as high as those of today's marijuana.
- Passive or unknowing exposure: Passive inhalation may occur if a person is in the vicinity of a smoker and inhaling secondhand or sidestream smoke. Unknowing inhalation is relatively rare because most adults are aware of the odor of smoked marijuana. Passive inhalation is more significant in the case of children in a household where smoking occurs. Unknowing ingestion of marijuana may occur by adults, children, or pets when an edible product containing marijuana is consumed without knowledge of the contents. A Massachusetts poison control center recently reported the more than doubling of cannabis-related calls following the implementation of medical marijuana [33]. Of interest is that the increase in calls was not in young children but in the 15–19 year age group, indicating that additional efforts must be made by adults, caregivers, and others to prevent access to marijuana by teens.

Metabolism

The absorption, metabolism, and pharmacokinetic profile of the THC vary with route of administration and the formulation; the time course of drug effects and metabolism for THC is quite different than for sublingual and edibles. Smoked or dabbed THC has a more immediate effect than THC consumed as an edible.

As shown in Fig. 1.1, the active THC is metabolized to the primary inactive metabolite delta-9-tetrahydrocannabinol-9-carboxylic acid (THC-COOH) and to a psychoactive substance 11-hydroxy-delta-9-tetrahydrocannabinol (11-OH-THC) and other metabolites, as well. The THC-COOH is more polar than the THC and can be excreted in the urine, although the excreted THC-COOH makes up a relatively small percentage of the total dose of THC administered. Approximately one third of the smoked THC dose is eliminated in the feces [34]. The presence of THC-COOH in the urine cannot be used to show impairment, but can only be used to demonstrate exposure of the individual to THC.

Synthetic Cannabinoids and Cannabimimetics

There are two classes of synthetic cannabinoids. One class includes substances such as dronabinol and nabilone that are created by chemical methods and approved for use as pharmaceuticals; both have been commercially available since 1985. Dronabinol is structurally identical to THC; nabilone is related to the THC structure and is more efficacious than dronabinol. Dronabinol is used to treat anorexia (as in AIDS conditions) and both dronabinol and nabilone are used to treat severe nausea and vomiting caused by chemotherapy, usually after traditional medications have been tried without success. The second class of the synthetic cannabinoids (cannabimimetics) are being used as alternatives to marijuana and are marketed as "incense" or similar product with no list of contents or active components. The packages are often marked as "not for human consumption." These materials are advertised as legal and are thought to achieve the effects of THC but are of concern due to their potential toxicity. The origin of this second class of cannabinoids began with pharmaceutical research to find substances with medical benefit, such as analgesia, but without the psychotropic effects of THC [35]. Auwarter et al. [36] identified a series of cannabimimetics in various "Spice" products and did not find THC in the products. The synthetic cannabimimetics are included in Schedule I of the CSA.

Hemp

Traditionally hemp has been grown for fiber and seeds; Canada, China, and North Korea are the world leaders in hemp production. The seeds may be pressed for oil that is polyunsaturated and used in cooking or for food for humans and animals or processed into cosmetics. The seed cake is protein rich and included in animal feed and fiber is used for paper or animal bedding. Recent technological advances use the fiber for production of plastics, 3D printer filaments, oil absorbent materials, and construction concrete. Hemp has become a crop of increasing interest, and Colorado is currently the leading producer of hemp in the U.S. The primary purpose of hemp in the U.S. is the production of CBD and the price is dependent on the concentration and varies from around $2.50/g to $10.00/g for CBD in flower materials [37].

Extracts of hemp will generally contain both CBD and THC. For example, an extract of 1000 pounds of hemp containing 0.3% THC (as allowed) and 6.0% CBD will contain 3 pounds of THC, 60 pounds of CBD, other phytocannabinoids, and oils and waxes from the plant. In this example, the THC represents about a 5% contamination of the CBD since these organic type molecules are extracted in an essentially similar manner. The significant point is that an extract of hemp that is not purified will certainly contain some concentration of THC. The THC may be removed; however, of interest in Colorado is that no regulation appears to control the THC that is removed from the hemp in the production of CBD. Colorado is in the process of developing a hemp advancement and management plan to be published in 2020 [38].

Hemp seeds, in and of themselves, do not contain THC or CBD [13, 18]; however, the processing often contaminates the seeds and produces great variability in the concentration of THC in the hemp seed oil. Yang et al. [39] found wide variation in the THC content of hemp seed oils, with a high of 125 ug/g hemp seed. This concentration raises the possibility of psychotropic effects of hemp seed oil and points out the requirement for appropriate analytical methods to be used before releasing hemp seed oil to the consumer. Other reports have reported on the potential presence of THC in hemp seed oil and the impact on consumers [40–43].

CBD

CBD is being widely advertised as a medication and a dietary supplement, although currently available CBD products do not meet normal expectations for a pharmaceutical [44]. The cannabis industry, having successfully legalized THC in many jurisdictions, has pivoted to the promotion of hemp and marketing of CBD. Many of the industry claims concerning quality, concentrations, and benefits of CBD are misleading or unsubstantiated [45]. Although the 2018 Farm Bill removed hemp and extracts of hemp from Schedule I of the CSA [46], the legislation specifically preserved the U.S. Food and Drug Administration's (FDA) responsibility over such products. The FDA has determined that CBD is to be treated as a drug [47] and has committed to assessing the science behind the use of CBD [48]. Also, the FDA has determined CBD does not meet the definition of a supplement for nutritional purposes [49]. On May 31, 2019, the FDA held a public hearing on CBD to begin the regulatory process and has published the full transcript of the hearings [50].

Following conversion of CBDA to CBD by heat, the CBD may be ingested in a variety of ways. The CBD is prepared as oils, tinctures, or edibles. The oils may be purchased as the full extract of the whole plant containing whatever substances were included in that hemp and extract by the particular company. The advantage as advertised by the industry is the potential entourage effect of interactions of the full spectrum of phytocannabinoids and terpenes substances extracted and included [51]. In addition, the industry offers "purified" and "THC-free" products. A quick internet search will find CBD products such as gummy candies, tinctures, protein bars, vape oils, dried fruit, and pet products [52]. The CBD, like THC, is metabolized and excreted in a variety of ways. Much of administered CBD is excreted unchanged or as a glucuronide. The metabolites produced by phase 1 metabolism are predominantly hydroxylated 7-COOH derivatives that are excreted intact or as glucuronides [2]. A recent study by Arkell et al. found that CBD content in vaporized cannabis does not prevent THC-induced impairment in driving [53].

Phytocannabinoids such as CBD are being appropriately investigated to identify and document actual benefits as medicinals. The benefit may come from the full extract of phytocannabinoids or just CBD. One example is Epidiolex® which was approved in 2018 by the FDA [54] as a pharmaceutical and is an essentially pure CBD oral formulation that is produced by GW Pharmaceuticals in the U.K. and marketed by their U.S. operating subsidiary, Greenwich Biosciences Inc. This CBD formulation was approved for the treatment of two rare, severe forms of epilepsy (Lennox-Gastaut Syndrome and Dravet Syndrome) [55]. As is appropriate for a medicine, the Epidiolex® is of known purity and concentration and the efficacy has been evaluated by studies presented to and approved by the FDA. For a CBD pharmaceutical to be included in Schedule V of the CSA, the pharmaceutical must contain no more than 0.1% THC and must be approved by the FDA as a drug [56]. The prescribing information warns of hepatocellular damage, suicidal ideation, and sedation, along with other concerns. These patients will be under the care of a physician that will monitor and determine efficacy of the treatment. Epidiolex® is also being evaluated as treatment for certain other medical diagnoses.

The hemp industry is working to have CBD approved as an additive to food or as a supplement, as well as FDA-approved medications. The use of CBD as a food additive is of concern. Although FDA has viewed CBD as a drug based on the initial investigations as a pharmaceutical, the FDA does have authority to provide an exemption to the drug status and allows the substance to be marketed as a food or supplement that is widely used. A significant concern is that many CBD products are widely advertised using unsubstantiated claims, improper labeling, and CBD concentration that are not correct. Two warning letters from FDA are informative as to types of claims that were made initially by companies producing CBD. In one case on October 31, 2017, the FDA, Division of Pharmaceutical Quality Operations IV, issued a warning letter to Stanley Brothers Social Enterprises to correct the claims that the products are drugs and intended to diagnose, cure, mitigate, treat, or prevent disease [57]. In addition to being new drugs, the products were misbranded. The second letter was issued to That's Natural, also a Colorado company, on the same date, concerning misbranding of CBD [58]. The FDA has issued similar letters concerning misbranding of CBD to other CBD producers.

Following the Letters of Warning, Colorado passed House Bill 18-1295 into law. This bill is significant because it is intended to establish, with no scientific analysis, that products are not (cannot be) adulterated or misbranded if they contain industrial hemp. HB 18-1295 defines "industrial hemp product" as a finished product containing industrial hemp that is a cosmetic, food, food additive, or herb and is for human use or consumption and contains … any part of the hemp plant (including extracts) but the finished product contains *THC at a concentration less than 0.3%* [59]. Of great significance is that the 0.3% limitation removes any restriction on a dose of THC per serving of product – that dose depends on the quantity of finished product consumed. For example, if a baked product weighing 1 ounce (28.3 g) contains the allowed concentration of 0.3% THC, the actual total dose of THC in the baked item is 85 mg. Having been baked, the THC would be in active form and is many times the dose that may cause impairment and is a danger to an unsuspecting consumer, since the product is sold as containing hemp or CBD and not THC. This law protecting edible hemp products is of particular significance in light of the prescribing information provided for Epidiolex® (essentially pure CBD) which warns of potential liver damage, developmental toxicity, and other adverse effects that should be monitored by a physician [55].

Conversion to THC

In recent years, the potential conversion of CBD to THC by gastric fluid has been investigated. That conversion has long been known to occur in acidic conditions in vitro [60, 61]; however, the in vivo conversion is a matter of interest. A study of metabolites of CBD in a single patient receiving a daily oral 600 mg dose found THC in the urine but did not identify the actual source [62]. The authors did not find the metabolite THC-COOH which argues against the in vivo conversion of CBD to THC. Additional study found delta-8-THC and delta-9-THC at 1.97 and 0.69% of extracted cannabinoids, respectively [63]. Watanabe et al. reported the conversion of CBD to delta-9-THC by artificial gastric fluid and that the metabolites demonstrated pharmacological effects in mice [64]. A similar conversion was also reported to occur over a 3-hour incubation in artificial gastric fluid, raising concerns about potential physiological responses to the products of degradation [65]. Grotenhermen et al. discount the conversion and the THC like effects of CBD being of clinical significance in humans [66]. Various studies have additional information on the conversion [67] and question the conversion of oral CBD to THC in humans [68].

CBD as a Quality Medicine

The view of CBD as a medicine that is demonstrated by the claims of the companies that are producing and selling CBD on a national scale is stunning. This acceptance of the wildly inflated claims of benefits, seemingly by a large percentage of the general population of this country, leads to the need for an assessment of the actual benefits and adverse consequences. The information for physicians prescribing Epidiolex® lists a number of potential adverse consequences, such as somnolence and sedation, suicidal ideation, hepatocellular injury, and drug-drug interactions [55]. In addition, a study of a CBD extract shows clear signs of hepatotoxicity [69].

A basic literature search of PUBMED displays numerous articles published in the last 25 years that propose a potential benefit of CBD as a medication for many purposes. That literature is too extensive to summarize here; however, a recent publication by S. Pisanti et al. provides extensive information and references pertaining to CBD [70]. A significant concern is the proposal to use CBD as medication to treat the opioid epidemic [71]. Colorado statistics show a concomitant increase in the opioid epidemic and the use of cannabinoids, but no decline in opioid use with the legalization of marijuana.

A 2017 study looking at market share of products by a cannabis investment group finds CBD is being used to replace traditional pharmaceuticals. The top conditions being treated included anxiety (67%), insomnia (60%), joint pain and inflammation (52%), and depression (43%). Respondents preferred CBD derived from cannabis to CBD derived from industrial hemp and only 9% of respondents indicated using hemp-derived CBD exclusively [72]. The preference for CBD from cannabis is significant because, without purification, the CBD extracted from cannabis will, most likely, contain a much higher percentage of THC than does CBD from hemp.

Discussion

Legalization of marijuana removes related criminal penalties and offers a new source of revenue with control expected from local and state government and collection of federal business and payroll taxes. The result has been the full commercialization of cannabis. Unfortunately, the legalization and liberalization of laws pertaining to marijuana have created a regulatory abyss that legislators appear unable or unwilling to fix, since control of production is very difficult. A second factor that is difficult to assess is the cost:benefit ratio of legalization. A state may tout the revenue; however, the costs to the state and to smaller jurisdictions within the state are not apparent and, in most cases, appear to not be considered. Only one report is available that completed any cost benefit analysis of legalization [73]. The report estimated costs as 4.5 times the benefits. The report may be subject to criticism; however, no other entity has attempted to assess the cost:benefit ratio. In any case, the real possibility is that the statewide costs of implementation and enforcement exceed the revenue. Every county, city, and town must establish marijuana rules and regulations and must cover the many social costs associated with legalization. These include law enforcement, social welfare, and medical care, in addition to the adverse effects on many individuals. The impact on generalized personal welfare and health cannot be assessed. In addition, the tax rates are fixed while costs of marijuana to consumers are not. As cannabinoid prices drop due to competition, sales volume must increase to maintain or increase state revenues. Marijuana, due to the ease of production, is quite different than tobacco and alcohol and is not easy to control and tax, especially when rules allow for growth by individuals at essentially any location. Cannabis growth by individuals and care givers is not taxed. In addition, the lax attitude toward marijuana has created a sanctuary for cartels and other illegal operations.

Many jurisdictions allow a long list of "medical" conditions to be treated with phytocannabinoids. In many cases the decisions have no basis in medical science or solid scientific evidence and there is significant evidence of acute negative outcomes [74]. A recent comprehensive review by the National Academy of Sciences (NAS) found conclusive or substantial evidence that cannabinoids have potential for treatment of chronic pain in adults, as anti-emetics for nausea from chemotherapy, and for improving multiple sclerosis spasticity symptoms. Of particular note is that the NAS report on chronic pain addressed neuropathic and cancer pain treated with synthetics or products not available in the U.S. (nabiximols), not with dispensary cannabis. Evidence for any other positive relationships to therapy with phytocannabinoids was only moderate, limited, or inconclusive. In addition, there was substantial evidence for negative outcomes such as worsening respiratory conditions, increased risk of motor vehicle crashes, lower birth-weight of offspring, and impairment of cognitive domains of learning [75]. The lack of scientific evidence supporting the many allowed medical uses is compounded by a variety of factors, for example:

- Medical care providers that lack understanding of how cannabinoids may impact a patient or medical treatment.
- Insufficient oversight by knowledgeable medical care providers of patients with critical illness that are using cannabinoids based on a recommendation.
- Variable individual responses to the therapeutic use of cannabinoids.
- Cannabis dispensary staff providing recommendations and assessment of medical conditions with no experience, training, or certification [76].
- Variability of quality and concentrations of the desired cannabinoid in non-pharmaceutical products.
- Improper labeling of products and contamination of the phytocannabinoid products by undesired or toxic constituents [77].

The quality and contents of both recreational and medical cannabis products are of concern. The intentional adulteration to enhance the psychotropic effects of THC with drugs such as opioids is recognized. Perhaps unrecognized are the problems of quality from contaminants in soil used to grow the cannabis, the improper use of pesticides, concentrations of phytocannabinoids that are either low or high and not consistent, the presence of many extracted natural products in the THC or CBD, and the presence of significant amounts of THC in CBD products. The involvement of many growers that have no knowledge of quality control in production of pharmaceuticals leads one to question how the plants are actually grown and how the products are treated during processing and marketing. Cannabis concentrates are of particular concern due to the potential concentrations of contaminants, along with the cannabinoid. A study of 57 concentrates from California found that over 80% were contaminated in some way including residual solvent and pesticides and had a very wide range in THC concentrations [78].

We have come to expect medications that are pure, of known and consistent efficacy, with a known mechanism, and from a manufacturer that is liable for the quality of the medication. Marijuana preparations are not consistent and vary from strain to strain and grower to grower or basement to basement. In addition, the effect and metabolism vary with the individual and the method of use [79].

All physicians must be aware of the potential impact of both THC and CBD on prescribed medications. The efficacy of THC or CBD for the many proposed therapeutic uses needs to be proven with legitimate, scientific, controlled studies. THC and CBD may place consumers, with no knowledge of the contents of the products, at risk. THC and CBD may also interact with or interfere in the metabolism of other medications [80] and may interfere with perioperative care [81]. In a recent address at the Institute of Cannabis Research, Dr. Di Marzo described research methods to assess the benefits of the phytocannabinoids as pharmaceuticals [82]. Pharmaceutical preparations of CBD may ultimately be useful; however, current motivation appears to be the financial reward to the CBD industry rather than the health and well-being of the consumer. The analysis of THC and CBD preparations for contaminants in the products being marketed to unsuspecting consumers is of great importance; however, that analysis is required to guarantee purity, safety, and the lack of psychotropic or intoxicant influences on other medications and human health.

Summary

THC has been widely investigated while the therapeutic potential of CBD has only come to the attention of the scientific community in more recent years. A quick search of PUBMED identified over 30,000 articles containing the word marijuana and 2300 articles containing the word cannabidiol that were published over the past decades [83]. The conclusions of the recent National Academy of Sciences review that there are few, if any, conditions that uniquely benefit from administration of THC indicate that the primary interest in THC is for the psychotropic effect. CBD, on the other hand, may be proven to be the phytocannabinoid of greatest pharmaceutical benefit; however, many persons are self-medicating with either or both THC and CBD products that are of suspect quality, concentration, and benefit. Few persons would choose to use pharmaceuticals from a drug company that were of questionable quality; however, many will obtain and use phytocannabinoids based on advice of persons with no scientific or medical training and with no assurance of quality or concentration. This creates a concern for the user, as well as any medical care provider. The impact of the use of THC and CBD on our society and, in particular, the practice of medicine remains to be understood. In addition, the absence of a true cost benefit analysis completed by an objective governmental agency is a critical issue that must be addressed. Regulatory decisions made without the benefit of actual costs results in inappropriate decisions and regulations.

Acknowledgments   The author would like to thank Ms. Kyong Smith, Library Technician, Evans Army Community Hospital, Lane Medical Library, Fort Carson, Colorado, for exceptional assistance with literature searches.

References

1. United Nations Office on Drugs and Crime [Internet]. World drug report 2016, p. 43. [Cited 2019 Aug 15]. Available from: https://www.unodc.org/doc/wdr2016/WDR_2016_Chapter_1_Cannabis.pdf.
2. Ujvary I, Hanus L. Human metabolites of cannabidiol: a review on their formation, biological activity, and relevance in therapy. Cannabis Cannabinoid Res. 2016;1(1):90–101.
3. ElSohly M, Gul W. Constituents of *Cannabis sativa*. In: Pertwee RG, editor. Handbook of Cannabis. Oxford: Oxford University Press; 2014. p. 3–22.
4. Drug Enforcement Administration [Internet]. Denial of petition to initiate proceedings to reschedule marijuana [Cited 2019 Aug 11]. Federal Register 2016; 81(156):5368853-766. Available from: https://www.govinfo.gov/content/pkg/FR-2016-08-12/pdf/2016-17954.pdf.

5. Hemp Industries Association [Internet]. U.S. Court of Appeals for the Ninth Circuit. [Cited 2019 May 30]. Available from: https://hempindustrydaily.com/wp-content/uploads/2018/05/HIA-decision-042018.pdf.

6. Drug Enforcement Administration [Internet]. Establishment of a new drug code for marijuana extract. [Cited 2019 May 30]. Available from: https://www.federalregister.gov/documents/2016/12/14/2016-29941/establishment-of-a-new-drug-code-for-marihuana-extract.

7. H.R. 2 (115th): Agricultural Improvement Act of 2018 (Farm Bill) p. 529 [Internet]. [Cited 2019 Jul 9]. Available from: https://www.govinfo.gov/content/pkg/BILLS-115hr2enr/pdf/BILLS-115hr2enr.pdf.

8. SAMHSA [Internet]. Key substance use and mental health indicators in the United States: results from the 2018 National Survey on Drug Use and Health, Figure 12. [Cited 2019 Aug 21]. Available from: https://www.samhsa.gov/data/report/2018-nsduh-annual-national-report.

9. SAMHDA [Internet]. Interactive NSDUH State Estimates. [Cited 2019 Jun 18]. Available from: https://pdas.samhsa.gov/saes/state.

10. Adams R, Hunt M, Clark JH. Structure of cannabidiol, a product isolated from the marihuana extract of Minnesota wild hemp. J Am Chem Soc. 1940;62:196–200.

11. Gaoni Y, Mechoulam R. Isolation, structure and partial synthesis of an active constituent of hashish. J Am Chem Soc. 1964;86:1646–7.

12. U.S. Departments of Agriculture, Justice, and Health and Human Services [Internet]. Statement of principles on industrial hemp. Notices, Federal Register 2016 81;156:53395-6.

13. Citti C, Pacchetti B, Vandelli MA, Forni F, Cannazza G. Analysis of cannabinoids in commercial hemp seed oil and decarboxylation kinetics studies of cannabidiolic acid (CBDA). J Pharm Biomed Anal. 2018;149:532–40.

14. DeMeijer EPM, van der Kamp HJ, van Eeuwijk FA. Characterization of cannabis accessions with regard to cannabinoid content and relation to other plant characters. Euphytica. 1992;62(3):187–200.

15. U.S. Department of Agriculture [Internet]. Industrial hemp in the United States: status and market potential. p 2. [Cited 2019 Jun 2]. Available from: https://www.ers.usda.gov/publications/pub-details/?pubid=41757.

16. Cirovic N, Kecmanovic M, Keckarevic D, Markovic MK. Differentiation of cannabis subspecies by THCA synthase gene analysis using RFLP. J Forensic Legal Med. 2017;51:81–4.

17. Ross SA, ElSohly MA. The volatile oil composition of fresh and air-dried buds of *Cannabis sativa*. J Nat Prod. 1996;59:49–51.

18. Potter DJ. Cannabis horticulture. In: Pertwee RG, editor. Handbook of Cannabis. Oxford: Oxford University Press; 2014. p. 65–88.

19. Growweedeasy [Internet]. How to grow cannabis in 10 easy steps. [Cited 2019 Jun 18]. Available from: https://www.growweedeasy.com/10-step-cannabis-grow-guide.

20. Colorado Department of Revenue [Internet]. Report on market size and demand for marijuana in Colorado 2017:market update. [Cited 2019 Jun 18]. Available from: https://www.colorado.gov/pacific/sites/default/files/MED%20Demand%20and%20Market%20%20Study%20%20082018.pdf.

21. Mehmedic Z, Chandra S, Slade D, Denham H, Foster S, Patel AS, et al. Potency trends of delta(9)–THC and other cannabinoids in confiscated cannabis preparations from 1993-2008. J Forensic Sci. 2010;55:1209–17.

22. ElSohly MA, Ross SA, Mehmedic Z, Arafat R, Yi B, Banahan BF. Potency trends of delta-9–THC and other cannabinoids in confiscated marijuana from 1980-1997. J Forensic Sci. 2000;45:24–30.

23. Chandra S, Radwan MM, Majumdar CG, Church JC, Freeman TP, ElSohly MA. New trends in cannabis potency in USA and Europe during the last decade (2008-2017). Eur Arch Psychiatry Clin Neurosci. 2019;269:5–15.

24. Code of Colorado Regulations [Internet]. 1 CCR 212-1 Medical Marijuana Rules. [Cited 2019 Jul 9]. Available from: https://www.sos.state.co.us/CCR/DisplayRule.do?action=ruleinfo&ruleId=3089&deptID=19&agencyID=185&deptName=Department%20of%20Revenue&agencyName=Marijuana%20Enforcement%20Division&seriesNum=1%20CCR%20212-1.

25. McLaren J, Swift W, Dillon P, Allsop S. Cannabis potency and contamination: a review of the literature. Addiction. 2008;103:1100–9.
26. Wall ME, Sadler BM, Brine D, Taylor H, Perez-Reyes M. Metabolism, disposition, and kinetics of delta-9-tetrahydrocannabinol in men and women. Clin Pharmacol Ther. 1983;34:352–63.
27. Maertens RM, White PA, Rickert W, Levasseur G, Douglas GR, Bellier PV, et al. The genotoxicity of mainstream and sidestream marijuana and tobacco smoke condensates. Chem Res Toxicol. 2009;22:1406–14.
28. California Environmental Protection Agency [Internet]. Evidence on the carcinogenicity of marijuana smoke. August 2009. 2019. Available from: https://oehha.ca.gov/media/downloads/proposition-65/chemicals/finalmjsmokehid.pdf.
29. Loflin M, Earleywine M. A new method of cannabis ingestion: the dangers of dabs? Addict Behav. 2014;39:1430–3.
30. Moir D, Rickert WS, Levasseur G, Larose Y, Maertens R, White P, et al. A comparison of mainstream and sidestream marijuana and tobacco cigarette smoke produced under two machine smoking conditions. Chem Res Toxicol. 2008;21:494–502.
31. Huestis MA, Smith ML. Cannabinoid pharmacokinetics and disposition in alternative matrices. In: Pertwee RG, editor. Handbook of Cannabis. Oxford: Oxford University Press; 2014. p. 296–316.
32. Cone EJ, Bigelow GE, Herrmann ES, Mitchell JM, LoDico C, Flegal R, et al. Non-smoker exposure to secondhand cannabis smoke. I. Urine screening and confirmation results. J Anal Toxicol. 2015;39:1–12.
33. Whitehill JM, Harrington C, Lang CJ, Chary M, Bhutta WA, Burns MM. Incidence of pediatric cannabis exposure among children and teenagers aged 0 to 19 years before and after medical marijuana legalization in Massachusetts. JAMA Network Open. 2019;2(8):e199456. Epub 2019 Aug 16.
34. Huestis MA. Cannabis (marijuana) – effects on human behavior and performance. Forensic Sci Rev. 2002;14:15–60.
35. Rosenbaum CD, Carreiro SP, Babu KM. Here today, gone tomorrow...and back again? A review of herbal marijuana alternatives (k2, spice), synthetic cathinones (bath salts), kratom, salvia divinorum, methoxetamine, and piperazines. J Med Toxicol. 2012;8:15–32.
36. Auwarter V, Dresen S, Weinmann W, Muller M, Putz M, Ferreiros N. "Spice" and other herbal blends: harmless incense or cannabinoid designer drugs. J Mass Spectrom. 2009;44:832–7.
37. Schluttenhofer C, Yuan L. Challenges towards revitalizing hemp: a multifaceted crop. Trends Plant Sci. 2017;22:917–29.
38. Colorado Department of Agriculture [Internet]. Colorado Hemp Advancement and Management Plan (CHAMP). 2019. Available from: https://www.colorado.gov/pacific/agplants/champ-initiative.
39. Yang Y, Lewis MM, Bello AM, Wasilewski E, Clarke HA, Kotra LP. *Cannabis sativa* (hemp) seeds, delta-9-tetrahydrocannabinol and potential overdose. Cannabis Cannabinoid Res. 2017;2:274–81.
40. Fortner N, Fogerson R, Lindman D, Iversen T, Armbruster D. Marijuana-positive urine test results from consumption of hemp seeds in food products. J Anal Toxicol. 1997;21:476–81.
41. Alt A, Reinhardt G. Positive cannabis results in urine and blood after consumption of hemp food products. J Anal Toxicol. 1998;22:80–1.
42. Chinello M, Scommegna S, Shardlow A, Mazzoli F, De Giovanni N, Fucci N, et al. Cannabinoid poisoning by hemp seed oil in a child. Pediatr Emerg Care. 2017;33:344–5.
43. Bozy TZ, Cole KA. Consumption and quantitation of delta9-tetrahydrocannabinol in commercially available hemp seed oil products. J Anal Toxicol. 2000;24:562–6.
44. Hilderbrand R. Hemp and Cannabidiol: what is a medicine? Mo Med. 2018;115(4):306–9.
45. Bonn-Miller MG, Loflin MJE, Thomas BF, Marcu JP, Hyke T, Vandrey R. Labeling accuracy of cannabidiol extracts sold online. Research Letter. JAMA. 2017;318:1708–9.
46. National Institute of Food and Agriculture [Internet]. Industrial hemp. [Cited 2019 Jun 2]. Available from: https://nifa.usda.gov/industrial-hemp.
47. Food and Drug Administration [Internet]. Statement from FDA Commissioner Scott Gottlieb, M.D., on signing of the Agricultural Improvement Act and the agency's regulation of products

containing cannabis and cannabis-derived products. [Cited 2019 May 30]. Available from: https://www.fda.gov/news-events/press-announcements/statement-fda-commissioner-scott-gottlieb-md-signing-agriculture-improvement-act-andagencys.

48. Food and Drug Administration [Internet]. FDA is committed to sound, science-based policy on CBD. [Cited 2019 Jul 8]. Available from: https://www.fda.gov/news-events/fda-voices-perspectives-fda-leadership-and-experts/fda-committed-sound-science-based-policy-cbd.

49. Food and Drug Administration [Internet]. FDA regulation of cannabis and cannabis-derived products: Questions and Answers. Question 9. [Cited 2019 Jun 3]. Available from https://www.fda.gov/news-events/public-health-focus/fda-regulation-Cannabis-and-Cannabis-derived-products-questions-and-answers.

50. Food and Drug Administration [Internet]. Scientific data and information about products containing cannabis or cannabis-derived compounds; public hearing. [Cited 2019 Aug 20]. Available from: https://www.fda.gov/news-events/fda-meetings-conferences-and-workshops/scientific-data-and-information-about-products-containing-cannabis-or-cannabis-derived-compounds.

51. Russo EB. Taming THC: potential cannabis synergy and phytocannabinoid-terpenoids entourage effects. Br J Pharmacol. 2011;163:1344–64.

52. JustCBD [Internet]. Our products. [Cited 2019 Jul 15]. Available from: https://www.just-cbdstore.com/.

53. Arkell TR, Lintzeris N, Kevin RC, Ramaekers JG, Vandrey R, Irwin C, et al. Cannabidiol (CBD) content in vaporized cannabis does not prevent tetrahydrocannabinol (THC)-induced impairment of driving and cognition. Psychopharmacology. 2019;236:2713–24.

54. Food and Drug Administration [Internet]. FDA approves first drug comprised of an active ingredient derived from marijuana to treat rare, severe forms of epilepsy. [Cited 2019 Aug 11]. Available from: https://www.fda.gov/news-events/press-announcements/fda-approves-first-drug-comprised-active-ingredient-derived-marijuana-treat-rare-severe-forms.

55. Greenwich Biosciences [Internet]. Full prescribing information for Epidiolex® oral solutions. 2018. [Cited 2019 Jun 27]. Available from: https://www.epidiolex.com/sites/default/files/EPIDIOLEX_Full_Prescribing_Information.pdf.

56. Department of Justice, DEA [Internet]. Schedules of controlled substances: placement in schedule V of certain FDA-approved drugs containing cannabidiol; corresponding change to permit requirements. [Cited 2019 Aug 11]. Available from: https://www.govinfo.gov/content/pkg/FR-2018-09-28/pdf/2018-21121.pdf.

57. 57. Food and Drug Administration [Internet]. Warning Letter: Stanley Brothers Social Enterprises 31 Oct 2017. [Cited 2019 Jun 21]. Available from: https://www.fda.gov/inspections-compliance-enforcement-and-criminal-investigations/warning-letters/stanley-brothers-social-enterprises-llc-490089-10312017.

58. Food and Drug Administration [Internet]. Warning Letter: That's Natural 31 Oct 2017. [Cited 2019 Jun 21]. Available from: https://www.fda.gov/inspections-compliance-enforcement-and-criminal-investigations/warning-letters/thats-natural-513302-10312017.

59. Colorado Revised Statutes [Internet]. HB18-1295. 2018. [Cited 2019 Jun 27]. Available from: https://leg.colorado.gov/sites/default/files/2018a_1295_signed.pdf.

60. Adams R, Pease DC, Cain CK, Clark JH. Structure of cannabidiol. VI. Isomerization of cannabidiol to tetrahydrocannabinol, a physiologically active product. Conversion of cannabidiol to cannabinol. J Am Chem Soc. 1940;62:2402–5.

61. Gaoni Y, Mechoulam R. Hashish-VII, the isomerization of cannabidiol to tetrahydrocannabinols. Tetrahedron. 1966;22:1481–8.

62. Harvey DJ, Mechoulam R. Metabolites of cannabidiol identified in human urine. Xenobiotica. 1990;20:303–20.

63. Harvey DJ, Samara E, Mechoulam R. Urinary metabolites of cannabidiol in dog, rat and man and their identification by gas chromatography–mass spectrometry. J Chromatogr. 1991;562:299–322.

64. Watanabe K, Itokawa Y, Yamaori S, Funahashi T, Kimura T, Kaji T, et al. Conversion of can-nabidiol to delta-9-tetrahydrocannabinol and related cannabinoids in artificial gastric juice, and their pharmacological effects in mice. Forensic Toxicol. 2007;25:16–21.
65. Merrick J, Lane B, Sebree T, Yaksh T, O'Neill C, Banks SL. Identification of psychoactive degradants of cannabidiol in simulated gastric and physiological fluid. Cannabis Cannabinoid Res. 2016;1:102–12.
66. Grotenhermen F, Russo E, Zuardi AW. Even high doses of oral cannabidol do not cause THC-like effects in humans: comment on Merrick et al. Cannabis Cannabinoid Res. 2016;1:102–12. Cannabis Cannabinoid Res. 2017;2:1–4.
67. Bonn-Miller MO, Banks SL, Sebree T. Conversion of cannabidiol following oral administra-tion: authors response to Grotenhermen et al. Cannabis Cannabinoid Res. 2017;2(1):5–7.
68. Nahler G, Grotenhermen F, Zuardi AW, Crippa JAS. A conversion of oral cannabidiol to Delta9-Tetrahydrocannabinol seems to not occur in humans. Cannabis Cannabinoid Res. 2017;2(1):81–6.
69. Ewing LE, Skinner CM, Quick CM, Kennon-McGill S, McGill MR, Walker LA, et al. Hepatoxicity of a cannabidiol-rich cannabis extract in the mouse model. Molecules. 2019;24:1694–710.
70. Pisanti S, Malfitano AM, Ciaglia E, Lamberti A, Ranieri R, Cuomo G, et al. Cannabidiol: state of the art and new challenges for therapeutic applications. Pharmacol Ther. 2017;175:133–50.
71. Hurd YL. Cannabidiol: Swinging the marijuana pendulum from "weed" to medication to treat the opioid epidemic. Trends Neurosci. 2017;40(3):124–7.
72. New Cannabis Ventures [Internet]. Study shows CBD is replacing traditional pharmaceuti-cals. 2017. [Cited 2019 Jun 26]. Available from: https://www.newcannabisventures.com/study-shows-cbd-is-replacing-traditional-pharmaceuticals/.
73. Centennial Institute, Colorado Christian University [Internet]. Economic and social costs of legalized marijuana. [Cited 2019 Aug 20]. Available from: http://www.ccu.edu/centennial/policy-briefs/marijuana-costs/.
74. Monte AA, Shelton SK, Mills E, Saben J, Hopkinson A, Sonn B, et al. Acute illness associated with cannabis use by route of exposure. Ann Intern Med. 2019;170:531–7.
75. National Academies of Science, Engineering, and Medicine. The health effects of Cannabis and Cannabinoids: the current state of evidence and recommendations for research. Washington, DC: The National Academies Press; 2017. p. 13–22.
76. Haug NA, Kieschnick D, Sottile JE, Babson KA, Vandrey R, Bonn-Miller MO. Training and practices of cannabis dispensary staff. Cannabis Cannabinoid Res. 2016;1:244–51.
77. Vandrey R, Raber JC, Raber ME, Douglass B, Miller C, Bonn-Miller MO. Cannabinoid dose and label accuracy in edible medical cannabis products. Research Letter. JAMA. 2015;313:2491–3.
78. Raber JC, Elzinga S, Kaplan C. Understanding dabs: contamination concerns of cannabis con-centrates and cannabinoid transfer during the act of dabbing. J Toxicol Sci. 2015;40:797–803.
79. Atakan Z. Cannabis, a complex plant: different compounds and different effects on individu-als. Ther Adv Psychopharmacol. 2012;2:241–54.
80. Rong C, Carmona NE, Lee YL, Ragguett RM, Pan Z, Rosenblat JD, et al. Drug-drug interac-tions as a result of co-administering Δ^9-THC and CBD with other psychotropic agents. Expert Opin Drug Saf. 2018;17(1):51–4.
81. Echeverria-Villalobos M, Todeschini AB, Stoicea N, Fiorda-Diaz J, Weaver T, Bergese SD. Perioperative care of cannabis users: a comprehensive review of pharmacological and anesthetic considerations. J Clin Anesthesia. 2019;57:41–9.
82. Di Marzo V. Institute of Cannabis Research 2018 Mechoulam Lecture. [Internet]. The phy-tocannabinoidome and the endocannabinoidome: how close are they? [Cited 2019 Jul 9]. Available from: https://www.csupueblo.edu/institute-of-cannabis-research/past-confer-ences/2018/index.html.
83. PUBMED searched May 20, 2019 by Endnote software.

Chapter 2
Cannabinoid and Marijuana Neurobiology

Bertha K. Madras

Introduction

The convergence of political, financial, medical, and basic science interests is transforming the field of marijuana science. In three decades from 1930 to 1960, a scant 109 marijuana-related reports were published in the biomedical literature. Fifty years later, in a single decade from 2011 to fall of 2019, a staggering 15,269 marijuana manuscripts were published. This 140-fold increase in the scientific literature was catalyzed by changes in our perception of marijuana and by the discovery of an entirely new signaling system, the endocannabinoid system, in living organisms. Shortly after this discovery, revelations appeared on how plant-based cannabinoids (phytocannabinoids) and de novo synthetically produced cannabinoids target and modulate this system in the brain and other organs. The current phase of this near-exponential growth in scientific inquisitiveness focuses on the biological mechanisms by which cannabinoids contribute to pathophysiology or the potential of cannabinoids for treating diseases. Endocannabinoids and their receptors are now recognized as significant modulators of human physiology and pathophysiology. This signaling system is among the most dense, widely distributed, and versatile in animals and humans.

B. K. Madras (✉)
Department of Psychiatry, Harvard Medical School, Boston, MA, USA

McLean Hospital, Belmont, MA, USA
e-mail: bertha_madras@hms.harvard.edu

© Springer Nature Switzerland AG 2020
K. Finn (ed.), *Cannabis in Medicine*,
https://doi.org/10.1007/978-3-030-45968-0_2

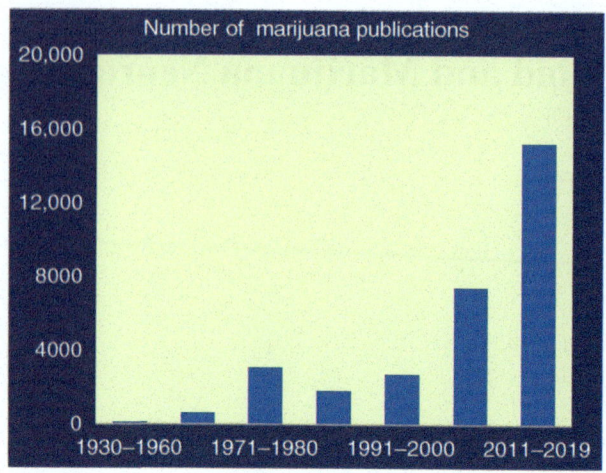

The review summarizes the endocannabinoid system and actions of exogenous cannabinoids on this system, but with a caveat: The composition of marijuana has changed dramatically with medicalization, legalization, and commercialization [1]. Marijuana is a complex plant [2] with over 700 identified constituents, including more than 100 cannabinoids. The most prominent of these are THC (Δ9-tetrahydrocannabinol) and CBD (cannabidiol). For most of the 20th century, research on marijuana biology was based on low-potency (low THC) botanical marijuana converted into crude smokable preparations of crushed plant parts and stems containing ~1–3% THC. Findings from this period require tempering or are obsolete, with the advent of high-potency strains of the plant (~20% THC), extreme potency of marijuana concentrates (as high as 90% THC), high THC:CBD ratios (>100), an expanding repertoire of synthetic cannabinoids [3], new routes of administration (e.g., vaping, edibles), and increased daily use. These parameters can influence the pharmacological actions of cannabinoids.

Discovery, Evolutionary Origins, and Function of the Endocannabinoid System

Cell-cell communication Among the many insights provided by the human genome project was the discovery of an abundance of genes implicated in cell-cell communication. Signaling between cells is a critical mechanism to coordinate the activities of multicellular organisms, enabling development, repair, immunity, homeostasis, and response to environmental cues. In general, communication systems are complex and comprise at least five components: a mechanism to synthesize, store, and release a signaling molecule (neurotransmitter or hormone) by the signaling cell; transport or diffusion of the signaling molecule to its target; binding and activation of a specific receptor (target); initiation of a signal transduction pathway to amplify or diminish the signal; and a mechanism to inactivate the signal. *Signaling molecules* can belong to different chemical classes, to include lipids, amino acids, monoamines, proteins, or gases. *Receptors* are proteins embedded in cell surface membranes, or function intracellularly, or mobilize and circulate between the two environments. At least 4% of our genome encodes G protein-coupled receptors, which are crucial for vision, smell, taste, immune response, water balance, blood pressure, and higher brain functions. Spanning the full thickness of cell membranes, G protein-coupled receptors are activated by a signaling molecule (e.g., dopamine) to undergo a conformational change. The change transfers the signal to the cell interior by enabling the receptor to bind to G proteins (guanine nucleotide-binding proteins), molecular switches inside cells that transmit signals generated by cell surface receptors. They activate effectors (e.g., enzymes such as adenylate cyclase or phospholipase C or RhoGEFs) to produce transducing molecules, e.g., cAMP, that amplify or depress signals to trigger a cascade of signaling events that change cell function.

Communication is the core activity of the brain. It has the most highly developed and complex system of cell-cell communication dynamics: ~80 billion nerve cells (neurons), each of which can make a few or 10,000+ connections to other neurons for signaling, with neurons supported by ~1 trillion glia (non-neuronal cells). G protein-coupled receptors are abundant in the brain (over 100 types) and include adrenergic, dopaminergic, muscarinic cholinergic, metabotropic glutamate, opioid, and other peptide receptors, olfactory, and light-sensitive photoreceptors. It is now established that the endocannabinoid signaling system is comprised of G protein-coupled receptors, the principal targets of THC in brain and peripheral organs, endocannabinoids, and enzymes that synthesize and degrade endocannabinoids.

The age of discovery Discovery of an endocannabinoid system was driven by scientific curiosity: how do marijuana, THC, and other exogenous cannabinoids so profoundly modulate behavioral, cognitive, motor, and physiological functions of living organisms? It was evident early on that THC, the principal and psychoactive constituent of marijuana, did not target any known receptor system in the brain, such as dopamine, serotonin, glutamate, cholinergic, adrenergic, or GABAergic receptors. Did it target a novel, as yet undiscovered signaling system? Isolation of THC and CBD from marijuana [4], [5], [6] and synthesis of an array of high-potency cannabinoids preceded and were essential for the discovery of the endocannabinoid system.

The search began by probing for a receptor. The first breakthrough came indirectly, by finding that cannabinoids inhibited cyclic AMP accumulation in neuronal cells [7]. As described above, cAMP translates receptor activity into a cascade of intracellular events, by amplifying or depressing G protein receptor signals. cAMP modulation was followed by the discovery that THC effects were stereoselective, another incentive to seek a receptor. Stereoselective or three-point (three-dimensional) binding of signaling molecules (ligands) is a common feature of receptors [8]. These leads drove the next stage of discovery. Using a radiolabeled, potent analog of THC as a ligand, Howlett identified a receptor in brain tissue that displayed appropriate pharmacological specificity for cannabinoids [9]. A radiolabeled probe was also used to map this newly discovered cannabinoid receptor in the brain [10]. Intriguingly, the brain distribution coincided with the brain map of an unknown, newly cloned receptor gene from a cDNA library [11, 12]. Confirmation was swift, as the gene encoded a protein with the same pharmacological properties as the receptor characterized in brain tissues. The existence of a brain cannabinoid receptor was indisputable. Intriguingly, the brain distribution of this receptor also corresponded to the known pharmacological actions of THC, with high to moderate expression levels in regions implicated in coordination, learning, memory, cognition, executive function, reward, and emotional state. With one receptor (CB1) now confirmed and a second cloned receptor (CB2) discovered shortly afterwards by structural homology [13], the field was ripe for discovering endocannabinoids, signaling molecules in the brain that would activate CB1 and CB2 receptors. As THC is a lipophilic molecule, it was assumed that an endogenous cannabinoid would probably be lipid-like. Indeed, using methods to isolate lipids, the discovery of the first endogenous cannabinoid signaling molecule, anandamide (AEA or N-arachidonoylethanolamine), followed shortly thereafter [14]. AEA is derived from arachidonic acid, a precursor of prostaglandins, leukotrienes, and others. Another arachidonic acid derivative which activates cannabinoid receptors, 2-AG (2-arachidonoylglycerol), was subsequently isolated [15]. 2-AG is now recognized as a primary cannabinoid transmitter in the brain. Other receptors implicated in cannabinoid signaling, but not proven definitively are GPR18 and GPR55. They exhibit limited sequence homology with CB1 and CB2 cannabinoid receptors, but their pharmacology overlaps [16]. The enzymes N-acyl phosphatidylethanolamine phospholipase D (NAPE-PLD), fatty acid amide hydrolase (FAAH), diacylglycerol lipase (DAGL), monoacylglycerol lipase (MAGL), and α/ß-hydrolase domain 6 (ABHD6) were shown to be critical for synthesizing, degrading, and regulating availability of endocannabinoids [17].

In conformity with other signaling systems, it is now established that the endocannabinoid system is composed of at least two receptors, CB1 and CB2, which are activated by endocannabinoid neurotransmitters 2-AG and AEA, to elicit physiological responses. Endocannabinoid availability is regulated by synthetic (e.g., diacylglycerol lipase alpha) and degradative enzymes (fatty acid amide hydrolase or FAAH).

Evolutionary Origins From an evolutionary perspective, the cannabinoid signaling system is ancient [18]. Comprehensive reviews of cannabinoid signaling show that invertebrates and advanced vertebrate organisms express cannabinoid signaling proteins. Although CB1 and CB2 receptors are unique to chordates, enzymatic synthesis and inactivation of endocannabinoids occur throughout the animal kingdom, even in the absence of CB1 or CB2 receptors. Accordingly, other receptors, e.g., transient receptor potential vanilloid-type ion channels, may also be used by endocannabinoids for signaling, with endocannabinoids binding to other proteins to elicit signaling responses. 2-AG is generated by diacylglycerol lipase alpha and acts via presynaptic CB1 cannabinoid receptors to inhibit neurotransmitter release. This retrograde signaling mechanism occurs throughout the vertebrate animal tree, with endocannabinoid signaling implicated in learning, locomotion, and feeding. Even though the endocannabinoid system is not unique to humans, certain human responses to cannabinoids (e.g., marijuana drug-seeking) are challenging to replicate in preclinical animal studies. For example, Western hemisphere squirrel monkeys, but not old-world monkeys, can be trained to self-administer THC [19, 20]. Squirrel monkeys will even self-administer an inhibitor of anandamide transport [21]. Conditioned place preference (animals prefer to spend time in a chamber associated with liking an administered drug) is another measure of drug liking/seeking. THC does not elicit conditioned place preference in rodents, except in those primed with prior exposure to cigarettes via smoke or vaping [22, 23]. Other drugs with abuse liability (cocaine, heroin) are readily self-administered by various species and engender robust conditioned place preference. Conceivably, the endocannabinoid system in humans is unique and elicits interoceptive effects (subjective responses) that may not be replicable in other mammalian species.

Endocannabinoid System in the Brain

The endocannabinoid system has four main components: (1) G protein-coupled cannabinoid CB1 and CB2 receptors, (2) endocannabinoids that target cannabinoid receptors and possibly other receptors, (3) enzymes that catalyze endocannabinoid biosynthesis and metabolism, and (4) mechanisms involved in cell modulation of specific endocannabinoids. Within the endocannabinoid system, cannabinoid receptors, enzymes, and genes represent putative therapeutic targets for addressing metabolic and behavioral dysfunctions.

Localization and function of cannabinoid receptors The endocannabinoid system is widespread throughout the brain. Endocannabinoids have a major role as retrograde transmitters in many brain regions, although often with region-specific specialization. A synapse is a small aqueous gap between neuronal extensions (axons, dendrites) across which transmitters diffuse. Most transmitters are released from presynaptic nerve terminals when the nerve is excited and activate receptors postsynaptically. In contrast to this general principle, the highest levels of CB1 receptors are found presynaptically in most brain regions, while endocannabinoid synthesizing enzymes are postsynaptic. AEA and 2-AG are made and released postsynaptically, diffuse to presynaptic neurons expressing cannabinoid receptors, and activate the receptors. Receptor activation modulates release of other neurotransmitters in the same cell.

The CB1 receptor is expressed in the brain and peripheral tissues, producing multiple physiological responses. In the brain, it is among the most abundant of the G protein-coupled receptors and mediates most if not all the psychoactive effects of THC in marijuana. Its brain distribution is strikingly consistent with the pharmacology of marijuana: CB1 receptors are enriched in the cerebellum (cognition, coordination), hippocampus (learning and memory), cortex (cognitive function, executive function and control, integration of sensory input), basal ganglia (motor control, planning), ventral striatum (prediction and feeling of reward), amygdala (anxiety, emotion, fear), hypothalamus (appetite, hormone levels, sexual behavior), brain stem, and spinal cord (vomiting, pain). CB1 is also found on vasculature and in some astrocytes and microglia. In peripheral tissues, CB1 receptors have been localized to the adrenal gland, heart, lung, prostate, liver, uterus, ovary, testes, vas deferens, bone marrow, thymus and tonsils myocardium, adipocytes, smooth muscle, and preganglionic sympathetic neurons. The CB2 receptor is expressed in peripheral blood mononuclear cells (macrophages, B cells, and natural killer cells), myocardium, vascular endothelium, smooth muscle, spleen, tonsils, thymus, and leukocytes, as well as the lung, testes, and sparsely in brain neurons. In brain microglia, it may regulate neuroinflammatory responses. CB2 receptors modulate the release of chemical signals primarily engaged in immune system functions (cytokines, immune cell migration) and may play a role in depression and substance abuse [24]. In contrast to CB1 receptors, the relevance of CB2 to problem and compulsive marijuana use is unknown. Anandamide and 2-arachidonoylglycerol function as full agonists at CB1 and CB2 receptors. CB2 receptors are of considerable interest because THC activation of CB2 does not produce psychoactive effects, as does THC on the CB1 receptor. Accordingly, it is a promising target for therapeutics that can circumvent the adverse effects promulgated by marijuana/THC via CB1 receptors. Accumulating evidence suggests that other receptors may be activated by cannabinoids to engender a broader and more divergent range of physiological and pharmacological effects. Several orphan G protein-coupled receptors, GPR18, GPR55, and GPR119, interact with cannabinoids. There may be others.

Five structurally distinct classes of cannabinoid compounds have been identified that bind CB1 receptors: the classical cannabinoids (e.g., THC); bicyclic cannabinoids (e.g., CP-55,940); indole-derived cannabinoids (e.g., WIN 55,212); eicosanoids (e.g., endogenous ligands AEA, 2-AG); indazole agonists (e.g AB-PINACA) and antagonist/inverse agonists (e.g., SR141716A for CB1, SR145528 for CB2) [25]. While few agonists show selectivity for the CB1 or CB2 receptors, antagonist compounds have been synthetized that are highly selective. Structural differences between CB1 and CB2 receptors are reflected in the actions of THC: THC binds CB1 and CB2 receptors with similar affinities, but THC is a partial agonist for CB1 receptors and a weak partial agonist or antagonist at CB2 receptors.

Polymorphisms of cannabinoid receptors CB receptor molecular genetics and CB regulation and functional consequences are complex [26]. Numerous polymorphic forms of the CB1 receptor have been identified, with sequences comprised of either single nucleotide polymorphisms (SNPs) or large changes in the number of repeat sequences. Polymorphisms in the untranslated region of the genes can affect splicing and promoter activity. Some of the SNPs are silent, while others lead to amino acid substitutions in the receptor protein. Many of the known genetic polymorphisms of the endocannabinoid system have been linked to pathophysiology of substance abuse, mental disorders, and energy metabolism. Specifically,

CB1 receptor gene variants have been associated with osteoporosis, ADHD, post-traumatic stress disorder, drug dependency, obesity, and depression. Functional variants of cannabinoid receptor genotypes may be associated with disturbances of the brain involving emotional and social stimuli, such as autism and depression. Polymorphisms in the CB2 gene are frequent and manifest as reduced function of the CB2. CB2 receptors reportedly are associated with disease phenotypes, including osteoporosis, schizophrenia, bipolar disease, depression, and immune-related and eating disorders [23].

Endocannabinoid synthesis, metabolism, regulation, and pharmacological relevance Endocannabinoids AEA and 2-AG play a fundamental role in regulating pleasure, memory, thinking, concentration, body movement, awareness of time, appetite, pain, sensory processing (taste, touch, smell, hearing, and sight), and immune response in the brain. They are produced "on demand" from membrane lipid precursors by biosynthetic pathways and are metabolized through distinct routes (see below). AEA and 2-AG can also be oxidized by cyclooxygenase-2, distinct lipoxygenases, or cytochromes P450, and these products likely have different biological activities arising from activation of other non CB1 or CB2 receptors. Endocannabinoids act at CB1 and CB2 receptors with different affinities [27] and may have other targets such as orphan receptors (e.g., GPR55), the transient receptor potential vanilloid 1 (TRPV1) ion channel, and the peroxisome proliferator-activated receptors (PPAR). AEA and 2-AG modulate and "fine-tune" signaling in most brain regions, to enable the brain to adapt to signals generated by multiple sources. Fundamental differences between endocannabinoid with phytocannabinoid signaling have been reported. Isoforms of sn-1-diacylglycerol lipases and N-acyl-phosphatidylethanolamine selective phospholipase D generate 2-AG and AEA, respectively. Endocannabinoids are released on demand in small quantal amounts in discrete brain regions. The process is tightly regulated; it is short-lasting and terminated rapidly by enzymatic degradation, with monoacylglycerol lipase and fatty acid amide hydrolase inactivating 2-AG and AEA, respectively [28]. THC and CBD are not substrates for these enzymes, and therefore signals cannot be rapidly cleared. If metabolic degradation of 2-AG is blocked artificially by genetic disruption of its degradative enzyme, CB1 receptors desensitize and downregulate. In a system designed to respond rapidly and reversibly to stimuli, phytocannabinoid levels and signaling are uncontrolled. Repeated dosing of THC causes the brain to adapt by altering endocannabinoid function, receptor response, promoting CB1 receptor downregulation and engendering a range of other molecular changes.

Endocannabinoid System Function in Early and Adolescent Brain Development

The brain is particularly susceptible to disruptions during the maturational process. A few clues indicate the wisdom of avoiding marijuan use during pregnancy, to enable brain development in utero to proceed undisturbed during this critical phase

[29]. Endocannabinoids play a critical role in neuronal and glial development in the brain, guiding neural stem cell survival, fate, proliferation, migration, and differentiation of neuronal and glial cells [39]. The endocannabinoid 2-AG also enhances proliferation and differentiation of oligodendrocyte progenitor cells (a subtype of glia), regulating essential steps in oligodendrocyte development [30]. Developmental endocannabinoid signaling, from fetus to young adult, may be susceptible to marijuana use during pregnancy and adolescence, possibly affecting brain structure and function. Exposure to marijuana in utero can influence neuropsychiatric outcomes in offspring. As a component of the ABCD study [31], a small sample of children exposed to marijuana in utero displayed higher scores on a 21-point rating scale for psychosis proneness [32]. The data suggest that prenatal marijuana exposure may be associated with later psychosis proneness in offspring only when fetal CB1 receptor expression is adequate, which may not occur until after mothers learn they are pregnant. CB1 receptors have been identified in the midgestational fetal human forebrain, in the amygdala, and in the hippocampus [33]. Decreased D2 dopamine receptor mRNA expression in the basal amygdala correlated with the amount of maternal marijuana intake and was specific to this brain region and not to the hippocampus or striatum [34]. Since these brain regions are involved in behavioral and mood disorders, altered dopamine receptor expression could contribute to depressive symptoms and impaired social behaviors, as reported in children upon longitudinal follow-up [35, 36]. These and other findings suggest that use of marijuana during pregnancy should be discouraged.

Initially functioning to determine cell fate prenatally, the endocannabinoid system switches to a different role, homeostatic regulation of synaptic neurotransmission, and bioenergetics in the mature nervous system [37]. In adolescents, marijuana use has been repeatedly shown to adversely impact brain structure and function [38], but with some potential for recovery. Notwithstanding the need for improved measures of use and longitudinal data, deleterious effects are more likely to occur with early age of use and continued use for decades. Adolescence is a vulnerable period because of rapid brain development [39]. The poorly understood mechanisms conceivably are shaped by age of onset, potency, frequency, duration of use, and other factors including polypharmacy and genetics. Dynamic changes in the development of corticolimbic structures occur during adolescence. Structures contributing to fear, stress responsivity, and anxiety-related behavioral regulation are regulated in part by the endocannabinoid system. During adolescence, endocannabinoid signaling modulates the maturation of local and corticolimbic circuit neurons, enhancing communication within and between brain regions and promoting brain development and plasticity. Not surprisingly, this period is sensitive to perturbations of endocannabinoid signaling as related to stress [40], potentially leading to altered developmental trajectories of neural circuits governing emotional behaviors. Perturbations of endocannabinoid signaling during adolescence conceivably hinder structural maturation of the prefrontal cortex and its circuitry [41]. Excess CB1 receptor stimulation alters dendritic arborization of specific cortical neurons. Conversely, blocking endocannabinoid activity during adolescence prevents normal developmental changes, as well [42].

Adolescents are vulnerable to environmental sources of stress and anxiety. Disturbances in endocannabinoid signaling disrupt discrete developmental changes in cortical-limbic circuit regions as manifest by altered emotional and stress responding [43]. Early cannabinoid, especially THC exposure, may increase vulnerability to adverse outcomes. Although CBD is considered safer for young patients, there are no long-term studies investigating CBD effects on brain development [44]. Endocannabinoids and marijuana-altered endocannabinoid signaling may contribute to neuropsychiatric diseases that are of developmental origins and in which modifications to signaling have been observed.

Overall Function of the Endocannabinoid System in the Brain [45]

Understanding the multiple functions of endocannabinoid signaling in the brain offers insight into the pharmacological effects of marijuana and other exogenous cannabinoids, their therapeutic potential, and undesirable adverse effects. An overview by Kalant [46] describes in depth "on-demand" endocannabinoid modulation of excitatory and inhibitory synaptic transmission and regulatory functions in the brain [47].

Brain development, neurogenesis, and psychiatric disorders. Endocannabinoid signaling is crucial for brain development. It modulates generation and survival of neurons from embryonic to adult periods [48], guides neural stem cell survival and proliferation, cell fate decisions, motility and differentiation of ensuing neuronal and glial cells (section "Endocannabinoid System in Brain" above) [37]. Developmental endocannabinoid signaling, from fetus to young adult, may be susceptible to marijuana use during pregnancy and adolescence, possibly affecting brain structure and function. Endocannabinoids and marijuana-altered endocannabinoid signaling may contribute to neuropsychiatric diseases that are of developmental origins and in which modifications to signaling have been observed: autism [49], schizophrenia [50], bipolar disorder [51], and depression [52]. The central role of the cannabinoid system in promoting adult neurogenesis in the hippocampus and the lateral ventricles provides insight into the processes underlying post-developmental neurogenesis in the mammalian brain. Abnormal activity of cannabinoid receptors may alter neurogenesis in embryonic or adult nervous systems, possibly influencing the emergence of psychiatric and neurological disorders such as anxiety, depression, and schizophrenia. An understanding of the mechanisms by which cannabinoid signaling influences developmental and adult neurogenesis may accelerate the development of new therapeutic strategies for neurodevelopmental, psychiatric, and neurological disorders. Both THC [53] and CBD [54] inhibit neurogenesis in adolescent or adult rodent brain, a process of potential relevance to a wide range of marijuana-induced adverse events [55]. Systematic review of the current literature indicates that the evidence is scant for therapeutic benefit of cannabinoids in improving depressive disorders and symptoms, anxiety disorders, attention-deficit hyperactivity disorder, Tourette syndrome, post-traumatic stress disorder, or psychosis. The evidence is of low quality that pharmaceutical THC (with or without CBD) leads to a small improvement in symptoms of anxiety among individuals with other medical conditions [56]. Conversely, marijuana use is implicated in psychosis and schizophrenia [57] [58], and its use is associated with poorer recovery from a psychotic disorder, increasing the risk of relapse, rehospitalization, and lower social functioning [59].

Neuroprotection Cannabinoids and CB1 and CB2 receptors display neuroprotective effects in the brain by preventing or decreasing the severity of damage resulting from mechanical, blood flow, or other forms of injury. Genetic ablation of the CB1 receptor exacerbates ischemic stroke [60], with CB2 agonists providing anti-inflammatory properties and CB1 activation promoting hypothermia. The use of marijuana for this purpose is compromised by the psychoactive effects and other adverse events of THC, and the development of tolerance to its neuroprotective effects.

Cannabinoids and sensory function (olfaction, auditory, and pain) The endocannabinoid system contributes to olfactory, auditory, and pain sensations. A review of these functions is beyond the scope of this summary, but readers are referred to an excellent overview [46]. There is extensive anatomical overlap of the opioid and cannabinoid receptor systems, and it appears probable that functional interactions between them occur in the production of analgesia.

Appetite and nausea A number of nuclei in the medulla are involved in the regulation of appetite and nausea. These nuclei coordinate sensory input from the brain stem, vagal complex, vestibular organs, and peripheral organs. Endocannabinoids and CB1 agonists inhibit vagal fibers to promote eating and CB1 antagonists decrease or inhibit food intake [61]. Even though marijuana has been promoted as an antiemetic for chemotherapy-induced nausea, cannabis hyperemesis syndrome (intractable vomiting) has emerged in heavy marijuana users [62].

Sleep Endogenous and exogenous cannabinoids, including marijuana and THC, affect sleep patterns [63]. There is poor quality evidence that marijuana or cannabinoids have therapeutic benefit in sleep disorders [64].

Affective disorders The endocannabinoid system has mood-elevating, antidepressant, and anxiolytic effects. The anxiolytic response to marijuana is biphasic, implying that marijuana dosing is a critical factor in minimizing risk of anxiety and depression and maximizing benefit [65, 66]. Marijuana or THC at high doses increases the risk for depression or anxiety possibly by downregulating CB1 receptors [67–70].

Seizure activity The endogenous cannabinoid system inhibits seizure susceptibility. Accordingly, it is not surprising that exogenous marijuana has antiseizure activity. However, if THC levels are high or if marijuana is consumed by susceptible individuals, THC may promote seizures [71]. CBD has therapeutic antiseizure benefits for rare childhood forms of epilepsy: Dravet and Lennox-Gastaut syndromes [72]. CBD is effective without the psychoactive effects or potential for pro-seizure activity of whole-plant marijuana [71, 73]. However, CBD is not without risk. The adverse events of CBD in animal studies range from developmental toxicity, embryo-fetal mortality, central nervous system inhibition and neurotoxicity, hepatocellular injuries, spermatogenesis reduction, organ weight alterations, male reproductive system alterations, and hypotension, although at doses higher than recommended for human pharmacotherapies. In humans, the therapeutic benfit of CBD for epilepsy and psychiatric disorders reportedly may be compromised by drug-drug interactions, hepatic abnormalities, diarrhea, fatigue, vomiting, and somnolence [74].

Motor function The endocannabinoid system plays a complex role in regulating motor pathways, which conceivably are relevant to symptomatic relief, or to addressing the underlying pathology in a wide range of neurological diseases characterized by motor impairment [75]. CB1 receptors are abundant in brain regions that regulate motor function and coordination, including the basal ganglia and cerebellum. CB1 receptors are downregulated in several neurological conditions [76].

Cognitive function Cannabinoids can both facilitate and degrade learning processes dependent upon the process involved. Endocannabinoids apparently facilitate various forms of learning and memory processes in a number of brain regions. The endogenous cannabinoid system is also implicated in extinguishing learning of aversive situations. On the other hand, THC and marijuana decrease working memory, apparently by actions in the hippocampus, a brain region critical for learning and memory. The memory decrements induced by THC or marijuana resemble hippocampal lesions. These impairments may result from suppression of glutamate release in the hippocampus, which is responsible for the establishment of synaptic plasticity [77–79]

Endocannabinoids and pain The endocannabinoid system modulates pain sensations. There is anatomical overlap of the opioid and cannabinoid receptor systems, and it appears probable that functional interactions between them occur in the production of analgesia. The endocannabinoid system is localized along the pain pathways in the spinal cord and brain pain centers including the thalamus, the dorsal raphe nucleus, and the periaqueductal grey. Both CB1 and CB2 agonists reduce pain responses. CB2-selective agonists have produced analgesia or reduction of hyperalgesia in models of neuropathic and inflammatory pain. There also is extensive overlap between endocannabinoid systems and prostanoid systems. Accordingly, modulation of endocannabinoid metabolism will affect the prostanoid system and conversely. Arachidonic acid is produced with endocannabinoid hydrolysis and anandamide, and 2-arachidonoylglycerol can be converted into prostaglandin-ethanolamides and prostaglandin-glycerol esters. The therapeutic benefit of marijuana or THC for pain management is controversial, with meta-analyses concluding the therapeutic benefit outweighed by adverse events.

Endocannabinoid System in Peripheral Tissues

Endocannabinoid signaling systems are found nearly ubiquitously in the peripheral tissues, with their distribution possibly accounting for the myriad of effects and potential medical applications of individual cannabinoids [80]. Differences in CB1 and CB2 receptor function in the body are a focus of this segment, because THC in the marijuana plant activates both CB1 and CB2 receptors and could have detrimental effects in tissues in which CB1 receptor activity may contribute to pathophysiological states [81].

Endocannabinoids in the regulation of energy intake and storage: homeostasis Accumulating evidence supports endocannabinoid signaling as critical to increased consumption and storage of energy [82]. Endocannabinoids are mobilized during exercise and conceivably replenish energy stores and contribute to analgesic and mood-elevating effects of exercise.

Gastrointestinal (GI) tract Virtually all gut functions are regulated by endocannabinoids and coordinate CNS control of its metabolic and homeostatic functions. CB1 and CB2 receptors are highly expressed on enteric nerves and on enteroendocrine cells (CB2) throughout the intestinal mucosa, on immune cells (CB1 and CB2), and enterocytes (CB1 and CB2). This discovery was guided by marijuana effects in the GI tract. Endocannabinoid actions in the GI tract are largely mediated by CB2 receptors [81].

Cardiovascular system CB1, CB2, endocannabinoids, and their anabolic/catabolic enzymes are present in cardiovascular tissues, and CB1 may contribute to the development of common cardiovascular disorders [83]. In the heart, there is strong evidence supporting a pathologically overactive endocannabinoid system (mainly CB1) in cardiometabolic disease [84], with endocannabinoids and exogenous cannabinoids exerting *opposing* effects on cardiovascular injury and inflammation. A consistently reliable acute action of marijuana is mild tachycardia, with increases cardiac output and correspondingly increases myocardial oxygen requirement. The increased myocardial load is problematic, if there is underlying coronary insufficiency [85]. Peripherally restricted CB2 agonists and CB1 antagonists are promising targets in cardiovascular disease [86].

Liver Liver differentiation (but not heart, pancreas, or kidney differentiation) requires functional CB1 and CB2 receptor signaling. Cannabinoid receptor expression is normally low in the liver, with CB1 and CB2 receptors acting in opposite directions: CB2 receptors mediate several biological functions in various types of liver cells, and CB1 *blockade* contributes to beneficial metabolic effects [40]. CB1 expression increases in pathological states, and the receptor plays a critical role in liver disease. It promotes fibrogenesis, steatosis, and the cardiovascular complications of liver disease, whereas CB2 is protective, reducing these indices of liver dysfunction. Clinical studies of marijuana reveal its detrimental effects on the liver, presumably by activating the CB1. Peripherally restricted CB1 antagonists and CB2 agonists have therapeutic potential in the liver: activation of CB2 reduces proinflammatory cytokines, attenuates reperfusion injury, reduces fat accumulation, and is antifibrotic; CB2 agonists and peripherally restricted CB1 antagonists may benefit (non)alcoholic fatty liver diseases.

Immune system Endocannabinoids modulate the functional activities of immune cells, largely through CB2 receptors. Immune functions may be modulated through the interaction of ligands with the CB2 cannabinoid receptor, providing novel targets for therapeutic manipulation.

Muscle The endocannabinoid 2-AG controls skeletal muscle cell differentiation via CB1 receptor-dependent inhibition of Kv7 channels [87]. In adults, endocannabinoid signaling (largely through CB2 receptors) contributes to regulating energy metabolism in muscle and the formation of new muscle fibers.

Reproductive system Endocannabinoid signaling, primarily mediated by the CB2 receptor, regulates all critical stages of pregnancy and affects pregnancy events. Signaling is also involved in the preservation of normal sperm function and thus male fertility.

Skin Endocannabinoid signaling, through both CB1 and CB2, is involved in regulating skin functions such as proliferation, differentiation, cell survival, immune responses, and suppressing cutaneous inflammation. Exogenous modulators of the receptors would clarify the role of the endocannabinoid system in hyperproliferative skin conditions, allergic, and inflammatory skin diseases.

Bone Endocannabinoid signaling regulates bone elongation and bone remodeling by modulating bone cell proliferation, by communicating between bone cells, and by neuronal control of bone remodeling. THC has profound effects on murine bone growth.

Other organs The role of endocannabinoid signaling in respiratory tract and urinary system remains unclear. The recent vaping crisis in the United States has implicated THC in > 80% of the new cases of EVALI (e-vaping associated lung injury). It is well documented that pulmonary function is compromised by marijuana smoking. Whether THC alone or a different substance used in preparing vaping cartiges or pods is responsbile for the vaping crisis is unknown [88]. Preliminary evidence indicates that CB1 and CB2 receptors may contribute to kidney disease. Endocannabinoid signaling is also implicated in pancreatic development, with fetal endocannabinoids orchestrating the organization of pancreatic islet microarchitecture [89].

Circulating endocannabinoids Circulating endocannabinoids respond to or reflect stressful conditions, and their concentrations are may be modulated in stress disorders, e.g., PTSD. At present, physiological regulation that contributes to circulating concentrations is too complex for using blood levels as a biomarker for a specific disorder. Circulating concentrations of 2-arachidonoylglycerol are circadian and dysregulated when sleep is disrupted. Other conditions under which circulating endocannabinoids are altered include inflammation, pain, and psychosis.

Disturbances of the Endocannabinoid System in the Brain

Every analysis of endocannabinoid tone, signaling, and relevance to disease states should consider marijuana use as a critical, confounding variable.

Genetic variants of endocannabinoid system neurological disorders Rare genetic variants in the endocannabinoid system genes encoding the CB1 and CB2 receptors, as well as synthetic and metabolic enzymes (DAGLA, MGLL, FAAH), have been identified in genetic testing of a small number of patients (6032) with neurological disorders. Heterozygous rare coding variants in CNR1 gene (CB1 receptor) were significantly associated with pain sensitivity (especially migraine), sleep, and memory disorders – alone or in combination with anxiety – compared to controls without variants. These phenotypes are similar to those implicated in a "clinical endocannabinoid deficiency syndrome" theory. Heterozygous rare variants in DAGLA, which encodes diacylglycerol lipase alpha (synthesizes 2-AG), were significantly associated with seizures and neurodevelopmental disorders (autism, brain morphology abnormalities), compared to controls. The severe phenotypes associated with rare DAGLA variants underscore the critical role of rapid 2-AG synthesis and the endocannabinoid system in regulating neurological function and development [90].

Genetic variants of the endocannabinoid system in behaviors A variant of FAAH (A385), which metabolizes and inactivates endocannabinoids, leads to reduced FAAH activity, resulting in increased AEA. This FAAH polymorphism in humans has been linked to threat and stress responses, manifest as reduced amygdala reactivity to threat possibly due to enhanced signaling. Stress exposure rapidly mobilizes FAAH to deplete anandamide and increase neuronal excitability in the amygdala. The FAAH variant A385 may sustain higher levels of AEA under stressful conditions.

Endocannabinoid system anomalies in schizophrenia The relevance of the endocannabinoid system to schizophrenia is through: 1. the abnormal levels of endogenous cannabinoids or receptors, 2. the association between marijuana use and the onset, course of illness, dose-dependent symptom severity, and 3. therapeutic potential of cannabidiol, a potential antipsychotic that elevates endocannabinoids. This segment summarizes the evidence for 1. In 5 studies (226 patients, 385 controls), significantly higher concentrations of anandamide were found in the CSF of patients than controls. In 9 studies (344 patients, 411 controls), anandamide levels were higher in blood of patients compared with controls. In 3 studies (88 patients, 179 controls), higher expression of CB1 was found on peripheral immune cells in patients compared with controls. Higher endocannabinoid tone was found at an early stage of illness in individuals who were antipsychotic naïve or free and an inverse association with symptom severity and was normalized after successful treatment. Testing clinically relevant markers of the endocannabinoid signaling elements in blood and CSF of people with psychotic illness may eventually provide useful biomarkers for the psychotic disorder and even insight into pathophysiological processes. However, as not all studies accounted for important variables, such as marijuana use, it is premature to assume that endocannabinoid dysregulation is a state or trait of the disease [91]. Nonetheless, higher endocannabinoid tone at an early stage of illness showed an inverse association with symptom severity, but normalized after treatments. Children with autism spectrum disorder had lower serum levels of anandamide, 2-arachidonoylglycerol, and their related endogenous compounds, N-palmitoylethanolamine and N-oleoylethanolamine, which were not associated with or correlated with age, gender, BMI, and medications.

Marijuana and the Brain: Receptors and Changes in Endocannabinoid Signaling

A comprehensive review of marijuana effects in the brain and behavior is beyond the scope of this chapter [92–105]. Marijuana can affect the brain at multiple levels, by physically altering molecular, cellular, function, circuitry, and morphology; by compromising cognition, motivation, learning, memory, coordination, sleep, and affect; and by engendering addiction and psychosis. Unless laboratory based, or constructed as a randomized controlled trial, current human marijuana research is challenging: THC doses consumed are rarely known unless chemical composition of each consumed product is tested, including the ratio of THC to CBD which varies widely, resulting in additive, neutral, or antagonistic pharmacological effects [106, 107]. Conclusions drawn from consumption of retail "marijuana" and self-reporting patterns of use are valid but lack the rigor needed to quantify the consequences of marijuana based on potency, purity, composition of matter, frequency of use and route of delivery. Also, polypharmacy is common among marijuana users, representing another potential confounding variable [108, 109]. At present, molecular observations are insufficient to develop a comprehensive model of the mechanisms underlying the behavioral, psychiatric, cognitive and psychological sequelae engendered by marijuana.

CB1 receptor tolerance Cannabinoid synaptic adaptability is core to understanding the primary effects of marijuana in the brain and how these effects can trigger a cascade of biological changes that compromise learning, motor function, tolerance, and other brain functions. CB receptors are primary targets of THC, the principal cannabinoid in marijuana. Cannabinoid tolerance leading to diminished biological responses in isolated tissue develops over time and is attributable to loss of receptor function and CB1 receptor downregulation following chronic exposure to THC. CB1 receptor down-regulation has also been observed in a brain region-specific manner. In humans, non-invasive PET imaging has revealed CB1 receptor downregulation after chronic marijuana exposure [110]. Specificity of regions more responsive to downregulation was observed in marijuana-dependent subjects, with reductions largely in cortical areas. Receptor downregulation correlated with number of years marijuana was smoked but was reversible upon cessation. One possible interpretation of these findings is that receptor downregulation may function as a driver of compulsive marijuana use to restore equilibrium levels of CB1 activity. Adaptation is variable and can be as transient as modulation of endocannabinoid signaling or longer term, involving CB1 receptor internalization and downregulation or altered activity of enzymes involved in synthesis and metabolism of endocannabinoids. Longer time frame adaptive responses include the generation of new neurons from neural stem cells in the hippocampus of the adult brain, crucial functions attenuated by THC. CB2 downregulation is not as reproducible as CB1 and may be modulated similarly by both agonists and antagonists. At a more granular level not feasible for scrutiny in living human brain, THC induces expression of immediate early genes (zif268, pCREB, c-Fos) differentially in brain regions, primarily in the dopamine-rich striatum, hippocampus, and cortex [111]. Repeated THC exposure produces less induction of these factors in certain regions, possibly reflecting the development of tolerance. In contrast, CB1 receptors in the basal ganglia exhibit less plasticity than in other brain regions, possibly accounting for why humans show less tolerance to the subjective and motor effects of marijuana.

Other molecular changes In rodents, acute marijuana exposure increases dopamine and opioid peptide release and attenuates GABA and glutamate release in the nucleus accumbens, leading to a rewarding effect. Cognitive function likely is compromised by reduced acetylcholine release in the hippocampus and prefrontal cortex. Other brain regions are also affected by introduction of THC. After repeated THC administration, three key changes conceivably drive impaired cognition, dysphoria/stress, and marijuana-seeking behavior: (1) CB1 receptors and function decline in many brain regions, especially in human and rodent cortex, even though declinations are not parallel in the two species. Memory and cognitive impairment is likely associated with the decline in CB1 receptor and impaired signaling in regions critical for learning and memory; (2) repeated exposure to THC also affects the magnitude of reward, as it downregulates dopamine signaling; (3) stress-related signaling (e.g., dynorphin, corticotropin-releasing factor) rises in the "emotional" amygdala, conceivably elevating dysphoria and increasing the compulsion to use the drug [94, 112]. Conventional approaches to investigating the biological targets of marijuana have traditionally been focused on "known zones" of commonly accepted critical brain regions and biological targets. Future preclinical research should incorporate more advanced approaches, using RNA-Seq and corresponding proteomics in multiple brain regions and within single neurons to clarify pathways most affected by a range of THC doses, THC:CBD ratios of marijuana, used acutely or repeatedly, by various routes (smoking, vaping, edibles) for various periods of time and at different age ranges. Ultimately, a comprehensive view of the full spectrum of marijuana's biological consequences will be generated.

Conclusion

Marijuana is the third most commonly used drug in the United States among adults (after alcohol and tobacco) and the second most widely used substance by adolescents. The principal target of marijuana is the vastly influential endocannabinoid system, a signaling system that modulates a wide range of behavioral, cognitive, psychiatric, endocrine, and motor functions in the brain and peripheral tissues. Consumption of novel, high potency marijuana products has launched, a vast human experiment without informed consent.

References

1. Chandra S, Radwan MM, Majumdar CG, Church JC, Freeman TP, ElSohly MA. New trends in cannabis potency in USA and Europe during the last decade (2008-2017). Eur Arch Psychiatry Clin Neurosci. 2019;269(1):5–15.
2. Santiago M, Sachdev S, Arnold JC, McGregor IS, Connor M. Absence of entourage: Terpenoids commonly found in Cannabis sativa do not modulate the functional activity of Δ(9)-THC at human CB(1) and CB(2) receptors. Cannabis Cannabinoid Res. 2019;4(3):165–76.
3. Armenian P, Darracq M, Gevorkyan J, Clark S, Kaye B, Brandehoff NP. Intoxication from the novel synthetic cannabinoids AB-PINACA and ADB-PINACA: a case series and review of the literature. Neuropharmacology. 2018;134(Pt A):82–91.
4. Gaoni Y, Mechoulam R. Isolation, structure and partial synthesis of an active constituent of hashish. J Amer Chem Soc. 1964;86:1646–7.
5. Mechoulam R, Shani A, Edery H, Grunfeld Y. Chemical basis of hashish activity. Science. 1970;169(3945):611–2.
6. Mechoulam R, Shvo Y, Hashish I. The structure of cannabidiol. Tetrahedron. 1963;19(12):2073–8.
7. Howlett AC. Inhibition of neuroblastoma adenylate cyclase by cannabinoid and nantradol compounds. Life Sci. 1984;35(17):1803–10.
8. Howlett AC, Champion TM, Wilken GH, Mechoulam R. Stereochemical effects of 11-OH-delta 8-tetrahydrocannabinol-dimethylheptyl to inhibit adenylate cyclase and bind to the cannabinoid receptor. Neuropharmacology. 1990;29(2):161–5.
9. Bidaut-Russell M, Devane WA, Howlett AC. Cannabinoid receptors and modulation of cyclic AMP accumulation in the rat brain. J Neurochem. 1990;55(1):21–6.

10. Westlake TM, Howlett AC, Bonner TI, Matsuda LA, Herkenham M. Cannabinoid receptor binding and messenger RNA expression in human brain: an in vitro receptor autoradiography and in situ hybridization histochemistry study of normal aged and Alzheimer's brains. Neuroscience. 1994;63(3):637–52.

11. Matsuda LA, Lolait SJ, Brownstein MJ, Young AC, Bonner TI. Structure of a cannabinoid receptor and functional expression of the cloned cDNA. Nature. 1990;346:561–4.

12. Felder CC, Veluz JS, Williams HL, Briley EM, Matsuda LA. Cannabinoid agonists stimulate both receptor- and non-receptor-mediated signal transduction pathways in cells transfected with and expressing cannabinoid receptor clones. Mol Pharmacol. 1992;42(5):838–45.

13. Griffin G, Tao Q, Abood ME. Cloning and pharmacological characterization of the rat CB(2) cannabinoid receptor. J Pharmacol Exp Ther. 2000;292(3):886–94.

14. Devane WA, Hanus L, Breuer A, Pertwee RG, Stevenson LA, Griffin G, Gibson D, Mandelbaum A, Etinger A, Mechoulam R. Isolation and structure of a brain constituent that binds to the cannabinoid receptor. Science. 1992;258(5090):1946–9.

15. Mechoulam R, Ben-Shabat S, Hanus L, Ligumsky M, Kaminski NE, Schatz AR, Gopher A, Almog S, Martin BR, Compton DR, et al. Identification of an endogenous 2-monoglyceride, present in canine gut, that binds to cannabinoid receptors. Biochem Pharmacol. 1995;50(1):83–90.

16. Irving A, Abdulrazzaq G, Chan SLF, Penman J, Harvey J, Alexander SPH. Cannabinoid receptor-related orphan G protein-coupled receptors. Adv Pharmacol. 2017;80:223–47.

17. Hu SS, Mackie K. Distribution of the endocannabinoid System in the central nervous System. Handb Exp Pharmacol. 2015;231:59–93.

18. Elphick MR. The evolution and comparative neurobiology of endocannabinoid signaling. Philos Trans R Soc Lond Ser B Biol Sci. 2012;367(1607):3201–15.

19. John WS, Martin TJ, Nader MA. Behavioral determinants of cannabinoid self-administration in old world monkeys. Neuropsychopharmacology. 2017;42(7):1522–30.

20. Justinová Z, Redhi GH, Goldberg SR, Ferré S. Differential effects of presynaptic versus postsynaptic adenosine A2A receptor blockade on Δ9-tetrahydrocannabinol (THC) self-administration in squirrel monkeys. J Neurosci. 2014;34(19):6480–4.

21. Schindler CW, Scherma M, Redhi GH, Vadivel SK, Makriyannis A, Goldberg SR, Justinova Z. Self-administration of the anandamide transport inhibitor AM404 by squirrel monkeys. Psychopharmacology. 2016;233(10):1867–77.

22. Wakeford AG, Flax SM, Pomfrey RL, Riley AL. Adolescent delta-9-tetrahydrocannabinol (THC) exposure fails to affect THC-induced place and taste conditioning in adult male rats. Pharmacol Biochem Behav. 2016;140:75–81.

23. Ponzoni L, Moretti M, Braida D, Zoli M, Clementi F, Viani P, Sala M, Gotti C. Increased sensitivity to Δ(9)-THC-induced rewarding effects after seven-week exposure to electronic and tobacco cigarettes in mice. Eur Neuropsychopharmacol. 2019;29(4):566–76.

24. Onaivi ES, Ishiguro H, Gong JP, Patel S, Meozzi PA, Myers L, Perchuk A, Mora Z, Tagliaferro PA, Gardner E, Brusco A, Akinshola BE, et al. Functional expression of brain neuronal CB2 cannabinoid receptors are involved in the effects of drugs of abuse and in depression. Ann N Y Acad Sci. 2008;1139:434–49.

25. Howlett AC, Abood ME. CB(1) and CB(2) receptor pharmacology. Adv Pharmacol. 2017;80:169–206.

26. Onaivi ES. Cannabinoid receptors in brain: pharmacogenetics, neuropharmacology, neurotoxicology, and potential therapeutic applications. Int Rev Neurobiol. 2009;88:335–69.

27. Pertwee RG, Howlett AC, Abood ME, Alexander SP, Di Marzo V, Elphick MR, Greasley PJ, Hansen HS, Kunos G, Mackie K, Mechoulam R, Ross RA. International Union of Basic and Clinical Pharmacology. LXXIX cannabinoid receptors and their ligands: beyond CB1 and CB2. Pharmacol Rev. 2010;62:588–631.

28. Alpár A, Di Marzo V, Harkany T. At the tip of an iceberg: prenatal marijuana and its possible relation to neuropsychiatric outcome in the offspring. Biol Psychiatry. 2016;79(7):e33–45.

29. Alpár A, Tortoriello G, Calvigioni D, Niphakis MJ, Milenkovic I, Bakker J, Cameron GA, Hanics J, Morris CV, Fuzik J, Kovacs GG, Cravatt BF, Parnavelas JG, Andrews WD, Hurd

YL, Keimpema E, Harkany T. Endocannabinoids modulate cortical development by configuring Slit2/Robo1 signaling. Nat Commun. 2014;5:4421.

30. Sanchez-Rodriguez MA, Gomez O, Esteban PF, Garcia-Ovejero D, Molina-Holgado E. The endocannabinoid 2-arachidonoy glycerol regulates oligodendrocyte progenitor cell migration. Biochem Pharmacol. 2018;157:180–8.
31. https://abcdstudy.org/.
32. Fine JD, Moreau AL, Karcher NR, Agrawal A, Rogers CE, Barch DM, Bogdan R. Association of prenatal Marijuana exposure with psychosis proneness among children in the adolescent brain cognitive development (ABCD) study. JAMA Psychiat. 2019;76(7):762–4.
33. Wang X, Dow-Edwards D, Keller E, Hurd YL. Preferential limbic expression of the cannabinoid receptor mRNA in the human fetal brain. Neuroscience. 2003;118:681–94.
34. Wang X, Dow-Edwards D, Anderson V, Minkoff H, Hurd YL. In utero marijuana exposure associated with abnormal amygdala dopamine D2 gene expression in the human fetus. Biol Psychiatry. 2004;56:909–15.
35. Goldschmidt L, Day NL, Richardson GA. Effects of prenatal marijuana exposure on child behavior problems at age 10. Neurotoxicol Teratol. 2000;22:325–36.
36. Leech SL, Richardson GA, Goldschmidt L, Day NL. Prenatal substance exposure: effects on attention and impulsivity of 6-year olds. Neurotoxicol Teratol. 1999;21:109–18.
37. Maccarrone M, Guzmán M, Mackie K, Doherty P, Harkany T. Programming of neural cells by (endo)cannabinoids: from physiological rules to emerging therapies. Nat Rev Neurosci. 2014;15(12):786–801.
38. Lubman DI, Cheetham A, Yücel M. Marijuana and adolescent brain development. Pharmacol Ther. 2015;148:1–16.
39. Brumback T, Castro N, Jacobus J, Tapert S. Effects of marijuana use on brain structure and function: neuroimaging findings from a neurodevelopmental perspective. Int Rev Neurobiol. 2016;129:33–65.
40. Crowe MS, Nass SR, Gabella KM, Kinsey SG. The endocannabinoid system modulates stress, emotionality, and inflammation. Brain Behav Immun. 2014;42:1–5.
41. Dow-Edwards D, Silva L. Endocannabinoids in brain plasticity: cortical maturation, HPA axis function and behavior. Brain Res. 2017;1654(Pt B):157–64.
42. Meyer HC, Lee FS, Gee DG. The role of the endocannabinoid System and genetic variation in adolescent brain development. Neuropsychopharmacology. 2018;43(1):21–33.
43. Lee TT, Gorzalka BB. Evidence for a role of adolescent endocannabinoid signaling in regulating HPA Axis stress responsivity and emotional behavior development. Int Rev Neurobiol. 2015;125:49–84.
44. Schonhofen P, Bristot IJ, Crippa JA, Hallak JEC, Zuardi AW, Parsons RB, Klamt F. Cannabinoid-based therapies and brain development: potential harmful effect of early modulation of the endocannabinoid System. CNS Drugs. 2018;32(8):697–712.
45. Madras, BK. World Health Organization, Update of Marijuana and its Medical Use https://www.who.int/medicines/access/controlled-substances/6_2_marijuana_update.pdf.
46. Harold Kalant, Chapter Thirteen - Effects of Cannabis and Cannabinoids in the Human Nervous System, Editor(s): Bertha Madras, Michael Kuhar, The Effects of Drug Abuse on the Human Nervous System, Academic Press, 2014, Pages 387-422, ISBN 9780124186798, San Diego, CA
47. lger BE, Kim J. Supply and demand for endocannabinoids. Trends Neurosci. 2011;34(6):304–15.
48. de Oliveira RW, Oliveira CL, Guimarães FS, Campos AC. Cannabinoid signaling in embryonic and adult neurogenesis: possible implications for psychiatric and neurological disorders. Acta Neuropsychiatr. 2019;31(1):1–16.
49. Foldy C, Malenka RC, Sudhof TC. Autism-associated neuroligin-3 mutations commonly disrupt tonic endocannabinoid signaling. Neuron. 2013;78:498–509.
50. Eggan SM, Stoyak SR, Verrico CD, Lewis DA. Cannabinoid CB1 receptor immunoreactivity in the prefrontal cortex: comparison of schizophrenia and major depressive disorder. Neuropsychopharmacology. 2010;35:2060–71.

51. Minocci D, et al. Genetic association between bipolar disorder and 524A>C (Leu133Ile) polymorphism of CNR2 gene, encoding for CB2 cannabinoid receptor. J Affect Disord. 2011;134:427–30.

52. Monteleone P, Bifulco M, Maina G, Tortorella A, Gazzerro P, Proto MC, Di Filippo C, Monteleone F, Canestrelli B, Buonerba G, Bogetto F, Maj M. Investigation of CNR1 and FAAH endocannabinoid gene polymorphisms in bipolar disorder and major depression. Pharmacol Res. 2010;61(5):400–4.

53. Steel RW, Miller JH, Sim DA, Day DJ. Delta-9-tetrahydrocannabinol disrupts hippocampal neuroplasticity and neurogenesis in trained, but not untrained adolescent Sprague-Dawley rats. Brain Res. 2014;1548:12–9.

54. Schiavon AP, Bonato JM, Milani H, Guimarães FS, Weffort de Oliveira RM. Influence of single and repeated cannabidiol administration on emotional behavior and markers of cell proliferation and neurogenesis in non-stressed mice. Prog Neuro-Psychopharmacol Biol Psychiatry. 2016;64:27–34.

55. Prenderville JA, Kelly ÁM, Downer EJ. The role of cannabinoids in adult neurogenesis. Br J Pharmacol. 2015;172(16):3950–63.

56. Black N, Stockings E, Campbell G, Tran LT, Zagic D, Hall WD, Farrell M, Degenhardt L. Cannabinoids for the treatment of mental disorders and symptoms of mental disorders: a systematic review and metaanalysis. Lancet Psychiatry. 2019;12: 995-1010.

57. Hasan A, von Keller R, Friemel CM, et al. Cannabis use and psychosis: a review of reviews [published online ahead of print, 2019 Sep 28]. Eur Arch Psychiatry Clin Neurosci. 2019; https://doi.org/10.1007/s00406-019-01068-z

58. Di Forti M, Quattrone D, Freeman TP, Tripoli G, Gayer-Anderson C, Quigley H, Rodriguez V, Jongsma HE, Ferraro L, La Cascia C, La Barbera D, Tarricone I, Berardi D, Szöke A, Arango C, Tortelli A, Velthorst E, Bernardo M, Del-Ben CM, Menezes PR, Selten JP, Jones PB, Kirkbride JB, Rutten BP, de Haan L, Sham PC, van Os J, Lewis CM, Lynskey M, Morgan C, Murray RM, EU-GEI WP2 Group. The contribution of cannabis use to variation in the incidence of psychotic disorder across Europe (EU-GEI): a multicentre case-control study. Lancet Psychiatry. 2019;6(5):427–36.

59. Wright A, Cather C, Gilman J, Evins AE. The changing legal landscape of Cannabis use and its role in youth-onset psychosis. Child Adolesc Psychiatr Clin N Am. 2020;29(1):145–56.

60. Parmentier-Batteur S, Jin K, Mao XO, Xie L, Greenberg DA. Increased severity of stroke in CB1 cannabinoid receptor knock-out mice. J Neurosci. 2002;22(22):9771–5.

61. Izzo AA, Piscitelli F, Capasso R, Aviello G, Romano B, Borrelli F, Petrosino S, Di Marzo V. Peripheral endocannabinoid dysregulation in obesity: relation to intestinal motility and energy processing induced by food deprivation and re-feeding. Br J Pharmacol. 2009;158(2):451–61.

62. Patel RS, Patel J, Jaladi PR, Bhimanadham NN, Imran S, Tankersley WE. Burden of Persistent Vomiting With Cannabis Use Disorder: Report From 55,549 Hospitalizations in the United States. Psychosomatics. 2019;60(6):549–555.

63. Murillo-Rodríguez E. The role of the CB1 receptor in the regulation of sleep. Prog Neuro-Psychopharmacol Biol Psychiatry. 2008;32(6):1420–7.

64. Whiting PF, Wolff RF, Deshpande S, Di Nisio M, Duffy S, Hernandez AV, Keurentjes JC, Lang S, Misso K, Ryder S, Schmidlkofer S, Westwood M, Kleijnen J. Cannabinoids for medical use: a systematic review and meta-analysis. JAMA. 2015;313(24):2456–73.

65. Akirav I. The role of cannabinoids in modulating emotional and non-emotional memory processes in the hippocampus. Front Behav Neurosci. 2011;5:34.

66. Lazary J, Juhasz J, Hunyady L, Bagdy G. Personalized medicine can pave the way for the safe use of CB receptor antagonists. Trends Pharmacol Sci. 2011;32(5):270–80.

67. Hirvonen J, Goodwin RS, Li CT, Terry GE, Zoghbi SS, Morse C, Pike VW, Volkow ND, Huestis MA, Innis RB. Reversible and regionally selective downregulation of brain cannabinoid CB1 receptors in chronic daily marijuana smokers. Mol Psychiatry. 2012;17(6):642–9.

68. Silins E, Horwood LJ, Patton GC, Fergusson DM, Olsson CA, Hutchinson DM, Spry E, Toumbourou JW, Degenhardt L, Swift W, Coffey C, Tait RJ, Letcher P, Copeland J. Mattick RP; marijuana cohorts research consortium. Young adult sequelae of adolescent marijuana use: an integrative analysis. Lancet Psychiatry. 2014;1(4):286–93.

69. Shollenbarger SG, Price J, Wieser J, Lisdahl K. Poorer frontolimbic white matter integrity is associated with chronic marijuana use, FAAH genotype, and increased depressive and apathy symptoms in adolescents and young adults. Neuroimage Clin. 2015;8:117–25.

70. CHindley G, Beck K, Borgan F, et al. Psychiatric symptoms caused by cannabis constituents: a systematic review and meta-analysis. Lancet Psychiatry. 2020;7(4):344–353.

71. Katona I. Marijuana and endocannabinoid signaling in epilepsy. Handb Exp Pharmacol. 2015;231:285–316.

72. Samanta D. Cannabidiol: a review of clinical efficacy and safety in epilepsy. Pediatr Neurol. 2019;96:24–9.

73. Rosenberg EC, Tsien RW, Whalley BJ, Devinsky O. Cannabinoids and Epilepsy. Neurotherapeutics. 2015;12(4):747–768.

74. Huestis MA, Solimini R, Pichini S, Pacifici R, Carlier J, Busardò FP. Cannabidiol adverse effects and toxicity. Curr Neuropharmacol. 2019;17(10):974–89.

75. El Manira A, Kyriakatos A. The role of endocannabinoid signaling in motor control. Physiology (Bethesda). 2010;25(4):230–8.

76. Fernández-Ruiz J. The endocannabinoid system as a target for the treatment of motor dysfunction. Br J Pharmacol. 2009;156(7):1029–40.

77. Mechoulam R, Parker LA. The endocannabinoid system and the brain. Annu Rev Psychol. 2013;64:21–47.

78. Zanettini C, Panlilio LV, Alicki M, Goldberg SR, Haller J, Yasar S. Effects of endocannabinoid system modulation on cognitive and emotional behavior. Front Behav Neurosci. 2011;5:57.

79. Morena M, Campolongo P. The endocannabinoid system: an emotional buffer in the modulation of memory function. Neurobiol Learn Mem. 2014;112:30–43.

80. Joshi N, Onaivi ES. Endocannabinoid System components: overview and tissue distribution. Adv Exp Med Biol. 2019;1162:1–12.

81. Maccarone M, Bab I, Bíró T, Cabral GA, Dey SK, Di Marzo V, Konje JC, Kunos G, Mechoulam R, Pacher P, Sharkey KA, Zimmer A. Endocannabinoid signaling at the periphery: 50 years after THC. Trends Pharmacol Sci. 2015;36(5):277–96.

82. Ruiz de Azua I, Lutz B. Multiple endocannabinoid-mediated mechanisms in the regulation of energy homeostasis in brain and peripheral tissues. Cell Mol Life Sci. 2019;76(7):1341–63.

83. Pacher P, Kunos G. Modulating the endocannabinoid system in human health and disease--successes and failures. FEBS J. 2013;280:1918–43.

84. Rajesh M, et al. Cannabinoid-1 receptor activation induces reactive oxygen species-dependent and -independent mitogen-activated protein kinase activation and cell death in human coronary artery endothelial cells. Br J Pharmacol. 2010;160:688–700.

85. Jouanjus E, et al. Marijuana use: signal of increasing risk of serious cardiovascular disorders. J Am Heart Assoc. 2014;3:e000638.

86. Steffens S, Pacher P. Targeting cannabinoid receptor CB2 in cardiovascular disorders: promises and controversies. Br J Pharmacol. 2012;167:313–23.

87. Iannotti FA, Silvestri C, Mazzarella E, Martella A, Calvigioni D, Piscitelli F, Ambrosino P, Petrosino S, Czifra G, Bíró T, Harkany T, Taglialatela M, Di Marzo V. The endocannabinoid 2-AG controls skeletal muscle cell differentiation via CB1 receptor-dependent inhibition of Kv7 channels. Proc Natl Acad Sci U S A. 2014;111(24):E2472–81.

88. https://www.cdc.gov/tobacco/basic_information/e-cigarettes/severe-lung-disease.html..

89. Malenczyk K, Keimpema E, Piscitelli F, Calvigioni D, Björklund P, Mackie K, Di Marzo V, Hökfelt TG, Dobrzyn A, Harkany T. Fetal endocannabinoids orchestrate the organization of pancreatic islet microarchitecture. Proc Natl Acad Sci U S A. 2015;112(45):E6185–94.

90. Smith DR, Stanley CM, Foss T, Boles RG, McKernan K. Rare genetic variants in the endo-cannabinoid system genes CNR1 and DAGLA are associated with neurological phenotypes in humans. PLoS One. 2017;12(11):e0187926.
91. Minichino A, Senior M, Brondino N, et al. Measuring Disturbance of the Endocannabinoid System in Psychosis: A Systematic Review and Meta-analysis [published online ahead of print, 2019 Jun 5]. JAMA Psychiatry. 2019;76(9):914–923.
92. Manza P, Yuan K, Shokri-Kojori E, Tomasi D, Volkow ND. Brain structural changes in can-nabis dependence: association with MAGL [published online ahead of print, 2019 Nov 6]. Mol Psychiatry. 2019; https://doi.org/10.1038/s41380-019-0577-z.
93. Madras BK. Tinkering with THC-to-CBD ratios in marijuana. Neuropsychopharmacology. 2019;44(1):215–6.
94. Zehra A, Burns J, Liu CK, Manza P, Wiers CE, Volkow ND, Wang GJ. Marijuana addiction and the brain: a review. J Neuroimmune Pharmacol. 2018;13(4):438–52.
95. Manza P, Tomasi D, Volkow ND. Subcortical local functional Hyperconnectivity in mari-juana dependence. Biol Psychiatry Cogn Neurosci Neuroimaging. 2018;3(3):285–93.
96. Volkow ND, Compton WM, Wargo EM. The risks of marijuana use during pregnancy. JAMA. 2017;317(2):129–30.
97. Bloomfield MA, Ashok AH, Volkow ND, Howes OD. The effects of Δ(9)-tetrahydrocannabinol on the dopamine system. Nature. 2016;539(7629):369–77.
98. Wiers CE, Shokri-Kojori E, Wong CT, Abi-Dargham A, Demiral ŞB, Tomasi D, Wang GJ, Volkow ND. Marijuana abusers show Hypofrontality and blunted brain responses to a stimulant challenge in females but not in males. Neuropsychopharmacology. 2016;41(10):2596–605.
99. van de Giessen E, Weinstein JJ, Cassidy CM, Haney M, Dong Z, Ghazzaoui R, Ojeil N, Kegeles LS, Xu X, Vadhan NP, Volkow ND, Slifstein M, Abi-Dargham A. Deficits in striatal dopamine release in marijuana dependence. Mol Psychiatry. 2017;22(1):68–75.
100. Volkow ND, Swanson JM, Evins AE, DeLisi LE, Meier MH, Gonzalez R, Bloomfield MA, Curran HV, Baler R. Effects of marijuana use on human behavior, including cognition, moti-vation, and psychosis: a review. JAMA Psychiat. 2016;73(3):292–7.
101. Volkow ND, Wang GJ, Telang F, Fowler JS, Alexoff D, Logan J, Jayne M, Wong C, Tomasi D. Decreased dopamine brain reactivity in marijuana abusers is associated with negative emotionality and addiction severity. Proc Natl Acad Sci U S A. 2014;111(30):E3149–56.
102. Volkow ND, Compton WM, Weiss SR. Adverse health effects of marijuana use. N Engl J Med. 2014;371(9):879.
103. Muniyappa R, Sable S, Ouwerkerk R, Mari A, Gharib AM, Walter M, Courville A, Hall G, Chen KY, Volkow ND, Kunos G, Huestis MA, Skarulis MC. Metabolic effects of chronic marijuana smoking. Diabetes Care. 2013;36(8):2415–22.
104. Hirvonen J, Goodwin RS, Li CT, Terry GE, Zoghbi SS, Morse C, Pike VW, Volkow ND, Huestis MA, Innis RB. Reversible and regionally selective downregulation of brain cannabi-noid CB1 receptors in chronic daily marijuana smokers. MolPsychiatry. 2012;17(6):642–9.
105. Madras BK. Update of marijuana and its medical uses. 2015. https://www.who.int/medi-cines/access/controlled-substances/6_2_marijuana_update.pdf.
106. Freeman AM, Petrilli K, Lees R, Hindocha C, Mokrysz C, Curran HV, Saunders R, Freeman TP. How does cannabidiol (CBD) influence the acute effects of delta-9-tetrahydrocannabinol (THC) in humans? A systematic review. Neurosci Biobehav Rev. 2019;107:696–712.
107. Wall MB, Pope R, Freeman TP, Kowalczyk OS, Demetriou L, Mokrysz C, Hindocha C, Lawn W, Bloomfield MA, Freeman AM, Feilding A, Nutt D, Curran HV. Dissociable effects of marijuana with and without cannabidiol on the human brain's resting-state functional con-nectivity. J Psychopharmacol. 2019;33(7):822–30.
108. Roche DJO, Bujarski S, Green R, Hartwell EE, Leventhal AM, Ray LA. Alcohol, tobacco, and marijuana consumption is associated with increased odds of same-day substance co- and tri-use. Drug Alcohol Depend. 2019;200:40–9.

109. Park JY, Wu LT. Trends and correlates of driving under the influence of alcohol among different types of adult substance users in the United States: a national survey study. BMC Public Health. 2019;19(1):509.

110. D'Souza DC, Cortes-Briones JA, Ranganathan M, Thurnauer H, Creatura G, Surti T, Planeta B, Neumeister A, Pittman B, Normandin M, Kapinos M, Ropchan J, Huang Y, Carson RE, Skosnik PD. Rapid changes in CB1 receptor availability in marijuana dependent males after abstinence from marijuana. Biol Psychiatry Cogn Neurosci Neuroimaging. 2016;1(1):60–7.

111. Lazenka MF, Selley DE, Sim-Selley LJ. Brain regional differences in CB1 receptor adaptation and regulation of transcription. Life Sci. 2013;92(8–9):446–52.

112. Curran HV, Freeman TP, Mokrysz C, Lewis DA, Morgan CJ, Parsons LH. Keep off the grass? Marijuana, cognition and addiction. Nat Rev Neurosci. 2016;17(5):293–306.

Chapter 3
The Pharmacodynamics, Pharmacokinetics, and Potential Drug Interactions of Cannabinoids

Grace S. Chin, Robert L. Page II, and Jacquelyn Bainbridge

Drug-Drug Interaction with Cannabinoids

Similar to other plant-based supplements, cannabis, or marijuana, is a polypharmaceutical substance comprised of many compounds but primarily CBD and THC. As the political landscape has changed across the United States, cannabis is now becoming legal in several states, allowing for its potential use recreationally, medicinally, or both. Many Americans have viewed cannabis as a treatment option for chronic diseases and debilitating symptoms, and evidence suggests that it has immunomodulatory and anti-inflammatory properties. However, patients with multiple chronic conditions may also be receiving multiple prescription medications. As the number of prescription medications increases, so does the potential for adverse drug events and drug-drug interactions. Goldberg et al. found that patients taking at least two prescription medications had a 13% risk of an adverse drug-drug interaction, which increased to 38% for four medications and 82% with greater than

G. S. Chin
University of Colorado Anschutz Medical Campus, Skaggs School of Pharmacy and Pharmaceutical Sciences, Department of Clinical Pharmacy and Neurology, Aurora, CO, USA

St. Joseph's Hospital, Denver, CO, USA
e-mail: grace.chin@cuanschutz.edu

J. Bainbridge (✉)
University of Colorado Anschutz Medical Campus, Skaggs School of Pharmacy and Pharmaceutical Sciences, Department of Clinical Pharmacy and Neurology, Aurora, CO, USA
e-mail: jacci.bainbridge@cuanschutz.edu

R. L. PageII
University of Colorado Anschutz Medical Campus, Skaggs School of Pharmacy and Pharmaceutical Sciences, Department of Clinical Pharmacy, Aurora, CO, USA
e-mail: robert.page@cuanschutz.edu

© Springer Nature Switzerland AG 2020
K. Finn (ed.), *Cannabis in Medicine*,
https://doi.org/10.1007/978-3-030-45968-0_3

seven medications [1]. Unfortunately, few published data are available regarding the potential drug interactions associated with cannabinoids as cannabis remains a Schedule I controlled substance. Most of the information regarding drug-drug inter-actions rely on observational studies and case reports. However, in 2018, Epidiolex® became the first prescription drug derived from plant-based CBD approved by the Food and Drug Administration (FDA) allowing for a more formal pharmacokinetic and pharmacodynamic evaluation and profile of CBD [2]. Nevertheless, due to the paucity of data, an understanding of the pharmacokinetics and pharmacodynamics of cannabis and its constituents is clinically important in order to predict possible drug-drug interactions.

Pharmacokinetics/Pharmacodynamics of Cannabinoids

Pharmacodynamics

The body is comprised of an extensive endocannabinoid system, in which the main function is to restore and maintain homeostasis. Cannabinoid (CB) receptors are located throughout the body within the brain, major organs, connective tissues, glands, and immune cells. Anandamide, the naturally occurring cannabinoid in the body, is responsible for biological effects such as increasing appetite, decreasing nausea, decreasing pain sensitivity, and providing anti-inflammatory activity [3, 4]. The two major identified cannabinoid receptors in the body are CB_1 and CB_2, both of which are coupled through G proteins to affect the conversion of AMP to cyclic AMP [5, 6]. The distribution of CB_1 receptors is primarily within the central ner-vous system located on neurons in the brain and spinal cord, but CB_1 receptors are also within the peripheral nervous system and along keratinocytes [7]. CB_2 recep-tors are concentrated in immune cells, like leukocytes, and the spleen. CB_2 receptor agonists are targets of emerging research due to their potential analgesic, anti-inflammatory, and immune-modulating properties [4]. Although CB_1 are primarily concentrated in the nervous system, CB_2 receptors are found extensively throughout the body like the gastrointestinal tract, skeletal muscle, skin, cardiovascular system, reproductive system, and liver [8]. Peripheral CB receptors are responsible for mod-ulating several different physiological responses and signalling, which make them an appealing target for therapy.

Cannabinoids demonstrate variable affinity to CB_1 and CB_2 receptors. THC has equal affinity to both the receptors, while synthetic cannabinoids are highly selec-tive agonists or antagonists to one of the receptor types. Contrarily, CBD does not directly affect either CB receptor, but instead modifies the receptors' ability to bind endocannabinoids. For example, CBD enhances the activity of anandamide, the endogenous cannabinoid [6, 9]. Furthermore, CBD is thought to interact with sev-eral other receptors like the μ-receptor and serotonin (5-HT) receptors. The exact pharmacodynamic property of Epidiolex®, the FDA-approved plant-based CBD product, is unknown and still requires further research.

Pharmacokinetics

The pharmacokinetics of cannabinoids is greatly dependent on the route of administration, the specific cannabinoid, and physical characteristics of the cannabis user. Both THC and CBD are highly lipophilic and can be stored and accumulated in the adipose tissue of the body. THC-A and CBD-A are activated by decarboxylation through heat or light exposure to produce THC and CBD, which have the psychoactive effects [10]. The psychoactive effects differ between THC and CBD in that THC is the compound responsible for the euphoric effects (i.e. "high"), whereas CBD demonstrates its biological activity without the euphoric effects. When smoked, about 50% of the cannabis contents (THC) combust to smoke, of which 50% of inhaled smoke is exhaled again while some of the remaining smoke undergoes localized metabolism in the lungs. The bioavailability or the percentage which actually makes its way into the blood stream, of inhaled THC, is highly variable and ranges between 10% and 25% [11]. The THC content also varies on the method it is smoked. Cannabis cigarettes were found to have less THC content partially due to pyrolysis at higher temperatures and loss due to side smoke [12]. Cigarettes were also found to have higher tar compounds and other impurities as compared to vaporized cannabis. Vaporized cannabis, on the other hand, produced the highest content of THC being the more effective method to extract THC. The controlled temperature of the vaporization method also produced cleaner cannabinoid vapour when compared to cigarettes [12].

Perceived effects of smoking cannabis can occur within seconds and are fully apparent within minutes lasting about 3 hours [13]. The amount of THC absorbed from oral ingestion is dependent on a person's weight, body mass index (BMI), metabolism, gender, and eating habits. The bioavailability of THC and CBD after oral ingestion is also widely variable from 5% to 20% in the controlled environment of clinical studies [11]. The onset of oral formulations (edibles) is often delayed when compared to inhalation, taking 1–3 hours due to the slow absorption and metabolism in the gut. Though the data is very limited, the few studies that investigated the decarboxylation of THC suggests that the acid precursor of THC (THC-A) was not decarboxylated in vitro [14]. The metabolism of THC-A by liver enzymes, however, does produce another THC metabolite, nor-11-THCA-A carboxylic acid [10, 14, 15]. The data on the decarboxylation in the body of CBD-A is still an area needing to be investigated further. The effects are often prolonged compared to inhaled THC, lasting about 6–12 hours [11]. Compared to THC, CBD has similar plasma concentration-time profiles. However, due to its slow onset, extended duration of activity, and variability in absorption, the use of oral formulations poses an increased risk for potential toxicity. Additionally, THC and CBD content labelling may be inconsistent, leading to greater variability. The variability of different cannabis products was reported to be as high as 23% for under-labelling and 60% for over-labelling [16]. The elimination half-life of THC can also vary greatly as it has a fast initial half-life of about 6 minutes but a prolonged terminal half-life of about 22 hours [6]. Due to the high lipophilicity of THC, there is rapid penetration of THC into the brain, which is 60 percent fatty tissue and is highly vascularized [17]. THC absorbed into the brain allows tissue redistribution and slow redistribution from the brain fatty acid back to the plasma contributing to variations in elimination half-life [18]. Even longer elimination half-life is observed in chronic and heavy users of cannabis and can be attributed to redistribution from the adipose tissue to the systemic circulation after last cannabis use (>24 hours). Likewise, CBD also has a prolonged terminal elimination half-life of 24–31 hours depending on route of administration (IV vs inhalation) [6].

Most of the clinical pharmacokinetic data arises from studies conducted with Epidiolex. The pharmacokinetic profile of Epidiolex® showed a time to maximum plasma concentration (T_{max}) of 2.5–5 days at steady state. Foods containing high fat and high calories with Epidiolex® were shown to increase the maximum plasma concentration (C_{max}) by fivefold and the area under the curve (AUC) by fourfold. The elimination half-life of Epidiolex® in the plasma collected from healthy patients was 56–61 hours after twice daily dosing for 7 days [2].

In terms of metabolism, both THC and CBD are metabolized extensively by the liver and gut to both active and inactive metabolites primarily by the cytochrome P450 (CYP450) enzymes and Uridine 5′diphospho-glucuronosyltransferase (UGT) enzymes. Both CBD and THC are then excreted in the faeces with minor renal clearance [2, 19].

Drug-Drug Interactions

Worldwide, cannabis is the most commonly used illicit substance. In the United States, more states are decriminalizing and legalizing cannabis for both recreational and medicinal uses. With cannabis becoming more accessible and popular, there is an increasing trend in medical cannabis use and cannabis as complementary medicine. "Medical cannabis" refers to any part of the cannabis plant or plant material used for medical purposes (e.g. flowers, marijuana, hashish, extracts, etc.) [20]. The term "cannabis-based" medicines refers to registered medicinal cannabis extracts where the THC and THC/CBD contents are standardized (e.g. Epidiolex®, nabilone, dronabinol, etc.) [20]. The emerging data on cannabinoids suggests efficacy and promise as drug targets for various disease states. The cannabis plant contains over 400 different compounds and over 100 isolated cannabinoids with many of these compounds having biological effects. The most abundant cannabinoids are THC and CBD, which both have biological effects and make them susceptible to drug-drug interactions with other medications. The possible drug interactions have led to concern of increased adverse effects and the loss of efficacy of certain concomitant drugs.

Proposed mechanisms of drug interactions with cannabinoids are through competitive inhibition, allosteric interactions, biotransformation enzymes responsible for metabolism, and transport proteins. Most of the research being conducted for these drug interactions is with THC and CBD, but the potential drug interactions with other cannabinoids and other biologically active compounds within the cannabis plant are still unknown and need to be studied and assessed. Therefore, there is an increased risk of adverse effects and toxicity with cannabinoids and cannabis and its potential drug interactions.

Phase I Metabolism (Cytochrome P450)

The CYP450 isoenzymes are primarily responsible for the majority of drug metabolism including both THC and CBD and provide the predominant mechanism responsible for drug interactions with cannabinoids. Knowing the metabolism of concomitant drugs administered with cannabinoids is extremely important when determining potential drug-drug interactions, as medications can be metabolized by the same CYP isoenzymes potentiating drug interactions and increasing risks of adverse effects and toxicity. In terms of clinical relevance, the CYP2C9, CYP2C19, CYP2D6, and CYP3A4 are the most impacted by THC and CBD [19, 21, 22]. For example, CYP3A4 is responsible for metabolizing 60% of all medications contributing to many drug-drug interactions [23]. THC and CBD are believed to both inhibit CYP2D6. Additionally, CBD is a potent inhibitor of CYP2C8, CYP2C9, and CYP3A4 [21, 24]. Examples of medications metabolized through CYP2D6 are antidepressants (citalopram, amitriptyline), antipsychotics (haloperidol, clozapine), and opioids (codeine, morphine). Macrolides, azole antifungals, calcium channel blockers, benzodiazepines, cyclosporine, tacrolimus, sildenafil (and other phosphodiesterase-5 inhibitors), antihistamines, haloperidol, antiretrovirals, and some statins (atorvastatin and simvastatin, but not pravastatin or rosuvastatin) are all substrates for CYP3A4. Additionally, the macrolides, non-dihydropyridine calcium channel blockers (diltiazem and verapamil), protease inhibitors, amiodarone, dronedarone, valproate, and azole antifungals are CYP3A4 inhibitors. Contrarily, St. John's wort, rifampin, carbamazepine, and phenytoin are considered potent inducers. The CYP2D6 isoenzyme metabolizes many antidepressants such as the selective serotonin inhibitors and tricyclic antidepressants as well as antiseizure medications (valproate), antipsychotics, beta blockers, and opioids (including codeine and oxycodone). The CYP2C9 is involved in the disposition of warfarin as well as several oral diabetes drugs and can also be inhibited by valproate and phenobarbital. Table 3.1 summarizes the potential substrates, inhibitors, and inducers for the CYP isoenzymes and their effects upon the disposition of CBD and THC.

Table 3.1 Drug interactions with cannabis

	CBD effects	THC effects	Clinical intervention	Examples of interacting drugs
Phase-I metabolism				
CYP2C9				
Substrates	↑ Substrate concentration	Conflicting data (↕ substrate concentration)	Consider decreasing dose of substrates; monitor for adverse reactions	Buprenorphine, celecoxib, sulfonylureas, naproxen, phenobarbital, phenytoin, valproate, warfarin

(continued)

Table 3.1 (continued)

	CBD effects	THC effects	Clinical intervention	Examples of interacting drugs
CYP2D6				
Substrates	↑ Substrate concentration	↑ Substrate concentration	Consider decreasing dose of substrates; monitor for adverse reactions	Valproate, antidepressants (e.g. amitriptyline, citalopram, nortriptyline, etc.); antipsychotics (e.g. clozapine, haloperidol, risperidone); antiarrhythmics (e.g. flecainide, propafenone, etc.); beta blockers (e.g. carvedilol, metoprolol, etc.); opioids (e.g. codeine, morphine, tramadol, etc.)
CYP3A4				
Substrates	↑ Substrate concentration	↑ Substrate concentration	Consider decreasing dose of substrate; monitor for adverse effects	Cyclosporine, benzodiazepines, zolpidem, zaleplon, zopiclone, amlodipine, antivirals, etc.
Inhibitors	↑ CBD concentration	↑ THC concentration	Consider decreasing dose of Epidiolex®	Valproate, diltiazem, verapamil, ketoconazole, itraconazole, erythromycin, amiodarone, dronedarone, protease inhibitors, and tyrosine kinase inhibitors
Inducers	↓ CBD concentration	↓ THC concentration	Consider increasing dose of Epidiolex®	Carbamazepine, rifampin, phenytoin, phenobarbital, St. John's Wort
CYP2C19				
Substrates	↑ Substrate concentration	↑ Substrate concentration	Consider decreasing dose of substrate; monitor for adverse effects	Antidepressants (e.g. amitriptyline, citalopram, bupropion, etc.); antiseizure (e.g. phenytoin, phenobarbital, diazepam, clobazam); proton pump inhibitors (e.g. omeprazole, pantoprazole, etc.); antifungals (e.g. fluconazole, ketoconazole, etc.); cimetidine; warfarin
Inhibitors	↑ CBD concentration	↑ THC concentration	Consider decreasing dose of Epidiolex®	Felbamate, topiramate, fluoxetine, fluvoxamine, isoniazid, ritonavir, chloramphenicol
Inducers	↓ CBD concentration	↓ THC concentration	Consider increasing dose of Epidiolex®	Carbamazepine, rifampin, phenytoin

Table 3.1 (continued)

	CBD effects	THC effects	Clinical intervention	Examples of interacting drugs
Phase II metabolism				
UGT1A9				
Substrates	↑ Substrate concentration	Minimal data	Consider decreasing dose of substrate; monitor for adverse effects	Propofol, fenofibrate, diflunisal
UGT2B7				
Substrates	↑ Substrate concentration	Minimal data	Consider decreasing dose of substrate; monitor for adverse effects	Lorazepam, lamotrigine, morphine, gemfibrozil
Protein transporters				
P-gp				
Substrates	↑ Substrate concentration	↑ Substrate concentration	Consider decreasing dose of substrate; monitor for adverse effects	DOACS (e.g. apixaban, rivaroxaban, dabigatran, etc.); colchicine; substrates for CYP3A4 (see above)
BCRP				
Substrates	↑ Substrate concentration	↑ Substrate concentration	Consider decreasing dose of substrate; monitor for adverse effects	Anthracenes (e.g. mitoxantrone, bisantrene, etc.); camptothecin derivatives (topotecan, irinotecan, etc.); methotrexate; nucleoside analogues (AZT, lamivudine); prazosin, tyrosine kinase inhibitors; glyburide; sulfasalazine; rosuvastatin; pantoprazole; nitrofurantoin
OAT1A2				
Substrates	↑ Substrate concentration	Minimal data	Consider decreasing dose of substrate; monitor for adverse effects	Fexofenadine, statins, beta-antagonists
OAT2B1				
Substrates	↑ Substrate concentration	Minimal data	Consider decreasing dose of substrate; monitor for adverse effects	Fexofenadine, statins, beta-antagonists

Abbreviations: *CYP* cytochrome P450, *CBD* cannabidiol, *THC* 9-tetrahydrocannabinol, *UGT* uridine 5′diphospho-glucuronosyltransferase, *P-gp* P-glycoprotein, *BCRP* breast cancer resistance protein, *OAT* organic anion-transporting peptides, *DOAC* direct oral anticoagulants, *AZT* azidothymidine

Phase II Metabolism

In Phase II metabolism, drugs are conjugated, allowing for secretion into the bile or urine promoting their eventual excretion. Cannabinoids, specifically CBD, interact with the enzymes responsible for glucuronidation and excretion through the uridine 5'diphospho-glucuronosyltransferase (UGT) enzymes. CBD inhibits both UGT1A9 and UGT2B7 [19, 21, 24]. When CBD inhibits these UGT enzymes, the excretion of substrates is decreased and increases the risk of adverse effects as drugs are not being sufficiently cleared. The clinical significance of the inhibition or induction of UGT is not known; however, with the combination of Epidiolex® and valproate, there is a possibility of significant increases in liver function enzymes via this mechanism.

Transport Proteins

Drug transporters are proteins responsible for mediating drug and other xenobiotic movements into and out of the cell. These transport proteins are located throughout the body where drugs may come in contact with tissue such as the epithelial cells lining the colon, small intestine, pancreatic ductules, bile ductules, kidney proximal tubules, adrenal gland, and blood-brain barrier. Inhibition or induction of such transport proteins can increase or decrease substrate concentrations, respectively. Currently, the data on the effects CBD and its metabolites have on transporters is conflicting and limited. Some studies suggest that CBD and its metabolites have an impact on transport proteins [21, 24, 25], For example, the main metabolite of CBD, 7-OH-CBD, may inhibit the function of the breast cancer resistance protein (BCRP) and be a substrate of p-glycoprotein (P-gp). By inhibiting these efflux proteins, CBD excretion is decreased, and the risk of adverse effects and toxicity is increased due to accumulation of the CBD substrate [21, 24, 25]. However, other studies and the information on the package insert for Epidiolex® suggest that CBD and some of its metabolites are not anticipated to interact with nor are substrates for BCRP and with some of the organic anion transporting peptides (OAT) [2, 26, 27]. Much of the information regarding CBD and its metabolites on the transport system are conducted in animal models, thus limiting its application to humans. Therefore, further research on the relationship between CBD and the transport system are still much needed. Additionally, other compounds in cannabis were found to affect the transport system. For example, THC and terpenes also inhibit P-gp and BCRP function. Flavonoid glycosides can inhibit organic anion-transporting peptides (OAT1A2 and OAT2B1), affecting renal organic anion transport and ultimately decreasing the renal excretion of cannabinoids. This also leads to accumulation of cannabinoids in the body and increases the risk of adverse effects and toxicity [19]. Many of the substrates, inducers, and inhibitors of CYP3A4 are also the same for P-gp (see Table 3.1). Since cannabis is comprised of hundreds of cannabinoids, the effects of other compounds on the transport system are still not well-understood.

Epidiolex® Drug-Drug Interactions

Epidiolex® is the first plant-based prescription cannabinoid approved by the FDA for the treatment of Lennox-Gastaut Syndrome (LGS) and Dravet Syndrome (DS) in patients 2 years of age and older [28]. It was FDA-approved in 2018 and was categorized as a Schedule V drug originally; however, it is now de-scheduled by the DEA. The content of THC is < 0.1 % in the powder crystalline form and < 0.01% in the finished oral solution. The precise mechanism of action for Epidiolex® remains unknown, but it is effective in significantly decreasing number of seizures in these disorders [29]. Epidiolex® is a weight-based medication; initiation of Epidiolex® is recommended at a starting dose of 2.5 mg/kg twice daily and can be increased after 1 week to a maintenance dose of 5 mg/kg twice daily if tolerated. If needed and tolerated, the dose can be increased in weekly increments of 2.5 mg/kg twice daily to a maximum dose of 10 mg/kg twice daily [2]. Since Epidiolex® is an FDA-approved medication, its drug interactions are better characterized than some of the other cannabinoids and compounds found in cannabis. However, there still is a need for more thorough investigation into CBD's drug interactions. As mentioned above, CBD is one of the cannabinoids that has been identified to have drug interactions through metabolism and drug transport enzymes and proteins. Epidiolex®, as a pure CBD compound, has notable drug interactions with CYP3A4 and CYP2C19 inhibitors and inducers [2, 30]. The effects certain drugs have on Epidiolex® are dependent on whether the drug has any interaction with CYP induction, inhibition, or substrates of the enzymes.

Drugs which are moderate or strong inhibitors of CYP3A4 and CYP2C19 will increase CBD plasma concentrations and produce a greater risk for adverse reactions. A dosage reduction of Epidiolex® may be required if used concurrently with medications that inhibit CYP3A4 (e.g. valproate, ketoconazole) and CYP2C19 (e.g. antidepressants, ritonavir). Furthermore, close monitoring of adverse reactions associated with Epidiolex® like somnolence, fatigue, and elevated transaminase may be required [2, 31]. To monitor for adverse reactions and to ensure patient safety while receiving Epidiolex® with concomitant interacting CYP450 inhibitors, it is imperative to appropriately monitor drug levels. It is recommended that Epidiolex® be initiated and allowed to reach steady state (around 3 days) and then to check the drug levels of inhibitor drug, if obtainable, and reduce the Epidiolex® dose as necessary. Some notable adverse effects with Epidiolex® use are anaemia (30% occurrence), elevations of serum creatinine and hepatic transaminases, and behavioural/psychiatric changes (e.g. suicidal ideation), lethargy, dizziness, decreased appetite, diarrhea and sedation. Epidiolex® is also not recommended in pregnancy [2]. It is important to also note any signs or symptoms of adverse effects that the patient is experiencing, which could help determine necessary drug modifications.

For example, co-administration of clobazam and Epidiolex® leads to a significant and well-documented drug-drug interaction. Clobazam, a substrate of CYP2C19, produces a threefold increase in plasma concentrations of N-desmethylclobazam, the active metabolite of clobazam [32]. This substantial increase in plasma concentration may lead to an increase in clobazam-related adverse reactions, especially transaminase elevation, and sedation [2, 33]. In clinical trials, clobazam dose was decreased by 50% when co-administered with Epidiolex® [34]. Valproate, a CYP2C9 inhibitor, also increases the incidence of liver enzyme elevation with concomitant Epidiolex® use due to an increase in CBD plasma concentrations [2, 35]. Liver enzyme elevations can be important predictors of hepatic dysfunction, and when they occur, it is worth considering discontinuing or dose adjusting the interacting drug. Additionally, monitoring liver function and enzymes is recommended with Epidiolex® therapy. Detection of transaminase elevations of more than three times the upper normal limit (UNL), in combination with elevated bilirubin, without an alternative explanation for these abnormal liver tests may be predictors of severe liver injury [2]. Additional data also demonstrated that Epidiolex® could increase serum concentrations of other antiseizure medications like eslicarbazepine, rufinamide, and zonisamide [35]. The data for topiramate, however, was conflicting as some studies suggested no interaction with Epidiolex® and others saw an increase in topiramate serum levels [35]. Nonetheless, it is imperative to know the existing interactions with Epidiolex® and to monitor closely for adverse effects.

Contrarily, induction of certain CYP450 enzymes may cause a decrease in CBD concentrations. Concomitant use of strong inducers of CYP3A4 and CYP2C19 (e.g. phenytoin, carbamazepine, and rifampin) will decrease Epidiolex® plasma concentrations, which may decrease its efficacy and could potentiate seizure activity in LGS and DS [2]. Therefore, drug monitoring is also important with interactions caused by inducers. The same recommendations of initiating Epidiolex®, obtaining steady state (~3 days), and checking drug levels of the inducing drug, if obtainable, and for signs or symptoms of adverse reactions and/or seizures should be applied for interactions that decrease CBD plasma concentrations. It is essential to be cognizant of any comprehensive or alternative supplements that patients may be on as they can also propose potential drug interactions with Epidiolex®. For example, St. John's wort is an infamous inducer of CYP3A4 and will decrease the plasma concentration of Epidiolex® and may potentially decrease the efficacy of CBD [2].

There are special populations especially vulnerable for drug-drug interactions such as solid organ transplant patients and immunocompromised patients (e.g. HIV) in which potential drug-drug interactions with cannabinoids could lead to serious adverse consequences. A case report documented a significant CYP3A4 interaction between CBD and tacrolimus, where tacrolimus levels were increased by threefold when CBD was used concurrently [36]. This substantial increase in tacrolimus heightens the risk of adverse reactions, dosage modifications, and additional close monitoring. Additionally, by inhibiting both P-gp and CYP3A4, cannabinoids can increase calcineurin inhibitor concentrations leading to significant toxicity such as renal failure [37]. Due to many of the medications used in these special populations having narrow therapeutic indexes and higher risks of adverse effects, identifying potential drug interactions and monitoring for adverse interactions are especially recommended.

THC Drug-Drug Interactions

THC, the psychoactive cannabinoid in cannabis, shares many of the same drug-drug interactions as CBD. Much of the drug interaction data with THC and the other cannabinoids are based on in vitro studies and propose theoretical drug-drug interactions [38]. In vitro data demonstrates that THC is an inhibitor of CYP2C9, CYP2C19, and CYP3A4 and an inducer of CYP1A2 [24]. The CYP1A2 isoenzyme is responsible for the metabolism of clozapine, duloxetine, naproxen, cyclobenzaprine, olanzapine, haloperidol, and chlorpromazine. Interaction of THC and substrates of these CYP enzymes can increase concentrations of the substrate medication, potentiating the risk of adverse effects. Inhibition of these enzymes results in increasing THC plasma concentration as THC clearance is reduced, which also increases the risk of THC adverse effects. For example, the inhibition of CYP2C9 and CYP3A4 by valproate can enhance the euphoric effects of THC due to this decrease in THC plasma clearance. In addition, when THC and phenytoin are given concomitantly, THC acts as the inhibitor of this same enzyme (CYP2C9) and can increase the phenytoin concentrations, leading to an increased risk of phenytoin side effects and/or toxicity (e.g. nystagmus, ataxia, cerebral dysfunction, hepatic dysfunction, etc.) [13]. The drug interactions of THC and the enzymes responsible for Phase II metabolism are not well understood at this time. Based on the lack of definitive data on THC drug-drug interactions, further research and investigation into the types and extents of these interactions and their effect on the body is still a necessary area of research for not only THC but also for the other compounds in cannabis.

Conclusion

In summary, drug interactions do occur with cannabinoids and can be significant. It is important that individuals discuss all their prescription medications, over-the-counter medications, herbal supplements, and cannabis use with their healthcare practitioners, including their pharmacists, to determine if significant drug interactions may be present. Due to a paucity of data on drug interactions documented with cannabinoids, more research needs to be completed and documented in the literature so that interactions can be readily identified and adverse effects can be prevented to provide comprehensive care to patients. With the increased use of cannabis and with more emerging data on cannabinoids, healthcare providers hold an important responsibility to be continually educated on potential drug interactions with cannabinoids so that these drug interactions are identified for the comprehensive care of our patients.

References

1. Goldberg RM, Mabee J, Chan L, Wong S. Drug-drug and drug-disease interactions in the ED: analysis of a high-risk population. Am J Emerg Med. 1996;14(5):447–50.
2. Epidiolex (cannabidiol) [package insert]. Carlsbad, CA; Greenwich Biosciences Inc. 2020.
3. Frontiers in Pharmacology. http://norml.org/library/item/introduction-to-the-endocannabinoid-system\. Published 2014. Accessed 2 Mar 2015.
4. Borgelt LM, Franson KL, Nussbaum AM, Wang GS. The pharmacologic and clinical effects of medical cannabis. Pharmacotherapy. 2013;33(2):195–209.
5. Grotenhermen F. Pharmacokinetics and pharmacodynamics of cannabinoids. Clin Pharmacokinet. 2003;42(4):327–60.
6. Lucas CJ, Galettis P, Schneider J. The pharmacokinetics and the pharmacodynamics of cannabinoids. Br J Clin Pharmacol. 2018;84(11):2477–82.
7. Caterina MJ. TRP channel cannabinoid receptors in skin sensation, homeostasis, and inflammation. ACS Chem Neurosci. 2014;5(11):1107–16.
8. Zou S, Kumar U. Cannabinoid receptors and the endocannabinoid system: signaling and function in the central nervous system. Int J Mol Sci. 2018;19:833.
9. Pertwee RG. Ligands that target cannabinoid receptors in the brain: from THC to anandamide and beyond. Addict Biol. 2008;13(2):147–59.
10. Moreno-Sanz G. Can you pass the acid test? Critical review and novel therapeutic perspectives of Delta(9)-Tetrahydrocannabinolic acid A. Cannabis Cannabinoid Res. 2016;1(1):124–30.
11. Agurell S, Halldin M, Lindgren JE, et al. Pharmacokinetics and metabolism of delta 1-tetrahydrocannabinol and other cannabinoids with emphasis on man. Pharmacol Rev. 1986;38(1):21–43.
12. Pomahacova B, Van der Kooy F, Verpoorte R. Cannabis smoke condensate III: the cannabinoid content of vaporised Cannabis sativa. Inhal Toxicol. 2009;21(13):1108–12.
13. Strougo A, Zuurman L, Roy C, et al. Modelling of the concentration--effect relationship of THC on central nervous system parameters and heart rate – insight into its mechanisms of action and a tool for clinical research and development of cannabinoids. J Psychopharmacol. 2008;22(7):717–26.
14. Raikos N, Schmid H, Nussbaumer S, et al. Determination of Delta9-tetrahydrocannabinolic acid A (Delta9-THCA-A) in whole blood and plasma by LC-MS/MS and application in authentic samples from drivers suspected of driving under the influence of cannabis. Forensic Sci Int. 2014;243:130–6.
15. Jung J, Meyer MR, Maurer HH, Neususs C, Weinmann W, Auwarter V. Studies on the metabolism of the Delta9-tetrahydrocannabinol precursor Delta9-tetrahydrocannabinolic acid A (Delta9-THCA-A) in rat using LC-MS/MS, LC-QTOF MS and GC-MS techniques. J Mass Spectrom. 2009;44(10):1423–33.
16. Vandrey R, Raber JC, Raber ME, Douglass B, Miller C, Bonn-Miller MO. Cannabinoid dose and label accuracy in edible medical Cannabis products. JAMA. 2015;313(24):2491–3.
17. Chang CY, Ke DS, Chen JY. Essential fatty acids and human brain. Acta Neurol Taiwanica. 2009;18(4):231–41.
18. Sharma P, Murthy P, Bharath MM. Chemistry, metabolism, and toxicology of cannabis: clinical implications. Iran J Psychiatry. 2012;7(4):149–56.
19. Foster BC, Abramovici H, Harris CS. Cannabis and cannabinoids: kinetics and interactions. Am J Med. 2019;132(11):1266–70.
20. Hauser W, Finn DP, Kalso E, et al. European Pain Federation (EFIC) position paper on appropriate use of cannabis-based medicines and medical cannabis for chronic pain management. Eur J Pain. 2018;22(9):1547–64.
21. Brown JD, Winterstein AG. Potential adverse drug events and drug-drug interactions with medical and consumer Cannabidiol (CBD) use. J Clin Med. 2019;8(7).
22. Stott C, White L, Wright S, Wilbraham D, Guy G. A phase I, open-label, randomized, crossover study in three parallel groups to evaluate the effect of rifampicin, ketoconazole, and

omeprazole on the pharmacokinetics of THC/CBD oromucosal spray in healthy volunteers. Springerplus. 2013;2(1):236.

23. Yu J, Zhou Z, Tay-Sontheimer J, Levy RH, Ragueneau-Majlessi I. Risk of clinically relevant pharmacokinetic-based drug-drug interactions with drugs approved by the U.S. Food and Drug Administration between 2013 and 2016. Drug Metab Dispos. 2018;46(6):835–45.

24. Qian Y, Gurley BJ, Markowitz JS. The potential for pharmacokinetic interactions between Cannabis products and conventional medications. J Clin Psychopharmacol. 2019.

25. Zhu HJ, Wang JS, Markowitz JS, et al. Characterization of P-glycoprotein inhibition by major cannabinoids from marijuana. J Pharmacol Exp Ther. 2006;317(2):850–7.

26. Brzozowska N, Li KM, Wang XS, et al. ABC transporters P-gp and Bcrp do not limit the brain uptake of the novel antipsychotic and anticonvulsant drug cannabidiol in mice. PeerJ. 2016;4:e2081.

27. Iffland K, Grotenhermen F. An update on safety and side effects of Cannabidiol: a review of clinical data and relevant animal studies. Cannabis Cannabinoid Res. 2017;2(1):139–54.

28. Devinsky O, Cross JH, Laux L, et al. Trial of Cannabidiol for drug-resistant seizures in the Dravet syndrome. N Engl J Med. 2017;376(21):2011–20.

29. Devinsky O, Marsh E, Friedman D, et al. Cannabidiol in patients with treatment-resistant epilepsy: an open-label interventional trial. Lancet Neurol. 2016;15(3):270–8.

30. Jiang R, Yamaori S, Okamoto Y, Yamamoto I, Watanabe K. Cannabidiol is a potent inhibitor of the catalytic activity of cytochrome P450 2C19. Drug Metab Pharmacokinet. 2013;28(4):332–8.

31. Volkow ND, Baler RD, Compton WM, Weiss SR. Adverse health effects of marijuana use. N Engl J Med. 2014;370(23):2219–27.

32. Russell GR, Phelps SJ, Shelton CM, Wheless JW. Impact of drug interactions on Clobazam and N-Desmethylclobazam concentrations in pediatric patients with epilepsy. Ther Drug Monit. 2018;40(4):452–62.

33. Geffrey AL, Pollack SF, Bruno PL, Thiele EA. Drug-drug interaction between clobazam and cannabidiol in children with refractory epilepsy. Epilepsia. 2015;56(8):1246–51.

34. Thiele EA, Marsh ED, French JA, et al. Cannabidiol in patients with seizures associated with Lennox-Gastaut syndrome (GWPCARE4): a randomised, double-blind, placebo-controlled phase 3 trial. Lancet. 2018;391(10125):1085–96.

35. Gaston TE, Bebin EM, Cutter GR, Liu Y, Szaflarski JP. Interactions between cannabidiol and commonly used antiepileptic drugs. Epilepsia. 2017;58(9):1586–92.

36. Leino AD, Emoto C, Fukuda T, Privitera M, Vinks AA, Alloway RR. Evidence of a clinically significant drug-drug interaction between cannabidiol and tacrolimus. Am J Transplant. 2019;19(10):2944–8.

37. Hauser N, Sahai T, Richards R, Roberts T. Corrigendum to "high on Cannabis and Calcineurin inhibitors: a word of warning in an era of legalized marijuana". Case Rep Transplant. 2018;2018:7095846.

38. Anderson GD, Chan LN. Pharmacokinetic drug interactions with tobacco, cannabinoids and smoking cessation products. Clin Pharmacokinet. 2016;55(11):1353–68.

Part II
Clinical Evidence

Chapter 4
Cannabis and Neuropsychiatric Effects

David C. Rettew, Doris C. Gundersen, Erica Kirsten Rapp, Paula Riggs, Christine L. Miller, Monica C. Jackson, Kevin Sabet, Ben Cort, and LaTisha L. Bader

D. C. Rettew (✉)
Child, Adolescent, and Family Unit, Vermont Department of Mental Health, Psychiatry and Pediatrics, University of Vermont Larner College of Medicine, @Pedipsych, Burlington, VT, USA
e-mail: David.rettew@med.uvm.edu

D. C. Gundersen
Department of Psychiatry, University of Colorado, Colorado Physician Health Program, Boulder, CU, USA
e-mail: dgundersen@cphp.org

E. K. Rapp · P. Riggs
Department of Psychiatry, University of Colorado School of Medicine, Aurora, CO, USA
e-mail: erica.rapp@cuanschutz.edu; paula.riggs@cuanschutz.edu

C. L. Miller
MillerBio, Baltimore, MD, USA
e-mail: cmiller@millerbio.com

M. C. Jackson
Department of Mathematics and Statistics, American University, Washington, DC, USA

K. Sabet
Department of Psychiatry, Yale University, New Haven, CT, USA

B. Cort
Cort Consulting, Longmont, CO, USA
e-mail: ben@cortconsulting.com

L. T. L. Bader
Women's Recovery, Denver, CO, USA
e-mail: lbader@womensrecovery.com

© Springer Nature Switzerland AG 2020
K. Finn (ed.), *Cannabis in Medicine*,
https://doi.org/10.1007/978-3-030-45968-0_4

Blunted: The Effects of Cannabis on Cognition and Motivation

David C. Rettew

The recent political momentum to decriminalize, legalize, and commercialize cannabis has put a premium on the need for high-quality objective research on its neurobehavioral effects. Not only are scientists and healthcare professionals interested in cannabis research of late but also advocates, the media, venture capitalists, cannabis consumers, and government officials. Due to the different goals various groups have, messaging about cannabis use often leaves the public and many medical professionals increasingly confused as they hear what appears to be dueling science on the potential risks and benefits of cannabis use. Scanning the Internet today, it is not difficult to encounter the view that concerns over the negative effects of cannabis on cognitive skills are completely unfounded with cannabis even being cognitive enhancing. It is also easy to find sources claiming that even infrequent use of cannabis in adults can irrevocably rot the brain. Thus, the primary goal of this chapter is to provide a brief summary and synthesis on what is actually known scientifically about the associations between cannabis use and cognition: a domain that has been a concern to many for decades. Beyond the fundamental question of whether or not there is a causal link between cannabis and cognitive deficits, this chapter will also examine clinically relevant questions such as the magnitude of the link and impact of moderating factors. Secondarily, however, this chapter will attempt to describe how some of this scientific knowledge has been applied to the ongoing debate regarding cannabis legalization and commercialization with the hopes that readers will be better equipped to think through the current controversy for their own benefit and when speaking to interested patients, clients, and students.

Memory

Memory function encompasses a number of related but somewhat distinct domains and has been one of most heavily studied areas when it comes to its association with cannabis use. Verbal memory is often assessed through tasks that require the recalling of word lists at different time intervals. A number of studies have shown that cannabis can acutely impair verbal memory [1, 2] with intrusion errors (i.e., believing that a word that was not on a recall list actually was) being particularly prominent. Further, there is evidence that these effects cannot be solely accounted for by the effect of cannabis on attentional systems, which will be covered next [3]. Verbal learning and memory has also been consistently [4, 5], although not uniformly [6], associated with chronic cannabis use in the absence of acute intoxication. Poorer performance has been associated with higher frequency, duration, and quantity of use as well as an earlier age of onset [2]. Higher delta-9-tetra-hydrocannabinol

(THC) content of consumed cannabis has also been associated with stronger impairment [7]. A period of abstinence, perhaps as short as a few weeks, may help improve or even eliminate these differences between cannabis users and non-users [8–10], although other studies have shown evidence of continued impairment even after cannabis use has stopped [11, 12]. One methodological complication from some of these studies which has limited conclusions regarding the causal impact of cannabis has been a lack of cognitive testing prior to the cannabis use, although efforts have been made to match users and non-users on early cognitive ability in some studies [11].

Working memory refers to processes that involve the ability to store and use information for short period of time. It is assessed through a number of procedures including digit recall or n-back tests. Working memory has also been shown to be vulnerable to the effects of cannabis in studies of both humans [13] and animals [14, 15] although the evidence has been judged as not as strong as it is in more verbally oriented skills [2].

Like many other areas of cannabis research, being able to demonstrate that cannabis actually causes cognitive deficits has been challenging from naturalistic studies of human beings, even those using statistical methods to try to account for non-causal associations. "Correlation does not prove causation" has been a frequent mantra of cannabis advocates eager to minimize the evidence that has demonstrated a link between cannabis use and decreased cognitive functioning. Consequently, some individual studies deserve mention due to their ability to offer stronger conclusions regarding causality. Some of this work is also quite recent and has yet to be fully incorporated into consensus opinions and documents.

One of those studies by Morin and colleagues involved the testing of 3826 students in the Montreal area who, beginning in the seventh grade, had multiple assessments of both substance use (alcohol and cannabis) and cognition across 4 years [16]. This provision allowed the researchers to look at different models of association including the possibility of reverse causation (i.e., that cognitive deficits lead to substance use rather than the other way around), common factors (that a shared factor leads to both cognitive deficits and substance use) and a more causal route. The study found that cannabis use was more strongly related to cognitive deficits such in areas such as working memory than alcohol. Further, some of these differences were not minor with cannabis using tenth graders showing levels of inhibitory control on par with non-cannabis using seventh graders. When it came to testing models of association, the authors found that there was evidence both that there may be common factors that lead to substance use and cognitive problems but also, for cannabis only, there was evidence of more direct "neurotoxic" effects of cannabis on cognitive domains of working memory and inhibitory control. This study is important not only scientifically but also with regard to public policy, as it suggests that the frequent debate that cognitive problems associated with cannabis represent *either* the presence of an unrelated third factor or a more direct effect may be a false dichotomy and that both mechanisms could be operating simultaneously.

From a large study published in JAMA Internal Medicine from the Coronary Artery Risk Development in Young Adults (CARDIA) study that followed a large cohort of young adults for 25 years, a dose-dependent association was found between lifetime cannabis use and worsening verbal memory in middle age, even after controlling for potential confounds [17]. For every additional 5 years of cannabis exposure, there was a reduction in 0.13 standardized units of verbal memory score compared to individuals who never used cannabis. Poorer processing speed and executive functioning was also found to be associated with cannabis use, but this link was no longer statistically significant when adjusting for other variables.

Experimental studies with animals can also be very valuable in lending confidence about causation when it comes to cannabis and cognitive problems. While this research tends not to be as well publicized as human studies, there indeed is a fairly sizable literature on the subject. Overall, many studies have demonstrated that cannabis exposure, especially to adolescent mice, rats, and monkeys, does result in deficits in memory and other cognitive functions [18–21]. Some of this dysfunction can be long-lasting [22]. At the same time, however, there have also been animal studies suggesting that THC may have positive cognitive effects and may be neuroprotective in studies involving animal models of Alzheimer's disease [23]. While much more research is needed, it has been hypothesized that age and dose may be crucial factors with THC having generally negative effects on cognition for younger individuals (regardless of the dose) while perhaps showing more positive effects for people who are older when used at very low doses [24]. A small open trial of 10 people with dementia has been touted as evidence that cannabis should be considered as a treatment alternative, although it is important to point out that this study used an oral preparation that contained more cannabidiol than THC [25].

In summary, the research suggests that both acute and chronic cannabis use is related to non-trivial reductions in memory skills, particularly with regard to verbal memory. Some of these deficits, but perhaps not all, are recoverable with extended period of abstinence. Regarding the component parts of memory, it has been hypothesized that cannabis causes result in alterations in both the encoding and recall of information and may disrupt the process through which information is transferred into long-term memory [1]. Further discussion of the potential brain areas and neurobiological mechanisms affected are reviewed at the end of this chapter.

Attention

The domain of attention also encompasses a rather broad set of skills that allows someone to maintain a goal-directed focus on an individual stimulus while also being able to shift that focus in response to environmental demands. As with other cognitive abilities, the various aspects of attention are supported by interrelated but somewhat distinct neural pathways and substrates and can be assessed through a variety of tasks such as the continuous performance task (CPT), reaction time tests, and other attentional control tests.

A 2017 review from the National Academies of Sciences, Engineering, and Medicine concluded on the basis of four systematic reviews that there was good evidence that cannabis can acutely impair the ability to focus and sustain attention and can weaken performance in situations that require divided attention [2, 26–28]. These effects appear to progress in a dose-dependent manner. The case for more chronic deficits, however, particularly for cannabis users who have abstained for at least a month, is less compelling with the majority of studies indicating that attentional skills return to baseline within a matter of weeks [29, 30]. Interestingly, however, there is evidence from neuroimaging studies that chronic cannabis users, while having similar scores on attentional tasks as non-cannabis using individuals, recruit different neural networks and pathways as a possible compensatory strategy [26].

Executive Function

The term executive functioning is often applied to higher-order cognitive processes that involve skills such as organization, planning, inhibiting behaviors, overcoming interference, and problem-solving. As a group, these skills have been shown to be significantly related to improved mental health, well-being, and socioeconomic status.

Studies related to executive functioning and cannabis use have been fairly inconsistent relative to both acute affects and chronic use [31]. This inconsistency for acute effects may reflect some important moderating variables that have been identified such as earlier onset of use [32] and extent of cannabis use prior to testing [33]. While the critical role of various other factors with regard to the link between cannabis use and cognitive problems will be explored in more detail later in this chapter, the variable findings regarding chronic use have been hypothesized to be due to the fact that executive functioning skills are relatively slow to mature with deficits being harder to document until later in adulthood [2]. The review of cannabis effects on cognition by Broyd and colleagues points out that this theory is supported by some of the data on the recovery of executive functioning abilities with abstinence in which persistent alternations have been better documented for older [9, 34] compared to younger [12, 30] samples.

Intelligence and IQ

Given the fact that many of the previously mentioned cognitive domains such as working memory are a component of the broader area of intelligence, it would be surprising that overall intelligence would be spared by cannabis, and many studies have used overall intelligence and IQ as their primary variable of interest. Given the public familiarity and concern with the concept of intelligence and IQ along with its significance in other domains of functioning, these studies are also frequently cited and discussed in deliberations about the effects of cannabis decriminalization, legalization, and commercialization.

A study comparing adult twins who were discordant for regular marijuana use did show differences in intelligence [9], although only on the block design subtest of the Wechsler Adult Intelligence Scale. While no assessment of intelligence was done prior to the cannabis use, the cannabis-using twins in this study had been abstinent from use for at least 1 year with the average length of abstinence being approximately 20 years.

One of the most dramatic and often cited studies regarding cannabis and IQ comes from the well-known Dunedin study which has followed a cohort of over 1000 individuals from age 3 well into adulthood [35]. Subjects completed neuropsychological testing around the age of 13 and 38, while cannabis and other substance use was assessed at multiple waves between the ages of 18 and 38. The researchers found that those who were regular cannabis users during at least 3 waves of the study lost about 6 IQ points while those who never used experienced a slight increase in IQ. This decline was found across IQ domains, although was most apparent with regard to processing speed and executive functioning skills. Furthermore, cognition did not fully recover among participants who began using cannabis in adolescence but later stopped. This study was in contrast to a smaller and earlier study which also examined changes in IQ among youth before (between age 9 and 12) and after cannabis exposure (between age 17 and 20) [36]. While this report also showed that heavy cannabis users had declines in IQ (here 4.1 points) relative to light and non-users who gained IQ during this interval, the authors failed to find evidence of long-lasting deficits among previously heavy users who had become abstinent.

In 2016, another study by Jackson and colleagues reported contrasting findings from two samples of twins who were adolescents around the years 2003–2010 [37]. Like the Dunedin study, the researchers did find that cannabis users tested lower than their non-cannabis-using peers (around 4 IQ points difference) and, further, their scores declined between preadolescence and late adolescence. However, increased frequency of use was not related to greater cognitive declines. In addition, comparisons within twin pairs in which one twin used cannabis and another didn't (an analysis that controls for other genetic predispositions and shared environmental variables) did not consistently show differences between the twins.

As might be expected, advocates for and against the promotion of cannabis tend to favor one study over another, but is it possible to reconcile these investigations? One clear difference among the Dunedin and Jackson studies relates to the threshold of what was defined as heavier cannabis use. In the Dunedin study, the amount of use among individuals with the IQ loss was quite extensive with many individuals using for long periods of time and at levels that would qualify them for a diagnosis of dependence. In the Jackson study, by contrast, heavy use only required using more than 30 times in one's life. As will be discussed in more detail, differences in these important variables may help explain what otherwise appear as inconsistent findings and can offer clues about important factors that are highly relevant in understanding an individual's risk.

Motivation

While the stereotype of the person who regularly uses cannabis often includes the idea of someone who has lost the drive and interest to do much of anything other than use more cannabis, the scientific literature has been more mixed in supporting such a caricature [38]. The topic of motivation is not usually considered a core dimension of cognition, but its discussion here is important not only because of its critical role for overall well-being and success [39] but also because it has been hypothesized that perhaps some of the cognitive differences found among cannabis users may be attributed to reduced motivation during these tasks rather than a cognitive deficit per se [40].

The term "amotivational syndrome" has often been used to describe many habitual cannabis users for decades [41]. What is controversial is not the frequent correlation that has been found between cannabis use and reduced levels of persistence, self-efficacy, and goal-directed behavior but the direction of causality, with some arguing that the association is primarily driven by less motivated individuals seeking out cannabis rather than any direct effect of the drug on motivational systems in the brain [42]. More recent work with designs better equipped to assess the direction of causality, however, continue to suggest that cannabis use can indeed lead to reduced motivation and self-efficacy. Using cross-lagged panel modeling, Lac and Luk demonstrated that cannabis use, but not alcohol or tobacco use, prospectively predicted lower initiative and persistence in the future while finding no evidence for causality going in the opposite direction [39]. An experimental study also demonstrated that acute cannabis use was associated with reduced effort in a money earning task with cannabidiol (CBD) partially moderating this effect [43]. Findings related to chronic cannabis users who had abstained for at least 12 hours, however, were more complicated with no differences found in comparison to controls when it came to effort-related decision-making but with cannabis-dependent subjects showing weaker overall reward learning. Further, randomized studies in animals, including one with rhesus monkeys, have also documented that cannabis can produce an amotivational-type syndrome among exposed animals, providing further support for this theory [44]. Overall, there continues to be evidence of motivation impairment associated particularly with acute cannabis use, but the data regarding more chronic and persistent effects is inconsistent and not as extensive as some of the stereotypes of cannabis users suggest.

Mechanisms of Action

Many researchers have moved beyond the question of *if* cannabis causes cognitive deficits to examine the topic of *how* cannabis exerts these effects. THC is known to inhibit cholinergic activity in many parts of the brain including the limbic system and cortex [25]. Mechanisms related to memory impairment have understandably focused on brain regions such as the hippocampus and its interactions with other areas of interest. Once again, studies with animals have proven very useful in this line of inquiry and a number of studies have indeed demonstrated changes in the structure and function of important cognitive processing brain regions such as the hippocampus and prefrontal cortex [45–47]. In an older study, chronic exposure to THC in young rats resulted in nerve cell loss in the hippocampus in patterns that resembled accelerated changes associated with aging [48].

One previously mentioned study that showed memory deficits in adolescent rats exposed to THC found that the induced deficits appeared to be mediated through increased expression of 56 genes involved in inflammation of hippocampal astrocyte cells [18]. Of additional interest in this study was the fact these mice also had an allele of the DISC1 gene that has been implicated with severe mental illness in a Scottish family study [49]. Adding confidence to the researchers' conclusions was also the finding that the cognitive deficits could be counteracted when THC was given at the same time as some anti-inflammatory medications.

Studies that expose animals in earlier stages of development to THC have demonstrated alternations in the expression of genes related to glutaminergic and noradrenergic systems in the brain [22]. In one previously cited study demonstrating memory impairment with acute cannabis use, some of the effects were found to be reversible with rivastigmine but not vardenafil, suggesting a stronger role for acetylcholine over glutamate in these deficits [13]. At the cellular level, a relatively recent study published in *Nature* demonstrated that the cognitive effects of acute THC exposure operates, at least in part, through the depletion of energy production in the mitochondria of hippocampal neurons that also express the cannabinoid 1 (CB1) receptor [50]. Such changes in mitochondrial energy metabolism are also present in some neurodegenerative disorders and strokes.

With regard to motivation, much of the attention has predictably focused on the interaction between the brain's endocannabinoid system and striatal dopaminergic pathways involved in reward processing and motivated behavior [51]. THC is known acutely to boost dopamine release which makes the effect of reduced motivation somewhat counterintuitive and illustrates the need for more research [43]. Chronic cannabis use, however, has been found to be related to reduced dopamine synthesis [52]. Using crossed-lagged models from multiple assessments of both cannabis use and functional brain activity, increased cannabis use was found to be associated with blunted activation of the nucleus accumbens, a region well-known for its role in addiction and behavioral response to reward [53].

Moderating Factors

As has been documented in many of the aforementioned studies, several factors have been shown to have a major impact on the link between cannabis use and cognitive/motivational deficits. Indeed, the variable presence and presentation of these factors from study to study may help explain much of what otherwise appears as inconsistency in the cannabis literature. The risk of 40-year-old who occasionally uses low potency cannabis appears to be quite different from the risk of a 16-year-old adolescent who is a regular consumer of cannabis with high levels of THC. Moreover, the direction in which some of these moderating factors alter the relations between cannabis use and cognition may vary between acute and more chronic settings. More experienced cannabis users, for example, may show less of a reduction in cognitive capacity with acute cannabis exposure compared to cannabis-naïve individuals, possibly through tolerance of the drug [40]. Over the long term, however, more cognitive impairment has generally been associated with earlier age of onset, more frequent use, and shorter periods of abstinence. Two characteristics of cannabis itself, namely, the concentrations of THC and CBD, also may play a significant role with regard to cognitive effects. While there is accumulating evidence suggesting that the potency of cannabis being used may be a critical factor when it comes to psychiatric risk for disorders like schizophrenia [54], this potentially important dimension has not been as well studied with regard to cognition.

Summary and Future Directions

Looking broadly over the scientific evidence that currently exists on the relations between cannabis use and cognition, several conclusions can reasonably be reached. First, there is robust evidence that cannabis use can impair cognition and motivation both in the short- and long-term. The supporting data span multiple areas of cognition but are arguably strongest when it comes to memory and attention. Lending credence to the likelihood that the noted associations represent a true causal effect of cannabis are the accumulating number of positive studies that are more experimental in nature (using both humans and animals as subjects) as well as the employment of more sophisticated analyses such as cross-lagged models that are able to examine various mechanisms of association. Interestingly, these studies have often shown evidence for *both* a direct neurotoxic effect of cannabis on cognition in addition to the presence of other mechanisms, such as third factors leading to both cannabis use and cognitive deficits. Public debates about the risks of cannabis use often assume that direct causal mechanisms and shared third factors are mutually exclusive in explaining the association between cannabis and negative outcomes, but the emerging research suggests that both pathways can be at play simultaneously.

In appreciation of the strength and diversity of studies that have looked at the link between cannabis use and decreased cognitive ability, the popular retort by some cannabis advocates that the scientific literature on this important topic is purely "correlational" and thus dismissible appears to be a gross underestimation of the current state of evidence. At the same time, claims of severe brain damage associated even with episodic use among adults also exaggerate the state of research findings. Like most complex topics in neuroscience, the literature on cannabis and cognition is not wholly consistent, leaving plenty of room for people to cherry pick studies that fit their personal, political, or financial objectives.

Related to this point, a second conclusion that can be made is that moderating factors such as the timing and amount of cannabis use may be extremely important when it comes to a person's risk. These factors, combined with others such as underlying genetic vulnerabilities, can lead to very different outcomes following use. It is likely that a significant portion of the variability in findings that have been reported on this subject is due to the failure to completely sample and account for these important variables, and future research would benefit from a more comprehensive and uniform approach to these factors that interject a real "it depends" when it comes to answering questions about the cognitive risks of cannabis use. Varied and somewhat arbitrary definitions of what constitutes "heavy use" or "high potency," for example, increase the likelihood of studies reaching different answers for the same question. Being able to account for CBD and THC concentrations may also prove to be important as well. As many of the long range prospective studies currently available are derived from cohorts who consumed cannabis with much smaller THC concentrations than is used today, it is possible that the risks associated with cannabis use from these studies have been understated, should THC concentration prove to be as important when it comes to cognition as it appears to be in other areas such as risk of psychosis. One promising development in the effort to resolve some of the many remaining questions about the effects of cannabis on cognition is the launch in 2015 of the Adolescent Brain Cognitive Development (ABCD) study which will be following a group of approximately 10,000 children for at least a decade, starting at the age of 9 [55]. This study will represent the largest and most comprehensive effort to date to examine cognitive development through adolescence and the impact of many factors, including cannabis.

Finally, a third conclusion that can be made is that there is reason to be hopeful that any cognitive deficits that occur can be mitigated and even reversed with a sustained period of abstinence. With a few exceptions, the literature does not support the notion that the typical cannabis user will suffer a substantial and irrevocable loss of cognitive skills once a period of abstinence has been achieved. Such a perspective could be useful in motivating those who need it to seek appropriate treatment for cannabis abuse and dependence once, of course, the public and the medical community are fully appraised about the many risks associated with this drug.

Cannabis and Psychiatric Conditions

Doris C. Gundersen

Psychosis

The mechanisms by which psychoactive cannabinoids produce transient psychotic symptoms are unclear but may involve dopamine, GABA, and glutamate neurotransmission. Dose, length of exposure, and the age of first exposure to cannabinoids may be important factors as well. Genetic factors that interact with cannabinoid exposure to moderate or amplify the risk of psychosis are being examined. Neurobiological changes seen with cannabis use show similarities with those seen in patients with schizophrenia. However, the similarities do not establish a cause-effect relationship because not all cannabis users go on to develop schizophrenia. It is likely that multiple, non-neurobiological factors also play a role [56].

Many studies confirm that cannabis is definitively linked to the development of psychoses, including the thought disorder schizophrenia, especially in the context of pre-existing genetic vulnerability [57–60]. Cannabis use causes cognitive changes (discussed in another chapter) and dysfunction in dopamine transmission in genetically vulnerable subjects, which may be responsible for the psychotic-like experience.

Approximately 14% of psychotic outcomes in young people would not have occurred if cannabis had not been consumed. Heavy use of potent cannabis at a younger age in individuals at risk for developing schizophrenia exacerbates the course of the illness by advancing the time of a first psychotic break by 2–6 years. This has prognostic significance in that most individuals who develop schizophrenia do so at a later age, late teens to early twenties. With an earlier onset of illness, academic and social performance will be compromised, leading to a poorer prognosis compared with later onset of illness [61].

Among those who have used cannabis, the risk of developing psychosis increases by 40% and there appears to be a dose-response effect leading to an increased risk of psychosis up to 200% in the most frequent users [62, 63].

Cannabis use among adults with schizophrenia appears to be a double-edged sword. Low doses of cannabis consumption may improve frontal lobe function by acutely increasing blood flow to cortices concerned with cognition, mood, and perception, increasing the availability and utilization of dopamine. However continued use actually depresses cerebral flow and high consumption augments mesolimbic dopamine release, opposing the therapeutic effects of antipsychotic medications, thereby exacerbating psychosis. Finally, cannabis use in patients with schizophrenia suppresses prefrontal cortex dopamine utilization resulting in cognitive dysfunction [64].

In Australia, a sibling pair analysis within a prospective birth cohort was conducted. Of the 3801 studied, early cannabis use was associated with psychosis-related outcomes including non-affective psychosis, hallucinations, and delusions [65]. In London, a study of 780 people between the ages of 18 and 65 years with 410 experiencing a first episode of psychosis and 370 healthy controls demonstrated that high potency cannabis use was associated with a triple risk for psychosis [66]. Finally, 25 percent of patients diagnosed with schizophrenia meet the criteria for cannabis use disorder, making it one of the most commonly used drug among this patient population. Patients using cannabis experience more psychotic symptoms, respond poorly to antipsychotic medications, demonstrate poorer treatment compliance and worse clinical outcomes, and more relapses as well as more hospital admissions [62].

Depression and Anxiety

Several studies have demonstrated that cannabis use is associated with increased levels of anxiety and mood disorders [67–70], and it has been reported that heavier cannabis use in adolescents was associated with a heightened risk for developing an anxiety disorder [69].

Early-onset cannabis smoking is associated with an increased risk of depression [67]. One study conducted in Australia tracked 1600 girls over a 7-year period. Those who used cannabis daily were five times more likely to suffer from depression and anxiety than non-users. Additionally, teenage girls who used the drug at least weekly were twice as likely to develop depression compared to those who did not use [61]. At the UCSF Department of Psychiatry, 307 patients with depression were assessed at baseline and again at 3- and 6- month intervals for symptoms, functioning and cannabis use. Over 40 percent of the participants used cannabis within the 30 days of the start of the study. Cannabis use was associated with poor recovery. Those 50 years of age and older actually increased their cannabis use ($P < .001$) compared to the younger study participants. Cannabis use worsened depression ($P < .001$) as well as anxiety ($P < .025$) and led to poorer mental health functioning ($P < .010$) [71]. In addition to research showing that smoking cannabis exacerbates anxiety and depression, it has also been shown to worsen disorders of attention [72].

In Australia, 3239 young adults were followed from birth to the age of 21 years. Potential confounding factors were prospectively measured when the child was born and again at 14 years. After controlling for confounding variables, those who started using cannabis before the age of 15 years and used it frequently at 21 years were more likely to report symptoms of anxiety and depression in early adulthood than those who did not use cannabis (odds ratio 3.4; 95% CI 1.9–6.1) [73].

Cannabis-related visits to emergency and urgent care facilities by adolescents in Colorado increased dramatically between 2005 and 2015. In 2005, 161 visits were made, whereas in 2015, 777 visits were made. Behavioral health evaluations accounted for 67 percent of the contacts. Additionally, nearly three-fourths of the adolescents seen with diagnostic codes related to cannabis use were also diagnosed with depression, mood disorders, and anxiety. A large number of the patients also tested positive for alcohol, amphetamines, and opiate [74].

Many states legalizing cannabis for medicinal purposes have included post-traumatic stress disorder (PTSD) as a qualifying condition for treatment, despite the fact that little evidence exists evaluating the effect of whole plant cannabis use in PTSD. Whereas CBD may hold promise in helping REM sleep/behavioral disorders, mitigate hippocampal volume loss, and reduce symptoms of anxiety, THC does not appear to be therapeutic and, in fact, may aggravate the underlying disorder [75, 76].

Wilkinson et al. examined the association between cannabis use and PTSD symptom severity in a longitudinal, observational study of 2276 veterans over 4 months. The researchers concluded that cannabis use was significantly associated with worsened outcomes with regard to PTSD symptoms severity ($P < .01$). Specifically, more violent behavior was associated with cannabis use ($P < .01$) and, more alcohol and drug use was associated with cannabis use in PTSD patients ($P < .01$). The veterans participating in the study who had never used cannabis or had abstained from using cannabis during the study had the lowest PTSD symptoms at discharge ($P < .0001$). Finally, those who started using cannabis during the study exhibited the highest levels of violent behavior ($P < .0001$) [75]. The Veterans Affairs official site states clearly that any substance that is illegal on the federal level is *not* permitted to be used, recommended, prescribed, or endorsed by the Department of Veterans Affairs, up to and including the recommendation that veterans use cannabis to alleviate symptoms or pain. Any substance listed by the US Food and Drug Administration as a Schedule I controlled substance are subject to this prohibition at the VA level [77].

Addiction

Although historically cannabis has been thought to be less addictive than substances such as nicotine, cocaine, and heroin, the potency of THC in cannabis products obtained through interdiction seizures has increased from approximately 3 percent in the 1980s to 12 percent or higher in 2014 [78]. As a result, the cannabis available today may be more hazardous than earlier studies reflect. Whereas an average-sized cannabis "joint" contains 10–15 percent THC, butane hashish oil, a concoction of hashish oil infused with butane, can contain up to 90 percent THC [63]. Long-term cannabis users can develop dependence and withdrawal requiring chemical dependency treatment [63, 79, 80].

Historically, about 9 percent of regular cannabis users became addicted. By comparison, 15 percent of alcohol users, 32 percent of nicotine users, and 26 percent of opiate users become addicted [57, 63, 64, 81]. However with the advent of high potency cannabis products, cannabis use disorders are rising in prevalence. The National Institute on Drug Abuse recently released data that suggests that 30 percent of those who use cannabis may have some degree of cannabis use disorder [82].

Early cannabis exposure alters brain reward pathways, thus facilitating the subsequent use of other drugs. If cannabis use starts in childhood, one in six starters will become addicted. Daily users of cannabis are at the highest risk for developing cannabis dependence. Twenty-five to fifty percent of these users will become addicted [57]. While there has been controversy about this, cannabis is very likely a gateway drug because of the high potency of contemporary strains [57]. The earlier a child is exposed to cannabis, the greater the risk of cocaine and heroin use and drug dependence as an adult. Today, the number of adults with substance abuse disorders is increasing. Increasing access and availability of high potency cannabis products will only exacerbate this trend [63, 81].

Some reports have suggested that the legalization of cannabis products would curtail opiate use and opioid overdose death. However in Colorado, heroin-related deaths have doubled since 2011 when statewide; 79 deaths were observed compared to 2015 when 160 heroin-related deaths occurred. Pueblo County in particular was in the highest percentile of heroin use by county and also ranked as having statistically higher cannabis use [83].

Chronic users of cannabis who become dependent develop an uncomfortable withdrawal syndrome that can interfere with cessation of use, even when the user is motivated to quit. Withdrawal symptoms include irritability, nervousness, insomnia, restlessness, depression, decreased appetite and other physical discomfort [57].

Cannabis-Related Violence and Death

Death by suicide has also been observed among cannabis users. Multiple studies have documented a relationship between cannabis use and suicidality [67], and cannabis use is considered to be an important risk factor for suicidal behaviors [84].

The Veterans Administration conducted a cross-sectional, multisite study of 3233 Iraq/Afghanistan-era veterans. Cannabis use disorder was significantly associated with both current suicidal ideation ($P < .0001$) as well as a lifetime history of suicide attempts ($P < .0001$) compared to veterans with no lifetime history of having a CUD. This difference in those with CUD and those not diagnosed with CUD persisted even after adjusting for gender, PTSD, depression, alcohol use disorder, other drug use, childhood sexual abuse, and combat exposure [75, 85].

A large longitudinal study in Australia and New Zealand including over 2000 adolescents found an almost seven times increase in suicide attempts in daily cannabis users compared with non-users [86]. Dugre et al. studied 1136 recently discharged psychiatric patients followed at 4 and 10-week time intervals and evaluated them for cannabis, alcohol, and cocaine use as well as episodes of violence between 1992 and 1995. Persistency of cannabis use was associated with an increased risk of subsequent violence, significantly more so than with alcohol or cocaine [87].

Many proponents of the legalization of cannabis argued for the safety of the drug by noting no deaths were associated with it compared to opiates, cocaine, and alcohol. However, lethal consequences have been observed due to the increasing risk of psychosis. When recreational cannabis became legal, cannabis cookies, candies, and drinks infused with THC soon became popular. Many new consumers were not aware of the potent THC content in edibles [78]. In September 2012, an 18-year-old male smoked potent cannabis and subsequently fatally stabbed himself 20 times. In April 2014, a Wyoming college student jumped to his death from a Denver hotel balcony after eating more than the recommended serving of an edible product. That same month, a Denverite shot and killed his spouse in front of their three children after consuming edibles [78].

Studies show that the persistency of cannabis use following acute psychiatric discharge is predictive of violence [87]. Moulin et al. found cannabis use disorder to be a significant risk factor for violent behavior. In this study, 265 patients with early psychosis (dichotomized by presence or absence of violent behavior) were followed prospectively for 36 months. Cannabis use was linked to impulsivity and lack of insight. A cannabis use disorder diagnosis was made in 61 percent of subjects engaging in violence compared to 23 percent of non-users. Subjects who began using cannabis at a younger age, were more violent. Preventive strategies could be developed on the basis of such patient profiles [88].

Cannabis consumption has increased with its legalization as well as the perception that it is an innocuous substance. Hospital emergency departments continue to see a rise in patients presenting with cannabis-related adverse events. For example, the University of Colorado Hospital Emergency Department found a more than threefold increase in cannabis-associated emergency department visits from 2012 to 2016. This has placed a new burden on the healthcare system resulting from costly workups and hospitalizations [89].

Potential Psychiatric Benefits of CBD

Most of the psychiatric complications secondary to whole plant cannabis are related to the psychoactive cannabinoid THC and not CBD [90]. The expanding literature on CBD provides promising evidence that it is useful in the treatment of several psychological conditions. For example, the use of whole plant cannabis with high THC and low CBD concentrations has been associated with reduction of hippocampal volume, which increases the risk of impaired memory and new learning. Higher CBD to THC ratios may have a role in neuroprotection [91]. A number of studies have suggested that CBD may mitigate THC-induced psychosis [92–95]. CBD alone has antipsychotic effects. This was demonstrated in a study of healthy volunteers who experienced a reduction in ketamine-induced depersonalization with CBD treatment [96]. In a single case report of a patient with schizophrenia who could not tolerate conventional antipsychotics, a significant reduction in psychotic symptoms was observed after the patient received high-dose CBD for 4 weeks, with a recurrence of symptoms after the CBD was discontinued [97]. CBD given to patients with either acute paranoid schizophrenia or schizophreniform psychosis resulted in reduced psychotic symptoms, similar to what was observed with conventional antipsychotic drugs but with a significantly more tolerable side effect profile [98]. Finally, Gomes and colleagues demonstrated that CBD diminished the catalepsy induced by haloperidol, supporting its potential benefit as an adjuvant in the treatment of psychotic disorders [99]. These preliminary findings are promising and support the need for additional larger-scale randomized controlled trials in an effort to the establish efficacy of CBD in the treatment of psychotic disorders.

Zuardi and colleagues discovered that CBD has anxiolytic properties in study participants exposed to stressful situations [100]. CBD has also demonstrated superior efficacy compared to placebo in the treatment of generalized anxiety disorder [101]. Evidence also supports the potential benefit of CBD in the treatment of post-traumatic stress disorder. In one study, CBD reduced subjective anxiety and autonomic arousal, as measured by skin conductance response [102]. Another study involving the dual-step administration of the partial NMDA agonist D-cycloserine and CBD showed a disruption of reconsolidation of traumatic memories [103]. Finally, a double-blind, placebo-controlled trial demonstrated that CBD administration led to an enhanced consolidation of fear extinction when administered after extinction suggesting that CBD may be useful in the treatment of all anxiety disorders, including PTSD [104].

The role of CBD in the treatment of addictions has also been examined. Morgan and colleagues found that smokers treated with CBD reduced the number of cigarettes that they smoked by 40%. The number of cigarettes smoked by the placebo group was unchanged [105]. CBD may also have some utility in reducing opioid-seeking behavior and also diminish the reward-facilitating effects associated with opioid use [106]. However, much more research is required to fully determine CBD's role in addiction medicine. While the growing body of clinical studies support the efficacy of CBD as an adjuvant as well as a monotherapy for psychiatric conditions, a recent Cochrane review concluded that there were insufficient high-quality studies to draw a reliable conclusion regarding efficacy, despite no reports of adverse events. Currently, the lack of regulation, testing, and contamination of CBD products demands that practitioners exercise an abundance of caution when making clinical decisions for a vulnerable patient population. Furthermore, studies of Epidiolex, the first FDA-approved CBD product for the treatment of refractory seizures, have demonstrated other potential adverse reactions such as hepatic transaminase elevations and hepatocellular injury. Drug-drug interactions with CBD are also a concern. For example, concomitant use of valproate and CBD can synergistically elevate hepatic enzymes. CBD dosages should be adjusted when combined with strong inhibitors or inducers of CYP3A4 and CYP2C19 to ensure efficacy and avoid excessive amounts of CBD being absorbed. Somnolence and sedation can occur with its use and patients must not drive or operate machinery until they have gained sufficient experience with CBD dosing. Suicidal ideation and behavior have been reported with the use of CBD. Decreased appetite, diarrhea, fatigue, and insomnia are other identified side effects [107].

An abundance of caution must be exercised when making clinical decisions for a vulnerable patient population. Because most studies demonstrate more harm than benefit with regard to whole plant cannabis in the treatment of psychiatric conditions, the American Psychiatric Association has taken the position that there is currently no scientific evidence to support the use of cannabis as an effective treatment for any psychiatric illness [108].

Conclusion

Across the country, states are contending with a truly novel situation. Public opinion, expressed through ballot initiatives to amend state constitutions, has resulted in the introduction of a new treatment in the absence of well-designed research and FDA approval. This new treatment includes an unusual and likely unhealthy route of administration (i.e., smoking). Whole plant cannabis is consumed, despite the fact that it is composed of hundreds of individual compounds with various psycho-active and non-psychoactive properties.

In the absence of rigorous scientific data, dispensaries are now distributing cannabis and cannabis products to large numbers of individuals. Yet physicians, who are the gatekeepers of this process under state law, lack adequate information on which to base their judgment if they choose to discuss cannabis as a treatment option with their patients.

The practice of medicine must remain evidence-based under most circumstances. Physicians should carefully consider their ethical and professional responsibilities before issuing a cannabis recommendation to a patient. A physician should not advise a patient to seek a treatment option about which the physician has inadequate information regarding composition, dose, side effects, or appropriate therapeutic targets and patient populations.

With regard to psychiatric conditions, there remains limited evidence that cannabis is effective in treating serious mental illnesses [108]. In most states legalizing cannabis for medicinal purposes, tax revenue has been earmarked for research. Until this research yields reliable information about the safety and efficacy of individual cannabinoids, mental health professionals should largely avoid making recommendations for cannabis products and simply stay abreast of advancing science.

Cannabis Use and Psychosis, Mood, and Anxiety Disorders

Erica Kirsten Rapp and Paula Riggs

Introduction

In the past decade, more than two-thirds of US states and the District of Columbia have legalized medical marijuana, and more than one-third of these have also legalized cannabis for recreational use. This has significantly expanded availability and public access to an increasingly wide array of cannabis products that have significantly higher potency than the cannabis available pre-legalization [109–113]. A number of research studies have reported an association between cannabis use and psychotic disorders as well as mood and anxiety disorders [114]. In most of these studies, the associations were based on the use of much lower potency cannabis products available prior to legalization. Also, methodological limitations of most previous studies did not enable determination of whether the relationship between cannabis use and psychiatric disorders was causal. This chapter will briefly summarize results of previous studies examining the association between cannabis use and psychiatric disorders including a recent meta-analysis [115] and emerging research on the effects of higher potency cannabis use on mental health problems.

This chapter will first examine recent trends in the potency of available cannabis products and rates of use in the post-legalization environment in the United States.

We will then review studies addressing the association between cannabis use and psychotic, mood, and anxiety disorders. Conclusions regarding the relationship between cannabis use and psychiatric disorders are based on the weight of evidence drawn from current research.

Increasing Cannabis Potency Post-legalization

In the 1960s, both cannabis plant material (marijuana) and resin (hashish) contained 3% THC or less [109], with a very modest increase in potency through the mid-1990s. In 1995, the average THC content in samples confiscated by the DEA was 4%, and only 0.6% of the samples were high potency, containing more than 12% THC. In 2014, shortly after Colorado and Washington became the first two states to legalize recreational cannabis, the average THC content of DEA-confiscated samples was 11.8%, and 41.2% of the samples contained more than 12% THC [110]. Among samples of cannabis legally for sale in Washington State between 2014 and 2016, cannabis flower had an average THC content of 20.6% [111]. The cannabis industry also produces highly concentrated cannabis products including "shatter," "wax," and other concentrates, including butane hash oil (BHO) containing 70–90% THC [112], with some crystalline products advertised as 99.9% THC [113].

From a public health standpoint, it very concerning that the market share for concentrates has increased after legalization. In Washington state, the market share for concentrates, averaging 69% THC, increased by 150% in the 2 years after recreational cannabis sales began, reaching 21.2% of total cannabis sales in 2016 [111]. Concerns about the increasingly widespread access and availability of high potency cannabis products is further heightened, given how little is known about the health risks, including the potential impact on mental health, associated with their use.

Post-legalization Trends in the Prevalence and Frequency of Cannabis Use

In the United States, past-year cannabis use among a sample of over 36,000 adults rose from 4.1% in 2001 to 9.5% in 2013. The increase was most dramatic in the 18–29 age group, with past-year use increasing from 10.5% in 2001 to 21.2% in 2013 [116]. Among 12th grade students, annual use peaked at 51% in 1979. It dropped throughout the 1980s, and in 1992, only 22% of 12th graders reported using cannabis in the prior year [117]. Use then increased by the late 1990s, declined slightly through the mid-2000s, and increased gradually between 2008 and 2015 [117, 118]. Across all grade levels, there was no significant change in the rate of lifetime or current marijuana use between 2015 and 2017 [118]. In 2018, 36% of 12th graders reported past-year cannabis use [117].

The prevalence and frequency of use are also increasing in many other parts of the world, most notably in westernized countries, including Canada, Australia, New Zealand, and western Europe [119]. In New Zealand, nearly 80% of participants in one cohort reported using cannabis at least once by age 30, and 59% reported using before age 18 [120]. In a UK cohort, 27% of 16-year-olds reported ever using cannabis, and 3.3% reported using more than 60 times [121]. In the Australian Twin Registry (ATR), the percentage of participants who reported ever using cannabis rose from 30% in 1993 to 69% in 2009 [122]. Age of first use also decreased from 21 years to 18 years over the same time period, and the prevalence of frequent use (greater than 100 times) increased from 4.9% to 15.2% [122].

Impact of Medical Legalization

Recent data from Canada raises concerns that many individuals who use medical cannabis, even for legally authorized medical conditions, increase the amount and frequency of their use after obtaining medical authorization. Sixty-five percent of medical cannabis users in a 2011–2012 Canadian survey reported increasing their cannabis consumption after obtaining a medical marijuana license; half of these reported large increases in use [123]. In a 2017 survey, 22% of medical cannabis users reported that their cannabis use had increased "a lot" since obtaining legal access to medical cannabis [124].

Additional research is needed to determine factors that may be contributing to the reported increases in cannabis use. These may include greater addictive potential of high potency cannabis, development of tolerance, or other factors. Additional research is also needed to evaluate whether the use of high potency cannabis has a greater impact on pre-existing psychiatric disorders and/or a greater risk of causing mental health problems compared to lower potency cannabis. The following section examines results of studies that have addressed the relationship between cannabis use and psychiatric conditions. Although causation cannot be determined based on results of individual studies, causation can be inferred when (1) consistent findings from multiple reports show a strong association with a large effect size, (2) the exposure consistently precedes the outcome, (3) there is a dose-response relationship between the exposure and outcome, and (4) there is a plausible biological explanation tying the exposure to the outcome [125, 126]. Evidence comes from both cross-sectional epidemiological studies and longitudinal population studies.

These principles are used to evaluate the current body of research and determine what the weight of evidence tells us about the relationship between cannabis use and psychosis, mood, and anxiety disorders.

What Does Research Tell Us About Cannabis Use and Mental Illness?

Cannabis, Psychosis, and Schizophrenia

In 1987, Andreasson and colleagues famously published follow-up data from a survey of more than 45,000 Swedish men who had undergone a compulsory medical examination for conscription in 1969–1970. The men were followed in the national health register through 1983. Compared to non-users, people who reported using 11–50 times at conscription had a relative risk of 3.0 for later developing schizophrenia. Relative risk was doubled (RR = 6.0) in those who reported using more than 50 times, supporting a dose-response relationship [127]. Subsequent secondary analyses of these data also supported a strong dose-response relationship between cannabis use and later development of schizophrenia, both in subjects who used cannabis only and those who used cannabis plus other drugs. There was no relationship between cannabis use and the later development of other psychotic disorders [128]. A recent meta-analysis of more than 50 studies reported that more than 1/3 (34%) of individuals with a cannabis-induced psychosis later developed schizophrenia [115].

Most other studies have examined the relationship between cannabis use and psychosis more generally, not limited to the diagnosis of schizophrenia. The early developmental stages of psychosis (EDSP) study collected 4-year follow-up data on 2437 participants who were aged 14–24 at the time of recruitment. Participants who reported using cannabis five or more times at study entry had more than double the risk of having two or more psychotic symptoms at follow up, compared to those who had used 0–4 times [129]. This finding suggests that young people who start using cannabis under age 25 may be vulnerable to developing psychosis even at low levels of exposure. Additionally, this study found a statistically significant linear relationship between the amount of cannabis use at baseline and the subsequent risk of psychotic symptoms. Participants who used less than once a month had no greater risk of developing psychosis than non-users. A gradation of increasing risk was found in participants whose use ranged from approximately weekly (OR = 1.50) to 3–4 times per week (OR = 2.44) [129].

Another important finding of this study was the increased risk associated with cannabis use among participants who had mild psychotic symptoms at baseline. Among those with no psychotic symptoms at baseline, people who had used cannabis (≥5 times) had a 6% difference in risk of psychosis at follow-up compared to non-users. However, participants who did have mild psychotic symptoms at baseline and who used cannabis had a 25% difference in their risk of subsequent psychosis compared to those who had psychotic symptoms at baseline but did not use cannabis [129]. Other studies have had similar findings. One study in a population at ultra-high risk (UHR) for psychosis based on clinical criteria found that people with early-onset and frequent cannabis use were more likely than non-users to transition to psychosis. Those who started using before age 15 and used at least once per week were at the highest risk [130]. There is a plausible biological explanation for increased vulnerability in adolescents, given that THC binds to CB1 receptor and may interfere with CB1's regulatory role in the development of the prefrontal cortex during rapid brain development occurring throughout adolescence [131]. These findings indicate that youth who have *any* psychotic symptoms should avoid even infrequent cannabis use.

Cannabis use in people with a possible genetic predisposition to psychosis was examined in one study of siblings of patients with psychotic disorders. In this group, cannabis users had a fourfold increase in the odds of developing psychosis compared to non-users (OR 4.1) [132].

A 2007 meta-analysis, based on seven studies available at the time, confirmed concerns about cannabis use in both adolescents and adults. Compared to individuals who had never used cannabis, those reporting any cannabis use had increased risks for psychotic symptoms (OR = 1.41) and for a psychotic disorder (OR = 2.58). Furthermore, the six studies that analyzed the effect of frequency of use (with the highest frequencies defined as >50 times to daily, depending on the study) all found dose-response relationships between frequency of use and risk of psychosis [133]. Only one of the seven studies included collected data exclusively on adolescent cannabis use [134]; three more included young adults [128, 129, 135]. The remaining three studies reported primarily on adults [136–138], indicating that even in adulthood, cannabis use increases the risk of psychosis.

A more recent epidemiologic survey study was conducted on nearly 18,000 young adults in the Netherlands [139], where cannabis use was allowed in certain "coffee shops" beginning in 1976 [140] and where some of the highest-potency products in Europe are available [141]. This study found that both positive symptoms (such as hallucinations and paranoia) and negative symptoms (such as avolition and social withdrawal) of psychosis were worse in the heaviest cannabis users, who spent more than €25 per week on cannabis. For positive symptoms, ORs compared to non-users increased from 1.7 in light users to 3.0 in the heaviest users, and for negative symptoms these ORs were 1.3 and 3.4, respectively. This study also found an increased odds of positive symptoms in people who began using cannabis before age 12 (OR = 3.1). People who started using between ages 12 and 15 had a slightly increased risk that did not reach statistical significance, while people who started using between ages 15 and 18 had an equivalent risk to those who started after age 18. A similar trend was seen for negative symptoms, with subjects who started use before age 12 having an OR of 1.7 [139].

Cannabis use has been associated with a variety of poor outcomes when used by people with pre-existing psychotic disorders [142], including greater risk of relapse [143] and longer duration of hospitalizations [144]. Compared to people with psychotic disorders who do not use cannabis, those with regular ongoing cannabis use have more positive psychotic symptoms [145], greater thought disturbance [146], and more hostility [146]. Cannabis use among people with psychotic disorders has also been linked to increased risk of death from accidents (SHR = 1.59) and all-cause mortality (HR = 1.24) [147].

A prospective study of first episode psychosis patients in South London found former regular cannabis users who quit had the lowest relapse rate (24%), while people who continued to use high-potency cannabis had the highest rate (58%) [148]. There were also significant effects of cannabis use on number of relapses and time to relapse [148], as well as length of relapse [149]. Some of these effects were mediated by negative effects of cannabis use on medication adherence [149].

Clearly, much more research is needed to understand the relationship between risk of psychosis and cannabis potency, especially with regard to the extremely high THC concentrations found in cannabis concentrates (e.g., BHO, shatter, wax, etc.) increasingly available post-legalization, about which little is known. Some studies suggest that CBD may have a protective effect against elevated risk of psychosis driven by THC [150–153]. Post-legalization trends in commercially marketed cannabis have seen dramatic increases in THC concentration, while CBD content has been removed or significantly reduced in most commercial cannabis products [114].

Taken together, the body of current research addressing relationship between cannabis use and psychosis strongly suggests that cannabis use is causally related to risk of psychosis. This risk is particularly elevated in adolescents and young adults using high-potency products. This conclusion is based on the consistent findings from multiple studies reporting cannabis use preceding the onset of psychosis, many of which show a dose-response relationship. Given the strong evidence for a dose-response relationship between frequency of cannabis use and psychotic symptoms, it is not surprising that emerging data indicate a higher risk for psychosis with higher potency products [140]. Emerging data also support a growing clinical concern that heavy or regular cannabis use – especially during adolescence – may precipitate earlier onset of psychotic disorders [154, 155]. Results from a recent meta-analysis showed that more than a third of individuals who experience psychosis related to cannabis use go on to later develop schizophrenia [115]. In individuals with pre-existing psychotic symptoms, cannabis use may worsen the risk for chronic symptoms [148, 149].

In summary, there is considerable evidence that cannabis use, especially in young people, can increase risk of psychosis in a dose-related manner. There is currently insufficient evidence to determine whether cannabis plays a causal role in the development of schizophrenia. However, there is growing evidence that cannabis use may precipitate earlier onset of schizophrenia in those who have other risk factors for developing the disorder [114, 115].

Cannabis and Mood and Anxiety Disorders

Compared to the research on psychosis and cannabis use, the current body of research examining the relationship between cannabis use and mood and anxiety disorders is more modest.

The National Epidemiologic Survey on Alcohol and Related Conditions (NESARC) surveyed more than 43,000 adults in 2001–2002 and again 3 years later. Data were collected on multiple psychiatric disorders, including major depression, bipolar disorder, and several anxiety disorders. At the baseline assessment, past-year cannabis use frequency of weekly or greater was associated with an increased overall risk for bipolar disorder (OR 2.62), depression (OR 2.27), and anxiety disorders (OR 2.20), as well as each specific anxiety disorder examined [156]. An even larger population-based survey, the National Survey on Drug Use and Health (NSDUH), gathered data from over 527,000 adolescent and adult participants between 2006 and 2015. A study examining the relationship between cannabis use and major depressive episodes found that in both age groups, participants with past-year cannabis use had a higher rate of past-year major depressive episodes than non-using participants [157].

One cohort study, focusing on adolescent use, found an increased risk of depression and anxiety at age 21 for all cannabis users who used every few days or more, but those whose use started at age 14 or earlier had a threefold increased risk (OR 3.4), while those who started after age 14 had a lower risk (OR = 2.3). Symptoms of anxiety or depression at age 14 did not predict later cannabis use (between ages 14 and 21) [158]. Results from another cohort showed that for young women, cannabis use at age 14–15 predicted anxiety/depression at age 20–21. Adolescent depression/anxiety did not predict later cannabis use for either sex [159].

Several systematic reviews and meta-analyses have examined this relationship as well. An early systematic review, published in 2003, concluded that there was evidence for a modest association between adolescent cannabis use and later depression [160]. Another, several years later, included all age groups and found a modestly increased risk (OR = 1.49) for depressive symptoms in people who used weekly or more, compared to non-users, using pooled data [133]. A meta-analysis of 31 studies with prospective cohort or cross-sectional designs found increased risks for anxiety in cannabis users (OR = 1.24) and people with cannabis use disorders (OR = 1.68) [161]. A recently published meta-analysis showed that adolescent-onset cannabis users, compared to non-users, had modestly but significantly increased risk (OR = 1.37) of depression in young adulthood as well as increased risk for suicidal ideation (OR = 1.50) and suicide attempts (OR = 3.46). The pooled risk (OR = 1.18) for anxiety was not statistically significant [162].

A few studies have explored the relationship between cannabis use and specific anxiety disorders, with mixed results. One study using NESARC data analyzed rates of specific anxiety disorders (panic disorder with and without agoraphobia, social phobia, specific phobia, and generalized anxiety disorder). Each of the individual disorders was associated with cannabis use, with ORs ranging from 1.74 for social phobia to 3.57 for panic disorder with agoraphobia [156]. A retrospective secondary analysis of NESARC data examined the temporal relationships between cannabis use and anxiety disorders. Results showed that for both adolescent- and adult-onset cannabis users, generalized anxiety disorder and panic disorder emerged after cannabis use, while social phobia and specific phobia emerged prior to cannabis use [163].

A study examining the relationship between cannabis use and adult mental health outcomes also reported that regular cannabis use was associated with higher risk of developing generalized anxiety disorder, but not social phobia, in young adulthood

[164]. Similar findings were reported in another cohort study showing a twofold increase (OR = 2.2) in depression among participants who reported using cannabis more than 60 times lifetime, compared to non-users [121]. A longitudinal twin study found that adolescent identical twins who reported using cannabis more than 100 times were significantly more likely to develop major depressive disorder as young adults compared to the identical twin who reported less frequent or no use (OR 1.98) [122].

Although there is some variability across studies in definitions of "early onset" and "heavy use," the current weight of evidence, based on consistent, convergent findings from these studies taken together, provides substantial empirical evidence that regular or frequent cannabis use, especially during adolescence, significantly increases the risk of developing depression and/or generalized anxiety disorder by young adulthood [165–169]. Preliminary findings from at least two of these studies also suggest that adolescents who significantly reduce or discontinue cannabis use may reduce their risk of developing major depression or generalized anxiety disorder to a level of risk similar to non-users [164, 170].

There is also consistent evidence that cannabis users, compared to non-users, who have pre-existing mood (depression, bipolar disorder) and/or anxiety disorders generally have a more severe and chronic course of illness and poorer response to treatment. In a study of 300 psychiatric outpatients with depression, cannabis users had significantly less improvement in depression symptom severity at 6-month follow-up compared to non-users [171]. Another study gathered data from 330 young women who were using cannabis. Those who reduced or stopped using cannabis during treatment (for depression) had significantly greater improvement in depression severity based on Beck Depression Inventory (BDI) scores, compared to participants who continued using cannabis at baseline levels [172].

Although the literature on cannabis use and bipolar disorder is scant, one large epidemiologic survey study found that individuals with bipolar disorder who reported any past year cannabis use, compared to non-users, had persistently higher subscale scores for mania and hallucinations/delusions, but not depression, throughout the 12-month study [173]. A 2-year prospective study of patients with bipolar disorder showed that bipolar patients who continued to use cannabis three or more times per week had significantly less symptom improvement and lower rates of clinical remission compared to non-users and less frequent cannabis users [174]. A large 2-year prospective observational study of European adults reported significantly higher rate of suicide attempts among current cannabis users with bipolar disorder (6.9%) compared to those who had never used cannabis (3.0%) and previous cannabis users (4.4%) [175]. A nationwide Danish national registry study of individuals diagnosed with schizophrenia, bipolar disorder, unipolar depression, or personality disorder found that current cannabis use disorder was associated with an increased risk of completed suicide in people with bipolar disorder (HR = 1.86) [176].

In summary, the current body of research addressing the relationship between cannabis use and mood or anxiety disorders provides substantial evidence to support the following conclusions:

1. Regular cannabis use during adolescence significantly increases the risk of developing major depressive disorder and/or generalized anxiety disorder in young adulthood.
2. Among individuals with major depressive disorder and bipolar disorder, regular ongoing cannabis use may interfere with treatment response and reduce likelihood of clinical remission.
3. Regular cannabis use in individuals diagnosed with major depression, bipolar disorder, or schizophrenia is associated with increased suicidal ideation, suicide attempts, and completed suicides.

Conclusion

There is clearly a need for more methodologically rigorous studies to address research gaps in our scientific understanding of the relationship between cannabis use and psychiatric disorders. However, in the context of ongoing rapid national expansion of cannabis legalization, the main goal of this chapter has been to critically evaluate and interpret findings and clinical implications of existing studies which taken together comprise the current body of research. Preliminary conclusions regarding the nature of the relationship between cannabis use and psychiatric disorders are based on consistent and convergent findings from multiple studies. The clinical implications of key findings and recommendations for clinical practice are discussed below.

1. There is substantial evidence that cannabis use causally increases risk of psychosis in a dose-response fashion, especially in adolescents and individuals with pre-existing psychotic symptoms or risk factors including family history of schizophrenia. Adolescents in general should be educated about the neurotoxic effects of cannabis use during adolescence, including at least quadrupled risk of psychosis even in individuals without any family history of schizophrenia or other risk factors for developing psychosis. In part this is related to rapid brain development that occurs throughout adolescence from ages 10–24. Adolescents and young adults with any prior history of psychotic symptoms are at especially high risk and should be strongly discouraged from using cannabis. Although there is currently insufficient evidence to determine whether cannabis plays a causal role in the development of schizophrenia, there is growing evidence that cannabis use, especially during adolescence, may precipitate earlier onset of schizophrenia in individuals who have a family history or other risk factors for schizophrenia.
2. Among individuals diagnosed with major depression, bipolar disorder or schizophrenia, there is robust evidence that regular cannabis use is associated with a more severe and chronic course of illness, less robust response to treatment, and lower rates of remission. Individuals with these and other psychiatric conditions should be routinely screened for cannabis use and provided with research-based

psychoeducation about the aforementioned risks associated with ongoing cannabis use and potential benefits of discontinuing or significantly reducing cannabis use in terms of clinical improvement and response to treatment for a co-occurring psychiatric disorders and reduced risk of suicidality.

Marijuana and Suicide: Case-Control Studies, Population Data and Potential Neurochemical Mechanisms

Christine L. Miller, Monica C. Jackson, and Kevin Sabet

Introduction

Suicide is clearly one of the most complex outcomes in behavioral research. It is both multifactorial, involving a large number of independent variables, and unpredictably episodic. Whereas most behavioral disorders which qualify for a DSM-V diagnosis can exhibit patterns over time which facilitate monitoring of symptoms in affected individuals, day to day or year to year, suicidal thoughts have been known to appear spontaneously 1 day and be gone the next [177, 178]. Even a history of depression is not a reliable predictor of suicidal ideation in college age young adults [179]; thus, parsing out the pre-existing risk factors for completed suicides can be very difficult. Suicidal ideation itself is also not consistently predictive [180]; rather, it is a prior suicide attempt which is the single most reliable marker of suicide completion [181, 182] and, as such, is the focus of much research.

This chapter will examine case-control publications on marijuana's impact on suicide risk in the context of what is known about the typical impact of other recreational drugs, along with demographic variables known to influence suicidal outcomes. Population data will be presented for marijuana use and suicide rates, and the potential neurobiological mechanisms for marijuana's impact will be explored.

The Impact of Recreational Drugs on Suicide Risk

Almost all recreational drugs are associated with an increased risk of suicide attempts when used to excess, and marijuana is no exception to this theme. Wong et al. [183] found a significant association with suicidality in US youth for each of ten substances used (heroin, methamphetamine, steroids, cocaine, ecstasy, hallucinogens, inhalants, alcohol, tobacco, and marijuana). O'Boyle and Brandon [184] identified suicide attempters as being significantly more likely to abuse multiple drugs, including alcohol, than non-attempters. The increased risk has been estimated to increase significantly for each additional drug used [185].

As with most behavioral outcomes, the role of drug use in precipitating the behavior rather than being a response to an underlying psychiatric disorder must be evaluated. This relationship has not been clarified for all recreational drugs, though the elevated suicide risk for some are high enough to eclipse the risk typically conveyed by depression, for example. Thus, although heroin addicts most often die from accidental overdoses [186], suicide attempts have been self-reported by 42% of a very large cohort of heroin users. Their risk of completed suicide is elevated as much as 14-fold [187], whereas the risk conveyed by depression alone has been estimated to be 6.1-fold [188, 189]. Abstinence from heroin in former addicts has been shown to be protective and polydrug use enhanced the suicide risk [190]. For cocaine users, the risk of suicide has been reported to be as high as ninefold [191]. Fowler et al. [192] found that fully 53% of suicide cases in the San Diego Suicide Study had received a substance abuse diagnosis of one type of another. Binge alcohol use has appeared to increase the risk for suicide attempts by a somewhat more modest factor of 1.3–2.6-fold [193], but it is primarily CNS depressants like alcohol, opiates, barbiturates, and benzodiazepines, which significantly increase the risk of a suicide attempt on the day of use [194].

Case-Control Studies Specific to Marijuana

Research on marijuana's role in suicide has been building substantially over the past decade. Most published reports controlled for a variety of demographic variables known to impact suicide risk, but only one specifically corrected for a prior history of mood disorders [195], finding the risk for suicide attempts to be elevated by 7.5-fold in 168 Irish adolescent marijuana-users as compared to controls. A large prospective study (over 2500 subjects) launched in stages in New Zealand and Australia from 1977 to 1992 reported the risk of suicide attempts at some point in the teen or young adult years was elevated 6.9-fold in those who were using marijuana daily by age 17 [196]. Completed suicides was evaluated for 6445 subjects in Denmark [197], finding the risk for suicide was elevated 5.3-fold in those with a cannabis use disorder as compared to control subjects.

Earlier work was suggestive of a substantial impact, but the studies were often not conclusive because they were small (increasing marijuana use preceded suicides in the small Micronesian Island of Truk [198]), unadjusted for covariates [199], the association diminished to a nonsignificant trend after adjustment for covariates [200], or marijuana use was completely unrelated to suicide after adjusting for covariates, as seen in a study of adolescents in Switzerland [201]. Case-control data from the US National Mortality Followback Survey in 1993, revealed an increased risk of suicide in marijuana users, 2.3-fold for males and 4.8-fold for females [202]. Similarly, Pedersen et al. [203] reported that Norwegian subjects who used cannabis 11 or more times in the past year were 2.9-fold more likely to attempt suicide after adjusting for confounding covariates.

A lack of association was reported in 2009 by Price et al. [204] in a large study of mortality in Swedish transcripts, who found that correcting for potentially confounding variables, rendered an association between suicide and marijuana use nonsignificant. Here, it should be mentioned that the investigators corrected for smoking of cigarettes, which holds the potential for creating what is known as a collider variable [205], whereby two supposedly independent variables actually interact to obscure real associations with the dependent variable (the outcome). In this case, it was the tobacco versus marijuana use that created potential collider variables, since most cannabis users also smoke tobacco and cannabis use is known to have a reverse gateway effect by leading to a tobacco habit [206]. Correcting for tobacco use can therefore substantially reduce the apparent impact of marijuana.

In Nova Scotia, Rasic et al. [207] found that marijuana-only use was predictive of depression without suicidal features, possibly because the marijuana-only users were found to use it infrequently. Similarly, Arria et al. [179] found that cannabis use disorder was not predictive of suicide ideation in students attending college, although the trend of the association was positive and the study was not adequately powered to detect less than about a 3.5-fold relative risk.

One of the most effective means to adjust for genetic background and confounding environmental effects is to study the differential impact of marijuana in twins. Agrawal and colleagues [208] analyzed an updated Australian twin registry and found that members of identical and non-identical twin pairs who frequently used marijuana (defined as more than 100 times of use) were at a more than 3.6-fold increased odds of reporting suicidal ideation lasting more than 1 day and a more than sixfold odds of engaging in a suicide attempt (here, the non-identical twin comparison only, in part due to small sample size of identical twins) than their non-using twin. Because the impacts were generally similar in the non-identical and identical twin pairs (with an exception being a difference in attempts), they concluded that genetic factors played a relatively small role in mediating the effects seen.

A meta-analysis by Borges et al. [209] included the most well constructed of these studies and many others, finding the average increase in risk for suicide attempt was 3.2-fold for heavy users. The definition of heavy use in the meta-analysis varied from as low as less than once per month to daily or near-daily use. If the analysis had been restricted to near-daily or daily use, the effect size might have approached that of the Silins et al. [196] study of a 6.9-fold increased risk as seen from Fig. 4 in the Borges et al.'s meta-analysis. It should also be noted that the meta-analysis included studies of lower potency marijuana than that available today, as well as non-Caucasian ethnic groups. Chandra et al. [210] have documented the changing potency, from an average of 4% for the dry-leaf product in 1995 to an average of 17% in 2017. Other factors in the study-to-study variabilities seen in this meta-analysis are the differences in ethnic and gender vulnerability to suicide. Although recent publication of youth suicides in 21 low- and middle-income countries confirms that the impact of marijuana use to increase suicide risk extends across many ethnic group [211], Caucasian males of combined age groups exhibit more than double the risk for completed suicides of African-American males and more than triple the risk of Caucasian females, with African American female risk lower yet [212]. Individuals of Hispanic descent also have a notably lower risk than Caucasians (https://www.nimh.nih.gov/health/statistics/suicide.shtml). Yet, as reviewed by Sellers et al. [212], the data for suicide attempts in adolescents shows trends opposite to that of completed adult [213] suicides: females are more likely to attempt suicide than males; Latino and African American adolescents are more likely to attempt suicide than Caucasians.

A more recent meta-analysis by Gobbi et al. [214] restricted the inclusion of studies to those which were longitudinal, assessed marijuana use prior to age 18, and included a follow-up periods from 18–32 years. In those who began using marijuana before age 18, the adjusted odds ratio (OR) for attempting suicide by age 32 was found to be 3.46. No determination of the effect for degree of usage or strength of product was reported.

The impact of marijuana use on groups already at risk for suicide is a particular concern, and here, attention should first be focused on those with post-traumatic stress disorder (PTSD). Several investigators have demonstrated that among veterans and active duty personnel who suffer from PTSD, those who use marijuana make less progress overcoming their symptoms and have worse outcomes [215], including suicidal events [216–219]. Allan et al. [216] found that marijuana use in current and former military personnel with PTSD predicted suicidal thoughts within 1 month and suicide attempts within 11 months, in a model that incorporated age, sex, baseline opiate, and alcohol and marijuana use. The impact of marijuana was significant in those with elevated PTSD symptoms at baseline and was proportional to the number of days using marijuana per month. Because veterans and active duty personnel often have been exposed to potentially confounding variables of high impact, the adjustment factors should be noted here. One study which controlled for age, race, service sector, and combat exposure, found past 6-month cannabis use to be associated with severity of PTSD, depression, and suicidality in veterans [217]. In terms of the degree of risk posed, a diagnosed cannabis use disorder was found to be associated with a 3.1-fold increased risk of suicidal self-injury in a group of veterans, some with and some without a PTSD diagnosis, after adjusting for after adjusting for sex, age, sexual orientation, combat exposure, traumatic life events, traumatic brain injury, depression, alcohol use disorder, non-cannabis drug use disorder, and the baseline risk posed by posttraumatic stress disorder [218]. However, the risk for suicide attempts has also been reported to be higher, increased eightfold in post-deployment veterans with a cannabis use disorder, after controlling for PTSD severity, pre-deployment suicide attempts, depression, pain, non-cannabis drug use, and gender [219].

The importance of the timing of marijuana's use relative to suicide events was addressed by Sellers et al. [212], who found that "day-of" use was a risk factor for both suicidal ideation and attempts in adolescents. In contrast, Bagge and Borges [194] reported that acute use of marijuana in the 24-hour period prior to a suicide attempt showed a trend to be protective in their unadjusted model, though when adjusted for other drug use, was not associated with risk; whereas past 24-hour use of recreational and prescription drugs that have CNS depressant actions (sedatives/anxiolytics, opioids, and alcohol) increased risk for suicide attempt. Stimulants showed a similar timing effect to that of marijuana, but the co-use of stimulants and marijuana resulted in the loss of significance in the adjusted models. The discrepancy between the two studies could relate to any of the following likely factors that distinguish the Sellers et al. study [212]: the bias inherent through selecting only subjects who were part of a teen alcohol use study (all were users, though not daily users); the much younger average age of the subjects; the 78% Caucasian ethnic distribution; the 80% proportion of females; the 32% proportion of subjects who were transgender; or the fact that the average 90 day use of marijuana was 15 days, which would likely indicate the majority were not addicted to marijuana.

Because both cannabis use and stimulant use over the long term are clearly associated with risk for suicide, one interpretation of the work of Bagge and Borges [194] is that the withdrawal from one or the other class of drug is likely a period of risk. It also should be kept in mind that mini-withdrawal episodes can happen within the course of 1 day as concentrations of active drug levels fall when a user may be too busy with other activities to keep their blood levels up. Vandrey et al. [220] have shown that withdrawal symptoms are already fairly pronounced by the time 24 hr. have elapsed.

Population Data on Suicide and Marijuana Use

In contrast to case-control studies, analysis of population level data cannot control for variables specific to individuals, such as pre-existing mood disorders, and must instead examine demographic data for populations available from public databases. But the advantage of studying health outcomes in whole populations is to confirm that case-control results are discernable in larger, unselected groups. The general public and many scientists regard effects observable at the population level as the necessary confirmation of importance to public health. A good example of this perspective can be found in the schizophrenia field, where numerous case-control findings for the association of marijuana use with the development of schizophrenia have often been discounted in the absence of corroborating trends in whole population-level data for the nation [221–223].

Thus, when this country was faced with a remarkable increase in suicide rates from 2007 through 2015 (Fig. 4.1), the question became which population-level factors could possibly underlie this shift, and this might prove to be an example of the relevance of case-control studies to population-wide impacts.

Potentially Confounding Demographic Variables

Among the many well-studied associations, some have high impact but have not changed in a manner that could explain the increase in suicide rates over recent time. For example, the proportion of gun-owning households in a clear factor in completed suicides [224] but has not significantly changed during the 15-year period covered by this study [225], and non-firearm suicides has increased at a higher rate over the past 10 years than have firearm suicides (http://webappa.cdc.gov/sasweb/ncipc/dataRestriction_inj.html). The rate of treatment of depression with antidepressants is another potential factor but has been found by others to have no discernible impact on suicide rates [226], and the antidepressant treatment rate remained flat from 2007 through 2010 [227] a time period encompassing the significant upturn in the national suicide rate. Federal funding for suicide prevention is undoubtedly important [228], and the Substance Abuse and Mental Health Services Administration (SAMHSA) increased the funding significantly over the years 2000–2015, going up roughly tenfold since the year 2004 (www.hhs.gov). Divorce is a well-accepted risk factor, but divorce rates have been declining for the past 35 years, most notably from 2008 through 2011 [229] during which time the slope in the suicide rate changed direction to head higher (Fig. 4.1). Teen suicide attempts stemming from overuse of social media [230] and its attendant abusive content have definitely increased, but the proportion of teen suicides as a fraction of the total increase seen by the end of 2015 was small (10%, http://webappa.cdc.gov/sasweb/ncipc/dataRestriction_inj.html).

Certain other influential variables either exhibited no change over recent time or changed in a direction inconsistent with their effect on suicide, for example, the proportion of the population living at high altitude [231, 232] and pathological gambling [233–235]. Colorado, as the bell weather state for impacts of altitude effects, experienced most of its population growth in the relatively low altitude front range during the period 2007–2015, and pathological gambling did not change discernibly across the country over the same time period [235].

As much as many aspects of life in the countryside may seem protective for suicide, rural rates of suicide are nearly double the per capita rates in urban environments [236]. Examining the degree of urbanization revealed a net increase in urbanization from 2001 through 2011 [237]; thus a flight of citizens to rural residences could not explain the increase in suicides during this span of time. Furthermore, as the population shifted to more urbanization, a shift toward more marijuana and other drug use was occurring in rural areas, a trend which would be expected to diminish the urban/rural gradient in suicide. For both urban and rural populations, marijuana was the most common cause of a substance use disorder [238]. In fact, Habecker et al. [239] found that urban and rural populations in Nebraska had become similar in profile with respect to ease of access to marijuana and other drugs with the following exceptions: women had markedly better access in to marijuana and prescription pills in rural than in urban areas and less access to methamphetamine and heroin in rural than in urban areas; white non-Hispanics had markedly better access to methamphetamine and heroin in rural than in urban environments. In contrast, Bukky [240] found at the national level, an urban-rural distinction was not present for marijuana, other illicit drugs or prescription drugs. Regardless, the increasing suicide rate in our country is unlikely to be driven by urban-rural distinctions, because urbanization increased during this time period, and residing in urban centers carries a lower risk of suicide than rural areas, though it remains possible the factors which increase rural risk may interact more strongly with the drug use increases seen in rural areas over time.

Two factors that changed markedly from 2007 to 2015, and in a direction consistent with increasing suicide risk, are unemployment and marijuana use. A study in the United Kingdom during the economic recession of 2008 attributed 40% of the suicides there to being unemployed [241]. The case-control, register-based, and population data on unemployment affecting suicide risk [241–245] show an impact ranging from two- to fourfold on completed suicides, thus somewhat less than the impact of marijuana as reviewed above. Others have found that the impact of unemployment most is strongly felt when it is of longer duration, showing greatest association when mass layoffs are occurring and exerting greatest impact at about 15–26 weeks [246]. Unemployment benefits often cease after 26 weeks, so it may be the anticipation of this event that becomes particularly problematic. The recession of 2008 fulfilled most of the high impact criteria for unemployment.

The Data on Suicide and Marijuana Use Rates Nationally and in Select States, 2000–2015

Figure 4.1 illustrates the plots of suicide in the general population and in veterans, marijuana use, unemployment, binge use of alcohol, and other drug use rates. Although binge alcohol use and other drug use did not change in a manner consistent with the increase in suicide rates, including these variables is important in order to illustrate that marijuana use is not acting as a proxy measure for binge alcohol or other drug consumption, but rather exhibits its own unique profile over time and prevalence. For example, the daily or near-daily use rate of marijuana by those aged 12 and over was 3.5% by 2015 [247], as compared to 0.33% using heroin in the past year (NSDUH reports, www.SAMHSA.gov).

Multiple linear regression of these dependent and independent variables yields a highly significant regression coefficient estimate for marijuana use rate predicting suicide in the general population, to the exclusion of the other variables ($r = 0.925$, $p < 0.000$) and for unemployment predicting suicide in veterans ($r = 0.885, p < 0.000$). It should be noted that for a small proportion of veterans, it is clear the impact of unemployment on suicide did outlast the elevation of the unemployment (cross-marked curve versus light gray curve in Fig. 4.1). In other words, it remains possible that not only did impact of unemployment outlast the recession for this population; it may also have done so for a portion of the general population.

Equivalent plots for state-level data in Colorado (lower panel, Fig. 4.1) show more variation as would be expected for a smaller population, but the results are very similar: marijuana use rates predicted the suicide rate to the exclusion of other variables ($r = 0.828, p < 0.000$).

A drug policy change that may have impacted marijuana use rates is shown in Fig. 4.2, the Ogden memo which was issued by then Attorney General Holder and stipulated that the federal government would not prosecute medical marijuana dispensaries operating according to local state laws [248]. The notification of the release date for this memo, as well as other court decisions initiated a rapid expansion in the population of medical marijuana, seen in data available from the Colorado Department of Health and Environment (upper panel). The break in slope is significant for the marijuana use rate but does not quite reach significance for the suicide

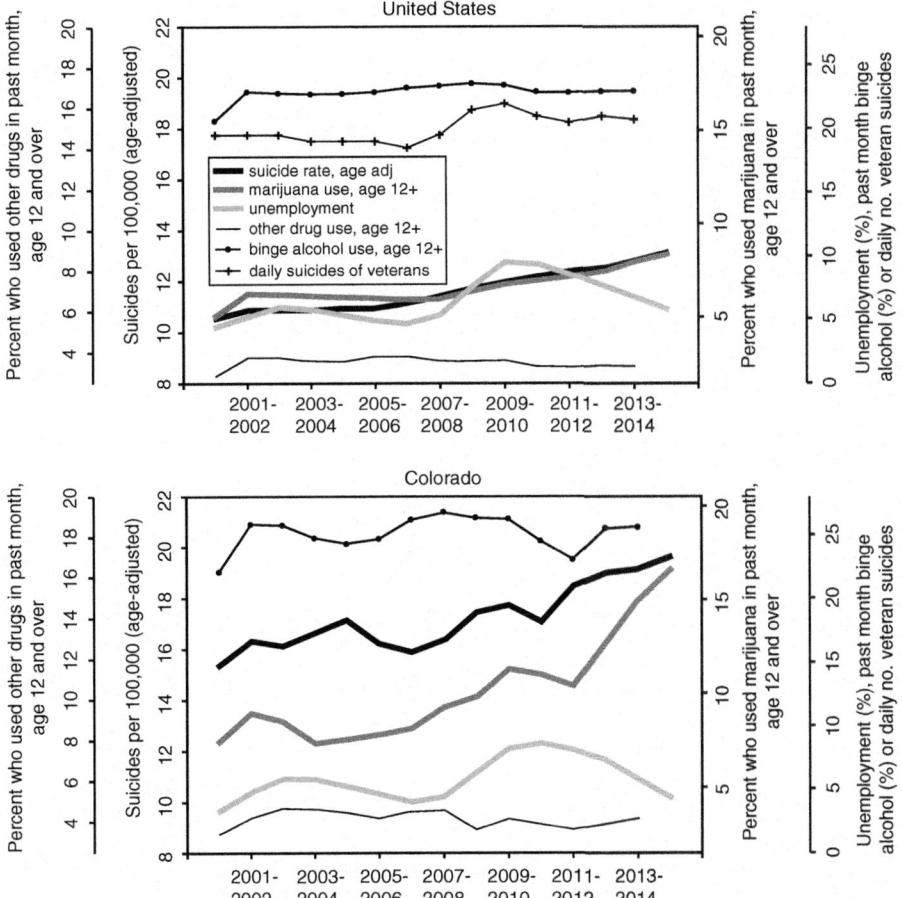

Fig. 4.1 Plots of age-adjusted suicide rates, unemployment rates, and percent who used marijuana, other drugs, or who engaged in binge drinking (on a monthly basis, age 12 and older) in the United States and Colorado for 2-year averages starting from the year 2000 through 2015. Daily veteran suicide rates are also shown for the United States (upper plot). The identification of the symbols and lines for the lower plot are the same as shown in the upper plot. Data for drug and alcohol use was obtained from NSDUH reports (www.SAMHSA.gov); for unemployment from the Bureau of Labor Statistics) http://beta.bls.gov; for suicide in the general population, from the CDC, www.CDC.gov and for veteran suicides, from a report issued by the Veterans Affairs Administration. Note that data for other drug use, binge drinking, and daily suicides of veterans were not available for 2015

rate in both the national and Colorado data. Strikingly, the timing of the break in slope of the curves for the national and Colorado suicides appears to coincide with the release of the Ogden memo (lower panel).

Examination of the 10-highest marijuana use states (Table 4.1) and the 10-lowest marijuana use states (Table 4.2) reveals the impact of marijuana is easier to discern in the highest use states, being the primary predictive variable for 6/10, versus 3/10

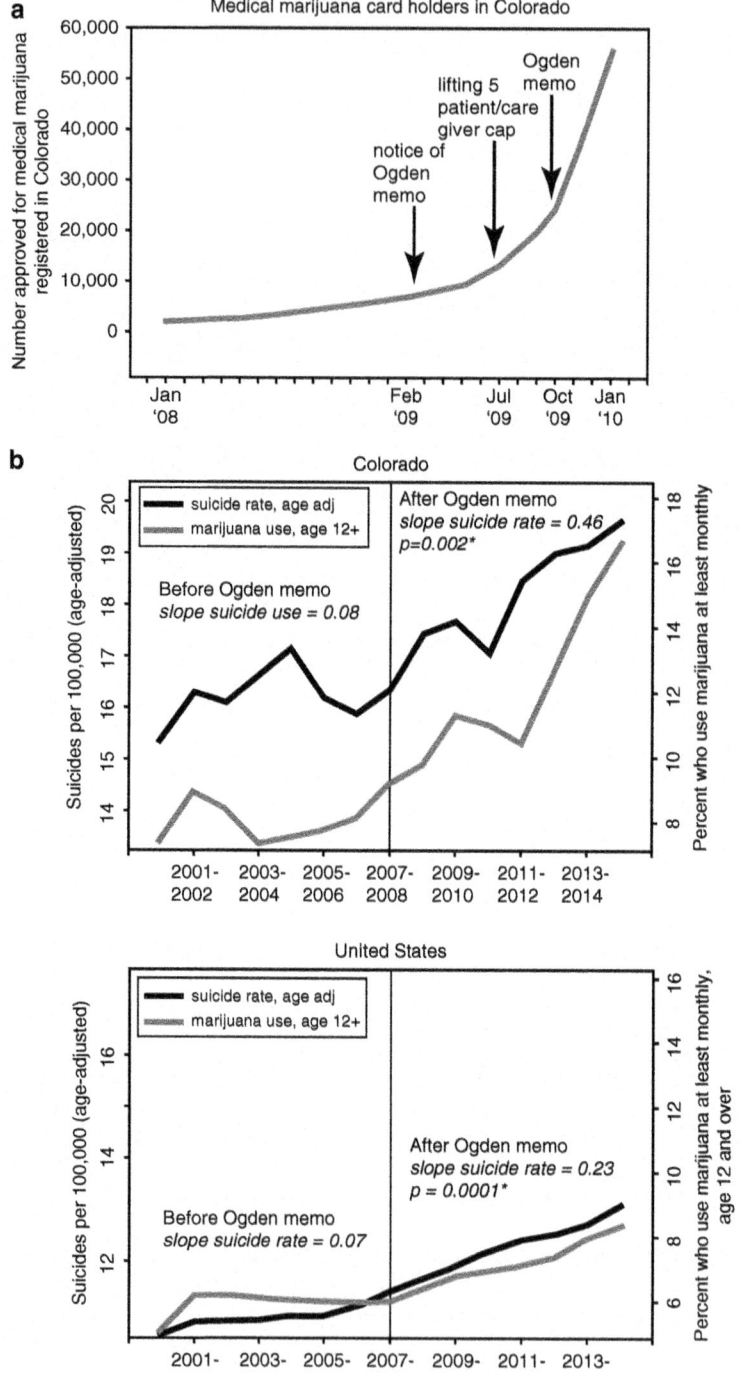

Fig. 4.2 Chronology of changes in marijuana drug policy, changes in marijuana use, and changes in suicide rates in Colorado and the United States. (**a**) The growth of registered medical marijuana users in Colorado during the year 2009, with key events depicted by the arrows. Colorado had legalized medical marijuana in 2001, but the regulations were stringent. The first easing of restrictions followed the news of the upcoming Ogden memo, which eventually would indicate the federal government would not enforce the law on medical marijuana dispensaries [248]. Next, the ruling of a district court lifting a five patient per caregiver cap was not contested. Finally, the Ogden memo was released in October 2009. By 2010, the adult medical marijuana users grew in number to represent ~ 1.4% of the total adult population. (**b**) An increase in the slope of regression for age-adjusted suicide rates and for the percent who used marijuana monthly (aged 12 and older), after the Ogden memo was issued. The scales of the graph for Colorado and the United States are the same, but the ranges depicted are different to allow for the enlargement and easier viewing of the change in slope. The data source for state suicides was www.CDC.gov and for marijuana use rates www.samhsa.gov.

◀──

of the lowest use states. This outcome is consistent with the concept that any increase in monthly marijuana use has a proportionally greater impact on daily marijuana use [249], the use frequency of most concern for suicide in some case-control studies [196].

Potential Mechanisms of Marijuana's Effect

Indirect Mechanisms

Marijuana increases risk for several behavioral disorders which themselves greatly increase the risk for suicide. The data are most strong for a causal role of marijuana use in the development of schizophrenia, showing a four- to fivefold increased risk [250, 251] with heavy use of products that are of moderate THC strength by today's standards (≤15%). Schizophrenia itself is associated with an increased risk for suicide of approximately 3.1-fold as compared to the general population (adjusted O.R. for age, etc.), a risk calculated based on proportion of suicides with schizophrenia versus the general population [252], with a lifetime risk of committing suicide of about 5% [253, 254]. The risk is highly dependent upon the age group and time since first diagnosis [255], decreasing markedly for those who survive 5 years past diagnosis and are beyond their 20s, as compared to the rates in the general population for the same age. Consistent with a mechanism involving the psychotic disorder itself, Waterreus et al. [256] found that once psychosis is activated, cannabis use does not further increase the risk for suicide.

The research on marijuana triggering bipolar disorder is not yet as extensive as the literature on its relationship with schizophrenia, though a large study conducted in the United State shows weekly use of low to moderate strength marijuana raises the risk for bipolar disorder by 2.6-fold when corrected for covariates [257], very similar to the 2.7-fold increased risk with weekly use seen for psychotic disorders

Table 4.1 High marijuana use states (arranged in order from lower to higher use)

	Montana		Massachusetts		Maine		Washington		D.C.	
	Estimate	P-value	Estimate	P-value	Estimate	P-value	Estimate	P-value	Estimate	P-value
Marijuana use rate	0.834	0.000	0.464	0.018	0.563	0.006	0.717	0.000	ex	
Unemployment rate	ex		0.535	0.008	0.478	0.015	0.341	0.031	ex	
Binge alcohol use rate	ex		ex		ex		ex		0.599	0.024
R^2	0.673		0.733		0.675		0.823		0.359	
Power	0.999		0.999		0.995		0.999		0.662*	

	Oregon		Alaska		Vermont		Rhode Island		Colorado	
	Estimate	P-value	Estimate	P-value	Estimate	P-value	Estimate	P-value	Estimate	P-value
Marijuana Use	0.912	0.000	0.477	0.085	0.886	0.000	ex		0.828	0.000
Unemployment rate	ex		ex		ex		0.836	0.000	0.222	0.093
Binge alcohol use rate	ex		ex		ex		ex		ex	
R^2	0.831		0.227		0.769		0.676		0.836	
Power	1.000		0.493*		0.999		0.999		0.998	

Multiple linear regression results from the final model using backward elimination method for variables potentially related to suicide in individual states

Note: This table presents the ten highest marijuana use states (past 30 day use) from NSDUH data (www.SAMHSA.gov) based on the average for 2012–2015. The variable other drug use was a priori excluded from all final regression models due to theoretical considerations concerning its negative coefficient (see text) and multicollinearity; "ex" represents variables that exited the model during the backward elimination method; the power analyses assumed the number of remaining independent variables as per the final model; the *D.C. and *Alaska results were underpowered (i.e., power < 0.8). The program SPSS was applied in this analysis. The results presented are from the final model using backward elimination method

Table 4.2 Low marijuana use states (arranged in order from lower to higher use)

	Utah Estimate	Utah P-value	Alabama Estimate	Alabama P-value	Iowa Estimate	Iowa P-value	North Dakota Estimate	North Dakota P-value	Kansas Estimate	Kansas P-value
Marijuana use rate	0.794	0.004	ex		0.733	0.003	0.452	0.091	ex	
Unemployment rate	0.591	0.023	ex		ex		ex		ex	
Binge alcohol use rate	ex		0.905	0.000	ex		ex		ex	
R^2	0.526		0.818		0.537		0.204			
Power	0.903		1.000		0.970		0.443*			

	Mississippi Estimate	Mississippi P-value	Louisiana Estimate	Louisiana P-values	Texas Estimate	Texas P-value	South Dakota Estimate	South Dakota P-value	Tennessee Estimate	Tennessee P-value
Marijuana use rate	ex		ex		0.939	0.000	ex		0.505	0.000
Unemployment rate	0.468	0.047	ex		ex		0.527	0.043	0.804	0.000
Binge alcohol use rate	0.454	0.053	ex		ex		ex		ex	
R^2	0.609				0.882		0.278		0.882	
Power	0.973				1.000		0.604*		1.000	

Multiple linear regression of variables potentially related to suicide in individual states

Note: This table presents the ten lowest marijuana use states (past 30 day use) from NSDUH data (www.SAMHSA.gov) based on the average for 2012–2015. The variable other drug use was á priori excluded from all final regression models due to theoretical considerations concerning its negative coefficient (see text) and multicollinearity; "ex" represents variables that exited the model during the backwards elimination method; the power analyses assumed the number of remaining independent variables as per the final model; *the analyses for North Dakota and South Dakota were underpowered (i.e., power < 0.8). There were concerns with the model predicating suicide rates in Utah as the residuals indicated a slight deviation from normality. The program SPSS was applied in this analysis. The results presented are from the final model using backward elimination method like schizophrenia [250]. Bipolar disorder is reported to be associated with a sixfold risk of suicide versus the general population in a meta-analysis [258], and a similar risk when compared to the risk of unaffected siblings in a large Swedish study (6.8-fold, see Fig. 4.1 of publication) [259].

The risk for major depression with marijuana use is less than for schizophrenia and bipolar disorder, with ≥100 times of use (about equivalent to weekly use over a 2 year period) approximately doubling the risk in a study of twins [208]. Major depression itself is associated with a 6.1-fold increased risk for suicide [188, 189] and variously reported to carry a lifetime risk of completed suicides of 3.4–8.6% in the United States [260, 261].

Obviously, all of the studies cited above are influenced by the efficacy of psychopharmacological treatment in normalizing behavior and the proportion of patients who comply with treatment. The direction of the effect is not always as expected in that antidepressants are variously reported to increase suicide risk in adolescents [262]; increase risk of attempts in a wide age group, but not completed suicides [263]; increase risk primarily in the first several days after commencing a prescription [264, 265]; and decrease in the overall risk, but with a warning about monitoring the initial period of treatment [266]. In general, antipsychotic treatment is regarded as offering modest protection from suicide and suicidal behaviors [267–270], with clozapine being the most effective and approved by the FDA for suicidal indications in patients with schizophrenia [271], but there are also some reports of negative impacts of antipsychotic drugs on suicide risk in the short term [272]. Lithium and valproic acid may be the most successful examples of the psychopharmacological agents for preventing suicide when used to treat bipolar disorders [273–275].

Direct Mechanisms, Both Chronic and Acute

Studies of a more direct mechanism for marijuana's impact on neurobiology have pointed towards a role for dopamine. Dunlop and Nemeroff [276] concluded that dopamine is important to a wide variety of pleasurable experiences and almost all abused drugs increase dopamine extracellular levels in the nucleus accumbens, long considered an integral part of the mesolimbic reward circuitry (reviewed by Ikemoto and Panksepp [277]). Dopamine, along with other stress-related biochemicals elevated by drug use, may exacerbate emotional distress and sensitivity to stressful stimuli [278]. Cocaine exerts similar effects on dopamine release in both animal and human models (as reviewed by Francis et al. [279]). Similar trends have also been reported for specific cannabinoid receptor-1 (CB1) agonists in animal models [280, 281] and in humans [282]. Even endogenous cannabinoids can upregulate dopaminergic neurotransmission in the striatum [283].

Indeed, chronic elevation of extracellular dopamine is thought to underlie the process of addiction (reviewed by Uhl et al. [284]), and therefore, extended use of marijuana can be expected to lead to depletion of dopamine in the reward centers of the brain [285], an outcome that would be consistent with loss of pleasure in everyday life. Paradoxically, there is inconsistent evidence that this long-term dopamine depletion from abuse of recreational drugs mirrors what happens in major depression, as reviewed in 2009 by Martin-Soelch [286]. More recently, Schneier et al. [287] found that extracellular dopamine in the ventral striatum does not appear to be lower in those with major depression.

Despite inconsistent parallels in dopamine levels between the anhedonia of drug addiction and depression, psychological testing coupled with fMRI data shows patterns in marijuana users that are consistent with depression. Zimmermann [288] demonstrated lower emotion regulation capacity in cannabis users (abstinent for 28 days) arising from increased prefrontal activation and diminished prefrontal-amygdala connectivity while expressing negative affect. In particular, marijuana users show decreases in regulation of emotion when the craving is strong, illustrating how poorly regulated motivational urges overwhelm cognitive control. Blum et al. [289] examined the question of experiencing pleasure derived from natural rewards such as social interaction and found a blunting of the reward experienced by users. All of these impacts, while not directly studied as a putative mechanism of marijuana's impact on suicide, are known to influence suicidal ideation and urges.

Both the indirect hypothetical mechanisms, via the chronic mental illnesses the use triggers, and the direct mechanism of dopamine depletion, require chronic use to see an effect. Is there any evidence of an acute impact of marijuana use, and if so, what mechanism could possibly explain such an effect?

Acute onset of suicidal ideation has most often been seen following oral ingestion Δ^9- THC ([290]; reviewed by Koppel et al. [291]). Suicidal ideation was observed in 1 out of 14 subjects administered with a liquid form of pure Δ^9- THC (20 mg doses) over a period of 3 days in a clinical setting [292]. This unexpected outcome preceded their subsequent testing of the CB1 "inverse agonist" Rimonobant, but Rimonobant was withdrawn from the market before the study was completed because it had also been linked to an increased risk for suicidal ideation in prior studies [293]. This side effect of an inverse agonist should not be interpreted as being contradictory to the results for the direct agonist effects of Δ^9- THC. Being a partial agonist, Δ^9- THC [294] could theoretically interfere with the full agonist action of endogenous cannabinoids, potentially leading to a neurophysiologic end result similar to Rimonobant's.

Why oral ingestion may be associated with suicidal urges more frequently could have something to do with first-pass metabolism by the liver following ingestion but not following smoking. The most striking difference in metabolites is the production by liver enzymes of significant amounts of 11-hydroxy-THC [295], a metabolite reported to be more psychoactive than Δ^9- THC itself. Some reports have even suggested that Δ^9- THC may in part be a pro-drug and it is 11-hydroxy-THC which is the primary psychoactive agent, based on the potency of its effect and the rapid onset of psychiatric and cardiac symptoms with its administration [296]. A percentage of the subjects studied by Lemberger et al. (66%, [297]) found the first exposure to 11-hydroxy-THC was quite unpleasant at its peak effect, while none reported that Δ^9- THC in the same dose was unpleasant. It is the unpleasant nature of the high reported which would obviously be a concern for suicidal behaviors. In point of fact, Favrat et al. [298] reported that higher levels of 11-hydroxy-THC were associated with more severe psychotic symptoms following oral ingestion of Δ^9- THC by two subjects.

The neurochemical basis for these acute effects on suicidal behaviors obviously requires much more research. One finding that holds promise to explain the rapid development of suicidal urges is the activation of the kynurenine pathway seen in postmortem samples of suicide victims or in blood samples from those who have attempted or contemplated suicide [298–302]. This activation is evident in ratios of the kynurenine, the first product of the pathway, to tryptophan, the initial substrate for the pathway [302]; is evident in the ratio of intermediate metabolites (quinolinate/picolinate) which could be indicated of higher flux through the pathway [301]; and is also evident in the elevation of a downstream metabolites, nicotinamide, in postmortem brain tissue of bipolar patients who have committed suicide [303] and quinolinate, in blood samples of those who have attempted suicide [304].

Cytokines which activate the kynurenine pathway have been shown to be elevated in those with suicidal behaviors [304], specifically IL6 [305] and TNF-α [306]. TNF-α is required for the induction of one of the two enzymes that initiate the kynurenine pathway, indoleamine 2,3-dioxygenase, IDO [307]. Although cannabinoids tend to depress the immune system [308, 309], including reductions in IL-6 and TNF-α that have been elevated by other agents [310, 311], administration of Δ^9- THC under basal conditions primes immune cells for a subsequent TH-2 response when stimulated; thus, IL-6 and TNF-α (as part of a TH-2 response) would be elevated. Another potential mechanism is via another initiating enzyme of the pathway, tryptophan 2–3-dioxygenase. Decades ago, biochemists Poddar and Gosh [312] discovered that Δ^9- THC activates tryptophan-2.3-dioxygenase (TDO2) in an animal model. This mode of activating of kynurenine synthesis would be unlikely to occur through cytokine signaling because unlike IDO, TDO2 is thought to be regulated independently of the cytokine system (reviewed by Miller et al. [296]).

Conclusions

The potential for suicidal behaviors is clearly the most severe mental health risk from marijuana use. Even unsuccessful suicides leave traumatic emotional scars on the individual and their loved ones. The circle of harm is wide. As a culture, we need to find routes to minimize suicidal thoughts and urges to begin with, and if minimizing the use of a drug associated with suicide risk is one strategy, it should be embraced as an easier route to prevention than attempting to solve many other complex social forces which increase suicide risk.

Preliminary evidence for marijuana's causal role in suicide can be seen in the acute onset in a clinical setting; in the significant increase in risk when a prior history of a mood disorder is corrected for; and in the existence of at least two plausible biological mechanisms. Thus, the continued rise in marijuana use across the broad age group of 12+ represents an ongoing public health concern. Suicide attempts may be most common in teens and young adults [313] but completed suicides in the United States peak in middle age or later [213]. Prevention goals should therefore be geared toward a widespread decrease in marijuana use across all age groups.

Cannabis Use Disorder, Treatment, and Recovery

Ben Cort and La Tisha L. Bader

Progression of the Disease

During an assessment or treatment, one of the common activities is to ask a patient to craft a timeline of their disease and its impact. This allows treatment professionals, patients, and families to understand the progressive nature of the disease as well as the parts of life that started to unravel because of use. For some, this begins a difficult conversation because life did not feel "unmanageable" for a lengthy period of time. An individual might have started using and continued to use cannabis without significant consequence, such as getting arrested, hangovers, fighting with family, overdose, or losing a lob. In some states, cannabis is legal for both recreational and medicinal use and might have slowed the impact of consequences. On average, adults seeking treatment have been daily users for more than 10 years and tried to quit more than six times [314].This would mean that use has become a daily way of life, integrated into the routines and patterns of life. Friends, family, and a person's social network may accept it as common place and find it difficult to consider needing treatment for cannabis.

Oftentimes to challenge a current stage of change (such as precontemplation), it might take a lengthy period of time or numerous negative situations or outcomes, to agree that one's life has become disorderly and requires intervention [315, 316]. Again, for cannabis, this might take longer because of legalization, a minimized perspective of the drug's impact, the role it plays in popular culture or less adverse feedback from friends and family.

Once an individual becomes open to the idea of treatment, at any level, the approach to treatment parallels that of other substances, it is imperative to use an objective evaluation of the disease and pursue placement in the appropriate level of care. The most respected criteria have been developed by the American Society of Addiction Medicine (ASAM) which cover six (6) dimensions that are affected by the disease.

ASAM's criteria uses six dimensions to create a holistic, biopsychosocial assessment of an individual to be used for service planning and treatment across all services and levels of care. The six dimensions are:

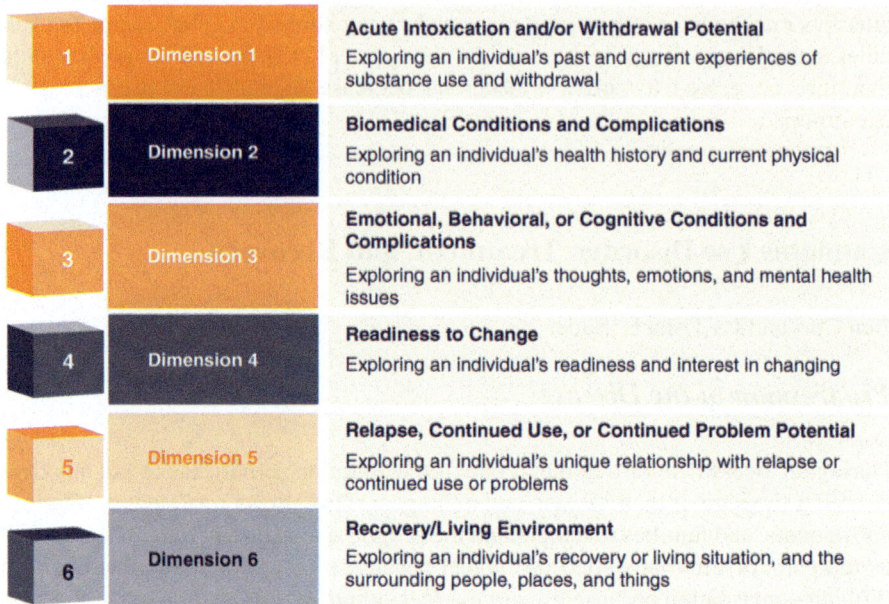

Acute Intoxication and/or Withdrawal Potential
Exploring an individual's past and current experiences of substance use and withdrawal

Biomedical Conditions and Complications
Exploring an individual's health history and current physical condition

Emotional, Behavioral, or Cognitive Conditions and Complications
Exploring an individual's thoughts, emotions, and mental health issues

Readiness to Change
Exploring an individual's readiness and interest in changing

Relapse, Continued Use, or Continued Problem Potential
Exploring an individual's unique relationship with relapse or continued use or problems

Recovery/Living Environment
Exploring an individual's recovery or living situation, and the surrounding people, places, and things

These criteria were developed in the 1980s so there could be a nationally standardized set of criteria to evaluate the care provided to treat addiction. Currently, it is used in 30 states [317] to assist in diagnosis and placement.

Once these dimensions are evaluated by a trained professional, an individual can be placed in an appropriate level of care, ranging from detoxification to outpatient treatment. The challenge with cannabis is that the potentially slower progression of the disease paired with minimization of consequences can cause people to underestimate the impact of use. This drug can be called a "dream killer," so sometimes measuring someone's lack of ambition is difficult versus the impairment in relationships, finances, and the repetitive return to use. This is usually expressed in their stage of change, as precontemplation ("it's not a problem for me")/Dimension 4, which can be a difficult perspective to challenge [315, 316].

Professionals refer to this mental state as "amotivational syndrome" which is associated with long-term cannabis use. It presents as detachment, blunted affect, and impaired executive functioning [318]. A person would have little desire to engage in activities, have a sense of apathy, and have poor concentration. If an individual has experienced significant mental health problems (i.e., psychosis, increased anxiety, or depression), they may be more likely to agree to an intervention or treatment.

Marijuana Anonymous is a mutual aid group, an organization and 12-step program for people with a common desire to maintain abstinence from marijuana. It is a fellowship of people who share experience, strength, and hope. Founded in 1989, teachings and meetings can be located on their website marijuana-anonymous.org

[319]. Groups such as this, can help challenge an individual's perspective that suggests cannabis use is "no big deal."

In the Marijuana Anonymous basic text questions like, "How did marijuana use keep me from realizing my potential?" or "How did my marijuana use keep me from doing what I wanted to do with my life?" suggest the nuanced concerns specific to long-term cannabis use [319]. As well as the distinctly different question of "Did I ever experience confusion, paranoia, and fear associated with my using?" A story told by a woman in treatment, suggested that she was waking at 4:30 am in order to clean the house and get high, then continued to use almost every 2 hours to stay high until she went to bed. The picture one might conjure of this type of user might not be a full-time working woman, wife, and mother of a one-year-old. She shared that she was unable to stop on her own, had been hiding her secret for months, and began questioning her partner's loyalty as well as job decisions.

> *We who are marijuana addicts know the answer to this question. Marijuana controls our lives! We lose interest in all else; our dreams go up in smoke. Ours is a progressive illness often leading us to addictions to other drugs, including alcohol. Our lives, our thinking, and our desires center around marijuana—scoring it, dealing it, and finding ways to stay high.*
>
> *Based on our own experiences, we who seek recovery in MA generally consider ourselves to be marijuana addicts. Whether or not our addiction is psychological, physical, or both, matters little. When it comes to the use of marijuana, we have lost the power of choice. It is strictly up to the individual to decide whether he or she feels addicted to marijuana. MA has no opinion about marijuana itself one way or another. Marijuana Anonymous exists solely to provide a means of recovery to the suffering addict who seeks help* [320].

In order to assess impairment or "unmanageablity" it might require referencing the law. For example, in states where the adult use of cannabis is legal, it is worthy to note that if an adult is found using in front of children, having children test positive for THC (at birth or through second hand smoke/contact) or break state safety laws pertaining to cannabis, they can be charged with child endangerment [321]. Most users would argue that because it is legal, they aren't breaking any laws. They are often mislead about the permitted parameters of possession, storage, and consumption. The cannabis industry goes as far to market its product to treat symptoms of pregnancy, such as nausea or pain, but fail to highlight that as soon as children, born or unborn, are involved, it becomes an illegal practice.

Mental Health

The use of cannabis can affect the mental health and thought patterns of an individual. Cannabis-induced psychosis typically refers to acute symptoms like paranoia, delusions, disorganized thinking, and hallucinations; however a growing body of evidence suggests that the higher-potency forms of cannabis such as "extracts" or "concentrates" can lead to these symptoms persisting even after use is discontinued, leading to a permanent shift in an individual's mental health and wellness. When and individual is in these states of impaired thinking, or if that impairment has become permanent, they are often times at a much higher risk of causing harm to self or others [322–325]. The most obvious example is impaired driving, but thought disorders can lead to violent behaviors to both self and others.

There has long raged a fierce debate about the link between cannabis and violence; we encourage our reader to move past this argument that is near impossible to fully prove in one way or another and to remember that impaired thinking/thought disorders are absolutely causal to acts of harming self and/or others. Since cannabis-induced psychosis is understood and can be severe, we must acknowledge the association between harmful and potentially harmful behaviors and cannabis use.

While we lack solid research at this early stage, those in the field of SUD treatment and professionals who work with the cannabis-dependent patient will often cite the increased potency and presence of THC (Tetrahydrocannabinol) in the marketplace as a major contributor to their patient's psychosis. To illustrate the radical shift, one must remember that the majority of our valid research relies on cannabis that contains under 10% THC and often some level of CBD (Cannabidiol) which is thought to mute the effects of THC on mental health. Products being produced as of this publication, such as "distillates" have been tested to be as pure as 99% THC with no trace of CBD. The majority of evidence we point to for "high-potency" marijuana comes from an ongoing study taking place in England and published regularly in *The Lancet* journal, this study, and most other countries, consider "high-potency" marijuana to be anything above 10% THC [326]. As the body of research grows, it does suggest that higher concentrations of THC are associated and or lead to higher instances of psychosis [326].

It is imperative to address potential barriers for effective treatment, like severe and pervasive illness including thought disorders. Treatment providers can use pharmacological interventions to treat as much of the symptomology as possible in order to begin and improve treatment outcomes. Examples could include the use of antipsychotics or mood stabilizers; even though symptoms might be a result of the effects of intoxication, it is helpful to stabilize an individual as quickly as possible so they can participate in their care. With this in mind, understand that treating mental health symptoms are made much more difficult if the patient continues their use. If the THC is causal or a contributing factor to the mental health conditions being treated, it should be removed in order to more successfully treat the symptoms of these conditions.

Money and Resources

Helping patients recognize the amount of money and time they are spending on cannabis also seems to be an effective way of helping them see the severity of their use. It is not uncommon to see individuals spending a concerning portion of their time and resources getting and using cannabis. Highlighting this can help them evaluate the importance of discontinuing use.

Behaviors

The cannabis-dependent individual often normalizes their use because they have cultivated a peer group for whom the same level of use is the norm. It is important to help them step back from this kind of sample group bias by helping them see destructive/concerning behaviors for what they are. The individual who waits outside of a dispensary for it to open at 9 am may easily justify this because they are there with friends doing the same and everyone just wants to take advantage of the "happy hour" sale being offered before noon. When asked to compare this to those waiting for a liquor store to open in the morning, they may be able to better see the concern.

Driving under the influence of cannabis is mistakenly considered by many users to improve their driving skills; this is categorically false. As a society, we recognize the harm caused by impaired driving under other substances and can draw this comparison to help them understand the severity of their actions. If patients are resistant to even this idea, which many are, a comparison to distracted driving may help to move them to a place of better understanding.

Citing examples of less socially unacceptable behaviors can be challenging but may help us build a case to the patient. Consuming cannabis in association with entertainment (concerts, movies, recorded music) is a long-standing past time that many report enhances the experience. Our concern for the dependent person is often an inability to enjoy these activities when not under the influence. For example, a glass of wine with dinner can contribute to the overall experience for some but an insistence that one be drunk to enjoy the same meal would be of concern. Discussing the ability to enjoy and engage without cannabis can often lead to important realizations for individuals. If they are unable to enjoy their favorite band, food, sex, the company of others, recreation, etc. without cannabis and if this can be pointed out, they will often see the flawed thinking and can open them up to treatment.

Cultural Considerations

The use of cannabis spans almost every culture and social group on earth, as does problem use. While there have long been religious groups for whom cannabis is a part of their tradition such as the Sandhu or Aghori in India or the Rastafarian tradition of the Jamaican islands to name a few, cannabis use is more prevalent in certain cultures outside of religious tradition.

For many in the Unites States, cannabis use has a long standing cultural and even familial tradition. When the dependent person is faced with treatment, it is important to remember that they are often being asked to remove themselves from their established culture, and this poses a unique challenge. Since few other mood-altering substances play such a large role in cultures and families, we often forget to address this specific barrier to treatment and recovery with patients. A comprehensive treatment and recovery plan will help patients learn to remain integrated with these important social groups without using cannabis. We suggest that the professional involved spend a good deal of time engaging and learning from the patient rather than dictating to them. It is important for the treatment provider to listen to their concerns in this area, recognize the cultural impact and collaborate for recovery focused solutions rather than give broad instructions that will often come across as dismissive and can impact therapeutic rapport. For providers who have little or no background inside of these social groups and or families in which cannabis use is the norm, it is very important to listen, learn, and engage.

Differences Between Adolescents and Adults

Adolescents may be able to recognize the severity of their use and need for interventions better than adults for several reasons. As there is extremely limited use for FDA-approved cannabis-derived medications in adolescents, almost all of their use is illicit and illegal. This simple reality often helps them understand that their use is not controlled. We also know a great deal about the negative consequences of youth use in regard to mental health, cognitive development, and even physical health and development. The simple reality is that delaying use in younger populations will lead to a much lower likelihood of problem use later in life. The younger the individual, the higher the level of concern and the more aggressive the intervention. This is reason enough to treat cannabis use early and for the appropriate length of time.

Detoxification

Many people decide to stop using because of life events, health concerns, challenges by friends, or family or work reasons. But a significant reason why people return to use of a substance is to avoid the experience of withdrawal. Cannabis withdrawal, which is now defined in the DSM 5 and ICD-10 Codes (F12.23), can represent an uncomfortable, drawn out experience [327, 328]. Symptoms of withdrawal include irritability, anger, or aggression; nervousness or anxiety; sleep difficulty; decrease in appetite or weight loss; restlessness; depressed mood; and at least one of the following symptoms that cause discomfort: abdominal pain, shakiness/tremors, sweating, fever, chills, or headache [327]. Note that many individuals who are dependent are doing so to "treat" the abovementioned conditions; this reality can pose a challenge to the provider. For example, the opiate, addict would be unlikely to report using their drug of choice to "treat" the vomiting associated with detoxification from opiates whereas the cannabis addict just "uses cannabis to help sleep." If an individual is not honest about their use with providers, these symptoms can frequently be misdiagnosed as other mood or medical disorders. This can lead to mistaking a diagnosable substance use disorder and/or encourage medical providers to add additional habit-forming medications to treat reported symptoms. Anecdotally, individuals in treatment report that sleep disturbances are the most frustrating symptom and can lead to a quick return to use of cannabis, if sleep is not addressed. This is one hallmark of cannabis treatment that is different than other substances; many of the symptoms of withdrawal do not have FDA-approved medications to help assist during the withdrawal period.

Acute withdrawal symptoms begin to present within the first 24 hours, peaking at 4 days and persisting for 16 days with long-term withdrawal lasting up to 1 month from the last use of cannabis [329]. Symptoms can include craving, restlessness, nervousness and sleeplessness, irritability, depression, anger, strange dreams, loss of appetite, and headache. Research indicates that withdrawal symptoms can be twice as difficult for women. Treatment studies suggest that if withdrawal symptoms can be reduced or alleviated, people will be less likely to resume cannabis use and could have better treatment outcomes.

Knowing that individuals have a better chance of recovery if they are being treated by professionals that understand specific concerns of cannabis intoxication and withdrawal, it is imperative that treatment be of the highest quality, with knowledgeable professionals and address specific cannabis withdrawal and common comorbid psychiatric disorders.

Treatment

The term treatment can range from inpatient detoxification to outpatient services, as well as mutual aid groups. Because of the uncomfortable, dysregulating, lengthy withdrawal period, it is best to have a person participate in an organized treatment plan. It does not mean that treatment has to be costly or remove an individual from their home environment, but it is imperative that the whole person be addressed within the care planning.

A recent study suggested that clinical trials of various treatments included psychotherapy, motivation enhancement therapy, cognitive behavioral therapy, and contingency management. Results suggested a combination of these produced the best abstinence outcomes, with modest rates of abstinence that decline post treatment [330].

Cognitive behavioral therapy (CBT) identifies thoughts, feelings, and behaviors that influence the use of substances. This treatment focuses on the pursuit of adaptive prosocial behaviors, cognitive restructuring, cost-benefit analysis, and modeling. It often includes the use of homework to improve coping skills and self-efficacy. Almost two decades ago, Stephens, Roffman, and Simpson conducted the first CBT treatment for cannabis use disorder [331]. Today, there are currently evidence-based programs that treat cannabis use disorder, both from an abstinence or harm-reduction [332].

Motivational enhancement therapy (MET) incorporates aspects of motivational interviewing (MI) and uses nonjudgmental feedback to challenge current thoughts and behaviors, decreasing ambivalence, and establishing collaborative goals. A hallmark of this approach is eliciting "change talk" to alter future behaviors. Researchers tested brief models (one or two sessions), gender-specific programs, and hybrid programs (9 sessions). Each demonstrating decreases in use, with better outcomes the longer an individual stayed in treatment [330, 333].

Contingency management (CM) targets a behavior and, based on operant conditioning, increases or decreases it using reinforcement. The use of vouchers, desired rewards for abstinence, negative UA, or attendance in groups is a regular practice [330, 333].

Results from clinical trials show moderate rates in reduction of use, but difficulty with sustained abstinence [330]. These rates are similar to other substances but surmised that a return to use of cannabis is often dismissed or minimized because "weed is no big deal," "it's medicine," or that it's "legal."

Presently and in the future, it will be important to develop effective treatment that incorporates appropriate technology. Suggesting what we know from recovery, the individual needing treatment will severely underestimate the need for treatment and we know that the longer an individual can stay in treatment the better the outcome. It is likely that given the prominent role that cannabis plays in popular culture and likely in the patient's daily life, that justification of a return to use will be easier for them than for those addicted to other substances. We must remember that there is significant societal pressure for many to return to use and to minimize it.

The most effective treatment includes not only the patient, but their social network. This can include family, friends, community members, employers, and/or any stakeholders in the individual's world. If approved with legal releases, these people can provide history, financial or emotional support, and accountability for the patient. Between 40% and 70% of a person's risk for developing a substance use disorder is genetic, but other risks include raised in a home with substance use, neighborhood where drug and alcohol are used, and associating with peers who use. One can see that these risks need to be addressed in order to support an individual's chances of recovery.

Substance Abuse Mental Health Association (SAMSHA) developed eight aspects of life that comprise the "whole person," and it is suggested that no matter what treatment is provided it address addiction; co-occurring and medical; grief, loss and trauma; social and relationships; financial, education, legal; spiritual; health, fitness and leisure; and recovery environment. If each of these aspects are addressed a person will have a chance of a rich and full recovery life.

Medication-assisted therapy (MAT) is one way that medical concerns, addiction, and mental health can be addressed. Currently, the FDA has not approved any medications for the treatment of cannabis use disorder. Although early research has indicated that pharmacological interventions, added to the previously described treatment modalities, may improve treatment outcomes [330]. This combination of treatment highlights biological, psychological and social aspects of care.

Lastly, there are no cost options of treatment such as Marijuana Anonymous (MA) which has a growing recovery environment. They follow similar recovery principles of Alcoholics Anonymous (AA) in their basic text "*Life with Hope: 12 Step Workbook*" (http://www.marijuana-anonymous.org).

Marijuana Anonymous is a fellowship of men and women who share our experience, strength, and hope with each other that we may solve our common problem and help others to recover from marijuana addiction.

They follow a process of identifying how their lives have become unmanageable and making a life worth living.

The Twelve Steps of Marijuana Anonymous

1. We admitted we were powerless over marijuana, that our lives had become unmanageable.
2. Came to believe that a Power greater than ourselves could restore us to sanity.
3. Made a decision to turn our will and our lives over to the care of God, as we understood God.

4. Made a searching and fearless moral inventory of ourselves.
5. Admitted to God, to ourselves, and to another human being the exact nature of our wrongs.
6. Were entirely ready to have God remove all these defects of character.
7. Humbly asked God to remove our shortcomings.
8. Made a list of all persons we had harmed and became willing to make amends to them all.
9. Made direct amends to such people wherever possible except when to do so would injure them or others.
10. Continued to take personal inventory and when we were wrong promptly admitted it.
11. Sought through prayer and meditation to improve our conscious contact with God, as we understood God, praying only for knowledge of God's will for us and the power to carry that out.
12. Having had a spiritual awakening as the result of these steps, we tried to carry this message to marijuana addicts and to practice these principles in all our affairs.

The most imperative aspect of seeking treatment is that it be trauma integrated, for those that have experienced adverse childhood experiences, or trauma as adults. This means that providers need to be aware of reactivity to trauma triggers and the brain's response. Many programs understand that substances are used to numb the effect of trauma and distract from emotional pain; cannabis use is no different than any other substance, in this way. It is often used as an analgesic for emotional pain. Programs must integrate addiction, mental health, and trauma treatment simultaneously.

Cultural Differences Between Cannabis and Other Substances

The role that cannabis plays in pop culture and even fashion is dramatically different than any other drug with the exception of alcohol, the most destructive of all addictive substance we know. It is difficult to believe the devastating aspects of alcohol because it is accepted and used at much higher rates than other substances; culture plays a significant role in shaping this message. It is easy to see the parallels with cannabis and alcohol, but harder for users to see this with cannabis and other drugs. There is an understanding that most other substances of abuse are potentially destructive and damaging; however, with cannabis this reality is challenged in popular culture. Consider the amount of entertainment that both normalizes and glorifies use of this specific substance and compare that to other substances; have you ever seen anyone wearing a methamphetamine hat, or an album cover with heroin pictured? There is even an entire genre of film defined as "stoner film" in which cannabis use and abuse is central to the theme and activities. Some of the most recognizable celebrities and role models in the country are involved in the cannabis industry and or promote its use.

Understand that this deep cultural integration poses additional challenges to treating cannabis addiction. While we are typically asking patients to move away from behaviors that are understood to be destructive with other substances, asking them to do the same with cannabis is in many ways asking them to move away from much of content of their lives from music to film to peers, in effect, their identity.

To an extent, cannabis differs from alcohol in this regard. While alcohol is much more widely used and accepted, it is still understood that alcoholism is a real threat to some people and that alcohol abuse and misuse can have devastating consequences. For many who live inside a culture of cannabis, they have seldom been exposed to messages about their drug of choice that are negative and when they are, their entire community tends to rally around the idea that the information must be false or dismiss the message as old-fashioned. Given the recent changes in cannabis laws, there has been a great deal of money spent to both normalize its use as well as counter arguments that threaten that use. Many of today's users believe cannabis to be a necessary and even life-giving part of their world and will push back on ideas contrary to that construct. With this in mind, know that for the addicted person to come to a point where they are willing to ask for help they have in effect stepped out of their entire world view and recognize the problem as serious enough that they are willing, at least in moments of desperation, to see that the lens through which they see almost everything might be fractured.

Stigma

Now that we understand how difficult it can be for the cannabis user to admit they have a problem and the immense social pressures not to seek help, we must consider what common reactions occur in the professional community as well as in circles of recovery. Many professionals remain uneducated on the severity of cannabis use disorder that is fueled by a MUCH more potent product than the plant of years past. As such, they underestimate the severity of the problem and can make it more difficult for the individual seeking help. It is commonly believed and repeated that "no one has ever died from weed." This factually untrue statement, in itself, draws a comparison to other substances and ranks the cannabis addicted person below other addicts. Statements from professionals that uphold this fallacy or contribute to them feeling "less than" can be extremely harmful. Saying things like "it's just weed," "there are no other serious drugs involved," or "you can't be physically addicted to marijuana" can be all the reason a potential patient might walk away from help.

Conversely, by acknowledging the courage it takes to ask for help and recognizing what a major shift in thinking is required to make this admission, professionals may be able to enhance their motivation.

Changing Perspective

There is an old adage inside of recovery circles; "all someone needs to do is change everything." While it might seem trite this simple bit of advice is the goal of the recovering person and everything we can do to help them work towards realizing it is helpful. For many of our patients working toward abstinence, we should remember that they very likely have not experienced or do not remember experiencing many daily situations that we all face and emotions we all feel without cannabis to mute or enhance those experiences. Remember that for many of our patients simply eating a meal without a ritual of cannabis use may feel impossible, not to mention listening to their favorite band, or watching a film. Since they were often engaged in their addiction throughout all aspects of daily life, it will be a learned skill to do so without cannabis. We can help by preparing them for this reality, listening as they process, and helping them identify and execute solutions. Things as simple as a poster on the wall, a shirt they see in public or a song that comes on might trigger their healing brains to crave cannabis starting a cycle that can often lead to relapse. Recognizing that these social cues will trigger them and developing action plans around those triggers can be very helpful. A patient in early recovery from cannabis addiction might tell us something that seems simple or absurd or unnecessary. People might clean out their music collection in order to avoid triggers, redecorate, and avoid certain foods or forms of entertainment. By recognizing the significant step that actions like these can represent, we will be better prepared to walk through these events and tasks with them. It is important to remember that for the cannabis addict triggers exist everywhere and old activities should be replaced by new ones that support their recovery and change. Helping them to identify the things that need to change and supporting those changes can help them in their journey to just "change everything" a daunting task when considered as a whole but one that is made much easier by putting one foot in front of the other, doing what they can in the moment and taking it one day at a time.

Summary

As the numbers of cannabis-dependent people increases, so does the number of those in recovery from cannabis addiction. This is good news for those working toward solutions with the addicted patient, we have more resources than ever before to aid in their assimilation into a community of recovery from cannabis addiction. As mentioned before, Marijuana Anonymous (MA) can be a powerful community to aid in one's recovery. Today, there are meetings taking place all over the world at all hours of the day; the closer one is to a metropolitan setting the more MA meetings exist as well a virtual meetings. It is crucial that those in early recovery find a community in which they can thrive without cannabis. For some that may be religious traditions, for others groups that base their recovery around sports or recreational activities. As of this writing there is a national group called SAFE entertainment (www.soberafe.com) that works to create safe sober zones at concerts, music festivals, and sporting events. Since the use of cannabis is heavily associated with live music events organizations like this allow individuals in recovery to still engage in activities, they are passionate about, in a safe way. It is important for professionals to remember that recovery isn't just the absence of substance, it can be the addition of a great deal and by adding social opportunities for those in early recovery we can aid in their efforts to remain abstinent.

References

Blunted: The Effects of Cannabis on Cognition and Motivation

1. Ranganathan M, D'Souza DC. The acute effects of cannabinoids on memory in humans: a review. Psychopharmacology. 2006;188(4):425–44.
2. Broyd SJ, van Hell HH, Beale C, Yucel M, Solowij N. Acute and chronic effects of cannabinoids on human cognition-a systematic review. Biol Psychiatry. 2016;79(7):557–67.
3. D'Souza DC, Perry E, MacDougall L, et al. The psychotomimetic effects of intravenous delta-9-tetrahydrocannabinol in healthy individuals: implications for psychosis. Neuropsychopharmacology. 2004;29(8):1558–72.
4. Harvey MA, Sellman JD, Porter RJ, Frampton CM. The relationship between non-acute adolescent cannabis use and cognition. Drug Alcohol Rev. 2007;26(3):309–19.
5. Solowij N, Jones KA, Rozman ME, et al. Verbal learning and memory in adolescent cannabis users, alcohol users and non-users. Psychopharmacology. 2011;216(1):131–44.
6. Lisdahl KM, Price JS. Increased marijuana use and gender predict poorer cognitive functioning in adolescents and emerging adults. J Int Neuropsychol Soc. 2012;18(4):678–88.
7. Morgan CJ, Gardener C, Schafer G, et al. Sub-chronic impact of cannabinoids in street cannabis on cognition, psychotic-like symptoms and psychological well-being. Psychol Med. 2012;42(2):391–400.
8. Hanson KL, Winward JL, Schweinsburg AD, Medina KL, Brown SA, Tapert SF. Longitudinal study of cognition among adolescent marijuana users over three weeks of abstinence. Addict Behav. 2010;35(11):970–6.
9. Lyons MJ, Bar JL, Panizzon MS, et al. Neuropsychological consequences of regular marijuana use: a twin study. Psychol Med. 2004;34(7):1239–50.
10. Tait RJ, Mackinnon A, Christensen H. Cannabis use and cognitive function: 8-year trajectory in a young adult cohort. Addiction. 2011;106(12):2195–203.
11. Winward JL, Hanson KL, Tapert SF, Brown SA. Heavy alcohol use, marijuana use, and concomitant use by adolescents are associated with unique and shared cognitive decrements. J Int Neuropsychol Soc. 2014;20(8):784–95.
12. Medina KL, Hanson KL, Schweinsburg AD, Cohen-Zion M, Nagel BJ, Tapert SF. Neuropsychological functioning in adolescent marijuana users: subtle deficits detectable after a month of abstinence. J Int Neuropsychol Soc. 2007;13(5):807–20.
13. Theunissen EL, Heckman P, de Sousa Fernandes Perna EB, et al. Rivastigmine but not vardenafil reverses cannabis-induced impairment of verbal memory in healthy humans. Psychopharmacology. 2015;232(2):343–53.
14. Castellano C, Rossi-Arnaud C, Cestari V, Costanzi M. Cannabinoids and memory: animal studies. Curr Drug Targets CNS Neurol Disord. 2003;2(6):389–402.
15. Collins DR, Pertwee RG, Davies SN. The action of synthetic cannabinoids on the induction of long-term potentiation in the rat hippocampal slice. Eur J Pharmacol. 1994;259(3):R7–8.
16. Morin JG, Afzali MH, Bourque J, et al. A population-based analysis of the relationship between substance use and adolescent cognitive development. Am J Psychiatry. 2019;176(2):98–106.
17. Auer R, Vittinghoff E, Yaffe K, et al. Association between lifetime marijuana use and cognitive function in middle age: the coronary artery risk development in young adults (CARDIA) study. JAMA Intern Med. 2016;176(3):352–61.
18. Jouroukhin Y, Zhu X, Shevelkin AV, et al. Adolescent delta(9)-tetrahydrocannabinol exposure and astrocyte-specific genetic vulnerability converge on nuclear factor-kappab-cyclooxygenase-2 signaling to impair memory in adulthood. Biol Psychiatry. 2019;85(11):891–903.
19. Verrico CD, Gu H, Peterson ML, Sampson AR, Lewis DA. Repeated delta9-tetrahydrocannabinol exposure in adolescent monkeys: persistent effects selective for spatial working memory. Am J Psychiatry. 2014;171(4):416–25.

20. Rubino T, Parolaro D. The impact of exposure to cannabinoids in adolescence: insights from animal models. Biol Psychiatry. 2016;79(7):578–85.
21. Sandler RA, Fetterhoff D, Hampson RE, Deadwyler SA, Marmarelis VZ. Cannabinoids disrupt memory encoding by functionally isolating hippocampal ca1 from ca3. PLoS Comput Biol. 2017;13(7):e1005624.
22. Campolongo P, Trezza V, Cassano T, et al. Perinatal exposure to delta-9-tetrahydrocannabinol causes enduring cognitive deficits associated with alteration of cortical gene expression and neurotransmission in rats. Addict Biol. 2007;12(3–4):485–95.
23. Ramirez BG, Blazquez C, Gomez del Pulgar T, Guzman M, de Ceballos ML. Prevention of alzheimer's disease pathology by cannabinoids: neuroprotection mediated by blockade of microglial activation. J Neurosci. 2005;25(8):1904–13.
24. Calabrese EJ, Rubio-Casillas A. Biphasic effects of thc in memory and cognition. Eur J Clin Investig. 2018;48(5):e12920.
25. Broers B, Pata Z, Mina A, Wampfler J, de Saussure C, Pautex S. Prescription of a THC/CBD-based medication to patients with dementia: a pilot study in Geneva. Med Cann Cannabinoids. 2019;2:56–9.
26. Batalla A, Bhattacharyya S, Yucel M, et al. Structural and functional imaging studies in chronic cannabis users: a systematic review of adolescent and adult findings. PLoS One. 2013;8(2):e55821.
27. Grant IR, Gonzales CL, Carey LN, Wolfon T. Non-acute (residual) neurocognitive effects of cannabis use: a meta-analytic study. J Int Neuropsychol Soc. 2003;9:679–89.
28. Schreiner AM, Dunn ME. Residual effects of cannabis use on neurocognitive performance after prolonged abstinence: a meta-analysis. Exp Clin Psychopharmacol. 2012;20(5):420–9.
29. National Academies of Sciences E, and Medicine. The health effects of cannabis and cannabinoids: the current state of evidence and recommendations for research. Washington, D.C.: The National Academies Press; 2017.
30. Hooper SR, Woolley D, De Bellis MD. Intellectual, neurocognitive, and academic achievement in abstinent adolescents with cannabis use disorder. Psychopharmacology. 2014;231(8):1467–77.
31. Oomen PP, van Hell HH, Bossong MG. The acute effects of cannabis on human executive function. Behav Pharmacol. 2018;29(7):605–16.
32. Gruber SA, Sagar KA, Dahlgren MK, Racine M, Lukas SE. Age of onset of marijuana use and executive function. Psychol Addict Behav. 2012;26(3):496–506.
33. Ramaekers JG, Kauert G, Theunissen EL, Toennes SW, Moeller MR. Neurocognitive performance during acute THC intoxication in heavy and occasional cannabis users. J Psychopharmacol. 2009;23(3):266–77.
34. Thames AD, Arbid N, Sayegh P. Cannabis use and neurocognitive functioning in a non-clinical sample of users. Addict Behav. 2014;39(5):994–9.
35. Meier MH, Caspi A, Ambler A, et al. Persistent cannabis users show neuropsychological decline from childhood to midlife. Proc Natl Acad Sci U S A. 2012;109(40):E2657–64.
36. Fried P, Watkinson B, James D, Gray R. Current and former marijuana use: preliminary findings of a longitudinal study of effects on iq in young adults. CMAJ. 2002;166(7):887–91.
37. Jackson NJ, Isen JD, Khoddam R, et al. Impact of adolescent marijuana use on intelligence: results from two longitudinal twin studies. Proc Natl Acad Sci U S A. 2016;113(5):E500–8.
38. Barnwell SS, Earleywine M, Wilcox R. Cannabis, motivation, and life satisfaction in an internet sample. Subst Abuse Treat Prev Policy. 2006;1:2.
39. Lac A, Luk JW. Testing the amotivational syndrome: marijuana use longitudinally predicts lower self-efficacy even after controlling for demographics, personality, and alcohol and cigarette use. Prev Sci. 2018;19(2):117–26.
40. Macher RB, Earleywine M. Enhancing neuropsychological performance in chronic cannabis users: the role of motivation. J Clin Exp Neuropsychol. 2012;34(4):405–15.
41. Smith DE. Acute and chronic toxicity of marijuana. J Psychoactive Drugs. 1968;2(1):37–48.
42. Volkow ND, Swanson JM, Evins AE, et al. Effects of cannabis use on human behavior, including cognition, motivation, and psychosis: a review. JAMA Psychiat. 2016;73(3):292–7.

43. Lawn W, Freeman TP, Pope RA, et al. Acute and chronic effects of cannabinoids on effort-related decision-making and reward learning: an evaluation of the cannabis 'amotivational' hypotheses. Psychopharmacology. 2016;233(19–20):3537–52.
44. Paule MG, Allen RR, Bailey JR, et al. Chronic marijuana smoke exposure in the rhesus monkey. Ii: effects on progressive ratio and conditioned position responding. J Pharmacol Exp Ther. 1992;260(1):210–22.
45. Rubino T, Realini N, Braida D, et al. The depressive phenotype induced in adult female rats by adolescent exposure to THC is associated with cognitive impairment and altered neuroplasticity in the prefrontal cortex. Neurotox Res. 2009;15(4):291–302.
46. Rubino T, Realini N, Braida D, et al. Changes in hippocampal morphology and neuroplasticity induced by adolescent THC treatment are associated with cognitive impairment in adulthood. Hippocampus. 2009;19(8):763–72.
47. Gleason KA, Birnbaum SG, Shukla A, Ghose S. Susceptibility of the adolescent brain to cannabinoids: long-term hippocampal effects and relevance to schizophrenia. Transl Psychiatry. 2012;2:e199.
48. Landfield PW. Hippocampal neurobiological mechanisms of age-related memory dysfunction. Neurobiol Aging. 1988;9(5–6):571–9.
49. Brandon NJ, Sawa A. Linking neurodevelopmental and synaptic theories of mental illness through disc1. Nat Rev. 2011;12(12):707–22.
50. Hebert-Chatelain E, Desprez T, Serrat R, et al. A cannabinoid link between mitochondria and memory. Nature. 2016;539(7630):555–9.
51. Bossong MG, Mehta MA, van Berckel BN, Howes OD, Kahn RS, Stokes PR. Further human evidence for striatal dopamine release induced by administration of 9-tetrahydrocannabinol (THC): selectivity to limbic striatum. Psychopharmacology. 2015;232(15):2723–9.
52. Bloomfield MA, Morgan CJ, Egerton A, Kapur S, Curran HV, Howes OD. Dopaminergic function in cannabis users and its relationship to cannabis-induced psychotic symptoms. Biol Psychiatry. 2014;75(6):470–8.
53. Martz ME, Trucco EM, Cope LM, et al. Association of marijuana use with blunted nucleus accumbens response to reward anticipation. JAMA Psychiat. 2016;73(8):838–44.
54. Di Forti M, Quattrone D, Freeman TP, et al. The contribution of cannabis use to variation in the incidence of psychotic disorder across europe (eu-gei): a multicentre case-control study. Lancet Psychiatry. 2019;6(5):427–36.
55. Garavan H, Bartsch H, Conway K, Decastro A, Goldstein RZ, Heeringa S, et al. Recruiting the ABCD sample: design considerations and procedures. Dev Cogn Neurosci. 2018;32:16–22.

Cannabis and Psychiatric Conditions

56. Shrivastava A, Johnston M, Terpstra K, Bureau Y. Cannabis and psychosis: neurobiology. Indian J Psychiatry. 2014 [cited 2014 Feb 13]; 56:8–16. Available from: http://www.indianj-psychiatry.org/text.asp?2014/56/1/8/124708.
57. Volkow ND, Baler RD, Compton WM, Weiss SRB. Adverse health effects of marijuana use. N Engl J Med. 2014;370:2219–27.
58. Seth A, Sheryl R, William PA. The impact of cannabis policies on youth clinical research and legal update. American Academy of Pediatrics. Denver, Colorado: 2015.
59. Joseph M, Pierre MD. Risks of increasingly potent Cannabis: the joint effects of potency and frequency. Curr Psychiatr Ther. 2017;16:14–20.
60. Strougo A, Zuurman L, Roy C, Pinquier JL, van Gerven JMA, Cohen AF, Schoemaker C. Modelling of the concentration—effect relationship of THC on central nervous system parameters and heart rate — insight into its mechanisms of action and a tool for clinical research and development of cannabinoids. J Psychopharmacol. 2008;22:717–26.
61. Arseneault L, Cannon M, Poulton R, Murray R, Caspi A, Moffit TE. Cannabis use in adolescence and risk for adult psychosis: longitudinal prospective study. BMJ. 2002;325:1212. Available from https://doi.org/10.1136/bmj.325.7374.1212.

62. Cohen M, et al. Cannabis, cannabinoids and schizophrenia: integration of the evidence. Aust N Z J Psychiatry. 2008;42:357–68.
63. Doris C, Gundersen MD. The legalization of marijuana: implications for regulation and practice. J Nurs Regul. 2015;6:3. Available from www.journalofnursingregulation.com
64. de Shazo RD, et al. Marijuana's effects on brain structure and function: what do we know and what should we do? A brief review and commentary. Am J Med. 2019;132(3):281–5.
65. McGrath J, et al. Association between cannabis use and psychosis-related outcomes using sibling pair analysis in a cohort of young adults. Arch Gen Psychiatry. 2010;67(5):440–7.
66. Di Forti M, et al. Proportion of patients in south London with first-episode psychosis attributable to use of high potency cannabis: a case-control study. Lancet Psychiatry. 2015;2:233–8.
67. Copeland J, et al. Changes in cannabis use among young people: impact on mental health. Curr Opin Psych. 2013;26(4):325–9.
68. Crippa J, Zuardi AW, Martin-Santos R, et al. Cannabis and anxiety: a critical review of the evidence. Hum Psychopharmacol Clin Exp. 2009; https://doi.org/10.1002/hup.104.
69. Cheung J, et al. Anxiety and mood disorders and Cannabis use. Am J Drug Alcohol Abuse. 2010;36(2):118–22.
70. Degenhardt L, et al. The Persistence of the association between adolescent cannabis use and common mental disorders into young adulthood. Addiction. 2013;108(1):124–33.
71. Bahorik AL et al, Patterns of marijuana use among psychiatry patients with depression and its impact on recovery. J Affect Disord 2017;312: 168–171.
72. Ho H, Hewitt J, Hopfer C. Temporal relationship between cannabis use and depression among adolescents in the United States. [Poster presentation]. American Psychiatric Association Annual Conference. Institute of Medicine; 2015.
73. Hayatbakhsh MR, et al. Cannabis and anxiety and depression in young adults: a large prospective study. J Am Acad Child Adolesc Psychiatry. 2007;46(3):408–17.
74. Wang GS, et al. Impact of marijuana legalization in Colorado on adolescent emergency and urgent care visits. J Adolesc Health. 2018;63(2):239–41.
75. Wilkinson ST, et al. Marijuana use is associated with worse outcomes in symptom severity and violent behavior in patients with posttraumatic stress disorder. J Clin Psychiatry. 2015;76(9):1174–80.
76. Bitencourt R, Takahash R. Cannabidiol as a therapeutic alternative for post traumatic stress disorder: from bench research to confirmation in human trials. Front Neurosci. 2018;12:502.
77. https://militarybenefits.info/va-medical-marijuana.
78. Rocky Mountain High Intensity Drug Trafficking Area (RMHIDTA) Investigative Support Center. The legalization of Marijuana in Colorado: the impact, vol 2. Denver, Colorado: 2014.
79. Anthony JC, Warner LA, Kessler RC. Comparative epidemiology of dependence on tobacco, alcohol, controlled substances, and inhalants: basic findings from the national comorbidity survey. Exp Clin Psychopharmacol. 1994;2(3):244–68.
80. Matochik JA, Eldreth DA, Cadet JL, Bolla KI. Altered brain tissue composition in heavy Cannabis users. Drug Alcohol Depend. 2005;77(1):23–30.
81. Gundersen DC. Medical Cannabis—a prescription for trouble? CPHP News. 2010. Retrieved from www.cphp.org/documents/CPHPnews-summer-2010.pdf.
82. https://www.drugabuse.gov/publications/research-reports/marijuana/marijuana-addictive.
83. Prescription drug abuse prevention: a colorado community reference 2018. www.corxconsortium.org/heroin-response-work-group/.
84. Buckner D, et al. Cannabis use and suicidal ideation: test of the utility of the interpersonal-psychological theory of suicide. Psychiatry Res. 2017;253:256–9.
85. Kimbrel NA, et al. Cannabis use disorder and suicide attempts in Iraq/Afghanistan-era veterans. J Psychiatr Res. 2017;89:1–5.
86. Silins E, et al. Young adult sequelae of adolescent cannabis use: an integrative analysis. Lancet Psychiatry. 2014;1(4):286–93.
87. Dugre JR, et al. Persistency of cannabis use predicts violence following acute psychiatric discharge. Front Psychiatry. 2017;8:176.

88. Moulin V, et al. Cannabis, a significant risk factor for violent Behavior in the early phase of psychosis. Two patterns of interaction of factors increase the risk of violent behavior: cannabis use disorder, lack of insight and treatment adherence, frontiers of psychiatry 2018. Available from https://doi.org/10.3389/fpsyt.2018.00294.

89. Volkow ND, Baler R. Emergency department visits from edible versus inhalable Cannabis. Ann Intern Med. 2019;170:569–70.

90. Niesink RJ, van Laar MW. Does cannabidiol protect against adverse psychological effects of THC? Front Psych. 2013;4:130.

91. Demirakca T, Sartorius A, Ende G, et al. Diminished gray matter in the hippocampus of cannabis users: possible protective effects of cannabidiol. Drug Alcohol Depend. 2011;114:242–5.

92. Morgan CJ, Curran HV. Effects of cannabidiol on schizophrenia-like symptoms in people who use cannabis. Br J Psychiatry. 2008;192:306–7.

93. Morgan CJ, Schafer G, Freeman TP, Curran HV. Impact of cannabidiol on the acute memory and psychotomimetic effects of smoked cannabis: naturalistic study [corrected]. Br J Psychiatry. 2010;197:285–90.

94. Bhattacharyya S, Morrison PD, Fusar-Poli P, et al. Opposite effects of delta-9-tetrahydrocannabinol and cannabidiol on human brain function and psychopathology. Neuropsychopharmacology. 2010;35:764–74.

95. Schubart CD, Sommer IE, van Gastel WA, Goetgebuer RL, Kahn RS, Boks MP. Cannabis with high cannabidiol content is associated with fewer psychotic experiences. Schizophr Res. 2011;130:216–21.

96. Hallak JE, Dursun SM, Bosi DC, et al. The interplay of cannabinoid and NMDA glutamate receptor systems in humans: preliminary evidence of interactive effects of cannabidiol and ketamine in healthy human subjects. Prog Neuro-Psychopharmacol Biol Psychiatry. 2011;35:198–202.

97. Zuardi AW, Morais SL, Guimarães FS, Mechoulam R. Anti-psychotic effect of cannabidiol. J Clin Psychiatry. 1995;56:485–6.

98. Leweke FM, Koethe D, Gerth CW, et al. Cannabidiol as an antipsychotic. A double-blind, controlled clinical trial on cannabidiol vs. amisulpride in acute schizophrenia. Eur Psychiatry. 2007;22:S14.02.

99. Gomes FV, Del Bel EA, Guimarães FS. Cannabidiol attenuates catalepsy induced by distinct pharmacological mechanisms via 5-HT1A receptor activation in mice. Prog Neuro-Psychopharmacol Biol Psychiatry. 2013;46:43–7.

100. Zuardi AW, Cosme RA, Graeff FG, Guimarães FS. Effects of ipsapirone and cannabidiol on human experimental anxiety. J Psychopharmacol. 1993;7(1 Suppl):82–8.

101. Crippa JA, Derenusson GN, Ferrari TB, et al. Neural basis of anxiolytic effects of cannabidiol (CBD) in generalized social anxiety disorder: a preliminary report. J Psychopharmacol. 2011;25:121–30.

102. Fusar-Poli P, Crippa JA, Bhattacharyya S, et al. Distinct effects of {delta}9-tetrahydrocannabinol and cannabidiol on neural activation during emotional processing. Arch Gen Psychiatry. 2009;66:95–105.

103. Gazarini L, Stern CA, Piornedo RR, Takahashi RN, Bertoglio LJ. PTSD-like memory generated through enhanced noradrenergic activity is mitigated by a dual step pharmacological intervention targeting its reconsolidation. Int J Neuropsychopharmacol. 2014;18

104. Das RK, Kamboj SK, Ramadas M, et al. Cannabidiol enhances consolidation of explicit fear extinction in humans. Psychopharmacol (Berl). 2013;226:781–92.

105. Schatman ME. Medical marijuana: the state of the science, medscape psychiatry. 2015.

106. Morgan CJ, Das RK, Joye A, Curran HV, Kamboj SK. Cannabidiol reduces cigarette consumption in tobacco smokers: preliminary findings. Addict Behav. 2013;38:2433–6.

107. file:///C:/Users/dorisg/Documents/EPIDIOLEX_Full_Prescribing_Information.pdf.

108. American Psychiatric Association Resource Document on opposition to cannabis as medicine, approved by the Joint Reference Committee, October 2018.

Cannabis Use and Psychosis, Mood, and Anxiety Disorders

109. Murray RM, Englund A, Abi-Dargham A, Lewis DA, Di Forti M, Davies C, et al. Cannabis-associated psychosis: neural substrate and clinical impact. Neuropharmacology. 2017;124:89–104.
110. ElSohly MA, Mehmedic Z, Foster S, Gon C, Chandra S, Church JC. Changes in Cannabis potency over the last 2 decades (1995–2014): analysis of current data in the United States. Biol Psychiatry. 2016;79(7):613–9.
111. Smart R, Caulkins JP, Kilmer B, Davenport S, Midgette G. Variation in cannabis potency and prices in a newly legal market: evidence from 30 million cannabis sales in Washington state. Addiction. 2017;112(12):2167–77.
112. Leafly Staff. A Guide to Cannabis Concentrates: Part 4, Cannabis Concentrates for Experts [Internet]. [updated 2019 June 14; cited 2019 Sept 6]. Available from: https://www.leafly.com/news/strains-products/marijuana-extracts-dabs-for-experts.
113. Bennett P. THCA and CBD Crystalline: Cannabinoids at Their Purest 2018 [Internet]. [updated 2018 Mar 22; cited 2019 Sept 6]. Available from: https://www.leafly.com/news/strains-products/what-are-thca-cbda-crystalline-cannabinoids.
114. Sideli L, Quigley H, La Cascia C, Murray RM. Cannabis use and the risk of psychosis and affective disorders. J Dual Diagn. 2019;16:22–42.
115. Murrie B, Lappin J, Large M, Sara G. Transition of substance-induced, brief, and atypical psychoses to schizophrenia: a systematic review and meta-analysis. Schizophr Bull. 2019;16:sbz102.
116. Hasin DS, Saha TD, Kerridge BT, Goldstein RB, Chou SP, Zhang H, et al. Prevalence of marijuana use disorders in the United States between 2001–2002 and 2012–2013. JAMA Psychiat. 2015;72(12):1235–42.
117. Johnston LD, Miech RA, O'Malley PM, Bachman JG, Schulenberg JE, Patrick ME. Monitoring the future National Survey Results on drug use, 1975–2018. Ann Arbor: Institute for Social Research, University of Michigan; 2019.
118. Kann L, McManus T, Harris WA, Shanklin SL, Flint KH, Queen B, et al. Youth risk behavior surveillance - United States, 2017. MMWR Surveill Summ. 2018;67(8):1–114.
119. Wilson J, Freeman TP, Mackie CJ. Effects of increasing cannabis potency on adolescent health. Lancet Child Adolesc Health. 2019;3(2):121–8.
120. van Ours JC, Williams J, Fergusson D, Horwood LJ. Cannabis use and suicidal ideation. J Health Econ. 2013;32(3):524–37.
121. Gage SH, Hickman M, Heron J, Munafo MR, Lewis G, Macleod J, et al. Associations of cannabis and cigarette use with depression and anxiety at age 18: findings from the Avon longitudinal study of parents and children. PLoS One. 2015;10(4):e0122896.
122. Agrawal A, Nelson EC, Bucholz KK, Tillman R, Grucza RA, Statham DJ, et al. Major depressive disorder, suicidal thoughts and behaviours, and cannabis involvement in discordant twins: a retrospective cohort study. Lancet Psychiatry. 2017;4(9):706–14.
123. Walsh Z, Callaway R, Belle-Isle L, Capler R, Kay R, Lucas P, et al. Cannabis for therapeutic purposes: patient characteristics, access, and reasons for use. Int J Drug Policy. 2013;24(6):511–6.
124. Turna J, Simpson W, Patterson B, Lucas P, Van Ameringen M. Cannabis use behaviors and prevalence of anxiety and depressive symptoms in a cohort of Canadian medicinal cannabis users. J Psychiatr Res. 2019;111:134–9.
125. Smit F, Bolier L, Cuijpers P. Cannabis use and the risk of later schizophrenia: a review. Addiction. 2004;99(4):425–30.
126. Henquet C, Murray R, Linszen D, van Os J. The environment and schizophrenia: the role of cannabis use. Schizophr Bull. 2005;31(3):608–12.
127. Andreasson S, Allebeck P, Engstrom A, Rydberg U. Cannabis and schizophrenia. A longitudinal study of Swedish conscripts. Lancet. 1987;330(8574):1483–6.

128. Zammit S, Allebeck P, Andreasson S, Lundberg I, Lewis G. Self reported cannabis use as a risk factor for schizophrenia in Swedish conscripts of 1969: historical cohort study. BMJ. 2002;325(7374):1199.

129. Henquet C, Krabbendam L, Spauwen J, Kaplan C, Lieb R, Wittchen HU, et al. Prospective cohort study of cannabis use, predisposition for psychosis, and psychotic symptoms in young people. BMJ. 2005;330(7481):11.

130. Valmaggia LR, Day FL, Jones C, Bissoli S, Pugh C, Hall D, et al. Cannabis use and transition to psychosis in people at ultra-high risk. Psychol Med. 2014;44(12):2503–12.

131. Jacobus J, Tapert SF. Effects of cannabis on the adolescent brain. Curr Pharm Des. 2014;20(13):2186–93.

132. van Nierop M, Janssens M, Genetic Risk OoPI, Bruggeman R, Cahn W, de Haan L, et al. Evidence that transition from health to psychotic disorder can be traced to semi-ubiquitous environmental effects operating against background genetic risk. PLoS One. 2013;8(11):e76690.

133. Moore TH, Zammit S, Lingford-Hughes A, Barnes TR, Jones PB, Burke M, et al. Cannabis use and risk of psychotic or affective mental health outcomes: a systematic review. Lancet. 2007;370(9584):319–28.

134. Arseneault L, Cannon M, Poulton R, Murray R, Caspi A, Moffitt TE. Cannabis use in adolescence and risk for adult psychosis: longitudinal prospective study. BMJ. 2002;325(7374):1212–3.

135. Fergusson DM, Horwood LJ, Swain-Campbell NR. Cannabis dependence and psychotic symptoms in young people. Psychol Med. 2003;33(1):15–21.

136. Tien AY, Anthony JC. Epidemiological analysis of alcohol and drug use as risk factors for psychotic experiences. J Nerv Ment Dis. 1990;178(8):473–80.

137. Wiles NJ, Zammit S, Bebbington P, Singleton N, Meltzer H, Lewis G. Self-reported psychotic symptoms in the general population: results from the longitudinal study of the British National Psychiatric Morbidity Survey. Br J Psychiatry. 2006;188:519–26.

138. van Os J, Bak M, Hanssen M, Bijl RV, de Graaf R, Verdoux H. Cannabis use and psychosis: a longitudinal population-based study. Am J Epidemiol. 2002;156(4):319–27.

139. Schubart CD, van Gastel WA, Breetvelt EJ, Beetz SL, Ophoff RA, Sommer IE, et al. Cannabis use at a young age is associated with psychotic experiences. Psychol Med. 2011;41(6):1301–10.

140. Mosher CJ, Akins S. Medical and recreational marijuana legalization process. In: In the weeds: demonization, legalization, and the evolution of US marijuana policy. Philadelphia: Temple University Press; 2019.

141. Di Forti M, Quattrone D, Freeman TP, Tripoli G, Gayer-Anderson C, Quigley H, et al. The contribution of cannabis use to variation in the incidence of psychotic disorder across Europe (EU-GEI): a multicentre case-control study. Lancet Psychiatry. 2019;6(5):427–36.

142. Barbeito S, Vega P, Ruiz de Azua S, Saenz M, Martinez-Cengotitabengoa M, Gonzalez-Ortega I, et al. Cannabis use and involuntary admission may mediate long-term adherence in first-episode psychosis patients: a prospective longitudinal study. BMC Psychiatry. 2013;13:326.

143. Wade D, Harrigan S, Edwards J, Burgess PM, Whelan G, McGorry PD. Substance misuse in first-episode psychosis: 15-month prospective follow-up study. Br J Psychiatry. 2006;189:229–34.

144. Dervaux A, Laqueille X, Bourdel MC, Leborgne MH, Olie JP, Loo H, et al. Cannabis and schizophrenia: demographic and clinical correlates. Encéphale. 2003;29(1):11–7.

145. Grech A, Van Os J, Jones PB, Lewis SW, Murray RM. Cannabis use and outcome of recent onset psychosis. Eur Psychiatry. 2005;20(4):349–53.

146. Caspari D. Cannabis and schizophrenia: results of a follow-up study. Eur Arch Psychiatry Clin Neurosci. 1999;249(1):45–9.

147. Hjorthoj C, Ostergaard ML, Benros ME, Toftdahl NG, Erlangsen A, Andersen JT, et al. Association between alcohol and substance use disorders and all-cause and cause-specific mortality in schizophrenia, bipolar disorder, and unipolar depression: a nationwide, prospective, register-based study. Lancet Psychiatry. 2015;2(9):801–8.

148. Schoeler T, Petros N, Di Forti M, Klamerus E, Foglia E, Ajnakina O, et al. Effects of continuation, frequency, and type of cannabis use on relapse in the first 2 years after onset of psychosis: an observational study. Lancet Psychiatry. 2016;3(10):947–53.
149. Schoeler T, Petros N, Di Forti M, Klamerus E, Foglia E, Murray R, et al. Poor medication adherence and risk of relapse associated with continued cannabis use in patients with first-episode psychosis: a prospective analysis. Lancet Psychiatry. 2017;4(8):627–33.
150. Morgan CJ, Curran HV. Effects of cannabidiol on schizophrenia-like symptoms in people who use cannabis. Br J Psychiatry. 2008;192(4):306–7.
151. Schubart CD, Sommer IE, van Gastel WA, Goetgebuer RL, Kahn RS, Boks MP. Cannabis with high cannabidiol content is associated with fewer psychotic experiences. Schizophr Res. 2011;130(1–3):216–21.
152. Leweke FM, Piomelli D, Pahlisch F, Muhl D, Gerth CW, Hoyer C, et al. Cannabidiol enhances anandamide signaling and alleviates psychotic symptoms of schizophrenia. Transl Psychiatry. 2012;2:e94.
153. McGuire P, Robson P, Cubala WJ, Vasile D, Morrison PD, Barron R, et al. Cannabidiol (CBD) as an adjunctive therapy in schizophrenia: a multicenter randomized controlled trial. Am J Psychiatry. 2018;175(3):225–31.
154. Myles N, Newall H, Nielssen O, Large M. The association between cannabis use and earlier age at onset of schizophrenia and other psychoses: meta-analysis of possible confounding factors. Curr Pharm Des. 2012;18(32):5055–69.
155. Di Forti M, Sallis H, Allegri F, Trotta A, Ferraro L, Stilo SA, et al. Daily use, especially of high-potency cannabis, drives the earlier onset of psychosis in cannabis users. Schizophr Bull. 2014;40(6):1509–17.
156. Cougle JR, Hakes JK, Macatee RJ, Chavarria J, Zvolensky MJ. Quality of life and risk of psychiatric disorders among regular users of alcohol, nicotine, and cannabis: an analysis of the National Epidemiological Survey on Alcohol and Related Conditions (NESARC). J Psychiatr Res. 2015;66–67:135–41.
157. Carra G, Bartoli F, Crocamo C. Trends of major depressive episode among people with cannabis use: findings from the National Survey on drug use and health 2006-2015. Subst Abus. 2019;40(2):178–84.
158. Hayatbakhsh MR, Najman JM, Jamrozik K, Mamun AA, Alati R, Bor W. Cannabis and anxiety and depression in young adults: a large prospective study. J Am Acad Child Adolesc Psychiatry. 2007;46(3):408–17.
159. Patton GC, Coffey C, Carlin JB, Degenhardt L, Lynskey M, Hall W. Cannabis use and mental health in young people: cohort study. BMJ. 2002;325(7374):1195–8.
160. Degenhardt L, Hall W, Lynskey M. Exploring the association between cannabis use and depression. Addiction. 2003;98(11):1493–504.
161. Kedzior KK, Laeber LT. A positive association between anxiety disorders and cannabis use or cannabis use disorders in the general population–a meta-analysis of 31 studies. BMC Psychiatry. 2014;14:136.
162. Gobbi G, Atkin T, Zytynski T, Wang S, Askari S, Boruff J, et al. Association of cannabis use in adolescence and risk of depression, anxiety, and suicidality in young adulthood: a systematic review and meta-analysis. JAMA Psychiat. 2019;76(4):426–34.
163. Feingold D, Weiser M, Rehm J, Lev-Ran S. The association between cannabis use and anxiety disorders: results from a population-based representative sample. Eur Neuropsychopharmacol. 2016;26(3):493–505.
164. Guttmannova K, Kosterman R, White HR, Bailey JA, Lee JO, Epstein M, et al. The association between regular marijuana use and adult mental health outcomes. Drug Alcohol Depend. 2017;179:109–16.
165. Schoeler T, Theobald D, Pingault JB, Farrington DP, Coid JW, Bhattacharyya S. Developmental sensitivity to cannabis use patterns and risk for major depressive disorder in mid-life: findings from 40 years of follow-up. Psychol Med. 2018;48(13):2169–76.

166. Lev-Ran S, Roerecke M, Le Foll B, George TP, McKenzie K, Rehm J. The association between cannabis use and depression: a systematic review and meta-analysis of longitudinal studies. Psychol Med. 2014;44(4):797–810.

167. Rasic D, Weerasinghe S, Asbridge M, Langille DB. Longitudinal associations of cannabis and illicit drug use with depression, suicidal ideation and suicidal attempts among Nova Scotia high school students. Drug Alcohol Depend. 2013;129(1–2):49–53.

168. Degenhardt L, Coffey C, Romaniuk H, Swift W, Carlin JB, Hall WD, et al. The persistence of the association between adolescent cannabis use and common mental disorders into young adulthood. Addiction. 2013;108(1):124–33.

169. van Laar M, van Dorsselaer S, Monshouwer K, de Graaf R. Does cannabis use predict the first incidence of mood and anxiety disorders in the adult population? Addiction. 2007;102(8):1251–60.

170. Brook JS, Zhang C, Brook DW. Developmental trajectories of marijuana use from adolescence to adulthood: personal predictors. Arch Pediatr Adolesc Med. 2011;165(1):55–60.

171. Bahorik AL, Leibowitz A, Sterling SA, Travis A, Weisner C, Satre DD. Patterns of marijuana use among psychiatry patients with depression and its impact on recovery. J Affect Disord. 2017;213:168–71.

172. Moitra E, Anderson BJ, Stein MD. Reductions in Cannabis use are associated with mood improvement in female emerging adults. Depress Anxiety. 2016;33(4):332–8.

173. van Rossum I, Boomsma M, Tenback D, Reed C, van Os J, Board EA. Does cannabis use affect treatment outcome in bipolar disorder? A longitudinal analysis. J Nerv Ment Dis. 2009;197(1):35–40.

174. Kim SW, Dodd S, Berk L, Kulkarni J, de Castella A, Fitzgerald PB, et al. Impact of cannabis use on long-term remission in bipolar I and schizoaffective disorder. Psychiatry Investig. 2015;12(3):349–55.

175. Zorrilla I, Aguado J, Haro JM, Barbeito S, Lopez Zurbano S, Ortiz A, et al. Cannabis and bipolar disorder: does quitting cannabis use during manic/mixed episode improve clinical/functional outcomes? Acta Psychiatr Scand. 2015;131(2):100–10.

176. Ostergaard MLD, Nordentoft M, Hjorthoj C. Associations between substance use disorders and suicide or suicide attempts in people with mental illness: a Danish nation-wide, prospective, register-based study of patients diagnosed with schizophrenia, bipolar disorder, unipolar depression or personality disorder. Addiction. 2017;112(7):1250–9.

Marijuana and Suicide: Case-control Studies, Population Data and Potential Neurochemical Mechanisms

177. Nock MK, Banaji MR. Prediction of suicide ideation and attempts among adolescents using a brief performance-based test. J Consult Clin Psychol. 2007;75(5):707–15.

178. Silverman MM, Berman AL, Sanddal ND, O'carroll PW, Joiner TE. Rebuilding the tower of Babel: a revised nomenclature for the study of suicide and suicidal behaviors. Part 2: suicide-related ideations, communications, and behaviors. Suicide Life Threat Behav. 2007;37(3):264–77.

179. Arria AM, O'Grady KE, Caldeira KM, Vincent KB, Wilcox HC, Wish ED. Suicide ideation among college students: a multivariate analysis. Arch Suicide Res. 2009;13(3):230–46.

180. McHugh CM, Corderoy A, Ryan CJ, Hickie IB, Large MM. Association between suicidal ideation and suicide: meta-analyses of odds ratios, sensitivity, specificity and positive predictive value. BJPsych Open. 2019;5(2):e1.

181. Nordström P, Asberg M, Aberg-Wistedt A, Nordin C. Attempted suicide predicts suicide risk in mood disorders. Acta Psychiatr Scand. 1995;92(5):345–50.

182. Hawton K, Casañas I, Comabella C, Haw C, Saunders K. Risk factors for suicide in individuals with depression: a systematic review. J Affect Disord. 2013;147(1–3):17–28.

183. Wong SS, Zhou B, Goebert D, Hishinuma ES. The risk of adolescent suicide across patterns of drug use: a nationally representative study of high school students in the United States from 1999 to 2009. Soc Psychiatry Psychiatr Epidemiol. 2013;48(10):1611–20.

184. O'Boyle M, Brandon EA. Suicide attempts, substance abuse, and personality. J Subst Abus Treat. 1998;15(4):353–6.

185. Kokkevi A, Rotsika V, Arapaki A, Richardson C. Adolescents' self-reported suicide attempts, self-harm thoughts and their correlates across 17 European countries. J Child Psychol Psychiatry. 2012;53(4):381–9.

186. Conner KR, Britton PC, Sworts LM, Joiner TE. Suicide attempts among individuals with opiate dependence: the critical role of belonging. Addict Behav. 2007;32(7):1395–404.

187. Darke S, Ross J. Suicide among heroin users: rates, risk factors and methods. Addiction. 2002;97(11):1383–94.

188. Mykletun A, Bjerkeset O, Dewey M, Prince M, Overland S, Stewart R. Anxiety, depression, and cause-specific mortality: the HUNT study. Psychosom Med. 2007;69(4):323–31.

189. Zhang J, Li Z. The association between depression and suicide when hopelessness is controlled for. Compr Psychiatry. 2013;54(7):790–6.

190. Darke S, Ross J, Marel C, Mills KL, Slade T, Burns L, Teesson M. Patterns and correlates of attempted suicide amongst heroin users: 11-year follow-up of the Australian treatment outcome study cohort. Psychiatry Res. 2015;227(2–3):166–70.

191. Marzuk PM, Tardiff K, Lepn AC, Stajic M, Morgan EB, Mann JJ. Prevalence of cocaine use among residents of New York City who committed suicide during a one-year period. Am J Psychiatry. 1992;149(3):371–5.

192. Fowler RC, Rich CL, Young D. San Diego Suicide Study. II. Substance abuse in young cases. Arch Gen Psychiatry. 1986;43(10):962–5.

193. Glasheen C, Pemberton MR, Lipari R, Copello EA, Mattson ME. Binge drinking and the risk of suicidal thoughts, plans, and attempts. Addict Behav. 2015;43:42–9.

194. Bagge CL, Borges G. Acute substance use as a warning sign for suicide attempts: a case-crossover examination of the 48 hours prior to a recent suicide attempt. J Clin Psychiatry. 2017;78(6):691–6.

195. Clarke MC, Coughlan H, Harley M, Connor D, Power E, Lynch F, et al. The impact of adolescent cannabis use, mood disorder and lack of education on attempted suicide in young adulthood. World Psychiatry. 2014;13(3):322–3.

196. Silins E, Horwood LJ, Patton GC, Fergusson DM, Olsson CA, Hutchinson DM, et al. Young adult sequelae of adolescent cannabis use: an integrative analysis. Lancet Psychiatry. 2014;1(4):286–93.

197. Arendt M, Munk-Jørgensen P, Sher L, Jensen SO. Mortality following treatment for cannabis use disorders: predictors and causes. J Subst Abus Treat. 2013;44(4):400–6.

198. Hezel FX. Cultural patterns in Trukese suicide. Ethnology. 1984;23(3):193–206.

199. Garnefski N, Wilde EJ. Addiction-risk behaviours and suicide attempts in adolescents. J Adolescence. 1998;21(2):135–42.

200. Beautrais AL, Joyce PR, Mulder RT. Cannabis abuse and serious suicide attempts. Addiction. 1999;94(8):1155–64.

201. Gex CR, Narring F, Ferron C, Michaud P. Suicide attempts among adolescents in Switzerland: Prevalence, associated factors and comorbidity. Acta Psychiatr Scand. 1998;98(1):28–33.

202. Kung HC, Pearson JL, Liu X. Risk factors for male and female suicide decedents ages 15–64 in the United States. Soc Psychiatry Psychiatr Epidemiol. 2003;38(8):419–26.

203. Pedersen W. Does cannabis use lead to depression and suicidal behaviours? A population-based longitudinal study. Acta Psychiatr Scand. 2008;118(5):395–403.

204. Price C, Hemmingsson T, Lewis G, Zammit S, Allebeck P. Cannabis and suicide: longitudinal study. Br J Psychiatry. 2009;195(6):492–7.

205. Madigan D, Stang PE, Berlin JA, Schuemie M, Overhage JM, Suchard MA, et al. A systematic statistical approach to evaluating evidence from observational studies. Annu Rev Stat Appl. 2014;1:11–39.

206. Patton GC, Coffey C, Carlin JB, Sawyer SM, Lynskey M. Reverse gateways? Frequent cannabis use as a predictor of tobacco initiation and nicotine dependence. Addiction. 2005;100(10):1518–25.
207. Rasic D, Weerasinghe S, Asbridge M, Langille DB. Longitudinal associations of cannabis and illicit drug use with depression, suicidal ideation and suicidal attempts among Nova Scotia high school students. Drug Alcohol Depend. 2013;129(1–2):49–53.
208. Agrawal A, Nelson EC, Bucholz KK, Tillman R, Grucza RA, Statham DJ, Madden PA, Martin NG, Heath AC, Lynskey MT. Major depressive disorder, suicidal thoughts and behaviours, and cannabis involvement in discordant twins: a retrospective cohort study. Lancet Psychiatry. 2017;4(9):706–14.
209. Borges G, Bagge CL, Orozco R. A literature review and meta-analyses of cannabis use and suicidality. J Affect Disord. 2016;195:63–74.
210. Chandra S, Radwan MM, Majumdar CG, Church JC, Freeman TP, ElSohly MA. New trends in cannabis potency in USA and Europe during the last decade (2008–2017). Eur Arch Psychiatry Clin Neurosci. 2019;269(1):5–15.
211. Carvalho AF, Stubbs B, Vancampfort D, Kloiber S, Maes M, Firth J, Kurdyak PA, Stein DJ, Rehm J, Koyanagi A. Cannabis use and suicide attempts among 86,254 adolescents aged 12–15 years from 21 low and middle-income countries. Eur Psychiatry. 2019;56:8–13.
212. Sellers CM, Diaz-Valdes Iriarte A, Wyman Battalen A, O'Brien KHM. Alcohol and marijuana use as daily predictors of suicide ideation and attempts among adolescents prior to psychiatric hospitalization. Psychiatry Res. 2019;273:672–7.
213. Conwell Y, Van Orden K, Caine ED. Suicide in older adults. Psychiatr Clin North Am. 2011;34(2):451–68.
214. Gobbi G, Atkin T, Zytynski T, Wang S, Askari S, Boruff J, et al. Association of cannabis use in adolescence and risk of depression, anxiety, and suicidality in young adulthood: a systematic review and meta-analysis. JAMA Psychiat. 2019; https://doi.org/10.1001/jamapsychiatry.2018.4500. [Epub ahead of print]
215. Wilkinson ST, Stefanovics E, Rosenheck RA. Marijuana use is associated with worse outcomes in symptom severity and violent behavior in patients with posttraumatic stress disorder. J Clin Psychiatry. 2015;76(9):1174–80.
216. Allan NP, Ashrafioun L, Kolnogorova K, Raines AM, Hoge CW, Stecker T. Interactive effects of PTSD and substance use on suicidal ideation and behavior in military personnel: increased risk from marijuana use. Depress Anxiety. 2019; https://doi.org/10.1002/da.22954. [Epub ahead of print]
217. Gentes EL, Schry AR, Hicks TA, Clancy CP, Collie CF, Kirby AC, Dennis MF, Hertzberg MA, Beckham JC, Calhoun PS. Prevalence and correlates of cannabis use in an outpatient VA posttraumatic stress disorder clinic. Psychol Addict Behav. 2016;30(3):415–21.
218. Kimbrel NA, Meyer EC, DeBeer BB, Gulliver SB, Morissette SB. The impact of cannabis use disorder on suicidal and nonsuicidal self-injury in Iraq/Afghanistan-Era veterans with and without mental health disorders. Suicide Life Threat Behav. 2018;48(2):140–8.
219. Adkisson K, Cunningham KC, Dedert EA, Dennis MF, Calhoun PS, Elbogen EB, Beckham JC, Kimbrel NA. Cannabis use disorder and post-deployment suicide attempts in Iraq/Afghanistan-Era veterans. Arch Suicide Res. 2019;23(4):678–87.
220. Vandrey RG, Budney AJ, Hughes JR, Liguori A. A within-subject comparison of withdrawal symptoms during abstinence from cannabis, tobacco, and both substances. Drug Alcohol Depend. 2008;92(1–3):48–54.
221. Degenhardt L, Ferrari AJ, Calabria B, Hall WD, Norman RE, McGrath J, et al. The global epidemiology and contribution of cannabis use and dependence to the global burden of disease: results from the GBD 2010 study. PLoS One. 2013;8(10):e76635.
222. Agrawal A, Lynskey MT. Cannabis controversies: how genetics can inform the study of comorbidity. Addiction. 2014;109(3):360–70.
223. Walsh Z, Gonzalez R, Crosby K, Thiessen MS, Carroll C, Bonn-Miller MO. Medical cannabis and mental health: a guided systematic review. Clin Psychol Rev. 2017;51:15–29.

224. Kposowa A, Hamilton D, Wang K. Impact of firearm availability and gun regulation on state suicide rates. Suicide Life Threat Behav. 2016;46(6):678–96.
225. Smith TW, Son J. Trends in gun ownership in the United States, 1972–2014. General Social Survey final report. Chicago: University of Chicago: NORC; 2015.
226. Gibbons RD, Hur K, Bhaumik DK, Mann JJ. The relationship between antidepressant medication use and rate of suicide. Arch Gen Psychiatry. 2005;62(2):165–72.
227. Lu CY, Zhang F, Lakoma MD, Madden JM, Rusinak D, Penfold RB, et al. Changes in antidepressant use by young people and suicidal behavior after FDA warnings and media coverage: quasi-experimental study. BMJ. 2014;348:g3596.
228. Laido Z, Voracek M, Till B, Pietschnig J, Eisenwort B, Dervic K, et al. Epidemiology of suicide among children and adolescents in Austria, 2001–2014. Wien Klin Wochenschr. 2017;129(3–4):121–8.
229. Cohen PN. Recession and divorce in the United States, 2008–2011. Popul Res Policy Rev. 2014;33(5):615–28.
230. Twenge JM, Campbell WK. Media use is linked to lower psychological well-being: evidence from three datasets. Psychiatry Q. 2019;90:311. [Epub ahead of print].
231. Brenner B, Cheng D, Clark S, Camargo CA Jr. Positive association between altitude and suicide in 2584 US counties. High Alt Med Biol. 2011;12(1):31–5.
232. Kim J, Choi N, Lee YJ, An H, Kim N, Yoon HK, Lee HJ. High altitude remains associated with elevated suicide rates after adjusting for socioeconomic status: a study from South Korea. Psychiatry Investig. 2014;11(4):492–4.
233. Wray M, Miller M, Gurvey J, Carroll J, Kawachi I. Leaving Las Vegas: exposure to Las Vegas and risk of suicide. Soc Sci Med. 2001;67(11):1882–8.
234. Battersby M, Tolchard B, Scurrah M, Thomas L. Suicide ideation and behaviour in people with pathological gambling attending a treatment service. Int J Ment Health Addict. 2006;4(3):233–46.
235. Welte JW, Barnes GM, Tidwell MC, Hoffman JH, Wieczorek WF. Gambling and problem gambling in the United States: changes between 1999 and 2013. J Gambl Stud. 2015;31(3):695–715.
236. Kegler SR, Stone DM, Holland KM. Trends in suicide by level of urbanization – United States, 1999–2015. MMWR Morb Mortal Wkly Rep. 2017;66(10):270–3.
237. Bounoua L, Nigro J, Zhang P, Thome K, Lachir A. Mapping urbanization in the United States from 2001 to 2011. Appl Geogr. 2018;90:123–33.
238. Brooks B, McBee M, Pack R, Alamian A. The effects of rurality on substance use disorder diagnosis: a multiple-groups latent class analysis. Addict Behav. 2017;68:24–9.
239. Habecker P, Welch-Lazoritz M, Dombrowski K. Rural and urban differences in Nebraskans' access to marijuana, methamphetamine, heroin, and prescription pills. J Drug Issues. 2018;48(4):608–24.
240. Bukky M. Urban and rural adolescent drug use and its relationship with classic criminological theories [dissertation]. Columbus: Ohio State University; 2017.
241. Barr B, Taylor-Robinson D, Scott-Samuel A, McKee M, Stuckler D. Suicides associated with the 2008–10 economic recession in England: time trend analysis. BMJ. 2012;345:e5142.
242. Lewis G, Sloggett A. Suicide, deprivation, and unemployment: record linkage study. BMJ. 1998;317(7168):1283–6.
243. Kposowa AJ. Unemployment and suicide: a cohort analysis of social factors predicting suicide in the US National Longitudinal Mortality Study. Psychol Med. 2001;31(1):127–38.
244. Blakely TA, Collings SC, Atkinson J. Unemployment and suicide. Evidence for a causal association? J Epidemiol Community Health. 2003;57(8):594–600.
245. Mäki N, Martikainen P. A register-based study on excess suicide mortality among unemployed men and women during different levels of unemployment in Finland. J Epidemiol Community Health. 2012;66(4):302–7.
246. Classen TJ, Dunn RA. The effect of job loss and unemployment duration on suicide risk in the United States: a new look using mass-layoffs and unemployment duration. Health Econ. 2012;21(3):338–50.

247. Azofeifa A, Mattson ME, Schauer G, McAfee T, Grant A, Lyerla R. National estimates of marijuana use and related indicators – National Survey on Drug Use and Health, United States, 2002–2014. In: Morbidity and mortality weekly report. Centers for Disease Control and Preventaion, September 2, 2016.
248. HIDTA. Rocky mountain high intensity drug trafficking area report, The legalization of marijuana in Colorado: the impact, vol. 4. Denver: Rocky Mountain High Intensity Drug Trafficking Area Investigative Support Center; 2016.
249. Mohler-Kuo M, Wydler H, Zellweger U, Gutzwiller F. Differences in health status and health behaviour among young Swiss adults between 1993 and 2003. Swiss Med Wkly. 2006;136(29–30):464–72.
250. Di Forti M, Marconi A, Carra E, Fraietta S, Trotta A, Bonomo M, et al. Proportion of patients in south London with first-episode psychosis attributable to use of high potency cannabis: a case-control study. Lancet Psychiatry. 2015;2(3):233–8.
251. Marconi A, Di Forti M, Lewis CM, Murray RM, Vassos E. Meta-analysis of the association between the level of cannabis use and risk of psychosis. Schizophr Bull. 2016;42(5):1262–9.
252. Randall JR, Walld R, Finlayson G, Sareen J, Martens PJ, Bolton JM. Acute risk of suicide and suicide attempts associated with recent diagnosis of mental disorders: a population-based, propensity score-matched analysis. Can J Psychiatr. 2014;59(10):531–8.
253. Palmer BA, Pankratz VS, Bostwick JM. The lifetime risk of suicide in schizophrenia: a reexamination. Arch Gen Psychiatry. 2005;62(3):247–53.
254. Hor K, Taylor M. Suicide and schizophrenia: a systematic review of rates and risk factors. J Psychopharmacol. 2010;24(4 Suppl):81–90.
255. Mortensen PB, Juel K. Mortality and causes of death in first admitted schizophrenic patients. Br J Psychiatry. 1993;163:183–9.
256. Waterreus A, Di Prinzio P, Badcock JC, Martin-Iverson M, Jablensky A, Morgan VA. Is cannabis a risk factor for suicide attempts in men and women with psychotic illness? Psychopharmacology. 2018;235(8):2275–85.
257. Cougle JR, Hakes JK, Macatee RJ, Chavarria J, Zvolensky MJ. Quality of life and risk of psychiatric disorders among regular users of alcohol, nicotine, and cannabis: an analysis of the National Epidemiological Survey on Alcohol and Related Conditions (NESARC). J Psychiatric Res. 2015;66–67:135–41.
258. Chen YW, Dilsaver SC. Lifetime rates of suicide attempts among subjects with bipolar and unipolar disorders relative to subjects with other Axis I disorders. Biol Psychiatry. 1996;39(10):896–9.
259. Webb RT, Lichtenstein P, Larsson H, Geddes JR, Fazel S. Suicide, hospital-presenting suicide attempts, and criminality in bipolar disorder: examination of risk for multiple adverse outcomes. J Clin Psychiatry. 2014;75(8):e809–16.
260. Blair-West GW, Cantor CH, Mellsop GW, Eyeson-Annan ML. Lifetime suicide risk in major depression: sex and age determinants. J Affect Disord. 1999;55(2–3):171–8.
261. Bostwick JM, Pankratz VS. Affective disorders and suicide risk: a reexamination. Am J Psychiatry. 2000;157(12):1925–32.
262. Sharma T, Guski LS, Freund N, Gøtzsche PC. Suicidality and aggression during antidepressant treatment: systematic review and meta-analyses based on clinical study reports. BMJ. 2016;352:i65.
263. Tiihonen J, Lönnqvist J, Wahlbeck K, Klaukka T, Tanskanen A, Haukka J. Antidepressants and the risk of suicide, attempted suicide, and overall mortality in a nationwide cohort. Arch Gen Psychiatry. 2006;63(12):1358–67.
264. Jick H, Kaye JA, Jick SS. Antidepressants and the risk of suicidal behaviors. JAMA. 2004;292(3):338–43.
265. Björkenstam C, Möller J, Ringbäck G, Salmi P, Hallqvist J, Ljung R. An association between initiation of selective serotonin reuptake inhibitors and suicide – a nationwide register-based case-crossover study. PLoS One. 2013;8(9):e73973.

266. Leon AC, Solomon DA, Li C, Fiedorowicz JG, Coryell WH, Endicott J, et al. Antidepressants and risks of suicide and suicide attempts: a 27-year observational study. J Clin Psychiatry. 2011;72(5):580–6.
267. Herings RM, Erkens JA. Increased suicide attempt rate among patients interrupting use of atypical antipsychotics. Pharmacoepidemiol Drug Saf. 2003;12(5):423–4.
268. Haukka J, Tiihonen J, Härkänen T, Lönnqvist J. Association between medication and risk of suicide, attempted suicide and death in nationwide cohort of suicidal patients with schizophrenia. Pharmacoepidemiol Drug Saf. 2008;17(7):686–96.
269. Kiviniemi M, Suvisaari J, Koivumaa-Honkanen H, Häkkinen U, Isohanni M, Hakko H. Antipsychotics and mortality in first-onset schizophrenia: prospective Finnish register study with 5-year follow-up. Schizophr Res. 2013;150(1):274–80.
270. Reutfors J, Bahmanyar S, Jönsson EG, Brandt L, Bodén R, Ekbom A, et al. Medication and suicide risk in schizophrenia: a nested case-control study. Schizophr Res. 2013;150(2–3):416–20.
271. Kasckow J, Felmet K, Zisook S. Managing suicide risk in patients with schizophrenia. CNS Drugs. 2011;25(2):129–43.
272. Khan A, Khan SR, Leventhal RM, Brown WA. Symptom reduction and suicide risk among patients treated with placebo in antipsychotic clinical trials: an analysis of the food and drug administration database. Am J Psychiatry. 2001;158(9):1449–54.
273. Tondo L, Hennen J, Baldessarini RJ. Lower suicide risk with long-term lithium treatment in major affective illness: a meta-analysis. Acta Psychiatr Scand. 2001;104(3):163–72.
274. Yerevanian BI, Koek RJ, Mintz J. Lithium, anticonvulsants and suicidal behavior in bipolar disorder. J Affect Disord. 2003;73(3):223–8.
275. Toffol E, Hätönen T, Tanskanen A, Lönnqvist J, Wahlbeck K, Joffe G, et al. Lithium is associated with decrease in all-cause and suicide mortality in high-risk bipolar patients: a nationwide registry-based prospective cohort study. J Affect Disord. 2015;183:159–65.
276. Dunlop BW, Nemeroff CB. The role of dopamine in the pathophysiology of depression. Arch Gen Psychiatry. 2007;64(3):327–37.
277. Ikemoto S, Panksepp J. The role of nucleus accumbens dopamine in motivated behavior: a unifying interpretation with special reference to reward-seeking. Brain Res Brain Res Rev. 1999;31(1):6–41.
278. Koob GF, Le Moal M. Drug abuse: hedonic homeostatic dysregulation. Science. 1997;278(5335):52–8.
279. Francis TC, Gantz SC, Moussawi K, Bonci A. Synaptic and intrinsic plasticity in the ventral tegmental area after chronic cocaine. Curr Opin Neurobiol. 2019;54:66–72.
280. Lecca D, Cacciapaglia F, Valentini V, Di Chiara G. Monitoring extracellular dopamine in the rat nucleus accumbens shell and core during acquisition and maintenance of intravenous WIN 55,212-2 self-administration. Psychopharmacology. 2006;188(1):63–74.
281. Fadda P, Scherma M, Spano MS, Salis P, Melis V, Fattore L, et al. Cannabinoid self-administration increases dopamine release in the nucleus accumbens. Neuroreport. 2006;17(15):1629–32.
282. Bossong MG, Mehta MA, van Berckel BN, Howes OD, Kahn RS, Stokes PR. Further human evidence for striatal dopamine release induced by administration of Δ9-tetrahydrocannabinol (THC): selectivity to limbic striatum. Psychopharmacology. 2015;232(15):2723–9.
283. Silveira MM, Arnold JC, Laviolette SR, Hillard CJ, Celorrio M, Aymerich MS, et al. Seeing through the smoke: human and animal studies of cannabis use and endocannabinoid signalling in corticolimbic networks. Neurosci Biobehav Rev. 2017;76(Pt B):380–95.
284. Uhl GR, Koob GF, Cable J. The neurobiology of addiction. Ann N Y Acad Sci. 2019; 1451(1): 5–28.
285. Bloomfield MA, Ashok AH, Volkow ND, Howes OD. The effects of Δ9-tetrahydrocannabinol on the dopamine system. Nature. 2016;539(7629):369–77.
286. Martin-Soelch C. Is depression associated with dysfunction of the central reward system? Biochem Soc Trans. 2009;37(Pt 1):313–7.

287. Schneier FR, Slifstein M, Whitton AE, Pizzagalli DA, Reinen J, McGrath PJ, et al. Dopamine release in antidepressant-naive major depressive disorder: a multimodal [11C]-(+)-PHNO positron emission tomography and functional magnetic resonance imaging study. Biol Psychiatry. 2018;84(8):563–73.
288. Zimmermann K. Reward and affective dysregulation in cannabis users. Doctoral dissertation, University of Dusseldorf, 2018. 66 pp.
289. Blum K, Cull JG, Braverman ER, Comings DE. Reward deficiency syndrome. Am Scientist. 1996;84:132–45.
290. Russo M, Rifici C, Sessa E, D'Aleo G, Bramanti P, Calabrò RS. Sativex-induced neurobehavioral effects: causal or concausal? A practical advice! Daru. 2015;23(1):25.
291. Koppel BS, Brust JC, Fife T, Bronstein J, Youssof S, Gronseth G, et al. Systematic review: efficacy and safety of medical marijuana in selected neurologic disorders Report of the Guideline Development Subcommittee of the American Academy of Neurology. Neurology. 2014;82(17):1556–63.
292. Gorelick DA, Goodwin RS, Schwilke E, Schwope DM, Darwin WD, Kelly DL, et al. Antagonist-elicited cannabis withdrawal in humans. J Clin Psychopharmacol. 2011;31(5):603–12.
293. Robertson HT, Allison DB. Drugs associated with more suicidal ideations are also associated with more suicide attempts. PLoS One. 2009;4(10):e7312.
294. Mackie K. Cannabinoid receptors: where they are and what they do. J Neuroendocrinol. 2008;20(S1):10–4.
295. Huestis MA. Human cannabinoid pharmacokinetics. Chem Biodivers. 2007;4(8):1770–804.
296. Lemberger L, Martz R, Rodda B, Forney R, Rowe H. Comparative pharmacology of Delta9-tetrahydrocannabinol and its metabolite, 11-OH-Delta9-tetrahydrocannabinol. J Clin Invest. 1973;52(10):2411–7.
297. Favrat B, Ménétrey A, Augsburger M, Rothuizen LE, Appenzeller M, Buclin T, et al. Two cases of "cannabis acute psychosis" following the administration of oral cannabis. BMC Psychiatry. 2005;5:17.
298. Sublette ME, Galfalvy HC, Fuchs D, Lapidus M, Grunebaum MF, Oquendo MA, et al. Plasma kynurenine levels are elevated in suicide attempters with major depressive disorder. Brain Behav Immun. 2011;25(6):1272–8.
299. Bradley KA, Case JA, Khan O, Ricart T, Hanna A, Alonso CM, et al. The role of the kynurenine pathway in suicidality in adolescent major depressive disorder. Psychiatry Res. 2015;227(2):206–12.
300. Erhardt S, Lim CK, Linderholm KR, Janelidze S, Lindqvist D, Samuelsson M, et al. Connecting inflammation with glutamate agonism in suicidality. Neuropsychopharmacology. 2013;38(5):743–52.
301. Brundin L, Sellgren CM, Lim CK, Grit J, Pålsson E, Landen M, et al. An enzyme in the kynurenine pathway that governs vulnerability to suicidal behavior by regulating excitotoxicity and neuroinflammation. Transl Psychiatry. 2016;6(8):e865.
302. Messaoud A, Mensi R, Douki W, Neffati F, Najjar MF, Gobbi G, et al. Reduced peripheral availability of tryptophan and increased activation of the kynurenine pathway and cortisol correlate with major depression and suicide. World J Biol Psychiatry. 2018;23:1–9. https://doi.org/10.1080/15622975.2018.1468031. [Epub ahead of print].
303. Miller CL, Llenos IC, Cwik M, Walkup J, Weis S. Alterations in kynurenine precursor and product levels in schizophrenia and bipolar disorder. Neurochem Int. 2008;52(6):1297–303.
304. O'Donovan A, Rush G, Hoatam G, Hughes BM, McCrohan A, Kelleher C, et al. Suicidal ideation is associated with elevated inflammation in patients with major depressive disorder. Depress Anxiety. 2013;30(4):307–14.
305. Lindqvist D, Janelidze S, Hagell P, Erhardt S, Samuelsson M, Minthon L, et al. Interleukin-6 is elevated in the cerebrospinal fluid of suicide attempters and related to symptom severity. Biol Psychiatry. 2009;66(3):287–92.

306. Janelidze S, Mattei D, Westrin Å, Träskman-Bendz L, Brundin L. Cytokine levels in the blood may distinguish suicide attempters from depressed patients. Brain Behav Immun. 2011;25(2):335–9.
307. Braun D, Longman RS, Albert ML. A two-step induction of indoleamine 2,3 dioxygenase (IDO) activity during dendritic-cell maturation. Blood. 2005;106(7):2375–81.
308. Massi P, Fuzio D, Viganò D, Sacerdote P, Parolaro D. Relative involvement of cannabinoid CB(1) and CB(2) receptors in the Delta(9)-tetrahydrocannabinol-induced inhibition of natural killer activity. Eur J Pharmacol. 2000;387(3):343–7.
309. McKallip RJ, Lombard C, Martin BR, Nagarkatti M, Nagarkatti PS. Delta(9)-tetrahydrocannabinol-induced apoptosis in the thymus and spleen as a mechanism of immunosuppression in vitro and in vivo. J Pharmacol Exp Ther. 2002;302(2):451–65.
310. Li X, Kaminski NE, Fischer LJ. Examination of the immunosuppressive effect of delta9-tetrahydrocannabinol in streptozotocin-induced autoimmune diabetes. Int Immunopharmacol. 2001;1(4):699–712.
311. Kozela E, Pietr M, Juknat A, Rimmerman N, Levy R, Vogel Z. Cannabinoids delta(9)-tetrahydrocannabinol and cannabidiol differentially inhibit the lipopolysaccharide-activated NF-kappaB and interferon-beta/STAT proinflammatory pathways in BV-2 microglial cells. J Biol Chem. 2010;285(3):1616–26.
312. Poddar MK, Ghosh JJ. Effect of cannabis extract, Δ^9-tetrahydrocannabinol and lysergic acid diethylamide on rat liver enzymes. Biochem Pharmacol. 1972;21(24):3301–3.
313. Doshi A, Boudreaux ED, Wang N, Pelletier AJ, Camargo CA. National study of US emergency department visits for attempted suicide and self-inflicted injury, 1997–2001. Ann Emerg Med. 2005;46(4):369–75.

Cannabis Use Disorder, Treatment, and Recovery

314. Budney AJ, Roffman R, Stephens RS, Walker D. Marijuana dependence and its treatment. Addict Sci Clin Pract. 2007;4(1):4–16.
315. Prochaska JO, DiClemente CC, Norcross JC. In search of how people change: applications to the addictive behaviors. Am Psychologist. 1992;47:1102–14.
316. Prochaska JO, Redding CA, Evers K. The transtheoretical model and atages of change. In: Glanz K, Rimer BK, Lewis FM, editors. Health and behaviors and health education theory, research and practice. 3rd ed. San Francisco: Jossey-Bass, Inc.; 2002.
317. American Society of Addiction Medicine. Criteria: treatment criteria for addictive, substance-related, and co-occurring conditions. 3rd edn. Carson City, NV: The Change Companies. 2013.
318. Pacheco-Colón I, Limia JM, Gonzalez R. Nonacute effects of cannabis use on motivation and reward sensitivity in humans: a systematic review. Psychol Addict Behav. 2018;32(5):497–507.
319. Marijuana Anonymous World Service. 2019. http://www.marijuana-anonymous.org.
320. Marijusana Anonymous. Life with hope 12 step workbook: a return to living through the 12 steps and 12 traditions of marijuana anonymous.
321. Venice N, Tung G. Marijuana and child abuse and neglect: a health impact assessment. Aurora: Colorado School of Public Health; 2016.
322. Few L, et al. Cannabis involvement and nonsuicidal self-injury: a discordant twin approach. J Stud Alcohol Drugs. 2016;77(6):873–80.
323. Rossow I, Hawton K, Ystgaard M. Cannabis use and deliberate self-harm in adolescence: a comparative analysis of associations in England and Norway. Arch Suicide Res. 2009;13(4):340–8.
324. Yassa AH, George SM. Cannabis abuse and self-mutilation. J Forensic Sci Criminol. 2016;4(5). ISSN: 2348–9804.
325. Delteil C, et al. Death by self-mutilation after oral cannabis consumption. Legal Med Tokyo. 2018;30:5–9.

326. Di Forti M, Quattrone D, Freeman TP, et al. The contribution of cannabis use to variation in the incidence of psychotic disorder across Europe (EU-GEI): a multicentre case-control study. Lancet Psychiatry. 2019;6:427–36.

327. American Psychiatric Association. Diagnostic and statistical manual of mental disorders: diagnostic and statistical manual of mental disorders, 5th edn. Arlington, VA: American Psychiatric Association, 2013.

328. World Health Organization. International statistical classification of diseases and related health problems, tenth revision. 5th edn. 2015, 2016. Geneva: World Health Organization.

329. Hall W. What has research over the past two decades revealed about the adverse health effects of recreational cannabis use? s. 2015;110(1):19–35.

330. Sherman BJ, McRae-Clark AL. Treatment of cannabis use disorder: current science and future outlook. Pharmacotherapy. 2016;36(5):511–35.

331. Stephens RS, Roffman RA, Simpson EE. Treating adult marijuana dependence: a test of the relapse prevention model. J Consult Clin Psychol. 1994;1:92–9. [PubMed: 8034835].

332. Hoch E, Bühringer G, Pixa A, Dittmer K, Henker J, Seifert A, Wittchen HU. CANDIS treatment program for cannabis use disorders: findings from a randomized multi-site translational trial. Drug Alcohol Depend. 2014;134:185–93.

333. Stephens RS, Roffman RA, Fearer SA, Williams C, Burke RS. The marijuana check-up: promoting change in ambivalent marijuana users. Addiction. 2007;6:947–57. [PubMed: 17523990].

Chapter 5
Cannabis and the Impact on the Pediatric and Adolescent Population

George Sam Wang, Donald E. Greydanus, and Maria Demma Cabral

Cannabis and Young Pediatric Exposures

George Sam Wang

Adult recreational and medical use of marijuana and related products impacts the entire pediatric population, from prenatal through adolescents and young adulthood [1]. Exposures begin as early as the prenatal and postpartum time period, including pregnancy and breastfeeding exposures from both recreational and medical use to treat pregnancy-related conditions such as morning sickness, hyperemesis gravidarum, or postpartum pain, depression, or anxiety. Young children are subject to passive (secondhand) smoke exposures when caregivers use within the home or car environments. When marijuana products, such as edibles, are poorly stored, there are risks for unintentional ingestions leading to a spectrum of clinical symptoms. Besides alcohol and nicotine, marijuana is the most commonly abuse drug in the adolescent population [2]. Finally, marijuana is also used for medicinal indications in the pediatric population as in the adult population, with varying amount of evidenced-based literature to support its use. A recent review demonstrated the best evidence for use of marijuana in the pediatric population was for seizures and chemotherapy-induced nausea and vomiting, with insufficient evidence for spasticity, neuropathic pain, post-traumatic stress disorder, and Tourette syndrome [3].

G. S. Wang (✉)
Section of Emergency Medicine and Medical Toxicology, Department of Pediatrics, University of Colorado Anschutz Medical Campus, Aurora, CO, USA
e-mail: George.wang@childrenscolorado.org

D. E. Greydanus · M. D. Cabral
Department of Pediatric and Adolescent Medicine, Western Michigan University Homer Stryker M.D. School of Medicine, Kalamazoo, MI, USA
e-mail: Donald.Greydanus@med.wmich.edu; MariaDemma.Cabral@med.wmich.edu

© Springer Nature Switzerland AG 2020
K. Finn (ed.), *Cannabis in Medicine*,
https://doi.org/10.1007/978-3-030-45968-0_5

Medical indications vary by state but include chronic pain, anorexia/cachexia, nausea/vomiting, seizures, post-traumatic stress disorder, and autism [4].

The current regulatory environment of federally scheduled I status of marijuana while allowing states to legalize both medical and recreational use leads to several disparities and difficulties with healthcare providers and social services specific with the pediatric population. Most hospitals and providers abide by federal laws; thus, questions arise on liability, provider awareness, in hospital/clinic storage, and administration. However, healthcare providers should not alienate these patients as many are medical fragile and require subspecialty care and stable medical homes. Some hospitals serve large patient catchment areas where nearby states do not allow medical marijuana. Questions arise about mandatory reporting of unintentional marijuana exposures or use without medical oversight. Furthermore, concerns for mandatory reporting may discourage admitted use when interventions may be of benefit, such as in the setting of prenatal use. In states that do allow medical marijuana, many of the prescribers and marijuana dispensaries do not have medical training; however, the healthcare providers often lack the knowledge base to recommend treatment.

The American Academy of Pediatrics (AAP) has release a policy statement and accompanied technical report on the impact of marijuana on the pediatric population [5]. Among the recommendations/statements concluded from this report include (1) opposition of marijuana use in children and adolescents <21 years of age (2) opposing "medical marijuana" outside the regulatory process of the US Food and Drug Administration (3) rules and regulations that limit access and marketing/advertising to youth (4) supports research and development of pharmaceutical cannabinoids (5) child-resistant packaging, (6) decriminalization of marijuana use for both minors and young adults, (7) oppose smoked marijuana, and (8) discourage use by adults around minors.

Pediatric Unintentional Exposures (Ingestions)

Prior to state legalization of marijuana for recreational and medical purposes, unintentional pediatric exposures were rare events, mostly described in case reports [6–10]. The first state to legalize marijuana was California in 1996. In 2019, there are now 33 states that have passed medical marijuana legislation and 10 allowing for recreational use [11]. The increased presence of the medical marijuana industry did not begin until the Ogden Memo was released in 2009. The Ogden Memo allowed local states to regulate their marijuana industry and stated the federal government would not interfere as long as the industry abided to state laws [12]. This led to a large growth within the country, especially in Colorado where medical marijuana patient applications increased from <10,000 in January 2009 to over 160,000 in November 2011 [13]. This change in the landscape of medical marijuana use was associated with an increase in patients seen in the tertiary care children's hospital in Colorado. From January 2005 through September 2009, there were 0 marijuana exposures in children less than 12 years, while 14 were seen in the emergency department from October 2009 through December 2011 ($p < 0.001$) [13]. Colorado then allowed marijuana for recreational use in 2014. Again, another significant increase in marijuana hospital visits and poison center exposure calls in children 9 years and younger for the first 2 years of legalization of recreational marijuana [13]. These hospital visits and poison center calls have continued to increase in 2017, with 36 annual hospital visits and 67 poison center calls [14].

The observation of an increase in unintentional pediatric exposures has not been isolated to Colorado. A review of US National Poison Drug Center (NPDS) marijuana exposure calls in children found the call rate in states that have allowed medical marijuana increased by 30.3% from 2005 to 2011 calls per year, with a difference of 28.3% in states without any legalization [15]. Washington, another state that has allowed both retail and recreational marijuana, has seen an increase in hospital visits after legalization [16]. The costs associated with marijuana exposures in the ED can be significant. Without history of exposure, children with neurologic symptoms can undergo a significant workup, including laboratory workup and radiographic imaging. One study found the hospital costs were fourfold less when children presented with a known exposure, rather than no exposure [17].

The epidemiology of unintentional pediatric exposures is mostly seen in the young pediatric population, approximately 2 years of age [18]. The scenario often involves ingestion of a guardian or caregivers' marijuana products, including parents, grandparents, and babysitters [19]. Most common products that were ingested included cannabis resins and edible products (food that is THC infused). Most common symptoms included lethargy and ataxia, with several reports of intubation due to mental status and/or respiratory depression [18–20]. In general, pediatric patients who ingested edible products and other concentrated products have more severe symptoms with longer hospital lengths of stay [20, 21]. There is one reported case of a death due to myocarditis in the setting of detectable marijuana exposure in an infant [22]. Authors describe an 11 months male who presented with central nervous system depression after seizures, which progressed to cardiac arrest and died. Myocarditis was diagnosed postmortem, and cannabis exposure was noted on postmortem cardiac blood testing. Although no other findings of infectious etiologies of myocarditis were identified, the exact relationship between the marijuana exposures had on the condition is unclear.

There is limited data on the potential dose response effect after an ingestion of marijuana in a child. In a small population of children receiving low-dose THC cannabis extracts for epilepsy, THC peak plasma concentrations were achieved in most patients within 2 hours, while acute phase elimination half-life ranged from 1 to 5 hours [23]. In a small cohort (8) of children where an estimated THC dose ingested was determined, children ingesting 3.27 (± 0.35) mg/kg THC received no intervention, while those who ingested 9.45 (± 6.46) mg/kg THC received some medical intervention. Children who ingested 3.17 (± 0.38) mg/kg THC were observed, 7.18 ($=/-4.36$) mg/kg THC were admitted to an inpatient floor, and 13 (± 0.19) mg/kg THC were admitted to the intensive care unit [24]. None of the children had plasma concentrations obtained, and the doses were estimates based on the product concentration and amount ingested.

In order to decrease unintentional pediatric exposures, many states have passed significant rules and regulations [25]. For example, Colorado has required child-resistant packaging, dose limitations (10 mg in serving, 100 mg in an entire package), limitations on marketing, and appealing labels attractive to young children and adolescents [26, 27]. Other state has followed similar regulations, including Washington and Oregon [28, 29]. Although regulations such as child-resistant packaging have shown to impact and decrease exposures to pharmaceutical products, it is unclear the impact on marijuana exposures [30–32]. In Colorado, even after regulations, exposures have continued to increase, although the severity of illness appeared to be less, potentially a result of dose limitations [14]. Surveillance reports from the Colorado Department of Public Health and Environment Marijuana Health Advisory Committee found that as many as 20,000 household do not store marijuana properly, leading to this increased risk of pediatric exposures [33]. Continued surveillance and improvements in public education are warranted.

Other Pediatric Exposures: Passive (Secondhand) Smoke Exposures and Breastfeeding Exposures

The medical and public health impacts of secondhand marijuana smoke are beginning to be understood. Marijuana smoke can have similar particulates and carcinogens as tobacco smoke [34]. Current regulations in most state ban public use of marijuana, leaving adults to use it within the confines of their homes. However, this increases the risk of secondhand smoke exposure to surrounding bystanders, including children. Studies have shown secondhand tobacco smoke has a negative impact on childhood illness including respiratory sensitive conditions (viral infections, asthma exacerbations, otitis media), along with cognitive and behavioral health [35]. In a cohort of hospitalized children in Colorado, 46% had detectable THC-COOH metabolite in their urine, and 11% had detectable THC. These children had parents more likely to use marijuana daily, smoke vs other forms of use, and use in the home and even in another room unaccompanied by children [36–38]. Additional research has demonstrated children in the setting with both tobacco and marijuana smoke that increases their likelihood of emergency department visits, along with diagnosis of otitis media [36]. There are additional concerns on the potential for children to model adult behaviors when using marijuana around children, along with their ability to parent while intoxicated.

Another "alternative" source of marijuana exposures in children is through breastmilk. Marijuana is the most commonly used illicit substance during and after pregnancy. Estimated 2–5% of pregnant women report use of marijuana during pregnancy [39–43]. Rates of admitted self-use have significant increased from 2002 to 2014 [44]. There is public perception that use of marijuana in pregnancy is safe as a "natural" product. Research performed in Colorado found that 69% of 400 contacted marijuana dispensaries recommended marijuana for morning sickness

[45]. In Colorado, use of cannabis during pregnancy had a 50% increased likelihood of low birthweight [46]. The American College of Obstetricians and Gynecologists recommends screening women for drug use (including marijuana), counselling them about potential adverse health consequences, and discouraging marijuana use. Furthermore, they discourage use during breastfeeding due to the undetermined consequences on the child [47]. One study evaluating 50 breastfeeding women found measurable amounts of THC in breastmilk with a mean concentration of 9.47 ng/ml (range 1.01–323.00), with concentrations detectable up to 6 days after last reported marijuana use [48]. Another small cohort of eight women using smoked cannabis found concentrations ranging from 5.8 to 15.8 ng/ml from 20 minutes to 4 hours after discontinuing cannabis use for 24 hours [49]. It remains unclear the neurocognitive or other health impact of THC exposure in infants breastfeeding with these levels of THC exposure, along with the risk benefits of continued or cessation of breastfeeding.

Medical Use of Marijuana in the Pediatric Population

States with legalized marijuana for medical indications have varying regulations surrounding the use in the pediatric population. In Colorado, a minor and the primary parent must be Colorado resident, two board-certified physicians need to verify the need for medical marijuana, and then an application is submitted to the state for approval [50]. Certified conditions include cancer, glaucoma, HIV/AIDS, cachexia, persistent muscle spasms, seizures, severe nausea, severe pain, and post-traumatic stress disorder (PTSD). There are currently no rules or regulations on the type of practitioner; thus non-pediatric-trained medical professionals can recommend medical marijuana.

As of 2019, there are three Food and Drug Administration (FDA)-approved cannabis products in the USA. Dronabinol and Nabilone are synthetic THC that comes in an oral capsule or solution [3]. Dronabinol is a scheduled III controlled substance and Nabilone is schedule II. Both are indicated in pediatrics for chemotherapy-induced nausea and vomiting. Cannabidiol was recently FDA approved in 2018 for treatment refractory seizures from Dravet syndrome and Lennox-Gateaux syndrome [51]. All other cannabis products available in states that have legalized marijuana are not FDA approved and considered federally schedule I [52]. It is illegal to sell any cannabis (THC or CBD) product as hemp (THC < 0.3%) if it is not used for agricultural purposes. Cannabidiol and other marijuana and cannabinoid products cannot be marketed as dietary supplements [53]. These products are mostly unregulated and have been found with contaminants, inconsistencies or potency or content, or false claims [54, 55]. States who allow marijuana should have regulations to standardize practices on pesticide use, testing, and limitations for contaminants such as mold and heavy metals, shelf life duration, and other quality control measures.

In a systematic review of pediatric clinical trials using marijuana, there were only five randomized controlled trials, five retrospective chart reviews, five case reports, four open-label trials, two parent surveys, and one case series [3]. There was insufficient research to support use for spasticity, neuropathic pain, PTSD, and Tourette syndrome. Most research performed were severely limited in methodology, small sample size, poor design, and lack of standardization of marijuana products. These findings demonstrate the difficulties of performing research with marijuana in the regulatory setting of state legalization, while remaining a federally schedule I substance. Evaluating the efficacy in a vulnerable population such as pediatrics creates an additional barrier. There has also been increased use of CBD extracts in children with autism, with its use to alleviate symptoms associated with autism spectrum including psychosis, anxiety, and sleep. Current evidence is limited to in vivo/vitro studies and small human cohort studies with mixed results in improving behavioral outbreaks, rage, hyperactivity, sleep, and anxiety [56–60].

Summary

State legalization of marijuana in the USA has made a significant impact on many aspects of pediatric health. Unintentional pediatric exposures continue to rise, and there continues to be many unknowns regarding the impact of breastfeeding and passive smoke exposures. Evidence for the use of marijuana for many "allowed" medical conditions is limited, and more rigorous scientific research is needed to evaluate both the potential benefits and harms of use in the pediatric population. State and national regulatory and public health agencies must continue to advocate for rules and regulations that limit the impact on this vulnerable population.

Cannabis and the Teen Brain

Donald E. Greydanus and Maria Demma Cabral

Introduction

Adolescence is a critical period of biopsychosocial growth that begins with puberty and ends sometime in the third decade of life as formal adulthood commences [61–63]. As a general term, adolescence derives from the fifteenth century; also, as a term from the field of biology, it stems from the nineteenth century. Its development is multifactorial (i.e., physical, cognitive, moral, others) and is asynchronous.

As the child matures into an adult, numerous accomplishments are achieved that are termed "tasks of adolescence" based in part on the research of the twentieth-century Danish-German-American developmental psychologist, Erik Erikson

(1902–1994) [64]. These vital tasks include physical maturation, psychosocial maturation, independence (emancipation), and establishment of vital identities necessary for healthy adult functioning: sexual, vocational, social, and moral.

In the acquisition of a normal self at the end of adolescence, Erikson noted that this person should be in a normal process of emancipation and in a normal development (acquisition) of identify; as such this person understands who s/he is in relation to the world, has a normal sense of sexual identity, and also has a normal vocational identity. Another twentieth-century giant in the field of human development was the twentieth-century Swiss psychologist – Jean Piaget (1896–1980) – who taught many concepts including change in adolescents' concrete operational thinking to complex abstract thought [65].

Traditional classification of adolescence includes early, middle, and late adolescence that is driven by the critical development and maturation of the central nervous system (CNS). Studies from the late twentieth and early twenty-first centuries involving CNS magnetic resonance imaging (MRI) and PET scans have revealed increasing information on this CNS maturation – including that such changes are notably sensitive to various toxins which can induce irreversible CNS damage with major negative sequelae for the emerging adult [66, 67].

Early Adolescence

This period is usually from 10 to 13 years of age – though it can be earlier or later as it is driven by the initiation of puberty. The growing individual becomes preoccupied with these pubertal changes controlled by CNS maturation and typically becomes concerned with the normal question: "Am I normal with this rapidly changing body?" As these secondary sexual characteristics arise, the CNS develops concrete thinking skills ("here and now" cognitive skills) without appreciation for the future results of current actions.

As psychosocial changes arise, there can be emerging moral concepts, increasing need for privacy, heightened narcissistic thoughts, negative interactions with parents/guardians (reflecting ambivalence about independence), sexual orientation realization, and potential risk-taking behavior that includes sexual thoughts as well as potential sexual behavior and impulse control problems. CNS changes include growth of gray matter (unmyelinated cells) and others as noted below.

Middle Adolescence

This period is usually from 14 to 16 years of age with normal initiation of puberty leading to increasingly more adult-like secondary characteristics. This person becomes more interested in his/her peer group, is less focused on parents/guardians, and tends to have a more secure body image along with increased potential for high-risk behavior (i.e., sexual activity, drug experimentation, others).

Driving such transformations are continued dramatic CNS changes (maturation) leading to cognitive maturity (i.e., reality testing) and more complex reasoning abilities that are challenged by a false sense of invincibility as well as intensive impulsivity. There is a loss of some brain cells as the CNS prepares for adulthood with pruning of cells and intensification of brain connections such as seen in the prefrontal cortex (PFC); such maturation eventually allows for more understanding of "right versus wrong" and concern for the welfare of others versus only oneself. Such major CNS changes are vulnerable to various toxins with lifetime implications for the health and well-being of this person.

Late Adolescence

This period usually is from 17 years of age to young adulthood with normal initiation of puberty leading to establishment of "normal" independence from one's family, improved understanding of what the future holds, how to obtain needed education and/or experience, and an adult-like sexual identify. The "tasks of adolescence" are being obtained with continued CNS maturation that includes healthy myelination and proper brain development in key areas as the PFC to help this person navigate the complexities of adult life.

The PFC allows the person to achieve proper decision-making with mature logic/cognitive abilities, weigh consequences of one's actions, have mature executive functioning, and assume responsibility for one's actions. This allows the adolescent to change from concrete operational thinking to complex abstract thinking [65]. Such a vital maturation (i.e., the PFC) that usually finalizes in the early to mid-20s is needed for healthy functioning in the complex twenty-first-century milieu and is vulnerable to various toxins.

CNS Changes in Adolescence

The US NIMH Longitudinal Brain Imaging Project was launched in 1989 and has utilized MRI to provide ongoing imaging of children's and adolescents' brains without the potentially harmful effects of ionizing radiation [66]. Such a major research study allows growing data on the enormous CNS maturation that occurs in children and adolescents as they grow revealing increases in volumes of white matter throughout the brain as well as "U-shaped" changes in gray matter volumes in specific brain locations. This project continues to teach scientists and clinicians about the complex neuronal circuitry alternations that take place with pruning, changes in the suprachiasmatic nucleus of the anterior hypothalamus, and maturation of the PFC with resultant executive function emergence. Genetic and environmental factors are critical in this process for health and disease [66].

More information is being derived in the twenty-first century from the Human Connectome Project (HCP) which provides a 3D model of the brain with a Google

Maps-like guide of the human brain at different ages after initiating with young adults [67–69]. It is allowing unique understanding of the complex brain circuitry, mapping of brain connections, and brain links called the connectome. Again, we are learning the complexities of the human brain and how vulnerable it is to genetic and environmental factors including damage from various toxins.

Classic features of adolescence (i.e., emotional intensity as well as liability, need for risk-taking, novelty-seeking behavior among others) can be correlated with cerebral maturation characterized by profound changes in CNS neurochemical and molecular systems (models) that eventually lead to abilities to survive adulthood [70]. Changes in these profound neurobiological processes from toxins or other threats are dangerous for this person as they seek healthy adulthood [70]. This is also consistent with science data revealing that challenges to early brain development can result in later damage, as noted with research linking adverse experiences in early childhood (ACES) with increased risks for mental health problems (including substance use disorders) in adolescence and adulthood [71].

These complex patterns of brain connectivity in adolescence affect brain functionality at basic levels that have profound outcomes for this person in later life [72]. Axonal myelination by oligodendrocytes enhances neural conduction and neural communication. White matter continues to grow throughout adolescence into adulthood.

There are changes in CNS gray matter in primary sensorimotor areas, dorsolateral prefrontal cortex, and lateral temporal cortices. Critical, curvilinear changes in cortical volume occur in children, adolescents, and young adults with respect to brain cortical thickness and surface area as well as degree of cortical gyrification associated with such factors as age and sex of the person [73]. Sex differences also lead to puberty-induced differences in maturation of the medial temporal lobe that includes the amygdala and hippocampus; these are structures critical for long-term memory [74].

The well-known adolescent pursuit of high-risk behavior is based, in part, on the changing adolescent CNS system with an imbalance between reward and regulatory brain circuitry; the reward system involves the ventral medial PFC as well as the ventral striatum, while the control brakes are linked to the dorsal anterior cingulate cortex and the lateral PFC [75–78]. Damage to this system (i.e., PFC) from outside threats can be catastrophic for this youth, and the need for a healthy PFC with active, positive thought/logic processes is vital to successful life [79].

Mental illness can be found in all ages and involves various CNS structures, as, for example, seen with increased activation in the amygdala and insular cortex noted with anxiety disorders [80–82]. In addition to the amygdala's involvement in fear conditioning, the hippocampus is involved in contextual processing in anxiety and the extinction of fear responses in the PFC. Damage to these structures can be dangerous for children and youth with rapidly changing/maturing CNS.

Changes in white matter maturation in the right anterior callosum in males are linked with impulsivity – a classic feature of many adolescents [83]. Damage to the PFC in youth can lead to problematic decision-making linked with impulsivity and negative actions in youth leading to juvenile court evaluations [84]. Damage or injury to the anterior-medial PFC can lead to moral deficits in youth identified by researchers as early as 1948 and now in the twenty-first century as well based on functional magnetic resonance imaging (fMRI) research [85].

Changes in the nucleus accumbens and amygdala in youth lead to responses to reward processes; also involved in reward as well as stress processes are dopamine, opioid, glutamate, and GABAergic neurotransmitter systems in the CNS [61, 87–92]. Normal puberty stimulates CNS maturational changes that lead many adolescents to seek new dangers, new thrills, and new risk behaviors that can raise risks for dangerous motor vehicle accidents [86]. Many adolescents are programmed by puberty toward poor decision-making and impulsivity with potentially negative outcomes from sexual behavior, illicit drug use, unintentional injuries, and violence [87–90]. Thus, encouraging youth to experiment with various drugs is a dangerous concept.

Mental Illness in Youth

Substance use disorders (SUDs) contribute to the high prevalence of mental illness in the adolescent and adult populations [91, 92]. Anxiety disorders are found in 13% of children and adolescents, while mood disorders are seen in 6% of this population. Approximately 10% have disruptive disorders, while autism spectrum disorder is found in 2–6 per 1000, and schizophrenia is seen in approximately 1% or more of the general population of adults [91, 92].

In light of research identifying mental illness in at least 20% of adolescents and young adults, the influence of SUDs must be carefully considered with regard to the influence of these substances on the pediatric as well as adult populations. It can be difficult for the adolescent to avoid high-risk behaviors (i.e., drug use) because of CNS immaturity reducing the ability to delay gratification; individual variations, however, are found in this regard [93, 94]. The profoundly negative impact of cannabis consumption on youth is now considered.

Cannabis

As discussed elsewhere, the cannabis plant (*Cannabis sativa*; *C. indica*; *C. ruderalis*) contains >500 components including the 104 phytocannabinoids – the best known of which is THC or delta-9-tetrahydrocannabinol [95]. Though little is known about the health effects of these hundreds of chemicals in the cannabis plant, information is slowly emerging about the adverse effects of THC on human beings including the developing brain of the child, adolescent, and young adult.

Part of the negative effects of THC on the CNS is due to effects on the endocannabinoid system (ECS) which consists of CNS receptors (cannabinoid-1 [CB1] and cannabinoid-2 [CB2] receptors) and their endogenous ligands [95]. These ligands include anandamide and 2-AG (2-arachidonoyl glycerol). The physiologic interaction of anandamide and 2-AG on the CB1 and CB2 receptors is a normal function of the body [95–97]. The CB1 receptors are particularly found in the brain with the highest concentrations in such vital structures as the cerebral cortex, cerebellum, basal ganglia, and hippocampus. The CB2 receptors are predominantly found on immune cells and are involved with the immune system.

The interaction of the ligands (anandamide and 2-AG) with gamma-aminobutyric acid and glutamate neurotransmitter systems leads to important effect regarding moods (emotions), thinking ability (cognition), sleep, appetite, movement, and pain perception [96, 98]. THC interacts with the cannabinoid receptors inducing the classic cannabis euphoric effects and is part of the brain reward processes of the CNS that includes various neurotransmitter systems (i.e., GABAergic, dopamine, opioid, glutamate) and CNS regions (i.e., nucleus accumbens, cortex, amygdala) [95]. A common pathway of many drugs of abuse involves the altering of brain levels of endocannabinoids. Replacement of the normal ligands by THC with interactions with the cannabinoid receptors can lead to various adverse effects in the vulnerable, developing CNS of the child and adolescent.

Cannabis and Neurodevelopment Effects

Research studies in both animals and humans reveal that the brain has considerable neuronal plasticity and as such is potentially vulnerable to continuous contact with THC because of its effects on the cannabinoid receptors – replacing the endogenous normal endogenous ligands (i.e., anandamide and 2-AG) and causing its effects of euphoria as well as varying cognitive distortion/dysfunction of an acute and/or chronic nature [95, 99–105].

Cannabis and Pregnancy

Negative effects of cannabis on the developing brain are particularly noted in the perinatal/prenatal period and during early adolescence [61].

As considered elsewhere, exposure to exogenous cannabinoids via the mother smoking cannabis can lead to increased risks for neonatal complications (i.e., low birthweight, small for gestational age, neonatal intensive care unit management) and early childhood effects of executive function dysfunction with inattention difficulties, problem-solving issues, memory/processing dysfunction, depression, and/or aggression [61, 106–121].

Certainly, much more is needed to be understood in this regard including separating out various drugs consumed at the same time during pregnancy [61, 116]. However, clinicians, parents, and society must understand that smoking cannabis during pregnancy provides the highly vulnerable fetal brain to the first cannabis-induced "hit" of its ECS [121]. Women are strongly urged to avoid cannabis during pregnancy as well as before and after; this includes avoiding smoking cannabis during lactation as well [46, 49, 120–123].

Cannabis and Adolescence

Youth who start smoking cannabis during early adolescence and continue into adulthood have increased risks for cognitive dysfunction, psychosis, cannabis dependence, and continued use of additional illicit drugs [61, 101, 124, 125]. The actual effects depend on many factors, including the youth's genetics, potency of the THC, length of the years smoking cannabis, effects of other drugs, and other factors [61, 95].

As noted, cannabinoid receptors are widespread and plentiful in the CNS white matter in this age group, and continuous exposure to THC can lead to negative effects on these receptors that include damaged axonal fiber connectivity, altered CB1R signaling, potential short-term memory dysfunction via hippocampal changes, and increase risks for neurodevelopmental as well as neuropsychiatric conditions [102, 126].

This potential widespread CNS injury to vital and vulnerable neural tissue including the ECS can lead, over time, to interference with daily life activities in the home, school, work, and other milieu. Results can include additional drug use (polydrug dependence), depression, drop out of school and/or work activities, and evidence of widespread cognitive dysfunction [61, 102, 105].

More research is needed as various studies can differ in final results, research standards as well as protocols can vary, the acute versus chronic effects of cannabis consumption may not be clearly separated out, the potential variable of drug tolerance may not be considered, and other factors may emerge that prevent definitive as well as consistent conclusions from various studies [61, 103, 127–132].

Cannabis and ADHD

Many persons with attention-deficit/hyperactivity disorder (ADHD) are also cannabis smokers as noted by various studies [133–136]. For example, one study of 600 adolescents from 13 to 16 years of age receiving management for cannabis-related issues found that 38% had ADHD [135]. Though cannabis consumption can impair attention span, the preference for many with ADHD for cannabis smoking suggests ADHD and cannabis dependence reflect developmental conditions/disorders whose physiologic mechanisms have kindred or parallel natures [136, 137].

Attempts to self-medicate ADHD with cannabis represent an unhealthy, misguided solution to the triad difficulties of ADHD: impulsivity, hyperactivity, and limited attention span [95, 136, 138]. Some research concludes that persons with ADHD and SUDs have decreased density of striatal dopamine transporters in the CNS in comparison with those with ADHD but no comorbid SUDs [139, 140]. The impact of genetic influences in this regard remains understudy, and clinicians should understand that those with ADHD have an increased risk for a lifetime of cannabis use as well as use of other drugs [141–143].

Cannabis and Addiction

Youth smoking cannabis unknowingly face seriously negative CNS consequences because of the continuous distortion of the ECS by displacing normal ligands (i.e., anandamide and 2-AG) with THC along with direct damage to other critically important neurotransmitter systems (i.e., GABAergic, dopamine, glutamate, opioid) [92, 95, 96, 98, 144]. Dependence on cannabis and other drugs includes damage to the meso-accumbens reward circuitry and PFC dysfunction with fronto-striatal alteration [145–147].

Exposure, as noted, can begin in utero and continue in childhood, adolescence, and/or adulthood [92, 95, 120]. Chronic cannabis consumption can lead to classic cognitive dysfunction with varying negative effects on the exposed person – depending on many known and as of yet unknown factors (i.e., genetics, degree of THC concentration, exposure to other drugs, and others) [92, 95, 127, 148, 149].

Addiction to (dependence on) cannabis may occur and has been classified by the 2013 American Psychiatric Association's *Diagnostic and Statistical Manual of Mental Disorders, 5th Edition (DSM-5)* as cannabis-related disorders that include cannabis use disorder (CUD), cannabis intoxication, cannabis withdrawal, and others [149]. These disorders (CUD, cannabis intoxication, cannabis withdrawal) and their managements are considered elsewhere in this book [92, 95, 149–152].

With widespread legalization of recreational use of marijuana nationally and internationally, there will be notable increasing rates of young adult marijuana users with potential abusers particularly college students due to lower rates of perceived risk of use. This was demonstrated in one study done in Portland, OR, showing that patterns of marijuana use are impacted with changing public health policies [153].

Cannabis addiction (dependence) is identified in various rates in different groups [92, 95]. Some research has noted that approximately 9% of persons develop cannabis dependence in those utilizing this drug on a regular basis; approximately 17% of cannabis smokers who began smoking this drug as adolescents eventually become addicted to this drug, though a higher potential can be seen [92, 95, 154]. Complicating this scenario even further is that adolescents who use and/or have cannabis dependence also have increased risks for consuming other illicit drugs as well both as youth and as adults; this may occur in those with comorbid psychiatric conditions such as mood disorders [92, 95, 155–157]. Links of cannabis use and psychosis are considered below (vide infra).

Cannabis intoxication (poisoning) in a young child resulting in acute symptoms (i.e., altered consciousness, coma, and rarely death) from oral consumption is also discussed elsewhere in this text [6, 9, 95, 158–170]. Cannabis poisoning, however, can occur in any age from oral cannabis consumption [171].

Cannabis and Mood-Anxiety Disorders

Research suggests that adolescents consuming cannabis over time have an increased risk for mood disorders in their adult years – though there are various variables in such studies to make precise predictions in specific individuals quite difficult [92,

95, 172, 173]. The high rate of cannabis consumption by youth and young adults provides a worrisome stimulant for mood disorders over time [172]. Further research is needed in this area but clinicians caring for these age groups should be cognizant of such studies. Youth who consistently consume cannabis also have an increased risk for anxiety disorders as youth and adults; heavy use of cannabis is of particular concern in this regard [92, 95, 174, 175].

Cannabis and Psychosis

CNS damage from cannabis consumption also leads to an increased risk for psychosis in the adolescent and young adult [176–184]. Taken by susceptible persons at critically vulnerable periods in adolescence, cannabis smoking may induce prefrontal neurocircuitry abnormalities from dysfunction of glutamatergic transmission as well as disruption of the ECS; also, there can be volume loss of brain material in the prefrontal cortex, cingulate, cerebellum, and other CNS areas [92, 95, 176–178]. This risk for psychosis (two times or more) is also seen and increased with exposure to cannabis with high THC potency and with newer synthetic cannabis products [92, 95].

Susceptible youth who smoke cannabis may develop psychosis at a mean time of 7.0 ± 4.3 years between onset of cannabis use and onset of psychosis [180]. Most persons who smoke cannabis over time do not develop psychosis, and this may be due, in part, to the moderating effects of the cannabinoid and cannabidiol [185]. As research reveals, however, some youth and young adults are at increased risk for psychosis with continuous cannabis consumption [95, 129, 174, 186–195].

Adding to this disturbing dilemma is the concept that cannabis is commonly utilized by persons with schizophrenia (psychosis) perhaps, in part, to blunt negative features of psychosis such as depression and/or boredom [92, 95, 195]. Persons with psychosis who are smoking cannabis may develop paranoia and have increased risks for hospitalization versus those with psychosis not consuming cannabis [179, 183]. Persons with psychosis who smoke cannabis may not see improvement in the symptoms of psychosis after stopping the cannabis [196]. The dilemma of cannabis and psychosis is a traumatic phenomenon for all those involved in this vicious circle [91, 92, 95, 149, 183].

Summary

Adolescence is a critical period of biological-psychological-sociological changes in human life that influences much of the success or failure of adulthood [61–68]. The adolescent has a rapidly changing central nervous system that is very vulnerable to environmental toxins. Research over the past decades has revealed the potential CNS damage that exposure to cannabis may produce by interference with a normal ECS as well as other neurotransmitter systems (i.e., GABAergic, dopamine, opioid, glutamate) [95, 197].

The results of exposing the vulnerable CNS of children and adolescents to THC overtime can lead to variable levels of cognitive dysfunction, cannabis dependence, and neuropsychiatric disorders such as psychosis [91, 92, 95, 129, 135, 144, 149, 189]. Some youth become dependent on other illicit drugs as well. Prevention of such exposure is critical for the health of our youth as no level of cannabis use in youth is considered harmless; such measures of preventive medicine include education of society regarding these very real, research-based reasons for the strong recommendation to our children and youth about the avoidance of such dangerous drugs as cannabis [95, 197].

References

Cannabis and Young Pediatric Exposures

1. Wang GS. Pediatric concerns due to expanded cannabis use: unintended consequences of legalization. J Med Toxicol. 2017;13(1):88–105. PMID: 27139708.
2. Johnston LD, Miech RA, O'Malley PM, Bachman JG, Schulenberg JE, Patrick ME. Monitoring the future national survey results on drug use 1975–2018: overview, key findings on adolescent drug use. Ann Arbor: Institute for Social Research, University of Michigan; 2019.
3. Wong SS, Wilens TE. Medical cannabinoids in children and adolescents: a systematic review. Pediatrics. 2017;140(5):e20171818.
4. https://www.leafly.com/news/health/qualifying-conditions-for-medical-marijuana-by-state. Last accessed 1 Apr 2019.
5. Committee on Substance Abuse, Committee on Adolescence, Committee on Substance Abuse Committee on Adolescence. The impact of marijuana policies on youth: clinical, research, and legal update. Pediatrics. 2015;135(3):584–7.
6. Appelboam A, Oades PJ. Coma due to cannabis toxicity in an infant. Eur J Emerg Med. 2006;13(3):177–9.
7. Bonkowsky JL, Sarco D, Pomeroy SL. Ataxia and shaking in a 2-year-old girl: acute marijuana intoxication presenting as seizure. Pediatr Emerg Care. 2005;21(8):527–8.
8. Carstairs SD, Fujinaka MK, Keeney GE, Ly BT. Prolonged coma in a child due to hashish ingestion with quantitation of THC metabolites in urine. J Emerg Med. 2011;41(3):e69–71.
9. Macnab A, Anderson E, Susak L. Ingestion of cannabis: a cause of coma in children. Pediatr Emerg Care. 1989;5(4):238–9.
10. Weinberg D, Lande A, Hilton N, Kerns DL. Intoxication from accidental marijuana ingestion. Pediatrics. 1983;71(5):848–50.
11. http://www.ncsl.org/research/health/state-medical-marijuana-laws.aspx. Last accessed 1 Apr 2019.
12. https://www.justice.gov/archives/opa/blog/memorandum-selected-united-state-attorneys-investigations-and-prosecutions-states. Last accessed 2 Apr 2019.
13. Wang GS, Roosevelt G, Heard K. Pediatric marijuana exposures in a medical marijuana state. JAMA Pediatr. 2013;167(7):630–3.
14. Wang GS, Hoyte C, Roosevelt G, Heard K. The continued impact of marijuana legalization on unintentional pediatric exposures in Colorado. Clin Pediatr. 2018;5:114. https://doi.org/10.1177/0009922818805206.
15. Wang GS, Roosevelt G, Bucher-Bartelson B, Le Lait MC, Bronstein A, Heard K. Impact of decriminalizing marijuana on unintentional pediatric exposures in the US. Ann Emerg Med. 2014;63(6):684–9.

16. Thomas AA, Dickerson-Young T, Mazor S. Unintentional pediatric marijuana exposures at a tertiary care children's hospital in Washington state: a retrospective review. J Emerg Med. 2017;53(6):e119–23.
17. Bashqoy F, Heizer J, Reiter P, Wang GS, Borgelt L. Increased testing and health care costs for pediatric cannabis exposures. Pediatr Emerg Care. 2019. Epub ahead of print.
18. Richards JR, Smith NE, Moulin AK. Unintentional cannabis ingestion in children: a systematic review. J Pediatr. 2017;190:142–52.
19. Wang GS, Lelait MC, Deakyne S, Bronstein A, Bajaj L, Roosevelt G. Increase in unintentional pediatric exposures in a recreational marijuana state. JAMA Peds. 2016;170(9):e160971.
20. Noble MJ, Hedberg K, Hendrickson RG. Acute cannabis toxicity. Clin Toxicol (Phila). 2019;57(8):735–42.
21. Vo KT, Horng H, Li K, Ho RY, Wu AHB, Lynch KL, Smollin CG. Cannabis intoxication case series: the dangers of edibles containing tetrahydrocannabinol. Ann Emerg Med. 2018;71(3):306–13.
22. Nappe TM, Hoyte CO. Pediatric death due to myocarditis after exposure to cannabis. Clin Pract Cases Emerg Med. 2017;1(3):166–70.
23. Wang GS, Bourne DWA, Klawitter J, Sempio C, Chapman K, Knupp K, Wempe MF, Borgelt L, Christians U, Heard K, Bajaj L. Disposition of oral delta-9 tetrahydrocannabinol (THC) in children receiving cannabis extracts for epilepsy. Clin Toxicol (Phila). 2019;58:1–5.
24. Heizer J, Borgelt L, Bashqoy F, Wang GS, Reiter PD. Marijuana misadventures in children: exploration of a dose-response relationship and summary of clinical effects and outcomes. Pediatr Emerg Care. 2018;34(7):457–62.
25. https://marijuanapackaginglaws.com/. Last accessed 1 Apr 2019.
26. https://www.colorado.gov/pacific/marijuana/news/med-bulletin-new-packaging-and-labeling-rules-and-effective-dates. Last accessed 2 Apr 2019.
27. https://www.colorado.gov/marijuana/. Last accessed 2 Apr 2019.
28. https://lcb.wa.gov/laws/labeling-resources. Last accessed 1 Apr 2019.
29. https://www.oregon.gov/olcc/marijuana/pages/packaginglabelingpreapproval.aspx.   Last accessed 1 Apr 2019.
30. Breault HJ. Five years with 5 million child-resistant containers. Clin Toxicol. 1974;7(1):91–5.
31. Sibert JR, Craft AW, Jackson RH. Child-resistant packaging and accidental child poisoning. Lancet. 1977;2(8032):289–90.
32. Walton WW. An evaluation of the poison prevention packaging act. Pediatrics. 1982;69(3):363–70.
33. https://www.colorado.gov/pacific/marijuanahealthinfo/summary. Last accessed 24 Jun 2019.
34. Moir D, Rickert WS, Levasseur G, Larose Y, Maertens R, White P, Desjardins S. A comparison of mainstream and sidestream marijuana and tobacco cigarette smoke produced under two machine smoking conditions. Chem Res Toxicol. 2008;21(2):494–502.
35. https://www.cdc.gov/tobacco/data_statistics/fact_sheets/secondhand_smoke/health_effects/index.htm. Last accessed 2 Apr 2019.
36. Wilson KM, Torok MR, Wei B, Wang L, Robinson M, Sosnoff CS, Blount BC. Detecting biomarkers of secondhand marijuana smoke in young children. Pediatr Res. 2017;81(4):589–92.
37. Wilson KM, Torok MR, Wei B, Wang L, Lowary M, Blount BC. Marijuana and tobacco coexposure in hospitalized children. Pediatrics. 2018;142(6):e20180820.
38. Johnson AB, Wilson KM, Wang GS, Mistry RD. Prevalence and impact of second hand marijuana smoke exposure on Emergency Department visitation in children. Pediatric Academic Societies Annual Meeting. San Francisco. May 9, 2017.
39. El Marroun H, Tiemeier H, Jaddoe VW, Hofman A, Verhulst FC, van den Brink W, et al. Agreement between maternal cannabis use during pregnancy according to self-report and urinalysis in a population-based cohort: the generation R study. Eur Addict Res. 2011;17:37–43.
40. van Gelder MM, Reefhuis J, Caton AR, Werler MM, Druschel CM, Roeleveld N. Characteristics of pregnant illicit drug users and associations between cannabis use and

perinatal outcome in a population-based study. National Birth Defects Prevention Study. Drug Alcohol Depend. 2010;109:243–7.

41. Passey ME, Sanson-Fisher RW, D'Este CA, Stirling JM. Tobacco, alcohol and cannabis use during pregnancy: clustering of risks. Drug Alcohol Depend. 2014;134:44–50.

42. Beatty JR, Svikis DS, Ondersma SJ. Prevalence and perceived financial costs of marijuana versus tobacco use among urban low-income pregnant women. J Addict Res Ther. 2012;3:1000135.

43. Schempf AH, Strobino DM. Illicit drug use and adverse birth outcomes: is it drugs or context? J Urban Health. 2008;85:858–73.

44. Volkow ND, Han B, Compton WM, McCance-Katz EF. Self-reported medical and nonmedical cannabis use among pregnant women in the United States. JAMA. 2019;322(2):167–69.

45. Dickson B, Mansfield C, Maryam G, Allshouse A, Borgelt L, Sheeder J, Silver R, Metz T. Recommendations from cannabis dispensaries about first-trimester cannabis use. Obstet Gynecol. 2018;6(131):1031–8.

46. Crume TL, Juhl AL, Brooks-Russell A, Hall KE, Wymore E, Borgelt LM. Cannabis use during the perinatal period in a state with legalized recreational and medical marijuana: the association between maternal characteristics, breastfeeding patterns, and neonatal outcomes. J Pediatr. 2018;197:90–6.

47. https://www.acog.org/Clinical-Guidance-and-Publications/Committee-Opinions/Committee-on-Obstetric-Practice/Marijuana-Use-During-Pregnancy-and-Lactation?IsMobil eSet=false. Last accessed 2 Apr 2019.

48. Bertrand KA, Hanan NJ, Honerkamp-Smith G, Best BM, Chambers CD. Marijuana use by breastfeeding mothers and cannabinoid concentrations in breast milk. Pediatrics. 2018;142(3).

49. Baker T, Datta P, Rewers-Felkins K, Thompson H, Kallem RR, Hale TW. Transfer of inhaled cannabis into human breast Milk. Obstet Gynecol. 2018;131(5):783–8.

50. https://www.colorado.gov/pacific/marijuana/laws-and-youth. Last accessed 1 Apr 2019.

51. https://www.fda.gov/newsevents/newsroom/pressannouncements/ucm611046.htm. Last accessed 2 Apr 2019.

52. https://www.dea.gov/drug-scheduling. Last accessed 2 Apr 2019.

53. https://www.fda.gov/newsevents/publichealthfocus/ucm421168.htm. Last accessed 2 Apr 2019.

54. https://www.fda.gov/newsevents/publichealthfocus/ucm484109.htm. Last accessed 2 Apr 2019.

55. https://www.fda.gov/newsevents/newsroom/pressannouncements/ucm583295.htm. Last accessed 2 Apr 2019.

56. Barchel D, Stolar O, De-Haan T, Ziv-Baran T, Saban N, Fuchs DO, Koren G, Berkovitch M. Oral cannabidiol use in children with autism spectrum disorder to treat related symptoms and co-morbidities. Front Pharmacol. 2019;9:1521.

57. Aran A, Cassuto H, Lubotzky A, Wattad N, Hazan E. Brief report: cannabidiol-rich cannabis in children with autism spectrum disorder and severe behavioral problems-a retrospective feasibility study. J Autism Dev Disord. 2019;49(3):1284–8.

58. Karhson DS, Krasinska KM, Dallaire JA, Libove RA, Phillips JM, Chien AS, Garner JP, Hardan AY, Parker KJ. Plasma anandamide concentrations are lower in children with autism spectrum disorder. Mol Autism. 2018;9:18.

59. Pretzsch CM, Freyberg J, Voinescu B, Lythgoe D, Horder J, Mendez MA, Wichers R, Ajram L, Ivin G, Heasman M, Edden RAE, Williams S, Murphy DGM, Daly E, McAlonan GM. Effects of cannabidiol on brain excitation and inhibition systems; a randomised placebo-controlled single dose trial during magnetic resonance spectroscopy in adults with and without autism spectrum disorder. Neuropsychopharmacology. 2019;44(8):1398–405.

60. Wei D, Lee D, Cox CD, Karsten CA, Peñagarikano O, Geschwind DH, Gall CM, Piomelli D. Endocannabinoid signaling mediates oxytocin-driven social reward. Proc Natl Acad Sci U S A. 2015;112:14084.

Cannabis and the Teen Brain

61. Greydanus DE, Pratt HD, Patel DR, editors. Behavioral pediatrics. 4th ed. New York: Nova Science Publishers; 2015. p. 550.
62. Greydanus DE, Patel DR, Feucht C, Merrick J, editors. Adolescent medicine: pharmacotherapeutics in general, mental, and sexual health. Berlin: De Gruyter; 2012. p. 400.
63. Greydanus DE, Patel DR, Pratt HD, editors. Essential adolescent medicine. New York: McGraw-Hill; 2006. p. 600.
64. Erikson E. Childhood and Society. New York: WW Norton and Co.; 1950. p. 445.
65. Piaget J, Inhelder B. The growth of logical thinking from childhood to adolescence. New York: Basic Books; 1958.
66. Lenroot RK, Giedd JN. Brain development in children and adolescents: insights from anatomical magnetic resonance imaging. Neurosci Biobehav Rev. 2006;30(6):718–29.
67. Sporns O. The human connectome: origins and challenges. NeuroImage. 2013;80:53–61.
68. Glasser MF, Smith SM, Marcus DS, Andersson JL, Auerbach EJ, Behrens TE, et al. The human connectome project's neuroimaging approach. Nat Neurosci. 2016;19(9):1175–87.
69. Bookheimer SY, Salat DH, Terpstra M, Ances BM, Barch DM, Buckner RL, et al. The lifespan human connectome project in aging: an overview. NeuroImage. 2019;185:335–48.
70. Ernst M, Korelitz KE. Cerebral maturation in adolescence: behavioral vulnerability. Encéphale. 2009;35(Suppl 6):S182–9.
71. Attridge M, Ghali L. Linking early brain and biological development to psychiatry: introduction and symposia review. J Can Acad Child Adolesc Psychiatry. 2011;20(4):253–64.
72. Keulers EH, Goulas A, Jolles J, Stiers P. Maturation of task-induced brain activation and long range functional connectivity in adolescence revealed by multivariate pattern classification. NeuroImage. 2012;60(2):1250–65.
73. Raznahan A, Shaw P, Lalonde F, Stockman M, Wallace GL, Greenstein D, et al. How does your cortex grow? J Neuro Sci. 2011;31(19):7174–7.
74. Bramen JE, Hranilovich JA, Dahl RE, Forbes EE, Chen J, Toga AW, et al. Puberty influences medial temporal lobe and cortical gray matter maturation differently in boys than girls matched for sexual maturity. Cereb Cortex. 2011;21:636–46.
75. Van Leijenhorst L, Gunther Moor B, Op de Macks ZA, Rombouts SA, Westenberg PM, Crone EA. Adolescent risky decision-making: neurocognitive development of reward and control regions. NeuroImage. 2010;51(1):345–55.
76. Van Duijenvoorde AC, Op de Macks ZA, Overgaauw S, Gunther Moor B, Dahl RE, Crone EA. A cross-sectional and longitudinal analysis of reward-related brain activation: effects of age, pubertal stage, and reward sensitivity. Brain Cogn. 2014;89:3–14.
77. Qu Y, Galvan A, Fuligni AJ, Lieberman MD, Telzer EH. Longitudinal changes in prefrontal cortex activation underlie declines in adolescent risk taking. J Neurosci. 2015;35(32):11308–14.
78. Blankenstein NE, Schreuders E, Peper JS, Crone EA, van Duijenvoorde ACK. Individual differences in risk-taking tendencies modulate the neural processing of risky and ambiguous decision-making in adolescence. NeuroImage. 2018;172:663–73.
79. Shallice T, Cipolotti L. The prefrontal cortex and neurological impairments of active thought. Annu Rev Psychol. 2018;69:157–80.
80. Pine DS, et al. Functional magnetic response imaging and pediatric anxiety. J Am Acad Child Adolesc Psychiatry. 2008;47:1217–21.
81. Roozendaal B, McEwen BS, Chattarji S. Stress, memory and the amygdala. Nat Rev Neurosci. 2009;10(6):423–33.
82. Shin LM, Liberzon I. The neurocircuitry of fear, stress, and anxiety disorders. Neuropsychopharmacology. 2010;35:169–91.
83. Silveri MM, Rohan ML, Pimentel PJ, Gruber SA, Rosso IM, Yurgelun-Todd DA. Sex differences in the relationship between white matter microstructure and impulsivity in adolescents. Magn Reson Imaging. 2006;24(7):833–41.

84. Kambam P, Thompson C. Development of decision-making capacities in children and adolescents. Behav Sci Law. 2009;27(2):173–90.
85. Eslinger PJ, Robinson-Long M, Realmuto J, Moll J, deOliveira-Souza R, Tovar-Moll F, et al. Developmental frontal lobe imaging in moral judgment: Arthur Benton's enduring influence 60 years later. J Clin Exp Neuropsychol. 2009;31(2):158–69.
86. Dahl RE. Biological, developmental, and neurobehavioral factors relevant to adolescent driving risks. Am J Prev Med. 2008;35(3S):S278–84.
87. Casey BJ, Jones RM, Hare TA. The adolescent brain. Ann N Y Acad Sci. 2008;1124:111–26.
88. Geier CF. Adolescent cognitive control and reward processing: implications for risk taking and substance use. Horm Behav. 2013;64(2):333–42.
89. Fite JE, Goodnight JA, Bates JE, Dodge KA, Pettit GS. Adolescent aggression and social cognition in the context of personality impulsivity as a moderator of predictions from social information processing. Aggress Behav. 2008;34(5):511–20.
90. Romer D, Betancourt L, Giannetta JM, Brodsky NL, Farah M, Hurt H. Executive cognitive functions and impulsivity as correlates of risk taking and problem behavior in preadolescents. Neuropsychologia. 2009;47(13):2916–26.
91. Greydanus DE, Calles JL Jr, Patel DR, Nazeer A, Merrick J, editors. Clinical aspects of psychopharmacology in childhood and adolescence—second edition. New York: Nova Science Publishers; 2017. p. 325.
92. Greydanus DE, Kaplan G, Patel DR, Merrick J. Substance use disorders in adolescents and young adults: a manual for pediatric and primary care clinicians. New York: Nova Science Publishers; 2019. p. 420.
93. Romer D. Adolescent risk taking, impulsivity, and brain development: implications for prevention. Dev Psychobiol. 2010;52(3):263–76.
94. Romer D, Duckworth AL, Sznitman PS. Can adolescents learn self-control? Delay of gratification in the development of control over risk taking. Prev Sci. 2010;11(3):319–30.
95. Greydanus DE, Kaplan G, Baxter LE Sr, Patel DR, Feucht CL. Cannabis: the never-ending, nefarious nepenthe of the 21st century: what should be clinician know? Dis Mon. 2015;61(4):118–75.
96. Felder C, Dickason-Chesterfield A, Moore S. Cannabinoid biology, the search for new therapeutic targets. Mol Interv. 2006;6(3):149–61.
97. Malfitano AM, Basu S, Maresz K, Bifulco M, Dittel BN. What we know and do not know about the cannabinoid receptor 2 (CB2). Semin Immunol. 2014;26(5):369–79.
98. Fezza F, Bari M, Florio R, Talamonti E, Feole M, Maccarrone M. Endocannabinoids, related compounds and their metabolic routes. Molecules. 2014;19(11):17078–106.
99. Fattore L, Spano MS, Deiana S, Melis V, Cossu G, Fadda P, et al. An endocannabinoid mechanism in relapse to drug seeking: a review of animal studies and clinical perspectives. Brain Res Rev. 2007;53(1):1–16.
100. Dinieri JA, Hurd YL. Rat models of prenatal and adolescent cannabis exposure. Methods Mol Biol. 2012;829:231–42.
101. Schneider M. Puberty as a highly vulnerable developmental period for the consequences of cannabis exposure. Addict Biol. 2008;13(2):253–63.
102. Yücel M, Solowij N, Respondek C, Whittle S, Fornito A, Pantelis C, et al. Regional brain abnormalities associated with long-term heavy cannabis use. Arch Gen Psychiatry. 2008;65(6):694–701.
103. Harvey MA, Sellman JD, Porter RJ, Frampton CM. The relationship between non-acute adolescent cannabis use and cognition. Drug Alcohol Res. 2007;26(3):309–19.
104. Lichenstein SD, Musselman S, Shaw DS, Sitnick S, Forbes EE. Nucleus accumbens functional connectivity at age 20 is associated with trajectory of adolescent cannabis use and predicts psychosocial functioning in young adulthood. Addiction. 2017;112(11):1961–70.
105. Pacheco-Colón I, Limia JM, Gonzalez R. Nonacute effects of cannabis use on motivation and reward sensitivity in humans: a systemic review. Psychol Addict Behav. 2018;32(5):497–507.

106. Fried PA. Marihuana use by pregnant women and effects on offspring: an update. Neurotoxicol Teratol. 1982;4:451–4.
107. Goldschmidt L, Day NL, Richardson GA. Effects of prenatal marijuana exposure on child behavior problems at age 10. Neurotoxicol Teratol. 2000;22:325–36.
108. Gray KA, Day NL, Leech S, Richardson GA. Prenatal marijuana exposure: effect on child depressive symptoms at ten years of age. Neurotoxicol Teratol. 2005;27(3):439–48.
109. Goldschmidt L, Richardson GA, Willford J, Day NL. Prenatal marijuana exposure and intelligence test performance at age 6. J Am Acad Child Adolesc Psychiatry. 2008;47(3):254–63.
110. El Marroun H, Hudziak JJ, Tiemeier H, Creemers H, Steegers EA, Jaddoe VW, et al. Intrauterine cannabis exposure leads to more aggressive behavior and attention problems in 18-month-old girls. Drug Alcohol Depend. 2011;118(2–3):470–4.
111. Fried PA. Cannabis use during pregnancy: its effects on offspring from birth to young adulthood. Clin Dev Med. 2011;188:153–68.
112. Hayatbakhsh MR, Flenady VJ, Gibbons KS, Kingsbury AM, Hurrion E, Mamun AA, et al. Birth outcomes associated with cannabis use before and during pregnancy. Pediatr Res. 2012;71(2):215–9.
113. Jaques SC, Kingsbury A, Henshcke P, Chomchai C, Clews S, Falconer J, et al. Cannabis, the pregnant woman and her child: weeding out the myths. J Perinatol. 2014;34(6):417–24.
114. Grant KS, Petroff R, Isoherranen N, Stella N, Burbacher TM. Cannabis use during pregnancy: pharmacokinetics and effects of child development. Pharmacol Ther. 2018;182:133–51.
115. Henschke P. Cannabis: an ancient friend or foe: what works and doesn't work. Semin Fetal Neonatal Med. 2019;24(2):149–54.
116. Lamy S, Laqueille X, Thibaut F. Consequences of tobacco, cocaine and cannabis consumption during pregnancy on the pregnancy itself, on the newborn and on child development: a review. Encephale, 2015. 41(Suppl 1):S12–20. [French].
117. Schreiber S, Pick CG. Cannabis use during pregnancy: are we at the verge of defining a "fetal cannabis spectrum disorder"? Med Hypotheses. 2019;124:53–5.
118. Luke S, Hutcheon J, Kendall T. Cannabis use in pregnancy in British Columbia and selected birth outcomes. J Obstet Gynaecol Can 2019. pii: S1701-2163(18)30909-5. doi: https://doi.org/10.1016/j.jogc.2018.11.014.
119. Huizink AC. Prenatal cannabis exposure and infant outcomes: overview of studies. Prog Neuro-Psychopharmacol Biol Psychiatry. 2014;52:45–52.
120. Jansson LM, Jordan CJ, Velez JL. Perinatal marijuana use and the developing child. JAMA. 2018;320(6):545–6.
121. Richardson KA, Hester AK, McLemore GL. Prenatal cannabis exposure- the "first hit" to the endocannabinoid system. Neurotoxicol Teratol. 2016;58:5–14.
122. American College of Obstetricians and Gynecologists. Committee Opinion No. 722. Marijuana use during pregnancy and lactation. Obstet Gynecol. 2017;130:e205–9.
123. National Academies of Sciences, Engineering, and Medicine. Prenatal, perinatal and neonatal exposure to cannabis. In: The health effects of cannabis and cannabinoids: the current state of evidence and recommendations for research. Washington, D.C.: National Academies Press; 2017.
124. Ford TC, Hayley AC, Downey LA, Parrott AC. Cannabis: an overview of its adverse acute and chronic effects and its implications. Curr Drug Abuse Rev. 2017;10(1):6–18.
125. Chadi N, Levy S. What every pediatric gynecologist should know about marijuana use in adolescents. J Pediatr Adolesc Gynecol 2019. pii: S1083-3188(19)30167-6. doi: https://doi.org/10.1016/j.jpag.2019.03.004.
126. Caballero A, Tseng KY. Association of cannabis use during adolescence, prefrontal CB1 receptor signaling, and schizophrenia. Front Pharmacol. 2012;3:101–4.
127. Scott JC, Slomiak ST, Jones JD, Rosen AFG, Moore TM, Gur RC. Association of cannabis with cognitive functioning in adolescents and young adults: a systematic review and meta-analysis. JAMA Psychiatry. 2018;75(6):585–95.

128. Crippa JA, Lacerda AL, Amaro E, Busatto Filho G, Zuardi AW, Bressan RA. Brain effects of cannabis—neuroimaging findings. Rev Bras Psiquiatr. 2005;27(1):70–8.
129. Sundram S. Cannabis and neurodevelopment: implications for psychiatric disorders. Hum Psychopharmacol. 2006;21(4):245–54.
130. Martin-Santos F, Fagundo AB, Crippa JA, Atakan Z, Bhattacharyya S, Allen P, et al. Neuroimaging in cannabis use: a systemic review of the literature. Psychol Med. 2010;40(3):383–98.
131. Marmorstein NR, Iacono WG, McGue M. Associations between substance use disorders and major depression in parents and late adolescent-emerging adult offspring: an adoption study. Addiction. 2012;107(11):1965–73.
132. Colizzi M, Bhattacharyya S. Cannabis use and the development of tolerance: a systematic review. Neurosci Biobehav Rev. 2018;93:1–25.
133. Gordon SM, Tulak F, Troncale J. Prevalence and characteristics of adolescent patients with co-occurring ADHD and substance dependence. J Addict Dis. 2004;23:31–40.
134. Dennis M, Godley SH, Diamond G, Tims FM, Babor T, Donaldson J, et al. The cannabis youth treatment (CYT) study: main findings from two randomized trials. J Subst Abuse Treat. 2004;27(3):197–213.
135. Greydanus DE, Apple RA, Merrick J. Cannabis and ADHD: a Pandora's box of perpetual perplexity. Int J Child Health Hum Dev. 2017;10(2):1–3.
136. Brandt A, Rehm J, Lev-Ran S. Clinical correlates of cannabis use among individuals with attention deficit hyperactivity disorder. J Nerv Ment Dis. 2018;206(9):726–32.
137. Wallace AL, Wade NE, Hatcher KF, Lisdahl KM. Effects of cannabis use and subclinical ADHD symptomatology on attention based tasks in adolescents and young adults. Arch Clin Neuropsychol. 2018;26:34. https://doi.org/10.1093/arclin/acy080.
138. Fergusson DM, Boden JM. Cannabis use and adult ADHD symptoms. Drug Alcohol Depend. 2008;95(1–2):90–6.
139. Silva N Jr, Szobot CM, Shih MC, Hoexter MQ, Anselmi CE, Pechansky F. Searching for a neurobiological basis for self-medication theory in ADHD comorbid with substance use disorders: an in vivo study of dopamine transporters using (99m)Tc-TRODAT-1 SPECT. Clin Nucl Med. 2014;39(2):e129–34.
140. Pandolfo P, Vendruscolo LF, Sordi R, Takahkashi RN. Cannabinoid-induced conditional place preference in the spontaneously hypertensive rate-an animal model of attention deficit hyperactivity disorder. Psychopharmacology. 2009;205(2):319–26.
141. Distel MA, Vink JM, Bartels M, van Beijsterveldt CEM, Neale MC, Boomsma DI. Age moderates non-genetic influences on the initiation of cannabis use: a twin-sibling study in Dutch adolescents and young adults. Addiction. 2011;106(9):1658–66.
142. Soler Artigas M, Sánchez-Mora C, Rovira P, Richarte V, Garcia-Martínex I, Pagerols M, et al. Attention-deficit/hyperactivity disorder and lifetime cannabis use; genetic overlap and causality. Mol Psychiatry. 2019. https://doi.org/10.1038/s41380-018-0339-3.
143. Kolla NJ, van der Maas M, Toplak ME, Erickson PB, Mann RE, Seeley J, et al. Adult attention deficit hyperactivity disorder symptoms profiles and current problems with alcohol and cannabis: sex differences in a representative, population survey. BMC Psychiatry. 2016;16:50. https://doi.org/10.1186/s12888-016-0746-4.
144. Costentin J. Neuropsychopharmacology of delta-9-tetrahydrocannabinol. Ann Pharm Fr. 2008;66(4):219–31. [French].
145. Goldstein RZ, Volkow ND. Dysfunction of the prefrontal cortex in addiction: neuroimaging findings and clinical implications. Nat Rev Neurosci. 2011;12(11):652–69.
146. Goldstein RZ, Volkow ND. Drug addiction and its underlying neurobiological basis: neuroimaging evidence for the involvement of the frontal cortex. Am J Psychiatry. 2002;159(10):1642–52.
147. Feil J, Sheppard D, Fitzgerald PB, Yücel M, Lubman DI, Bradshaw JL. Addiction, compulsive drug seeking, and the role of frontostriatal mechanisms in regulating inhibitory control. Neurosci Biobehav Rev. 2010;35(2):248–75.

148. Bloomfield MA, Ashok AH, Volkow ND, Howes OD. The effects of Δ9-tetrahydrocannabinol on the dopamine system. Nature. 2016;539(7629):369–77.
149. American Psychiatric Association. Diagnostic and statistical manual of mental disorders, DSM-5. 5th ed. Washington, D.C.: American Psychiatric Association; 2013.
150. Brezing CA, Levin FR. The current state of pharmacological treatments for cannabis use disorder and withdrawal. Neuropsychopharmacology. 2018;43(1):173–94.
151. Patel J, Marwaha R. Cannabis use disorder. StatPearls [Internet]. Treasure Island: StatPearls Publishing; 2019.
152. Simpson AK, Magid V. Cannabis use disorder in adolescence. Child Adolesc Psychiatr Clin N Am. 2016;25(3):431–43.
153. Stormshak EA, Caruthers AS, Gau JM, Winter C. The impact of recreational marijuana legalization on rates of use and behavior: a 10-year comparison of two cohorts from high school to young adulthood. Psychol Addict Behav. 2019;33:595. https://doi.org/10.1037/adb0000508.
154. Freeman TP, Winstock AR. Examining the profile of high-potency cannabis and its association with severity of cannabis dependence. Psychol Med. 2015;45(15):3181–9.
155. Kmietowicz A. Teens who use cannabis show higher risk of taking other illicit drugs. BMJ. 2017;357:j2791. https://doi.org/10.1136/bmj.j2791.
156. De Luca MA, Di Chiara G, Cadoni C, Lecca D, Orsolini L, Papanti D, et al. Cannabis: epidemiological, neurobiological and psychopathological issues: an update. CNS Neurol Disord Drug Targets. 2017;16:598. https://doi.org/10.2174/1871527316666170413113246.
157. Lopez-Quintero C, Granja K, Hawes S, Duperrouzel JC, Pacheco-Colón I, Gonzalez R. Transition to drug co-use among adolescent cannabis users: the role of decision-making and mental health. Addict Behav. 2018;85:43–50.
158. Christozov C. The Moroccan aspect of cannabis poisoning from studies made in a psychiatric hospital for chronic diseases [article in French]. Maroc Med. 1965;44(483):630–42.
159. Debray H, Vidal F, Enjoiras M. Cannabis poisoning in a 13-month-old girl. Presse Med. 1987;16(36):1807.
160. Boros CA, Parsons DW, Zoanetti GD, Ketteridge D, Kennedy D. Cannabis cookies: a cause of coma. J Paediatr Child Health. 1996;32(2):194–5.
161. Spadari M, Glaizal M, Tichadou L, Blanc I, Drouet G, Aymard I, et al. Accidental cannabis poisoning in children: experience of the Marseille poison center. Presse Med. 2009;38(11):1563–7. [French].
162. Croche Santander B, Alonso Salas MT, Loscertales AM. Accidental cannabis poisoning in children: report of four cases in a tertiary care center from southern Spain. Arch Argent Pediatr. 2011;109(1):4–7. [Spanish].
163. Carstairs SD, Fujinaka MK, Keeney GE, Ly BT. Prolonged coma in a child due to hashish ingestion with quantification of THC metabolites in urine. J Emerg Med. 2011;41(3):e69–71.
164. Zarfin Y, Yefet E, Abozaid S, Nasser WM, Finkelstein Y. Infant with altered consciousness after cannabis passive inhalation. Child Abuse Negl. 2012;36(2):81–3.
165. Molly C, Mory O, Basset T, Patural H. Acute cannabis poisoning in a 10-month-old infant. Arch Pediatr. 2012;19(7):729–32.
166. Le Garrec S, Dauger S, Sachs P. Cannabis poisoning in children. Intensive Care Med. 2014;40(9):1494–5.
167. Pélissier F, Claudet I, Pélissier-Alicot AL, Franchitto N. Parental cannabis abuse and accidential intoxications in children: prevention by detecting neglectful situations and at-risk families. Pediatr Emerg Care. 2014;30(12):862–6.
168. Wang GS, Le Lait MC, Deakyne SJ, Bronstein AC, Bajaj L, Roosevelt G. Unintentional pediatric exposures to marijuana in Colorado, 2009-2015. JAMA Pediatr. 2016;170(9):e160971. https://doi.org/10.1001/jamapediatrics.2016.0971.
169. Pinedo-Painous I, Garrido-Romero R, Valls-Lafon A, Muñoz-Santanach D, Martínez-Sánchez L. Cannabis poisoning under the age of 3 years. Emergencias. 2018;30(6):408–11. [English, Spanish].

170. Noble MJ, Hedberg K, Hendrickson RG. Acute cannabis toxicity. Clin Toxicol (Phila). 2019;24:1–8. https://doi.org/10.1080/15563650.2018.1548708.
171. Zupan Mežnar A, Brvar M, Kralj G, Kovačič D. Accidental cannabis poisoning in the elderly. Wien Klin Wochenschr. 2016;128(Suppl 7):548–52.
172. Gobbi G, Atkin T, Zytynski T, Wang S, Askara S, Boruff J, et al. Association of cannabis use in adolescence and risk of depression, anxiety, and suicidality in young adulthood: a systemic review and meta-analysis. JAMA Psychiatry. 2019;76:426. https://doi.org/10.1001/jamapsychiatry.2018.4500.
173. Horwood LJ, Fergusson DM, Coffey C, Patton GC, Tait R, Smart D, et al. Cannabis and depression: an integrative data analysis of four Australasian cohorts. Drug Alcohol Depend. 2012;126(3):369–78.
174. Degenhardt L, Chiu WT, Sampson N, Kessler RC, Anthony JC, Angermeyer M, et al. Toward a global view of alcohol, tobacco, cannabis, ad cocaine use. Findings from the WHO World Mental Health Surveys. PLoS Med. 2008;5(7):e141. https://doi.org/10.1371/journal.pmed.0050141.
175. De Aquino JP, Sherif M, Radhakrishnan R, Cahill JD, Ranganathan M, D'Souza DC. The psychiatric consequences of cannabinoids. Clin Ther. 2018;40(9):1448–56.
176. Leweke FM, Koethe D. Cannabis and psychiatric disorders: it is not only addiction. Addict Biol. 2008;13(2):264–75.
177. Bossong MG, Niesink RJ. Adolescent brain maturation, the endogenous cannabinoid system, and the neurobiology of cannabis-induced schizophrenia. Prog Neurobiol. 2010;92(3):370–85.
178. Rapp C, Bugra H, Riecher-Rössler A, Borgwardt S. Effects of cannabis use on human brain structure in psychosis: a systematic review combining in vivo structural neuroimaging and post-mortem studies. Curr Pharm Des. 2012;18(32):5070–80.
179. Van Dijk D, Koeter MW, Hijman R, Kahn RS, van den Bring W. Effect of cannabis use on the course of schizophrenia in male patients: a prospective cohort study. Scizophr Res. 2012;137(1–3):50–7.
180. Galvez-Buccollini JA, Proal AC, Tomaselli V, Trachtenberg M, Coconcea C, Chun J, et al. Association between age at onset of psychosis and age at onset of cannabis use in non-affective psychosis. Schizophr Res. 2012;139(1–3):157–60.
181. Giovanni M, Giuseppe DI, Gianna S, Domenico DB, Luisa DR, Massimo DG. Cannabis use and psychosis: theme introduction. Curr Pharm Des. 2012;18(32):4991–8.
182. Decoster J, van Os J, Myin-Germeys I, De Hert M, van Winkel R. Genetic variation underlying psychosis-inducing effects of cannabis: critical review and future directions. Curr Pharm Des. 2012;18(32):5015–23.
183. Nazeer A, Calles JL Jr. Schizophrenia in children and adolescents. In: Greydanus DE, Calles Jr JL, Patel DR, Nazeer A, Merrick J, editors. Clinical aspects of psychopharmacology in childhood and adolescence. 2nd ed. New York: Nova Science Publishers Inc; 2017. p. 191–204.
184. Bagot KS, Chang A. Marijuana and psychosis: policy implications for treatment providers. J Am Acad Child Adolesc Psychiatry. 2018;57(8):613–4.
185. Zuardi AW, Crippa JA, Bhattacharyya S, Atakan Z, Martin-Santos R, et al. A critical review of the antipsychotic effects of Cannabidiol: 30 years of translational investigation. Curr Phar Des. 2012;18(32):5131–40.
186. Murray RM, De Forti M. Cannabis and psychosis: what degree of proof do we require? Biol Psychiatry. 2016;79(7):514–5.
187. Murray RM, Englund A, Abi-Dargham A, Lewis DA, Di Forti M, Davies C, et al. Cannabis-associated psychosis: neural substrate and clinical impact. Neuropharmacology. 2017;124:89–104.
188. Costentin J. Neurobiology of cannabis—recent data enlightening driving disturbances. Ann Pharm Fr. 2008;64(3):148–59.
189. Mizrahi R, Watts JJ, Tseng KY. Mechanisms contributing to cognitive deficits in cannabis users. Neuropharmacology. 2017;124:84–8. https://doi.org/10.1016/j.neuropharm.2017.04.018. Epub 14 Apr 2017.

190. Gomes FV, Rincón-Cortés M, Grace AA. Adolescence as a period of vulnerability and intervention in schizophrenia: insights from the MAM model. Neurosci Biobehav Rev. 2016;70:260–70.

191. Hamilton I. The need for health warnings about cannabis and psychosis. Lancet Psychiatry. 2016;3(4):322. https://doi.org/10.1016/S2215-0366(16)00086-9.

192. Nestoros JN, Vakonaki E, Tzatzarakis MN, Alegakis A, Skondras MD, Tsatsakis AM. Long lasting effects of chronic heavy cannabis abuse. Am J Addict. 2017;26(4):335–42.

193. D'Souza DC, Radhakrishnan R, Sherif M, Cortes-Briones J, Cahill J, Gupta S, et al. Cannabinoids and psychosis. Curr Pharm Des. 2016;22(42):6380–91.

194. Abush H, Ghose S, Van Enkevort EA, Clementz BA, Pearlson GD, Sweeney JA, et al. Associations between adolescent cannabis use and brain structure in psychosis. Psychiatry Res Neuroimaging. 2018;276:53–64.

195. Lev-Ran S, Aviram A, Braw Y, Nitzan U, Ratzoni G, Fennig S. Clinical correlates of cannabis use among adolescent psychiatric inpatients. Eur Psychiatry. 2012;27(6):470–5.

196. Barrowclough C, Emsley R, Eisner E, Beardmore R, Wykes T. Does change in cannabis use in established psychosis affect clinical outcome? Schizophr Bull. 2013;39(2):339–48.

197. Orr C, Spechler P, Cao Z, Albaugh M, Chaarani B, Mackey S, et al. Grey matter volume differences associated with extremely low levels of cannabis use in adolescence. J Neurosci. 2019;39(10):1817–27.

Chapter 6
Acute Emergency Department Presentations Related to Cannabis

Karen Randall, Brad Roberts, and John Cienki

Acute Marijuana Toxicity

The change in potency and methods of delivery during the time period of cannabis legalization has altered patient presentations seen with acute marijuana toxicity. Cannabis potency has dramatically increased [1]. Current commercialized cannabis is now over 20% tetrahydrocannabinol (THC), up from a concentration that was around 2% before 1990. This tenfold increase in potency does not take in to account other ways of using marijuana such as oils, edibles, waxes, and dabs, which can reach levels of 80–95% THC. These formulations are obtained when THC is extracted with a hydrocarbon solvent to create concentrated oils which can then be used in cooking to create edibles, further concentrated into waxes, and those waxes again heated and the vapor inhaled in the form of dabs. Vaping is able to generate higher drug potency and symptoms than smoking [2]. Edibles have been made to mimic products that people regularly consume such as chocolates or gummy bears. This gives a sense of safety that can lead to inadvertent overdose. First-pass metabolism often gives unpredictable onset of action. As a result, there has been a significant increase in the accidental exposure/overdoses, especially in children [3]. Young children and the elderly are more susceptible and frequently display more dramatic and life-threatening symptoms [4, 5].

K. Randall (✉)
Southern Colorado Emergency Medicine Associates, Pueblo, CO, USA

B. Roberts
Southern Colorado Emergency Medicine Associates, Pueblo, CO, USA

University of New Mexico, Albuquerque, NM, USA

J. Cienki
Jackson Memorial Hospital, Miami, FL, USA
e-mail: jcienki@jhsmiami.org

© Springer Nature Switzerland AG 2020
K. Finn (ed.), *Cannabis in Medicine*,
https://doi.org/10.1007/978-3-030-45968-0_6

Most common symptoms of acute toxicity continue to be psychologic: euphoria and disinhibition; anxiety, agitation; paranoid ideation; temporal slowing (a sense that time is passing very slowly, and/or the person is experiencing a rapid flow of ideas); impaired judgment; impaired reaction time; and auditory, visual, or tactile hallucinations with preserved orientation. However, presentations with increased severity of symptoms are rising [6]. Acute psychotic episodes after using high-potency THC and specifically "dabs" are well described [7, 8]. Mounting evidence suggest the risk of cannabis-induced psychosis is related to both dose and potency of tetrahydrocannabinol [9, 10]. Subjects with cannabis-induced psychosis had psychopathologic symptoms belonging to a neurotic profile (somatizations, obsessive-compulsive, interpersonal sensitivity, depression, anxiety, and phobic anxiety) than non-cannabis psychosis [11]. No literature exists to prove a superiority of benzodiazepines or antipsychotics to treat symptoms.

Cannabinoids are well-known to cause tachycardia. However other dysrhythmias including atrial fibrillation, ventricular tachycardia, and Brugada syndrome [12] have been attributed to marijuana [13, 14]. Multiple case reports exist of sudden cardiac death after smoking marijuana in previously healthy individuals [15]. The risk of acute myocardial infarction increases dramatically shortly after marijuana use independent of cardiovascular risk factors [16]. No literature exists to suggest a change in standard practice for managing these cardiac events. Marijuana has been associated with postural hypotension likely secondary to alterations of vasomotor reflex mechanisms [17].

Respiratory emergencies have been associated with the inhalation of combustion products of marijuana. Acute use can cause pneumothorax and pneumomediastinum especially in cigarette smokers [18, 19]. Recently, there have been reports of an increase in a vaping-associated pulmonary illness or EVALI in patient's vaping THC. The findings of pulmonary alveolar hemorrhage, neutrophil-predominant lavage, a reverse CD4/CD8 ratio, and organizing pneumonia in lung tissue biopsy specimens further support acute inhalational lung injury as the cause of this respiratory failure. Whether marijuana or the vaping process is causal, the provider needs to consider this diagnosis. It has also been postulated that unapproved pesticides, residual solvent contamination, additives with unknown inhalation effects, or heavy metal contamination inhaled from vaping can lead to lung injury [20].

Cannabis-Related Mental Health Disorders in the Emergency Department

Cannabis use has been associated with significant effects on mental health disorders. These disorders may include psychosis, depression, anxiety, suicide, and decrements in IQ, decision-making processes, social interactions, habits, and routines. These effects on mental health impact the emergency department, and states that have legalized recreational cannabis have seen increasing mental health visits related to cannabis use. This may affect emergency department overcrowding, cost of care, length of stay, and clinical provider job satisfaction [21–23].

Following cannabis legalization in Colorado, mental health visits with a marijuana-related billing code increased. A retrospective review reported Colorado Hospital Association hospitalizations and ED visits with marijuana-related billing codes. Between 2000 and 2015, hospitalization rates increased 116% from 274 to 593 per 100,000 hospitalizations. For primary diagnosis categories, the prevalence of mental illness was fivefold higher (5.07; 95% CI = 4.96–5.09) for ED visits and ninefold higher (9.67; 95% CI = 9.59–9.74) for hospital admissions for patients with marijuana-related billing codes compared to those without [24].

This increase in mental health visits had also been true for adolescents and young adults. A subsequent retrospective review by Wang et al. from 2005 to 2015 identified 4202 such visits for patients 13 to <21 years old to a tertiary care children's hospital system. Behavioral health evaluation was obtained for 2813 (67%), and a psychiatric diagnosis was made for the majority (71%) of the visits. ED/UC visits with cannabis-associated ICD codes or positive urine drug screens of all types increased almost 3 times from 1.8 per 1000 in 2009 to 4.9 per 1000 in 2015 (n = 161 in 2005 to 777 in 2015). Behavioral health consultations increased 2.7-fold from 1.2 per 1000 in 2009 to 3.2 per 1000 in 2015 (n = 84 in 2005 to 500 in 2015) [25].

These ED visits represent multiple diagnostic codes related to mental health. They correspond with changes seen on brain functional and structural MRI studies that correspond with mental health outcomes in cannabis users compared to nonusers [26–38]. They also correspond with changes to chemical neurotransmitters in the brain related to mental health with cannabis users compared to nonusers including disruptions in glutamate, dopamine, N-acetylaspartate, myoinositol, choline, and γ-aminobutyric acid (GABA) [39, 40]. These findings have been demonstrated in multiple epidemiological and observational studies. Common mental health emergency department presentations will be reviewed including acute psychosis with progression to schizophrenia, depression, anxiety, and suicidal ideation.

Acute Psychosis and Schizophrenia

Frequently, the acutely psychotic patients are brought to the ED for treatment and evaluation. Large reviews by the World Health Organization (WHO) and the National Academies of Sciences, Engineering, and Medicine (NASEM) have found substantial evidence of a statistical association between cannabis use and the development of schizophrenia or other psychoses, with the highest risk among the most frequent users [41, 42].

In a study of 45,570 Swedish men drafted into the military, the authors found that the men who had tried cannabis by age 18 were 2.4 times (95% CI = 1.8–3.3) more likely to be diagnosed with schizophrenia over the next 15 years than those who had not [43]. A follow-up study found a dose–response relationship between frequency of cannabis use at the age of 18 and the risk of schizophrenia. This effect persisted after controlling for confounding factors such as psychiatric diagnosis at enlistment, IQ score, personality variables concerned with interpersonal relationships, place of upbringing, paternal age, cigarette smoking, disturbed behaviors in childhood, history of alcohol misuse, family history of psychiatric illness, financial situation of the family, and father's occupation (the enlistment procedure included intelligence tests and non-anonymous self-reported questionnaires on family, social background, behavior during adolescence, and substance use – including first drug used, drug most commonly used, frequency of use, and direct questions regarding use of a list of specified drugs). The researchers estimated that 13% of cases of schizophrenia could have been averted if no one in the cohort had used cannabis [44]. These findings have been reproduced repeatedly and across the world [45–52].

In a double-blind, randomized, and counterbalanced study assessing behavioral, cognitive, and endocrine effects of THC, IV THC was administered at concentrations of 0, 2.5, and 5 mg in 22 healthy individuals. In all individuals in the study, IV THC produced transient effects of positive symptoms, negative symptoms, perceptual alterations, euphoria, anxiety, and deficits in working memory, recall, and the executive control of attention. The positive symptoms induced by THC included suspiciousness, paranoid and grandiose delusions, conceptual disorganization, and illusions. It also produced depersonalization, derealization, distorted sensory perceptions, altered body perception, feelings of unreality, and extreme slowing of time. Intravenous THC also produced negative symptoms which included blunted affect, reduced rapport, lack of spontaneity, psychomotor retardation, and emotional withdrawal. They concluded that THC produced a range of transient behavioral and cognitive effects in psychiatrically healthy individuals similar to those seen in schizophrenia and other endogenous psychoses [53].

Specific treatment for cannabis-induced psychosis has not yet been established. Current treatment is similar to other psychoses and consists of treatment with second-generation antipsychotics, benzodiazepines, and mood stabilizers [54]. However in a study in which patients were administered IV THC, haloperidol pretreatment to antagonize the psychotomimetic effects failed to ameliorate these effects, suggesting that the psychotic effects of THC are likely not mediated by the DA D2 receptor and that novel pharmacologic approaches will be needed [55]. It is the author's experience that both antipsychotics and benzodiazepines currently appear to be the most effective treatments until the acute effects of cannabis-induced psychosis have worn off. Early treatment strategies should minimize harm both to patients and staff and focus on adequate sedation, particularly when episodes may become violent. Caution should be taken to assess for rhabdomyolysis in cases in which patients have had prolonged restraint by EMS or police [56]. There are recent studies that may suggest treatment with cannabidiol (CBD) in chronic cannabis psychoses to be an effective treatment [57].

Depression

A large systematic review which ultimately reviewed 14 peer-reviewed studies for a total of 76,058 subjects found that the OR for cannabis users developing depression compared with controls was 1.17 [95% confidence interval (CI) 1.05–1.30]. The OR for heavy cannabis users developing depression was 1.62 (95% CI 1.21–2.16), compared with nonusers or light users [58]. A similar systematic review in the *Journal of the American Medical Association* reviewed 11 studies with 23,317 subjects and found similar results with the OR of developing depression for cannabis users in young adulthood compared with nonusers was 1.37 (95% CI 1.16–1.62; I2 = 0%) [59].

Anxiety

Frequent cannabis users consistently have a high prevalence of anxiety disorders, and patients with anxiety disorders have relatively high rates of cannabis use. However, it is unclear if cannabis use increases the risk of developing long-lasting anxiety disorders [60]. In general systematic reviews of cannabis use have demonstrated a minimal increase in anxiety disorders with an OR of 1.15 (95% CI 1.03–1.29). Cannabis use is likely only a minor risk factor for the development of elevated anxiety symptoms in the general population [61].

Suicide

Cannabis use has been correlated with an increased propensity for suicidal ideation, suicide attempts, and suicide completion. A literature review and meta-analysis found that any cannabis use had an OR of 1.43 (95% CI = 1.13–1.83) for suicidal ideation (OR = 2.53; 95% CI = 1.00–6.39 with heavy cannabis use). Suicide attempts had an OR = 2.23 (95% CI = 1.24–4.00) (OR = 3.20; 95% CI = 1.72–5.94) with heavy cannabis use. Suicide completion had an OR of 2.56; (95% CI = 1.25–5.27) for chronic cannabis use [62]. In Colorado, there was a 22% increase in the number of suicides (4822 suicides for 2004–2009 to 5880 for 2010–2015) following cannabis legalization, and the proportion of suicides with cannabis present in final toxicology rose by 5.5%. Following cannabis legalization in Colorado, there was a statistically significant 77.5% increase in the proportion of suicide victims with toxicology positive for marijuana for which toxicology data was reported [21].

Emergency providers need to ensure accurate substance abuse history, including cannabis, when assessing risk factors for depression, anxiety, and suicide. Patients should be advised to not use cannabis and informed regarding increased risk of these disorders with use. Emergency department management of these disorders remains similar to treatment of these disorders without cannabis involvement aside from informing patients of risk of exacerbation of symptoms with continued use.

Cannabinoid Hyperemesis Syndrome

Cannabinoid hyperemesis syndrome (CHS) symptoms include significant nausea, violent vomiting, and abdominal pain in the setting of chronic cannabis use. Cardinal diagnostic characteristics include regular cannabis use, cyclic nausea and vomiting, and compulsive hot baths or showers with resolution of symptoms after cessation of cannabis use [63]. CHS patients present similarly to cyclic vomiting syndrome patients with the exception that cannabis use is required to make the diagnosis. Following legalization of cannabis, the prevalence of cyclic vomiting presentations to the emergency department has increased [64]. From 2012 to 2016, there were 788 total cannabis gastrointestinal-related emergency department visits to a single hospital in Colorado, and the majority of these were for cannabinoid hyperemesis syndrome [65].

These patients often are evaluated with multiple imaging studies, lab work, endoscopies, and admissions to the hospital as well as antiemetic treatment. These studies are often nondiagnostic and treatment often ineffective [66]. Delayed diagnosis can lead to significantly increased overall cost of care, one study noting that on average the total combined cost for a single patient with multiple ED visits and radiological studies was $76,920.92. On average patients had 17.9 ED visits before the diagnosis of CHS was made [67]. Renal failure and electrolyte disturbances with cannabinoid hyperemesis syndrome have been reported [68]. Deaths attributable to cannabinoid hyperemesis syndrome, primarily secondary to renal and electrolyte disturbances, have also been reported [69].

Multiple treatment modalities for the acute symptoms CHS have been tried with varying degrees of success including topical capsaicin cream [70, 71], benzodiazepines [72], and haloperidol [73–75]. In general typical antiemetic treatments such as ondansetron, promethazine, prochlorperazine, metoclopramide, H2 blockers, or proton pump inhibitors are ineffective [76]. Chronic symptoms are best treated with cannabis cessation [63].

Acute Pulmonary and Cardiovascular Changes in the ED

There are known and emerging patterns of respiratory involvement. Chronic smoking, over time, produces a COPD-like presentation. Patients will present with wheezing, coughing, and prolonged expiratory phase. A recent small study in the *Radiology* journal showed that the act of just vaping alone impacts endothelial function in healthy nonsmokers [77].

There are many recent health advisories out that indicate a severe pulmonary disease associated with vaping. The cartridges of THC that are used in a vaping instrument are mixed with thickening substances. The thicker the concentrate, the better it is thought to be. Many of the THC concentrates have been mixed with vitamin E. A brief report in September of 2019 showed 53 affected individuals in Illinois and Wisconsin. The median age was 19 years. 32% underwent intubation. 84% specifically report using THC products [78]. This type of lung disease is being called e-cigarette/vaping-associated lung injury (EVALI). The substances associated with most EVALI cases recently reported are THC or THC + nicotine. At this time, the actual cause of acute pulmonary symptoms is not quite clear. There is thought that there are heavy metal contaminants, vitamin e contaminants, and other cutting products used in the THC vaping cartridges. Patients present with worsening cough, hypoxemia, and a vaping history. Other symptoms associated are cough (possible hemoptysis), pleuritic chest pain, fevers, night sweats, and possible vomiting and diarrhea. Health departments have listed criteria [79]: respiratory illness requiring hospitalization, poorly defined bilateral infiltrates on plain film or CT (ground-glass opacities), and absence of pulmonary infection on initial workup (negative influenza and viral panels). CBC may show a moderate leukocytosis. C-reactive protein may be mildly to moderately elevated. Findings in bronchoscope often show lipid-laden macrophages (pulmonary foam cells). Treatment for presumed EVALI is empiric antibiotics, supplemental oxygen, and steroids [80]. In a 1987 study, biopsies were performed on marijuana smokers, tobacco smokers, and nonsmokers. There was hyperplasia of goblet and basal cells in both marijuana and tobacco smokers. However here was greater hyperplasia of these cells in marijuana smokers, and cellular disorganization was present in over 50% of marijuana smokers. This was not noted in tobacco smokers. This was done during a time of lower-potency marijuana products [81].

Aspergillus fungi are frequently found on the marijuana plant. *Aspergillus fumigatus* is one known species. This has the additive risk in that it produces aflatoxins. These can survive for a long time on the cannabis plant and products (joints, blunts), as well as smoking items – bongs, rigs, etc. [82]. *Aspergillus* rarely causes illness in healthy individuals but can become life-threatening or cause death in those who are immunocompromised [83], with one known associated death being reported in California. Additionally, the aflatoxins produced by *Aspergillus fumigatus* can also have cardiovascular side effects. These include disruption of protein synthesis in myocytes, as well as disruption of mitochondria [84].

CB1 and CB2 receptors are activated by THC. CB1 receptors are located in the cardiovascular, central nervous system, and peripheral vasculature. THC causes an acute increase in blood pressure and heart rate [16]. There are numerous chemical additives to the THC being smoked/vaped ranging from heavy metals to pesticides/insecticides. Cardiovascular side effects such as transient hypertension, vasospasm, angina, sudden death, and arrhythmias have all been reported [85]. A review of the French Addictovigilance Network from 2006 to 2010 indicated that 1.8% of all cannabis-related reports (35/1979) were CV complications. Most were men (~85%) with an average age of about 34.3. There were 22 cardiac complications (20 acute coronary syndromes), 10 with peripheral vascular complications, and 3 with cerebral vascular complications. Nine led to death [86]. Cannabis-related cardiovascular complications increased from 1.1% in 2006 to 3.6% in 2010.

There is evidence from older literature from the 1970s which suggests that increased frequency of use led to increased risks for MI and cardiac arrhythmias [87, 88]. Again, literature from 2001 and 2009 suggests that the use of cannabis acutely increases the risks of myocardial infarction in younger patients [16, 89]. True incidence most likely is underreported and does not reflect the potency of marijuana products available currently.

Cannabis arteritis has also been described. This group of patients typically presents at a younger age than those with Buerger's disease [90] and the same clinical findings of peripheral vascular disease.

Finally, a brief mention of previously unreported findings. At least two cases of adult presentation of acute catatonia have been seen in a single ED. The patients were both adults over the age of 50 and had ingested a significant quantity of cannabis product (one was extract and one was THC butter). The patients both presented as a possible stroke. Workup was negative for both (including CT, MRI and labs), except each had a positive urine drug screen for cannabis. The patients were monitored. Ultimately in both cases, families mentioned a large ingestion of cannabis product. Patients were observed for a prolonged period of time and ultimately released to family members. No previous case reports exist for this phenomenon.

Emergency Department Sedations

The risk of sedation-anesthesia in cannabis users has been acknowledged since the 1970s [91]. Since that time, changes in ED utilization of sedation-anesthesia, as well as changes in cannabinoid use and concentration, necessitate an increased understanding of the potential complications.

Multiple case reports exist of patients suffering from significant respiratory distress due to isolated uvulitis, occurring after inhaling large quantities of cannabis within 6–12 hours of the onset of symptoms [92, 93]. Uvulitis is typically a disease of low incidence associated with infection or traumatic instrumentation of the airway. Care should be taken to examine the oropharynx in patients who are smoking marijuana prior to receiving sedation. Recommendations are that at the first signs of airway obstruction, dexamethasone should be used as the drug of choice, 1 mg/kg every 6–12 hours over the course of 1–2 days.

As a result of fat sequestration and subsequent slow elimination from the tissues, cannabinoids may be present to interact with multiple anesthetic agents long after last use. In a single-blind study, chronic marijuana users required significantly increased doses of propofol to facilitate successful insertion of the laryngeal mask, thus suggesting that chronic marijuana use may require larger doses to achieve sedation as well as airway reflex depression. Preclinical studies indicated that cannabinoids also prolong the action of some intravenous anesthetics such as pentobarbital, thiopental, and ketamine [94].

In a clinical trial in which patients were premedicated with THC, peak heart rate increased by 24.1% in surgical patients compared to those who did not receive surgery. In a randomized, double-blind trial, the patient population who underwent general anesthesia within 72 hours of marijuana use had a sustained postoperative tachycardia, a finding potentially due to an interaction between cannabinol metabolites and atropine administration during anesthesia. The authors thus concluded that THC may have a synergistic cardiovascular relationship with surgical stress [95]. This tachycardia has led to anesthesia recommendations that ketamine, pancuronium, atropine, and epinephrine, all drugs known to affect heart rate, should be avoided in patients with history of acute marijuana use.

With respect to muscle blockade, animal models show that cannabinoid administration decreased not only the release of acetylcholine at the neuromuscular junction but also the frequency and amplitude of miniature end-plate potentials [96]. Based on this premise, some authors inferred that cannabis may potentiate or prolong the effects of non-depolarizing neuromuscular blockers [97].

Often-cited literature reports on other synergistic effects of cannabis including potentiation of norepinephrine; the augmentation of any drug causing respiratory or cardiac depression, as well as a more profound response to inhaled anesthetics; and sensitization of the myocardium to catecholamines [98].

However much of the literature cites animal studies using isolated cannabinoids, each of which can have different effects and may even counteract each other. Human reports are almost all anecdotal. Complications from cannabinoid interactions can also vary between new and chronic users, amount and potency of marijuana, and time elapsed since last use. Therefore, caution should be taken when sedating any patient in the ED where cannabis use is suspected. Questions about illicit drug use should be a routine part of the preanesthetic assessment.

The rate of marijuana use via patient self-reporting was found to be 14% among surgical patients in 2003. This led the authors to conclude that, especially in patients that the anesthesiologist finds hard to settle, due to anxiety or other psychologic manifestations, care should be taken prior to anesthesia because of the potential anesthetic complications that may occur [99].

Conclusion

Much of the current literature reporting the harms of cannabis being seen in the emergency department is dated and involves low-potency cannabis products. As potency has increased and use is becoming more acceptable, the ED presentations are increasing in frequency and severity. Many of the acute issues include mental health, cannabinoid hyperemesis syndrome, respiratory and cardiovascular disease, and difficulties with conscious sedation. As the potency increases, emergency department visits for treatment of the acute side effects will also likely increase.

Costs related to the care of emergent presentations related to side effects of cannabis will continue to increase.

References

1. The health and social effects of non-medical cannabis use. 2016. http://apps.who.int/iris/bitstr eam/10665/251056/1/9789241510240-eng.pdf?ua=1.
2. Spindle TR, Cone EJ, Schlienz NJ. Acute effects of smoked and vaporized cannabis in healthy adults who infrequently use cannabis. A crossover trial. JAMA Netw Open. 2018;1(7):e184841.
3. Wang GS, et al. Unintentional pediatric exposures to marijuana in Colorado, 2009-2015. JAMA Pediatr. 2016;170(9):e160971.
4. Macnab A, Anderson E, Susak L. Ingestion of cannabis, a cause of coma in children. Pediatr Emerg Care. 1989;5:238–9.
5. Cao D, Srisuma S, Bronstein AC, Hoyate CO. Characterization of edible marijuana product exposures reported to United States poison centers. Clin Toxicol (Phila). 2016;54(9):840–6. Epub 15 Jul 2016.
6. Wang GS, Hall K, Vigil D, et al. Marijuana and acute health care contracts in Colorado. Prev Med. 2017;104:24–30.
7. DiForti M, Marconi A, Carra E, Fraietta S, Trotta A, Bonomo M, Bianconi F, Gardner-Sood P, et al. Proportion of patient in South London with first episode psychosis attributable to use of high potency cannabis: a case control study. Lancet Psychiatry. 2015;2(3):233–8.
8. Pierre JM, et al. Cannabis-induced psychosis associated with high potency "wax dabs". Schizophr Res. 2016;172:211–2.
9. Moore T, et al. Cannabis use and risk of psychotic or affective mental health outcomes: a systematic review. Lancet. 2007;370(9584):319–28.
10. DiForti M, Quattrone D. The contribution of cannabis use to variation in the incidence of psychotic disorder across Europe (EU-GEI): a multicentre case-control study. Lancet Psychiatry. 2019;6(5):427–36.
11. Rubioa G, Marin-Lozanod J, Ferreb F, Martinez-Grasa, et al. Psychopathologic differences between cannabis-induced psychoses and recent -onset primary psychoses with abuse of cannabis. Compr Psychiatry. 2012;53:1063–70.
12. Daccarett M, Freih M, Machado C. Acute cannabis intoxication mimicking brugada-like ST segment abnormalities. Int J Cardiol. 2007;119(2):235–6.
13. Aryana A, Williams MA. Marijuana as a trigger of cardiovascular events: speculation or scientific certainty. Int J Cardiol. 2007;118(2):141–4. Epub 26 Sep 2006.
14. Singh GK. Atrial fibrillation associated with marijuana use. Pediatr Cardiol. 2000;21(3):284.
15. Drummer OH, Gerostamoulos D, Woodford NW. Cannabis as a cause of death: a review. Forensic Sci Int. 2019;298:298–306. https://doi.org/10.1016/j.forsciint.2019.03.007. Epub 14 Mar 2019.
16. Mittleman MA, Lewis RA, Maclure M, Sherwood JB, Muller JE. Triggering myocardial infarction by marijuana. Circulation. 2001;103:2805–9.
17. Beaconsfield P, Ginsburg MA, Rainsbury R. Marihuana smoking – cardiovascular effects in man and possible mechanisms. NEJM. 1972;287:209–12.
18. Underner M, Urban T, Perriot J, Reiffer G, Harkia-Germaneau G, Jaafari N. Spontaneous pneumothorax and lung emphysema in cannabis users. Rev Pneumol Clin. 2018;74(6):400–15. https://doi.org/10.1016/j.pneumo.2018.06.003.
19. Weiss ZF, Gore S, Foderaro A. Pneumomediastinum in marijuana users: a retrospective review of 14 cases. BMJ Open Respir Res. 2019;6(1):e000391.
20. https://www.cdc.gov/mmwr/volumes/68/wr/mm6846e2.htm
21. Roberts BA. Legalized cannabis in Colorado emergency departments: a cautionary review of negative health and safety effects. West J Emerg Med. 2019;20(4):557–72.

22. Hall KE, Monte AA, Chang T, Fox J, Brevik C, Vigil DI, Van Dyke M, James KA. Mental health–related emergency department visits associated with cannabis in Colorado. Acad Emerg Med. 2018;25(5):526–37.
23. Salmore R, Finn K. The hidden costs of marijuana use in Colorado: one emergency department's experience. J Global Drug Policy Pract. 2016;10:1–26.
24. Wang GS, Hall K, Vigil D, Banerji S, Monte A, VanDyke M. Marijuana and acute health care contacts in Colorado. Prev Med. 2017;104:24–30.
25. Wang GS, Davies SD, Halmo LS, Sass A, Mistry RD. Impact of marijuana legalization in Colorado on adolescent emergency and urgent care visits. J Adolesc Health. 2018;63:239. Available online 30 Mar 2018.
26. Batalla A, Bhattacharyya S, Yücel M, Fusar-Poli P, Crippa JA, Nogué SS, Torrens M, Pujol J, Farré M, Martin-Santos R. Structural and functional imaging studies in chronic cannabis users: a systematic review of adolescent and adult findings. PLOS One. 2013;8(2):e55821.
27. Blanco-Hinojo L, Pujol J, Harrison BJ, Macià D, Batalla A, Nogué S, Torrens M, Farré M, Deus J, Martín-Santos R. Attenuated frontal and sensory inputs to the basal ganglia in cannabis users. Addict Biol. 2017;22(4):1036–47.
28. Cousijn J, Wiers RW, Ridderinkhof KR, van den Brink W, Veltman DJ, Goudriaan AE. Grey matter alterations associated with cannabis use: results of a VBM study in heavy cannabis users and healthy controls. NeuroImage. 2012;59(4):3845–51.
29. Camchong J, Lim KO, Kumra S. Adverse effects of cannabis on adolescent brain development: a longitudinal study. Cereb Cortex. 2017;27(3):1922–30.
30. Churchwell J, Lopez-Larson M, Yurgelun-Todd D. Altered frontal cortical volume and decision making in adolescent cannabis users. Front Psychol. 2010;1:225.
31. Filbey F, Yezhuvath U. Functional connectivity in inhibitory control networks and severity of cannabis use disorder. Am J Drug Alcohol Abuse. 2013;39(6):382–91.
32. Fischer AS, Whitfield-Gabrieli S, Roth RM, Brunette MF, Green AI. Impaired functional connectivity of brain reward circuitry in patients with schizophrenia and cannabis use disorder: effects of cannabis and THC. Schizophr Res. 2014;158(1):176–82.
33. Gruber SA, Yurgelun-Todd DA. Neuroimaging of marijuana smokers during inhibitory processing: a pilot investigation. Cogn Brain Res. 2005;23(1):107–18.
34. Lorenzetti V, Lubman DI, Whittle S, Solowij N, Yücel M. Structural MRI findings in long-term cannabis users: what do we know? Subst use Misuse. 2010;45(11):1787–808.
35. Rocchetti M, Crescini A, Borgwardt S, Caverzasi E, Politi P, Atakan Z, Fusar-Poli P. Is cannabis neurotoxic for the healthy brain? A meta-analytical review of structural brain alterations in non-psychotic users. Psychiatry Clin Neurosci. 2013;67(7):483–92.
36. Wrege J, Schmidt A, Walter A, Smieskova R, Bendfeldt K, Radue E, Lang U, Borgwardt S. Effects of cannabis on impulsivity: a systematic review of neuroimaging findings. Curr Pharm Des. 2014;20(13):2126.
37. Yücel M, Solowij N, Respondek C, Whittle S, Fornito A, Pantelis C, Lubman D. Regional brain abnormalities associated with long-term heavy cannabis use. Arch Gen Psychiatry. 2008;65(6):694–701.
38. Zalesky A, Solowij N, Yücel M, Lubman DI, Takagi M, Harding IH, Lorenzetti V, Wang R, Searle K, Pantelis C, et al. Effect of long-term cannabis use on axonal fibre connectivity. Brain. 2012;135(7):2245–55.
39. Colizzi M, McGuire P, Pertwee RG, Bhattacharyya S. Effect of cannabis on glutamate signalling in the brain: a systematic review of human and animal evidence. Neurosci Biobeh Rev. 2016;64:359–81.
40. Sami MB, Rabiner EA, Bhattacharyya S. Does cannabis affect dopaminergic signaling in the human brain? A systematic review of evidence to date. Eur Neuropsychopharmacol. 2015;25(8):1201–24.
41. National Academies of Sciences, Engineering, and Medicine. The health effects of cannabis and cannabinoids: current state of evidence and recommendations for research. Washington, D.C.: National Academies Press; 2017.

42. The health and social effects of non-medical cannabis use [Internet]. c2016 [cited 2016]. Available from: http://apps.who.int/iris/bitstream/10665/251056/1/9789241510240-eng. pdf?ua=1.
43. Andréasson S, Engström A, Allebeck P, Rydberg U. Cannabis and schizophrenia. A longitudinal study of Swedish conscripts. Lancet. 1987;330(8574):1483–6.
44. Zammit S, Allebeck P, Andreasson S, Lundberg I, Lewis G. Self reported cannabis use as a risk factor for schizophrenia in Swedish conscripts of 1969: historical cohort study. BMJ. 2002;325(7374):1199.
45. van Os J, Bak M, Hanssen M, Bijl RV, de Graaf R, Verdoux H. Cannabis use and psychosis: a longitudinal population-based study. Am J Epidemiol. 2002;156(4): 319–27.
46. Henquet C, Krabbendam L, Spauwen J, Kaplan C, Lieb R, Wittchen H, van Os J. Prospective cohort study of cannabis use, predisposition for psychosis, and psychotic symptoms in young people. BMJ. 2004;330(7481):11.
47. Arseneault L, Cannon M, Poulton R, Murray R, Caspi A, Moffitt TE. Cannabis use in adolescence and risk for adult psychosis: longitudinal prospective study. BMJ. 2002;325(7374): 1212–3.
48. Fergusson DM. Cannabis dependence and psychotic symptoms in young people. Psychol Med. 2003;33(1):15–21.
49. Stefanis NC, Dragovic M, Power BD, Jablensky A, Castle D, Morgan VA. The effect of drug use on the age at onset of psychotic disorders in an Australian cohort. Schizophr Res. 2014;156(2–3):211–6.
50. Moore TH, Zammit S, Lingford-Hughes A, Barnes TR, Jones PB, Burke M, Lewis G. Cannabis use and risk of psychotic or affective mental health outcomes: a systematic review. Lancet. 2007;370(9584):319–28.
51. Libuy N, Angel V, Ibáñez C. Risk of schizophrenia in marijuana users: findings from a nationwide sample of drug users in Chile. Natl Inst Drug Abuse. 2015.
52. Di Forti M, Sallis H, Allegri F, Trotta A, Ferraro L, Stilo SA, Marconi A, La Cascia C, Reis Marques T, Pariante C, et al. Daily use, especially of high-potency cannabis, drives the earlier onset of psychosis in cannabis users. Schizophr Bull. 2014;40(6):1509–17.
53. D'Souza DC, Perry E, MacDougall L, Ammerman Y, Cooper T, Wu Y, Braley G, Gueorguieva R, Krystal JH. The psychotomimetic effects of intravenous delta-9-tetrahydrocannabinol in healthy individuals: implications for psychosis. Neuropsychopharmacology. 2004;29(8):1558–72.
54. Gerlach J, Koret B, Geres N, Matic K, Prskalo-Cule D, Zadravec Vrbanc T, Lovretic V, Skopljak K, Matos T, Simunovic Filipcic I, et al. Clinical challenges in patients with first episode psychosis and cannabis use: mini-review and a case study. Psychiatr Danub. 2019;31 (Suppl 2):162–70.
55. D'Souza DC, Braley G, Blaise R, Vendetti M, Oliver S, Pittman B, Ranganathan M, Bhakta S, Zimolo Z, Cooper T, et al. Effects of haloperidol on the behavioral, subjective, cognitive, motor, and neuroendocrine effects of delta-9-tetrahydrocannabinol in humans. Psychopharmacology (Berl). 2008;198(4):587–603.
56. Strote J, Walsh M, Auerbach D, Burns T, Maher P. Medical conditions and restraint in patients experiencing excited delirium. Am J Emerg Med. 2014;32(9):1093–6.
57. Hahn B. The potential of cannabidiol treatment for cannabis users with recent-onset psychosis. Schizophr Bull. 2018;44(1):46–53.
58. Lev-Ran S, Roerecke M, Le Foll B, George TP, McKenzie K, Rehm J. The association between cannabis use and depression: a systematic review and meta-analysis of longitudinal studies. Psychol Med. 2014;44(4):797–810.
59. Gobbi G, Atkin T, Zytynski T, Wang S, Askari S, Boruff J, Ware M, Marmorstein N, Cipriani A, Dendukuri N, et al. Association of cannabis use in adolescence and risk of depression, anxiety, and suicidality in young adulthood: a systematic review and meta-analysis. JAMA Psychiatry. 2019;76(4):426–34.

60. Crippa JA, Zuardi AW, Martin-Santos R, Bhattacharyya S, Atakan Z, McGuire P, Fusar-Poli P. Cannabis and anxiety: a critical review of the evidence. Hum Psychopharmacol. 2009;24(7):515–23.
61. Twomey CD. Association of cannabis use with the development of elevated anxiety symptoms in the general population: a meta-analysis. J Epidemiol Community Health. 2017;71(8):811–6.
62. Borges G, Bagge CL, Orozco R. A literature review and meta-analyses of cannabis use and suicidality. J Affect Disord. 2016;195:63–74.
63. Sorensen C, DeSanto K, Borgelt L, Phillips K, Monte A. Cannabinoid hyperemesis syndrome: diagnosis, pathophysiology, and treatment – a systematic review. J Med Toxicol. 2017;13(1):71,71–87.
64. Hernandez JM, Paty J, Price IM. Cannabinoid hyperemesis syndrome presentation to the emergency department: a two-year multicentre retrospective chart review in a major urban area. CJEM.2018;20(4):550–55. https://doi.org/10.1017/cem.2017.381. Epub 2017 Aug 24.
65. Monte AA, Shelton SK, Mills E, Saben J, Hopkinson A, Sonn B, Devivo M, Chang T, Fox J, Brevik C, et al. Acute illness associated with cannabis use, by route of exposure: an observational study. Ann Intern Med. 2019;170:531.
66. Lapoint J, Meyer S, Yu CK, Koenig KL, Lev R, Thihalolipavan S, Staats K, Kahn CA. Cannabinoid hyperemesis syndrome: public health implications and a novel model treatment guideline. West J Emerg Med. 2017;19(2):380–6.
67. Zimmer DI, McCauley R, Konanki V, Dynako J, Zackariya N, Shariff F, Miller J, Binz S, Walsh M. Emergency department and radiological cost of delayed diagnosis of cannabinoid hyperemesis. J Addict. 2019;2019:1307345.
68. Habboushe J, Sedor J. Cannabinoid hyperemesis acute renal failure: a common sequela of cannabinoid hyperemesis syndrome. Am J Emerg Med. 2014;32(6):690.e1–2.
69. Nourbakhsh M, Miller A, Gofton J, Jones G, Adeagbo B. Cannabinoid hyperemesis syndrome: reports of fatal cases. J Forensic Sci. 2019;64(1):270–4.
70. Dezieck L, Hafez Z, Conicella A, Blohm E, O'Connor MJ, Schwarz ES, Mullins ME. Resolution of cannabis hyperemesis syndrome with topical capsaicin in the emergency department: a case series. Clin Toxicol (Phila). 2017;55(8):908–13.
71. Waterson Duncan R, Maguire M. Capsaicin topical in emergency department treatment of cannabinoid hyperemesis syndrome. Am J Emerg Med. 2017;35(12):1977–8.
72. Graham J, Barberio M, Wang GS. Capsaicin cream for treatment of cannabinoid hyperemesis syndrome in adolescents: a case series. Pediatrics. 2017;140(6). https://doi.org/10.1542/peds.2016.3795. Epub 9 Nov 2017.
73. Kheifets M, Karniel E, Landa D, Vons SA, Meridor K, Charach G. Resolution of cannabinoid hyperemesis syndrome with benzodiazepines: a case series. Isr Med Assoc J. 2019;21(6):404–7.
74. Witsil JC, Mycyk MB. Haloperidol, a novel treatment for cannabinoid hyperemesis syndrome. Am J Ther. 2017;24(1):e64–7.
75. Hickey JL, Witsil JC, Mycyk MB. Haloperidol for treatment of cannabinoid hyperemesis syndrome. Am J Emerg Med. 2013;31(6):1003.e5–6.
76. Inayat F, Virk HU, Ullah W, Hussain Q. Is haloperidol the wonder drug for cannabinoid hyperemesis syndrome? BMJ Case Rep. 2017. https://doi.org/10.1136/bcr-2016-218239.
77. Caporole A, Langham MC, Wensheng G, Joncola A, Chatterjee S, Wehrli F. Acute effects of electronic cigarette aerosol inhalation on vascular function detected at quantitative MRI. Radiology. 2019;293:97–106. https://pubs.rsna.org/10.1148/radiol.2019190562#d9977e1.
78. Layden J, Ghinai I, Pray I, Kimball A, et al. Pulmonary illness related to e-cigarette use in Illinois and Wisconsin - preliminary report. N Engl J Med. 2020;382:903–16. https://doi.org/10.1056/NEJMoa1911614.
79. State of California - Health and Human Services Agency, CA Dept of Public Health. Vaping associated pulmonary injury. 27 Aug 2019.
80. Farkas J. Vaping associated pulmonary injury. The internet book of critical care. 19 Aug 2019. emcrit.org/ibcc/vaping-associated-pulmonary-injury/.

81. Gong H, Fligiel S, Tashkin DP, Barbers RG. Tracheobronchial changes in habitual, heavy smokers of marijuana with and without tobacco. Am Rev Respir Dis. 1987;136:142–9.
82. Grotenhermen F. Cannabis and cannabinoids: pharmacology, toxicology, and therapeutic potential. Birmingham: The Hagworth Integrated Healing Process; 2002.
83. Hamadeh R, Ardehali A, Locksley RM, York MK. Fatal aspergillosis associated with smoking contaminated marijuana, in a marrow transplant recipient. Chest. 1988;94(2):432–3.
84. Bbosa GS, Lubega A, Kyegombe DB, Kitya D, Ogwal-Okeng J, Anokbonggo WW. Review of the biological and health effects of aflatoxins on body organs and body systems: INTECH Open Access Publisher; 2013.
85. Goyal H, Awad H, Ghali J. Role of cannabis in cardiovascular disorders. J Thorac Dis. 2017;9(7):2079–92.
86. Jouanjus E, Lapeyre-Mestre M, Micallef J, et al. Cannabis use: signal of increasing risk of serious cardiovascular disorders. J Am Heart Assoc. 2014;3:e000638.
87. Prakash R, Aronow WS, Warren M, Laverty W, Gottschalk LA. Effects of marijuana and placebo marijuana smoking on hemodynamics in coronary disease. Clin Pharmacol Ther. 1975;18:90–5.
88. Benowitz NL, Rosenberg J, Rogers W, Bachman J, Jones RT. Cardiovascular effects of intravenous delta-9-tetrahydrocannabinol: autonomic nervous mechanisms. Clin Pharmacol Ther. 1979;25:440–6.
89. Jouanjus E, Leymarie F, Tubery M, Lapeyre-Mestre M. Cannabis-related hospitalizations: unexpected serious events identified through hospital databases. Br J Clin Pharmacol. 2011;71:758–65.
90. Disdier P, Granel B, Serratrice J, Constans J, Michon-Pasturel U, Hachulla E, Conri C, Devulder B, Swiader L, Piquet P, Branchereau A, Jouglard J, Moulin G, Weiller PJ. Cannabis arteritis revisited - ten new case reports. Angiology. 2001;52:1–5.
91. Gregg JM, Campbell RL, Levin KJ, Ghia J, Elliott RA. Cardiovascular effects of cannabinol during oral surgery. Anesth Analg. 1976;55(2):203–13.
92. Gaurisco JL, Cheney ML, LeJeune FE, Reed HT. Isolated uvulitis secondary to marijuana use. Laryngoscope. 1988;98:1309–10.
93. Boyce SH, Quigley MA. Uvulitis and partial upper airway obstruction following cannabis inhalation. Emerg Med. 2002;14(1):106–8.
94. Frizza J, Chesher G, Jackson D, Malor R, Starmer G. The effect of delta 9 cannabidiol, and cannabinol on the anesthesia induced by various anaesthetic agents in mice. Psychopharmacology. 1977;55(1):103–7.
95. Gregg JM, Campbell RL, et al. Cardiovascular effects of cannabinol during oral surgery. Anesth Analg. 1976;55(2):203–13.
96. Sanchez-Pastor E, Trujillo X, Huerta M, Andrade F. Effects of cannabinoids on synaptic transmission i the frog neuromuscular junction. J Pharmacol Exp Ther. 2007;321(2):439–45.
97. Karam K, Abbasi S, Khan FA. Anaesthetic consideration in a cannabis addict. J Coll Physicians Surg Pak. 2015;25(suppl 1):S2–3.
98. Dickerson SJ. Cannabis and its effect on anesthesia. AANA J. 1980;48:526–8.
99. Mills PM, Penfold N. Cannabis abuse and anaesthesia. Anaesthesia. 2003;58:1125.

Chapter 7
Evidence of Cannabinoids in Pain

Peter R. Wilson and Sanjog Pangarkar

Evidence of Cannabinoids in Pain

Cannabinoids and opioids have had worldwide use for millennia. They were renowned for analgesic, sedative, and euphoriant properties. Both were typically smoked in individual or community settings such as opium dens and hash clubs. Both have come under legislative scrutiny in the United States and elsewhere [1]. Opioids are generally accepted as valid medical agents (DEA Schedule II), while marijuana is generally illegal (DEA Schedule I).

There is increasing interest in potential interactions between the two groups of drugs, raising the following complex questions [2, 3]:

1. Do opioids have limitations in their analgesic properties?
2. How addictive are opioids when used for analgesia short and long term?
3. What are the analgesic properties of the cannabinoids?
4. How addictive are the cannabinoids?
5. Are opioids and cannabinoids potentiators of each other's analgesia?
6. Do cannabinoids "protect" from opioid addiction?
7. Is there any role for "medical marijuana"?

P. R. Wilson (✉)
Pain Medicine, Mayo Clinic College of Medicine, Rochester, MN, USA

S. Pangarkar
Greater Los Angeles VA Healthcare Service, Department of Medicine, David Geffen School of Medicine at UCLA, Los Angeles, CA, USA

© Springer Nature Switzerland AG 2020   171
K. Finn (ed.), *Cannabis in Medicine*,
https://doi.org/10.1007/978-3-030-45968-0_7

1. Do Opioids Have Limitations in Their Analgesic Properties?

Opioids and opiates have a generally accepted clinical place in the comprehensive management of acute and cancer pain. Their effect is primarily from inhibiting neurotransmitter release and activating descending inhibition within the nervous system at multiple levels. Their pharmacology is well described in standard textbooks and is beyond the scope of this chapter [4]. When used for acute pain, opioids produce significant dose-dependent adverse effects including nausea and vomiting, urinary retention, respiratory depression, hyperalgesia, pruritis, acute tolerance, and chronic dependence. Opioids may have greater effect depending on patient genotype, physiology, route of administration, and the type of pain. There is usually no ceiling effect of these effects or adverse effects. However, clinical adverse effects may limit dosage.

A significant contributor to the misuse of opioids has been liberal prescribing practices related to acute pain. The longer the duration of the "acute" prescription, the more likely the subsequent misuse of the opioid medication. According to the Centers for Disease Control and Prevention (CDC) guideline [5], when opioids are used for acute pain, clinicians should prescribe the lowest effective dose of immediate-release opioids. They should prescribe no greater quantity than needed for the expected duration of pain severe enough to require opioids. Three days or less will often be sufficient; more than 7 days will rarely be needed according to the CDC. In 2016, Mudumbai et al. looked at postsurgical opioid use in US Veterans. The median duration for stopping opioids after surgery in opioid-naïve individuals was 15 days. For any patient on regular or intermittent opioids before surgery, the median day for stopping was much longer [6].

However, the role of opioids in the management of chronic and neuropathic pain is under increasing scrutiny [1]. Part of this renewed interest is the result of increasing knowledge and precision surrounding chronic and neuropathic pain.

Chronic pain was originally defined as pain that lasted for more than 3 months or beyond the normal healing time. This was found to be an inadequate categorization. Chronic pain has been subsequently recognized as a symptom or a disease by the IASP [7]. An issue of the journal *Pain* was dedicated to this (Volume 160, Number 1, January 2019). The IASP classification for chronic pain was expanded to include nine chronic categories for the purposes of inclusion in ICD-11.

- Chronic primary pain
- Chronic cancer-related pain
- Chronic postsurgical pain
- Chronic posttraumatic pain
- Chronic neuropathic pain
- Chronic secondary headache
- Chronic orofacial pain
- Chronic secondary visceral pain
- Chronic secondary musculoskeletal pain

This apparent heterogeneity of a previously simplistic diagnosis indicates that there can be no rational guideline for "chronic pain management." Therefore, no meaningful guidelines can be formulated for overall management of chronic pain.

The long-term use of opioids in chronic pain was generally believed to be safe and efficacious. The "opioid crisis" has focused attention and questions on this assumption [8–10]. There is increasing evidence that opioids may not be as effective for long-term use as previously believed. A recent systematic review and meta-analysis of opioids for chronic noncancer pain [11] concluded that opioid use was associated with statistically significant but only small but probably not meaningful clinical improvements in pain and physical functioning compared with placebo. Comparisons of opioids with non-opioid alternatives suggested that the benefit for pain and functioning may be similar for both approaches.

The data above refers to full opioid agonists. Partial agonists have a ceiling effect in both analgesia and adverse effects [4]. Their long-term use for pain conditions seems less well documented than for management of opioid misuse situations [12].

2. How Addictive Are Opioids when Used for Analgesia Short- and Long-Term?

A recent publication by the National Institute on Drug Abuse [13] stated that in the late 1990s pharmaceutical companies reassured the medical profession that patients would not become addicted to prescription opioid pain relievers. This is felt to be a major factor in increased prescription rates for opioids.

The NIDA stated in January 2019 that more than 130 people die each day in the United States after overdosing on opioids. These include prescription analgesics, but perhaps more importantly heroin and fentanyl.

Data that the NIDA published in January 2019 include the following:

- Roughly 21–29 percent of patients prescribed opioids for chronic pain misuse them.
- Between 8–12 percent develop an opioid use disorder.
- An estimated 4–6 percent who misuse prescription opioids transition to heroin.
- About 80 percent of people who use heroin first misused prescription opioids.

It should be noted, however, that these data are from individual publications, some retrospective, and not from reviews or meta-analyses. They should be interpreted with caution. Nevertheless, they might appear to have some medicolegal appeal in an adversarial situation.

It must be concluded that there is a real risk in prescribing and using opioids for chronic pain [14. 15].

The Guideline was carefully evaluated by a panel of pain medicine specialists under the auspices of the American Academy of Pain Medicine [16]. This panel commended the CDC clinical reminders to:

- Know that opioids are not first-line therapy for chronic pain
- Discuss risks, benefits, and availability of non-opioid treatments with patients
- Establish and measure goals for pain and function
- Emphasize patient-centeredness and individualized care
- Evaluate risk factors for opioid-related harms specific to the individual
- Avoid concurrent benzodiazepine and opioid prescribing
- Prescribe opioids only in needed quantities and durations
- Initiate opioids at the lowest effective dose with frequent follow-up and monitoring
- Ensure opioids, when indicated, are part of a comprehensive, multimodal pain treatment plan
- Use prescription drug monitoring programs and urine drug testing to monitor patient adherence to the treatment plan
- Reduce opioid dose or taper and discontinue if risks outweigh benefits or if benefits do not outweigh harms
- Arrange treatment for opioid use disorder if indicated

However, the panel noted some challenges in clinical and policy issues related to potential misapplication of the guidelines:

- Inflexible application of recommended ceiling or prescriptions as hard limits
- Abrupt opioid taper or cessation in physically dependent patients
- Lack of availability and coverage for recommended comprehensive multimodal care
- Difficulty of opioid use disorder diagnosis and barriers to treatment
- Underutilization of naloxone
- Incomplete data in reporting of overdose death statistics

As a result, the panel made several proposals (their Box A4) under five general headings:

- Appropriate opioid tapering
- Prescription dose and duration limits
- Toward comprehensive multimodal care
- Protecting patients from unintended consequences
- Toward naloxone and opioid use disorder treatment optimization

This panel report, if widely accepted, will take time to be tested and have results published. In the meantime, it should act as a valuable resource for practitioners contemplating the initiation or maintenance of long-term opioid therapy for chronic pain patients.

Prescribing guidelines for chronic opioids have been promulgated by numerous other entities, such as the Federation of State Medical Boards [17], Drug Enforcement Administration, Colorado Department of Regulatory Agencies [18], Veterans Administration/Department of Defense [19], and the Washington State Agency Medical Directors' Group [20]. These guidelines carry the same general message as the CDC – be cautious and document carefully.

It is just as important when discussing prescribing decisions as it is to discuss exit strategies [12]. It may become necessary to reduce, stabilize, transition, or discontinue opioid therapy for one or more reasons:

1. Failure to produce adequate analgesia
2. Development of tolerance
3. Development of physiologic dependence or pseudoaddiction
4. Development of unacceptable adverse effects
5. Evidence of misuse of opioids or other substances
6. Evidence of non-compliance with agreed-upon interventions (such as physical therapy, work hardening, urinalyses, etc.)
7. Problematic use of other substances (alcohol, cannabis)

The patient must not be abandoned but must have suitable transitions to alternative therapies, perhaps even under the care of a different healthcare provider.

3. What Are the Analgesic Properties of the Cannabinoids?

The US Department of Justice Drug Enforcement Administration was petitioned on December 17, 2009, for removal of marijuana from Schedule 1 of the Controlled Substances Act [21]. This Schedule contains drugs with no currently accepted medical use and a high potential for abuse. Some examples of Schedule I drugs are heroin, lysergic acid diethylamide (LSD), marijuana (cannabis), 3,4-methylenedioxymethamphetamine (ecstasy), methaqualone, peyote, and psilocybin.

This reschedule application was denied by a letter dated July 19, 2016. The Department considered the available literature and tabulated 11 reference papers in the report.

They tabulated the "five elements both necessary and sufficient to establish a prima facie case of currently accepted medical use":

- The drug's chemistry must be known and reproducible.
- There must be adequate safety studies.
- There must be adequate and well-controlled studies proving efficacy.
- The drug must be accepted by qualified experts.
- Scientific evidence must be widely available.

The FDA has not approved cannabis for the treatment of any disease or condition (FDA FAQ accessed 7/18/2019). It has approved Epidiolex® for certain seizures and Marinol® and Syndros® (dronabinol) for nausea and anorexia under certain conditions. Cesamet® (nabilone) is also approved.

This makes both animal and human studies very difficult in the United States.

However, Vučkovic and her colleagues recently published a comprehensive review of cannabinoids and pain with new insights from old molecules [22]. This followed several other reviews of clinical data [23–26].

- Pharmacodynamics
  These papers point out that cannabis and cannabinoids act on multiple pain targets. These include both central and peripheral targets, not only CB1/CB2 receptors but also GPCR55 and other GPCRs such as opioid and serotonin receptors. There are several nuclear receptors and transient receptor (TRPV1) channels which may interact. TRPV1 and CB1Or CB2 may be co-localized at peripheral and/or central neurons. Interaction between these receptors is being demonstrated as a component of pain modulation.
- Phytocannabinoids
  Although the main psychoactive component of the cannabis plant is delta-9-tetrahydrocannabinol, there are more than 100 different cannabinoids so far identified.
  Cannabidiol (CBD) is a non-psychoactive analog of THC, and the other main putative active compound. The FDA has approved this as Epidiolex® for treatment of two rare and severe forms of epilepsy (Lennox-Gastaut Syndrome (LGS) and Dravet Syndrome (DS)) [27].
  The FDA notes liver toxicity as a potential adverse effect of CBD. In controlled studies on Epidiolex®, the incidence of ALT elevation 3 times that of normal values was 13%, compared with 1% for placebo in patients with LGS and DS. As such, periodic LFT monitoring is suggested. The most common cause for discontinuing the medication was LFT elevations. Other common adverse reactions include somnolence, reduced appetite, diarrhea, fatigue, malaise, asthenia, rash, insomnia, sleep difficulty, and infection. At this time, there are no documented cases reported of fatal cannabis overdosage. It is clear that more and better clinical studies are needed to demonstrate whether CBD has clinically significant analgesic effects and to define adverse effect profiles.
- Endocannabinoid System
  Current evidence suggests that the CB1 and CB2 are involved in multiple regulatory functions:

  - Learning and memory
  - Mood and anxiety
  - Drug addiction
  - Feeding behavior
  - Modulation of pain and certain cardiovascular functions

  The CB1 receptor is localized in regions of the peripheral and central nervous systems where pain signaling, transmission, and modulation occur.
  The CB2 receptor is predominantly peripheral and appear to inhibit cytokine/chemokine inflammatory processes. It may also stimulate the release of beta-endorphin from keratinocytes.
- Synthetic Cannabinoids
  Dronabinol is the oral preparation of THC. It is approved for nausea and vomiting associated with chemotherapy and anorexia associated with AIDS.
  Nabilone is a synthetic structural analog of THC, with similar approved indications. However, studies of these have shown minimal, if any benefit in reducing morbidity or mortality [28].

The off-label use of these medications for pain management is likely to be expensive and ineffective. No reliable data exist.

- Cannabinoids in Animal Models of Pain
  Animal data show that cannabinoids are effective in some models of acute/nociceptive pain, chronic neuropathic pain, and chronic inflammation. Certain animal cancer pain models also suggest cannabinoid efficacy. On the other hand, Delta-9-THC has been shown to preferentially increase dopamine transmission in the shell of the nucleus accumbens, similar to heroin [29]. Though this observation was found Sprague-Dawley rats, it suggests activation of dopamine transmission may be involved in Delta-9-THCs affective and motivational properties. In addition, activation of specific cannabinoid receptors may activate dopamine transmission in the nucleus accumbens through activation of an endogenous opioid system affecting Mu1 opioid receptors of the ventral tegmental area. Neuroimaging studies have suggested hypodopaminergia with regular cannabis use, which may reduce reward sensitivity and amotivation [30].
  It has been difficult to translate animal data to the clinical situation.

- Cannabinoids in Clinical Pain Research and Therapy
  It is expected that human volunteer subjects will respond to experimental pain stimuli quite differently than patients with diagnosable pathological pain generators, whether acute or chronic [31]. Of note, endogenous opioids, endocannabinoids, and dopamine transmission may be involved in the placebo effect. Enhanced dopamine release in the nucleus accumbens correlated to placebo responsiveness and financial reward [32]. More recent evidence suggests that the endocannabinoid system and the endogenous opioid system contribute to analgesic placebo response [33].

- Cannabinoids and Acute Clinical Pain
  Data are presently inconclusive on the efficacy of cannabinoids in acute clinical pain, whether postoperative or traumatic [34]. There may be a window of efficacy, with "moderate" doses being somewhat effective.
  There is evidence that chronic cannabinoid use increases opioid requirements after polytrauma [34].

- Cannabinoids and Clinical Neuropathic Pain
  Several systematic reviews of cannabinoids and neuropathic pain have shown moderate strength evidence of potential benefit, but better research is necessary to clearly define dose-response characteristics [35, 36].

- Nabiximols (Trade Name Sativex) and Cancer Pain
  Sativex (50% THC, 50% CBD) had been thought to improve pain in advanced cancer and to be associated with decreased opioid use. However, data are presently inconclusive. Sativex has failed two Phase III clinical trials in cancer pain patients who maximized opioids [37].

- Cannabis and Chronic Pain
  Although cannabis appears to be widely used for chronic pain management, there is often little medical input [37, 38]. There are a few data supporting cannabis safety and efficacy, despite more than 30 US states enacting "medical marijuana" legislation [39]. This deficit is widely recognized [40].

- Cannabis is rarely the first drug chosen by the patient for the management of pain. Pain can obviously occur in chronic cannabis users, who revert to usual medical pain management.

  It was also hoped that medical marijuana legislation would produce a reduction in community use of prescribed opioids [41]. This has not become evident. It was also hoped that the legalization of recreational marijuana would mitigate the opioid crisis. This has also not occurred [42]. The data showed that in 2017, among 70,237 drug overdose deaths, 47,600 (67.8%) involved opioids. From 2013 to 2017, synthetic opioids (heroin and illegally manufactured fentanyl) contributed to increases in drug overdose death rates in several states, including Washington and Colorado.

4. How Addictive Are the Cannabinoids?

Cannabis use disorder is a diagnosis in DSM-5 under Substance-Related and Addictive Disorders. DSM-5 eliminated Cannabis Abuse and Cannabis Dependence in lieu of a single category, which includes all of the problems previously discussed in the separate categories. The diagnosis is made by defining at least 2 of 11 criteria occurring within a 12-month period. Further, the severity of the problem can be indicated as mild, moderate, or severe, based on the number of symptoms exhibited.

It is worth noting that as potency of cannabis products has increased, so has progression to cannabis use disorders [43]. For further details, please refer to the corresponding chapter in this book.

5. Do Cannabinoids and Opioids Potentiate Each Other's Analgesia?

A multi-institutional pilot study of marijuana uses and acute pain management following traumatic injury suggested that marijuana use may affect pain response to injury by requiring greater use of opioid analgesia. This effect was less pronounced with other drugs [34].

6. Do Cannabinoids "Protect" Users from Opioid Addiction?

This question has been difficult to address for reasons given earlier. The definitive review of the current state of knowledge appears as a draft dated June18, 2019, by Larkin PJ and Madras BK [2].

Individuals using marijuana for pain relief do not exhibit a reduction or elimination of opioid use [2]. Indeed, there is some evidence that cannabis users increase their opioid use without obtaining increased pain relief. In another study cannabis users appeared to be at increased risk of prescription opioid misuse [38].

In addition, the concomitant use of marijuana and opioids appears to interfere with treatment of opioid use disorder [44, 45].

7. Is There Any Role for "Medical Marijuana"?

The DEA is unequivocal that marijuana cannot be considered a drug under its charter [21]. The reasons are many and include:

- No smoked substance can be considered a drug.
- No plant can be considered a drug.
- Active ingredients cannot be defined or quantitated.
- It is a Schedule I substance.

Smoking the plant delivers active compounds and contaminants rapidly, avoiding a first pass effect. Pulmonary absorption depends on numerous individual factors which might include:

- Volume of smoke/aspirate
- Depth of inspiration
- Duration of inspiratory hold

These obviously cannot be standardized from one individual to another.

Because of the issues listed above and elsewhere in this paper, it does appear that the science presently fails to support the concept of "medical marijuana" [46].

Nevertheless, as noted above, more than 30 states have enacted "medical marijuana" or "medical cannabis" statutes. For example, Washington State [47] defines qualifying conditions for cannabis authorization as:

- Cancer, HIV, multiple sclerosis, epilepsy or other seizure disorder, or spasticity disorders.
- Intractable pain, limited for the purpose of this chapter to mean pain unrelieved by standard medical treatments or medications
- Glaucoma
- Crohn's disease
- Hepatitis C with debilitating nausea or intractable pain
- Diseases, including anorexia
- Chronic renal failure requiring hemodialysis
- Posttraumatic stress disorder
- Traumatic brain injury

Practitioners in Washington State who may authorize medical marijuana are defined as:

- Medical doctor (MD)
- Physician assistant (PA)
- Osteopathic physician (DO)
- Osteopathic physician assistant (DOA)
- Naturopathic physician
- Advanced registered nurse practitioner

Guidelines for documentation before authorization should include:

- Complete health history
- Comorbidities
- History of substance abuse
- Complete physical examination
- Review of medications
- Written treatment plan
- Treatment options
- Determination of need for marijuana
- Risks of marijuana
- Periodic reevaluation
- Maintenance of health records
- Written consent

Such requirements are consistent with prescribing regulations and practice guidelines for opioids. They should surely discourage both "pill mills" and "pot shops." Time will tell, but more than 39,000 medical marijuana cards have been issued to Washington state residents by April 25, 2019. There seem to be no data on the impact on any aspect of public health of this legislation. Opioid prescriptions and overdoses have continued to rise nationally [42] in an apparently inexorable manner, with no respite from either recreational or medical marijuana legislation.

The role of patient advocacy groups in the opioid/cannabis crisis is unclear. There was no question that these groups were strong supporters of the concept of pain as the "fifth vital sign" [48]. They also helped improve access to opioids for acute, chronic, and terminal pain. There is a question, reflected in opioid overdose mortality data, that the pendulum might have swung too far in the direction of permissive prescribing of opioids [48, 49]. Again, there are few data available.

The American Chronic Pain Association (www.theapca.org) has published a thoughtful, scientifically valid informational booklet for patients and, I hope, providers. It contains a very useful section on opioids (pp. 75–102). This should be required reading for patients and prescribers of opioids [3].

Summary

Cannabis and opiates have been used for millennia for their euphoriant effects. However, with the advent of cannabinoids and opioids within the last century, there has been increasing attention paid to the putative analgesic effects.

Cannabis use disorder has increased in the United States. Many states (but not the federal government) have enabling legislation. Growth of more potent strains of cannabis has increased. Cannabis itself does not produce analgesia and paradoxically might interfere with opioid analgesia. Cannabis users have been shown to increase their opioid use without an increase in analgesia.

Opiates and opioids have physiological effects, including analgesia, respiratory depression, nausea and vomiting, hyperalgesia, pruritis, and tolerance and dependence. These effects are of relatively minor significance and controllable in acute use for analgesia. However, when tolerance and dependence occur, the analgesic effect is also reduced, and adverse effects become more important.

Opioid use disorder and overdosage have become significant public health problems in the United States. There are opioid prescribing guidelines at federal and state levels. Despite these, opioid overdoses account for nearly 70% of drug overdose deaths (47,600 in 2017). A significant proportion of these individuals were first exposed to prescription opioids.

It is clear that there needs to be more basic research on cannabinoids and opioids. It is also clear that the clinical use of these chemicals should be based on a more rational scientific basis than is available at present.

This chapter cannot address the particular medicolegal circumstances in each state. Each practitioner who has prescribing or authorizing capability for cannabinoids and/or opioids must conform to their own state guidelines. It must be recognized that cannabis is a federal Schedule I substance and illegal in that jurisdiction. State guidelines might therefore be in conflict with federal guidelines.

References

1. Gebhart GF. Intellectual milestones in our understanding and treatment of pain. In: Ballantyne JC, Fishman SM, Rathmell JP, editors. Bonica's management of pain. 5th ed. Philadelphia: Wolters Kluwer; 2019. p. 1–10.
2. Larkin PJ, Madras BK. Opioids, overdoses, and cannabis: is marijuana an effective response to the opioid abuse epidemic? Draft 6.18.19. Electronic copy available at: https://ssm.com/abstract=3275773. Accessed 25 July 2019.
3. American Chronic Pain Association. The opioid dilemma. https://www.theacpa.org/wp-content/uploads/2019/02/ACPA_Resource_Guide_2019.pdf. p. 75–100. Accessed 25 July 2019.
4. Inturrisi CE, Craig DS, Lipman AG. Opioid analgesics. In: Ballantyne JC, Fishman SM, Rathmell JP, editors. Bonica's management of pain. 5th ed. Philadelphia: Wolters Kluwer; 2019. p. 1333–51.
5. Dowell D, Haegerich TM, Chou R. CDC guideline for prescribing opioids for chronic pain – United States, 2016. Morbidity and Mortality Weekly Report. 18 Mar 2016. https://www.cdc.gov/drugoverdose/prescribing/guideline.html p. 1–49. Accessed 25 July 2019.
6. Mudumbai SC, Oliva EM, Lewis ET, et al. Time-to-cessation of postoperative opioids: a population-level analysis of the veterans affairs health care. Pain Med. 2016;17:1732–43.
7. Teede R-D, Rief W, Barke A, et al. Chronic pain as a symptom or a disease: the IASP classification of chronic pain for the international classification of diseases [ICD-11]. Pain. 2019;160(1):19–27.

8. Trigiero AA, Kirsh KL, Passik SD. Scope of the problem: intersection of chronic pain and addiction. In: Staats PS, Silverman SM, editors. Controlled substance management in chronic pain. Cham: Springer; 2016. p. 13–27.
9. Volkow ND, Jones EB, Einstein EB, et al. Prevention and treatment of opioid misuse and addiction. JAMA Psychiatry. 2019;76(2):208–16.
10. Finn K. Why marijuana will not fix the opioid epidemic. Missouri Med. 2018;115(3):191–3.
11. Busse JW, Wang L, Kamaledin M, et al. Opioids for chronic noncancer pain. A systematic review and meta-analysis. JAMA. 2018;320(23):2448–60. https://doi.org/10.1001/jama.2018.18472.
12. Silverman SM. Controlled substance management: exit strategies for the pain practitioner. In: Staats PS, Silverman SM, editors. Controlled substance management in chronic pain. Cham: Springer; 2016. p. 251–80.
13. National Institute on Drug Abuse. Opioid overdose crisis. https://www.drugabuse.gov/drugs-abuse/opioids/opioid-overdose-crisis. Accessed 25 Jul 2019.
14. Rosenquist EWK, Aronson MD, Crowley M. Overview of the treatment of chronic non-cancer pain. https://www.uptodate.com/contents/overview-of-the-treatment-of-chronic-non-cancer-pain.
15. Centers for Disease Control and Prevention. CDC guideline for prescribing opioids for chronic pain – United States, 2016. Morbidity and Mortality Weekly Report. 18 Mar 2016. Recommendations and Reports/Vol.65/No.1.
16. Kroenke K, Alford DP, Argoff C, et al. Challenges with implementing the centers for disease control and prevention opioid guideline: a consensus panel report. Pain Med. 2019;20(4):724–35.
17. Federation of State Medical Boards. Guidelines for the chronic use of opioid analgesics. Policy April 2017. https://www.fsmb.org/siteassets/advocacy/policies/opioid_guidelines_as_adopted_april-2017_final.pdf.
18. Colorado Department of Regulatory Agencies. Guidelines for the safe prescribing and dispensing of opioids. Revised 14 Mar 19. https://drive.google.com/file/d/19xrPqsCbaHHA9nTD1Fl3NeCn5kwK60zR/view.
19. Veterans Administration. https://www.healthquality.va.gov/guidelines/Pain/cot/VADoDOTCPG022717.pdf.
20. https://www.doh.wa.gov/ForPublicHealthandHealthcareProviders/HealthcareProfessionsandFacilities/OpioidPrescribing/HealthcareProviders/Toolkits.
21. Department of Justice. Drug Enforcement Administration. Denial of petition to initiate proceedings to reschedule marijuana. Federal Register/Vol. 81, No. 156/Friday, 12 Aug 2016/Proposed Rules. 53767-53845.
22. Vučkovic S, Srebro D, Vujovic KS, et al. Cannabinoids and pain. New insights from old molecules. Front Pharmacol. 2018;9:1259–91.
23. Hill KP, Palastro MD, Johnson B, et al. Cannabis and pain: a clinical review. Cannabis Cannabinoid Res. 2017;2(1):96–104. https://doi.org/10.1089/can.2017.0017.
24. Meng H, Johnston B, Englesakis M, et al. Selective cannabinoids for chronic neuropathic pain: a systemic review and meta-analysis. Anesth Analg. 2017;125(5):1638–52.
25. Stockings E, Campbell G, Hall WD, et al. Cannabis and cannabinoids for the treatment of people with chronic noncancer pain conditions: a systematic review and meta-analysis of controlled and observational studies. Pain. 2018;159:1932–54.
26. Häuser W, Finn DP, Kalso E, et al. European pain federation [EFIC] position paper on appropriate use of cannabis-based medicines and medical cannabis for chronic pain management. Eur J Pain. 2018;22:1547–64.
27. https://www.drugs.com/newdrugs/fda-approves-epidiolex-cannabidiol-lennox-gastaut-syndrome-dravet-syndrome-4769.html.
28. Lutge EE, Gray A, Siegfried N. The medical use of cannabis for reducing morbidity and mortality in patients with HIV/AIDS. Cochrane Database Syst Rev. 2013;(4):CD005175. https://doi.org/10.1002/14651858.CD005175.pub3.
29. Tanda G, Pontieri FE, Di Chiara G. Cannabinoid and heroin activation of mesolimbic dopamine transmission by a common mu1 opioid receptor mechanism. Science. 1997;276:2048–50.

30. Van Hell HH, Vink M, Ossewaarde L, et al. Chronic effects of cannabis use on the human reward system: an fMRI study. Eur Neuropsychopharmacol. 2010;20:153–63.
31. Van de Donk T, Niesters M, Kowal MA, et al. An experimental randomized study on the analgesic effects of pharmaceutical-grade cannabis in chronic pain patients with fibromyalgia. Pain. 2019;160:860–9.
32. Scott DJ, Stohler CS, Egnatuk CM, et al. Individual differences in reward responding explain placebo-induced expectations and effects. Neuron. 2007;55:325–36.
33. Peciña M, Bohnert AS, Avery ET, et al. Association between placebo-activated neural systems and antidepressant responses: neurochemistry of placebo effects in major depression. JAMA Psychiat. 2015;72:1087–94.
34. Salottolo K, Peck L, Tanner A II, Carrick MM. The grass is not always greener: a multi-institutional pilot study of marijuana use and acute pain management following traumatic injury. Patient Saf Surg. 2018;12–6. https://doi.org/10.1186/s13037-018-0163-3.
35. Meng H, Johnston B, Englesakis M, et al. Selective cannabinoids for chronic neuropathic pain: a systematic review and meta-analysis. Anesth Analg. 2017;125:1638–52.
36. Mücke M, Phillips T, Radbruch L, et al. Cannabis-based medicines for chronic neuropathic pain in adults (Review). Cochrane Database Syst Rev. 2018;(3):CD012182.
37. Fallon MT, Albert LE, McQuade R, et al. Sativex oromucosal spray as adjunctive therapy in advanced cancer patients with chronic pain unalleviated by optimized opioid therapy: two double-blind, randomized, placebo-controlled phase 3 studies. Br J Pain. 2017;11(3):119–33.
38. Nugent SM, Yarborough BJ, Smith NX, et al. Patterns and correlates of medical cannabis use for pain among patients prescribed long-term opioid therapy. Gen Hosp Psychiatry. 2018;50:104–10.
39. www.ncsl.org/research/health/state-medical-marijuana-laws.aspx.
40. Dowell D, Haegerich T, Chou R. No shortcuts to safer opioid prescribing. N Engl J Med. 2019;3380:2285–7.
41. Chan NW, Burkhardt J, Flyr M. The effects of recreational marijuana legalization and dispensing on opioid mortality. Econ Inq. 2019;58:589–606. https://doi.org/10.1111/ecin.12819.
42. Scholl L, Seth P, Karilsa M, et al. Drug and opioid-involved overdose deaths – United States, 2013 – 2017. CDC MMWR Weekly. 2019;67:1419–27. https://www.cdc.gov/mmwr/volumes/67/wr/mm675152e1.htm?s_cid=mm675152e1_w.
43. Arterberry BJ, Padovano HT, Foster KT, et al. Higher average potency across the United States is associated with progression to first cannabis use disorder symptom. Drug Alcohol Dep. 195:186. https://doi.org/10.1016/j.drugalcdep.2018.11.012.
44. Lee DC, Schlienz NJ, Peters EN, et al. Systematic review of outcome domains and measures used in psychosocial and pharmacological treatment trials for cannabis use disorder. Drug Alcohol Depend. 194:500. https://doi.org/10.1016/j.drugalcdep.2018.10.020.
45. Shover CL, Davis CS, Gordon SC, et al. Association between medical cannabis laws and opioid overdose mortality has reversed over time. Proc Nat Acad Sci. 2019;116(26):12624–6.
46. Segura LE, Mauro CM, Levy NS, et al. Association of US medical marijuana Laws with nonmedical prescription opioid use and prescription opioid use disorder. JAMA Netw Open. 2019;2(7):e197216.
47. Washington State Department of Health. Medical marijuana (cannabis) authorization guidelines. DOH 631-053 July 2018. https://www.doh.wa.gov/YouandYourFamily/Marijuana/MedicalMarijuana/PatientInformation/QualifyingConditions.
48. Washington State Department of Health Medical Marijuana Authorization Form. doh.wa.gov/Portals/1/Documents/Pubs/623123.pdf.
49. Levy N, Sturgess J, Mills P. "Pain as the fifth vital sign" and dependence on the "numerical pain scale" is being abandoned in the US: why? Br J Anaesth. 2018;120:435–8.

Chapter 8
Cannabis in Pulmonary Medicine

Christopher M. Merrick and Jesse J. LeBlanc III

Cannabinoids and the Respiratory System

Christopher M. Merrick

Introduction

Marijuana use is steadily on the rise in the United States for both medical and recreational indications. This has been largely driven by increasing legalization and direct to consumer mass marketing. According to recent survey data, there is not only increased prevalence of marijuana use – up to 13% – but also decreased concern that marijuana use poses any threat for health risks or negative impact [1, 2].

Current data on the respiratory impact of marijuana inhalation is incomplete. However, the pulmonary manifestations of disease related to cannabis use are of utmost importance since inhalation is the most popular form of use. This chapter seeks to discuss known literature and clinical experience.

Lung Cancer

An area of concern and active investigation is the potential carcinogenicity of inhaled marijuana. The risk of inhaled cigarette smoke and the development of pulmonary malignancy have been well established [3]. This is also something that is

C. M. Merrick (✉)
Pulmonary Associates, PC, Memorial Hospital, Colorado Springs, CO, USA
e-mail: cmerrick@pulmassoc.com

J. J. LeBlanc III
Engineering Advisor-Ret., League City, TX, USA

© Springer Nature Switzerland AG 2020
K. Finn (ed.), *Cannabis in Medicine*,
https://doi.org/10.1007/978-3-030-45968-0_8

well understood by the general public and well advertised on product packaging and additional avenues such as online and television public service announcement style advertising.

There are currently a limited amount of published data evaluating cannabis use and development of pulmonary malignancy. Retrospective databases have been evaluated. According to database review in the United States, Canada, the United Kingdom, and New Zealand, there is a suggestion for increased risk of adenocarcinoma with increased daily use of inhaled marijuana. However, there was no distinct risk with increased number of years. The authors note that the confidence intervals on the accumulated data were very wide due to small sample sizes of the retrospective cohorts [4].

Additional data point to an increased risk of development of pulmonary malignancy with increased frequency and intensity of inhaled marijuana use. Among a cohort of men from North Africa, an odds ratio of 2.4 was found after correcting for multiple variables including tobacco smoke. Of note, in this study all cannabis users were also tobacco smokers. The study suggested that lung cancer risk increased with increasing joint-years. A "joint-year" is quantified by the number of marijuana products (joints, bowls, bongs, etc.) smoked per day for the course of a year. However, the authors note that the residual effects of tobacco smoking remain a significant confounding factor [5].

Other studies appear to come down more firmly on the risk that marijuana smoke poses for malignancy. One retrospective cohort in New Zealand demonstrated an 8% increase in lung cancer risk for each joint-year of cannabis smoking even after adjusting for cigarette smoking. These data are especially compelling as all 79 individuals with lung cancer in the cohort were under the age of 55, which represents a demographic characterized by a low prevalence of primary pulmonary malignancy [6].

Another retrospective case control study containing over 300 subjects found a significant link between current lung cancer and past cannabis smoking. The risk for development of pulmonary malignancy was significantly increased in the cohort of cigarette smokers with prior cannabis use than for cigarette smokers who had never smoked cannabis (OR 65.0 vs 15.3) [7].

A recent large meta-analysis that included over 20 studies and a total of over 13,000 individuals with cancer of any type demonstrated a significant association between cannabis smoke and development of both lung and testicular cancer. For testicular cancer, there was a notable relationship of risk for individuals who smoked cannabis for greater than 10 years [8].

There are striking case reports regarding chest malignancy in cannabis smokers. One such report is that of a 26-year-old man with extensive cannabis smoking history but negligible cigarette smoking history that was diagnosed with small cell lung cancer. This patient was aggressively treated but unfortunately ultimately succumbed to his disease [9].

In summary, the net effect of cannabis smoke on risk for chest malignancy remains incompletely understood due to limited prospective data as well as significant overlap of tobacco smoking among individuals who smoke marijuana [10]. However, multiple observational studies have demonstrated an elevated risk of cancer development as it relates to cannabis smoking. This area certainly requires ongoing investigation especially in light of those data, which do suggest a causative role of cannabis in the development of pulmonary malignancies.

Finally, healthcare professionals should educate their patients on the potential carcinogenic risk of cannabis smoke exposure.

Lung Function

Inhalation of combustible substances and small particles is known to have ramifications for pulmonary function. However, the effects of smoking cannabis on pulmonary function remain poorly understood.

Lung function is complex and dynamic. It is affected by the ability of air to flow unobstructed through the tracheobronchial tree in order to reach the distal alveolar sacs. From the alveolar space, gas must be able to diffuse efficiently into the capillary bed where oxygen is bound by hemoglobin within red blood cells and carbon dioxide is diffused from the blood back into the alveolar space in order that it might be exhaled into the environment. This process of ventilation is delicate and can be affected by many variables and disease states. Environmental exposures such as dust, smoke, and ozone – to name a few – play a vital role in disease within the lung.

Pulmonary function can be assessed by multiple dynamic tests such as spirometry, plethysmography, and diffusion limitation of carbon monoxide. These tests evaluate the different aspects of ventilation and oxygenation as described above and give the clinician a view into rapid cellular processes that would otherwise be indiscernible.

Early data on the effects of smoking marijuana point to an acute improvement of airflow through the tracheobronchial tree. Marijuana smoke with 1–2% THC results in an acute increase in airway conductance that remains present for as long as 60 min. Ingested THC of 10–20 mg has been shown to result in a similar acute increase in airway conductance that lasts for as long as 6 h. This is in contrast to the effects of inhaled tobacco smoke, which results in an acute decrease in airway conductance [11]. Of note, the concentration of THC in inhaled products has significantly increased with the evolution of the industry. In Colorado, THC content now routinely pushes 30% for smoked flower and in other types of inhalation such as butane hash oil (BHO) – discussed further later in the chapter – the THC content has been seen to surpass 60%. The pulmonary physiologic effects of high-dose THC are currently an area of much needed investigation [12, 13].

More recent data evaluating the effects of chronic inhaled marijuana use demonstrate similar findings. This data was contained in a large study using NHANES cohort data wherein individuals underwent a standardized questionnaire regarding cannabis and also underwent standardized spirometry. Marijuana use duration was measured in joint-years. In the 1–5 joint-year and 6–20 joint-year cohorts, a statistically significant increase in FVC was found. There appeared to be no significant influence on FEV1. In the 6–20 joint-year cohort, a decrease in FEV1/FVC ratio to less than 70% was detected; however this was felt to be more likely attributable to a rise in FVC than a decrease in FEV1. A finding in this study which deserves mentioning is that although there appeared to be no decrement in pulmonary physiologic indices, researchers found that "current marijuana smokers were more likely to be male, younger, of lower socioeconomic and education levels, to concurrently smoke tobacco, to have first tried marijuana at an earlier age, and have a history of a chronic respiratory illness" [14]. This at-risk nature of current marijuana smokers will be further discussed later in this chapter.

Multiple other studies have demonstrated similar pulmonary function testing results, which are notable for a persistently elevated FVC in cannabis smokers, which is not demonstrated in tobacco smokers [15, 16].

There are non-spirometric data suggesting that marijuana affects the pulmonary endothelium in ways similar to tobacco use. One study demonstrated a decrease in exhaled nitric oxide (eNO) in active or recent cannabis smokers. Spirometry was also performed in these individuals, but similar to other studies, these individuals were found to have an increase in FVC. This study was not powered to show a dose-response relationship. The authors of this study contend that given the vital role of NO in vascular and immune response pathways a better understanding of the clinical role of decreased NO would be beneficial [17].

Finally, a finding that deserves mentioning and will be further addressed in the next section: chronic cannabis smokers develop a heavier burden of pulmonary disease when compared to the general population. According to a large retrospective analysis of cannabis smokers, in spite of the early bronchodilation demonstrated on spirometry, there was a late development of chronic bronchitis symptoms. These symptoms were increased cough, wheeze, and sputum production, all of which are suggestive of obstructive lung disease [18].

COPD/Emphysema

Whether or not inhaled cannabis use results in chronic lung disease is incompletely understood. Many professional respiratory societies discourage smoking marijuana due to the sparse data on long-term outcomes, but very real concern that its use leads to development of worsening respiratory symptoms of cough, sputum production, and wheeze [19, 20].

One study noted that inhaled cannabis use resulted in a decreased FEV1/FVC ratio, but it had no direct effect on FEV1 – very similar to the data described above. However, this study did suggest hyperinflation as demonstrated by increases in both FVC and TLC with inhaled marijuana. In addition, standardized cross-sectional imaging was performed and demonstrated increased apical lucency in the lung fields of cannabis smokers. There was not a distinct association with inhaled cannabis use and presence of macroscopic emphysema. However, one cannabis only smoker with a greater than 400 joint-year smoking history did show evidence of macroscopic emphysema [21].

This finding was corroborated in a Dutch study of individuals under the age of 50 years who developed primary spontaneous pneumothorax. The 53 study subjects underwent high-resolution chest CT following treatment of their pneumothorax. Imaging findings were striking. Bullae were present in 87% of cannabis users, in contrast to 57% in tobacco-only smokers and none in nonsmokers [22]. There are also case reports of young individuals with minimal tobacco smoking histories that develop significant paraseptal emphysema. This is compelling because all of these individuals had significant cannabis smoking history. In addition, the demonstrated paraseptal pattern differs from the typical centrilobular pattern seen in individuals who develop pulmonary emphysema later in life as a result of chronic tobacco smoking [23].

Similar results were demonstrated in a Swiss study retrospectively evaluating spontaneous pneumothorax. The investigators observed a significant correlation between duration of cannabis smoking, development of emphysema and bullous disease, and incidence of spontaneous pneumothorax in young adults [24].

A key issue with inhaled cannabis and its currently poorly understood effects is the significant practice overlap of tobacco smoking with cannabis smoking. Recent data suggests that cannabis use is associated with tobacco smoking initiation, persistence, and relapse [25]. This is not only a confounding variable but also appears to have a synergistic effect in the development of chronic lung disease. A study in Canada evaluated the development of obstructive lung disease in individuals who smoked only cannabis, only tobacco, and those who smoked both cannabis and tobacco. Compared to never smokers, individuals who smoked tobacco cigarettes were more likely to have chronic lung disease and worse spirometric indices as well more symptoms of chronic respiratory disease such as cough, sputum production, wheezing, and dyspnea. In cannabis only smokers who had smoked at least 50 marijuana cigarettes, there was no significant risk for development of obstructive lung disease by pulmonary function testing or worsening respiratory symptoms. However, in those individuals who had smoked tobacco as well as cannabis, there was a significantly elevated risk of both outcomes. According to the authors, this suggests a synergistic effect between inhaled cannabis and tobacco smoke on the development of chronic lung disease [26].

Another study from the United Kingdom builds upon these data. This study also evaluated the development of COPD and chronic respiratory symptoms among tobacco and cannabis smokers. In the overlap group, when tobacco use was fully adjusted for, there remained a 0.3% increased prevalence in COPD attributable to cannabis smoke. In addition, COPD was found to be more prevalent at an earlier age among those who smoked both tobacco and cannabis. According to the study: "in the age range 25–34 years, 6% of tobacco-only users compared with 14% of tobacco and cannabis users met COPD criteria; in the 35–44 years age range, these proportions rose to 16% and 29%, respectively" [27].

A large retrospective review and meta-analysis of English language studies spanning from 1973 to 2018 concluded that there is insufficient evidence currently to establish a risk for COPD due to cannabis smoking alone. However, this analysis did demonstrate that there is at least low-strength evidence suggesting that individuals who smoke marijuana suffer more chronic pulmonary symptoms such as cough, wheezing, dyspnea, and sputum production [28].

This increased burden of respiratory symptoms due to cannabis smoke inhalation has been demonstrated in the primary care setting as well [29].

In summary, the data on cannabis smoking and chronic lung disease is inconclusive. Spirometric data is relatively sparse. However, from the data available, we can surmise that cannabis smoking, although not detrimental to spirometric indices, does appear to have a negative effect on the pulmonary system as represented by a higher burden of chronic respiratory symptoms of cough, wheeze, dyspnea, and sputum production. It is also evident that small particles result in the destruction of lung parenchyma as evidenced by findings of increased apical lucency, pulmonary bullae, and overt emphysema. This pattern is especially true in co-occurring tobacco and cannabis smokers.

Vaping

Electronic cigarettes came to market in 2007 and since then have continued to grow in popularity [30]. Vaping is the act of inhaling vapor produced by heating the oil within a cartridge or device of an electronic cigarette.

The pattern of use of cannabis from available literature and population data suggests that smoking is the most common means of ingestion followed by other forms such as edibles and vaporized products [31, 32].

Vaporized marijuana has gained in popularity due to the individual's ability to inhale a deodorized product as well as the popular opinion that using vaporized marijuana gives a more intense psychoactive experience [33].

This anecdotal information of its intense psychoactive effects is supported by the data. A clinical trial in healthy adults who infrequently use cannabis demonstrated that vaporized cannabis resulted in higher serum concentrations of THC as well as more pronounced psychoactive effects [34].

However, there is still much to be learned about the vaporized products inhaled by means of e-cigarettes. Vaping has begun to represent an underappreciated public health risk. This is due at least in part to the minimal standardization and oversight present in the vaporized product market. The electronic cigarette market has dramatically expanded in recent years and is fast outpacing the ability of appropriate biomedical research to ensure safety.

The vaporized product market is very broad due to a wide-ranging variety of flavors. These flavors are produced by the addition of synthetic flavoring agents, namely, diacetyl. This is very notable given diacetyl's known risk for causing bronchiolitis obliterans after a major outbreak of this disease among popcorn factory workers. This prompted development of the informal name "popcorn lung." This resulted in the removal of diacetyl from the flavoring process of popcorn. Unfortunately, diacetyl is known to be present in the flavoring of vaporized compounds for direct inhalation. In a recent study, diacetyl was detected in 39 of 51 flavors studied that are popular among teens and adolescents [35]. The Food and Drug Administration has taken notice of the damaging effects of these "kid-friendly" flavors and has start limiting their availability [36].

Additionally, another recent study demonstrated that dangerous carbonyl compounds formaldehyde and acetaldehyde were present in large amounts in the thinning agents used in vapor oil [37]. These compounds are formed during the heating process of the oil much as would be seen when the oil is heated to vapor and inhaled.

Still other studies have demonstrated contamination by microbial toxins. One study demonstrated significant contamination of electronic cigarette products with endotoxin and 1,3 B-D glucan. Concentrations of these microbial toxins were above the limit of detection in 23% and 81%, respectively, in a cohort of e-cigarette oil products sold in the United States [38].

Trace metals evaluations of electronic cigarette aerosols have demonstrated the presence of nickel at a higher concentration than is seen in traditional smoking modalities [39].

It is perhaps due to these toxic substances that e-cigarette-related acute lung disease has become so prominently noticeable. One such incidence was in Wisconsin and Illinois when 14 teens and young adults were hospitalized for acute respiratory failure after vaping. Several of the teens and young adults required intubation and mechanical ventilation [40].

There are reports of similar patterns of disease outbreak resulting in hospitalization in New Jersey, Texas, Colorado, and North Carolina among young adults without any significant history of lung disease or other respiratory exposures [41–43]. Of most concern, at the time of this manuscript, 48 individuals have died as a result of e-cigarette/vaping product-associated lung injury (EVALI) [44]. In response to this outbreak, the Centers for Disease Control and Prevention (CDC) released this statement: "The CDC recommends that people should not use THC-containing e-cigarette, or vaping, products, particularly from informal sources like friends, family, or in-person or online dealers" [45]. According to the CDC, THC-containing vaping products are the most commonly used vaping product used by individuals suffering from EVALI [45].

While the etiology of acute lung disease in the affected individuals has not yet been fully elucidated, there are specific pathologies known to be associated with vaping-induced acute lung injury. A recent case was reported wherein surgical lung biopsy samples of individuals suffering from vaping-induced lung injury demonstrated respiratory bronchiolitis interstitial lung disease (RB-ILD) [46].

Additionally, there are reports of vaping-induced lung injury due to diffuse alveolar hemorrhage, acute eosinophilic pneumonitis, and lipoid pneumonia [46–49]. Vitamin E acetate has been proposed as an etiologic agent as it has been isolated from bronchoalveolar lavage from many individuals suffering from EVALI [50].

One study evaluated the effects of single episode vaping on individuals with severe chronic obstructive pulmonary disease (COPD). Inhaling 35 mg of vaporized THC had no significant spirometric or symptomatic effects on individuals with severe COPD [51].

A major public health concern in the consideration of electronic cigarettes is the large prevalence of teenage and young adult users. Market research supports the role of aggressive advertising campaigns on social media platforms as being highly effective at dramatically increasing the use and popularity of electronic cigarettes in recent years [52]. The extreme popularity of certain brands such as JUUL among youth suggests a correlation between effective marketing campaigns and adolescent susceptibility to such trends [53]. Additionally, there are strong data to support that the "low risk" of electronic cigarettes is attracting youth to tobacco smoking who otherwise would not consider cigarette smoking [54].

Whereas the risks of electronic cigarettes and cannabis smoking are still poorly understood, the risks of tobacco smoking are well known. Electronic cigarettes have been trumpeted as a means to tobacco cessation and an alternative to cigarette use. Unfortunately, preliminary studies of teenagers demonstrate that electronic cigarette use is a substantial risk factor for future cigarette smoking as well as experimenting with other illicit substances including alcohol, prescription narcotics, and hallucinogenic drugs [31, 55]. There is equally as compelling data in adults that the use of inhalational cannabis significantly increases likelihood for concomitant tobacco abuse [25].

Vaping cannabis by means of electronic cigarette poses a major only recently appreciated public health crisis. This is due to its prevalence among young adults, its underreported ramifications for respiratory health due to both psychoactive substance (cannabis or nicotine) and contaminant, and finally its known overlap with initiation and persistence of tobacco smoking. In spite of clever marketing schemes and positioning itself as a "safe alternative" to smoking combustible substances, vaping has been recurrently found to be unsafe and a poor choice for lung health. It is for this reason that the American Lung Association takes a strong stance against electronic cigarettes and states that it is "very concerned that we are at risk of losing another generation to tobacco-caused diseases as the result of e-cigarettes" [56].

Lung Health

The effects of cannabis smoke on respiratory airflow and lung cancer development remain incompletely understood. However, its effects on general lung health have been adequately demonstrated to be overall deleterious.

Individuals who smoke marijuana on a regular basis have been found to demonstrate a bronchitic phenotype with increased wheeze, cough, and sputum production [57]. As discussed above, this has not yet been associated with an increased incidence of obstructive lung disease. These findings of bronchitic phenotype have been reproduced in multiple studies [58].

Marijuana inhalation has been demonstrated to have a negative impact on mucociliary clearance and immune cell function. This results in decreased host defenses and increased propensity for infection and likely contributes to the chronic bronchitis frequently observed in individuals who chronically use marijuana [59, 60].

Not only does inhaled marijuana alter host respiratory defense but has also been demonstrated to increase infectious risk in community clusters due to microbial contamination. Case report evidence documents infectious outbreaks of *Aspergillus* spp. and Mycobacterium tuberculosis directly related to marijuana use [61–63].

Cannabis smoking has also been associated with acute lung diseases such as recurrent necrotizing bronchiolitis and hemoptysis [64, 65]. There is an increasing recognition of cannabis inhalation resulting in acute pleural disorders such as pneumothorax and pneumomediastinum. This is thought to be due to inhalational technique which often results in coughing against a closed glottis. In addition, there is an association with emesis, which is a known complication of marijuana use. Several studies evaluating etiology of spontaneous pneumothorax found a significant correlation between cannabis use in young adults, development of lung bullae, and subsequent development of spontaneous pneumothorax [22, 24, 66].

Alternate forms of cannabis inhalation have also been demonstrated to be damaging. Butane hash oil (BHO) refers to an extraction technique of concentrating THC to much higher levels through extraction with butane. In a process known colloquially as "dabbing," this extraction is then inhaled after being superheated and vaporized. Studies evaluating lung availability of phytocannabinoids such as THC and CBD have demonstrated THC concentrations in excess of 60% in dabbing versus 19–27% in marijuana flower smoking [13]. This form of inhalational use has been associated with acute lung injury, which mimics pneumonia. The BHO process results in residual butane as well as terpenes. When terpenes are heated, they degrade into methacrolein and benzene. It is hypothesized that high levels of these substances result in the acute lung injury, which has been observed in the dabbing process [67].

There are additional concerns regarding cannabis product contamination. Studies evaluating cannabis purity have demonstrated shockingly high recovery of pesticide residue within the cannabis smoke, which would be inhaled by the user. Recovery of permethrin from glass pipe smoked cannabis was found to be approaching 70% [68]. In dab preparations, over 80% of tested samples were found to have significant residual pesticide and solvent contamination [69]. One study evaluated self-identified cannabis smokers for the increased presence of toxic combustion by-products. In this study, cannabis smokers were found to have significantly elevated urinary concentrations of polycyclic aromatic hydrocarbons (PAHs) and volatile organic compounds (VOCs) when compared to nonusing control subjects [70]. Finally, there are firsthand reports from cannabis workers of industrial cannabis growers using illegal pesticides such as Eagle 20, which has a residue that is known to break down into hydrogen cyanide when it is heated and smoked [71].

Environmental Considerations

The environmental impact of rapidly increasing volume cannabis growth and use must be considered in regard to its implications for lung health. One recent study created leaf enclosures to replicate on a smaller scale the growing conditions inside of cannabis cultivation facilities. Ambient measurements of biogenic volatile organic compounds (BVOCs) were obtained and were demonstrated to be elevated above baseline. The authors of the study hypothesize that if the results of their data are extrapolated to the large scale, then the production of BVOCs from cannabis cultivation could result in a doubling of atmospheric BVOCs in a large production city such as Denver, Colorado [72]. This data is very meaningful because BVOCs are precursors to ozone and particulate matter. Volatile organic compounds have been demonstrated to increase airway inflammation in mouse models and have also been demonstrated to have a significant negative impact on the spirometric indices of elderly individuals [73, 74].

Additionally, vaping products have been shown to have detrimental effects on local indoor air quality. Electronic cigarette use results in aerosolization and distribution of significant volumes of multiple polluting substances such as 1,2-propanediol, glycerine, nicotine (in the setting of nicotine electronic cigarette use), $PM_{2.5}$, and carcinogenic PAH molecules [75, 76]. One quantitative study of air quality at an indoor vaping event demonstrated that the degree of air pollution and amount of particulate matter present were similar to that found in the setting of extreme air pollution such as wildfires or industrial pollution [77]. This level of air pollution is certainly detrimental to both the lung and general health of individuals and communities.

Cannabis has also been demonstrated to be a mild allergen, resulting in the development of allergic response both among users and secondhand exposed individuals. There are reports of children with uncontrolled asthma related to passive cannabis exposure. Disease was notably improved following removal of exposure [78]. There are case reports of lifelong nonusers who develop cannabis allergy due to second-hand exposure. Symptoms include rhinoconjunctivitis and ingestion-related allergies as evidence of cross-reactivity [79]. One report from a Colorado allergy practice found that up to 12% of individuals who have never smoked marijuana demonstrated evidence of cannabis allergy. This number increases to 26% for past smokers, and as much as 50% of current smokers that experience symptoms and demonstrate findings of cannabis allergy [80].

Secondhand cannabis smoke exposure is also an area of growing concern. Studies regarding secondhand smoke exposure in the home have demonstrated a significant trend toward increased respiratory morbidity for exposed children. These children were found to have a trend toward higher incidence of ear infection, asthma, bronchiolitis, and eczema and emergency department visit for cough or dyspnea [81]. Animal studies on brief passive smoke exposure have shown vascular endothelial dysfunction. The degree of dysfunction is similar to that caused by cigarette smoke [82]. Another study on nonsmoking individuals found that exposure in varying levels of room ventilation demonstrated inverse proportions of sedative effects, impaired cognitive performance, and detectable serum/urine THC concentration related to degree of ventilation (i.e., better ventilation results in lower adverse outcome detection) [83].

Air quality has become an area of increasing public interest due to its known impact on the health of communities. A recent report by the American Thoracic Society cited excess morbidity and mortality related to air quality. The American Thoracic Society has called for even more conservative reduction thresholds for ozone and particulate matter [84]. The respiratory impact of large-scale cannabis growth in communities, vaping, carcinogen and particulate matter production, as well as first- and secondhand cannabis allergy, and secondhand smoke exposure must be considered in discussions of lung health as it relates to air quality.

Conclusion

In summary, although cannabis has been propagated as safe for inhalation, it has been seen to have detrimental effects not only on individual lung health but also on community health given its impact on air quality. Cannabis smoke inhalation by any means puts its users at undue respiratory risk due to mitigation of respiratory immune defense, increase in respiratory secretions, and development of pulmonary syndromes such as bronchitis, COPD, emphysema, necrotizing bronchiolitis, pneumothorax, pneumomediastinum, fungal pneumonia, tuberculosis, and lung cancer. These illnesses are not due to cannabis alone but undoubtedly to the significant contaminant burden inhaled by its users. Enhanced awareness among the general public but also certainly among healthcare practitioners is absolutely necessary to decrease the unnecessary development of acute and chronic respiratory illnesses due to cannabis smoking. Healthcare providers should consider screening high-risk individuals for inhalational marijuana use and educating their patients on the above findings. Based on this body of evidence, patients should be counseled in accordance with the ALA position: "Due to the risks it poses to lung health, the American Lung Association strongly cautions the public against smoking marijuana" [85].

THC & CBD Decomposition and Terpene Hazards While Vaping or Dabbing

Jesse J. LeBlanc

Introduction

In order to solve a complex problem, sometimes the cause(s) and solution(s) are more easily discovered when one begins with the fundamentals. In light of the current vaping epidemic, some of the possible answers to this crisis may be found by simply beginning the investigation at the atomic level of matter.

Basic Chemistry-Organic Molecules and Compounds

Organic molecules are the building blocks of life and center around chains of carbon atoms. There are four main groups of organic molecules that combine and form compounds necessary for life to exist, namely, carbohydrates, proteins, lipids (fats, oils, and waxes), and nucleic acids. In addition to living matter, organic molecules are also found in non-living matter. Fossil fuels, derived from crude oil, which are formed from the remains of once living organisms, are comprised of organic molecules too [86]. In general, organic chemicals always contain carbon atoms, most contain hydrogen atoms, and many also contain oxygen atoms [87].

Decomposition of Organic Chemicals, Specifically Lipids

Lipids, a family of organic chemicals, are fat-like substances. Lipids are readily soluble in organic solvents, such as butane and ethanol (alcohol), but are not soluble in water [88]. Well-known examples of lipids are vegetable oils, such as olive oil [89]. It should be noted that when lipids are heated to a high enough temperature, decomposition will occur. Assuming a very high temperature and an adequate amount of air (made up of nitrogen and oxygen), all that will remain are trace amounts of elemental carbon, carbon dioxide (CO_2), nitrogen dioxide (NO_2), and water (H_2O) assuming almost complete combustion. However, if the temperature is not elevated enough for perfect combustion, there is a high probability that the atoms will rearrange and form a different compound, which in many cases will be harmful to human health. For example, if oil is heated above its "*smoke point*," it can react with oxygen and form free radicals, which can injure living cells and one's DNA. Further, it can also break down into HNE (4-hydroxynonenal), which is a compound linked to vascular diseases such as atherosclerosis, diabetes, and neuro-degenerative disorders [90]. It can also decompose and form a compound called acrolein, which is a known irritant to the nose, lungs, eyes, stomach, and skin [91, 92]. Heating any oil to its smoke point therefore produces chemical compounds that are harmful to healthy tissue. Table 8.1 lists the smoke points of commonly used cooking oils:

Incandescence (Emission of Visible Light as a Result of a Body's Temperature)

The Draper point is the approximate temperature where almost all solid materials visibly glow. This was discovered by John William Draper in 1847. The approximate temperature where this occurs is about 977°F or 525°C [94]. This principle

Table 8.1 Smoke point temperatures of various cooking oils [93]

Oil (lipid)	Temperature
Extra virgin olive oil	325–410°F (163–210°C)
Vegetable shortening	360–410°F (180–210°C)
Margarine	410–430°F (210–221°C)
Refined avocado oil (one of the highest smoke points)	520–570°F (271–299°C)

Table 8.2 Visible color of steel when heated [95]

Temperature color chart – Steel

°F	°C	Approx. color
1,112	600	Faint red
1,292	700	Dark red
1,472	800	Bright red
1,652	900	Dull orange
1,742	950	Orange
1,832	1,000	Dark yellow
1,922	1,050	Yellow
2,012	1,100	Bright yellow
2,192	1,200	White

was used to determine the temperature of steel by blacksmiths when doing metal-work before thermometers were available. Steel, when a bright red, is approximately 1,472°F or 800°C as noted in Table 8.2 [95]:
Table designed by J. LeBlanc and based on Ref. [95]

Nickel-chrome wire is widely used to manufacture the heating elements used in vape pens and e-cigarettes. It has a melting temperature of approximately 2,462°F (1,350°C) and a maximum operating temperature, when used as a heating element, of 1,652°F (900°C) [96]. For comparison purposes, steel has a melting temperature of approximately 2,500°F (1,370°C) [97]. In theory, regardless of the material, including ceramics and even titanium, any solid object will glow a similar color when heated to the respective temperature listed in Table 8.2.

THC and CBD

Delta 9-tetrahydrocannabinol or THC, the psychoactive component of the marijuana plant, is classified as a lipid and is therefore an organic chemical by definition. When extracted from the marijuana plant using a solvent such as butane (the resulting product is known as butane hash oil or BHO), ethanol (same as alcohol), or carbon dioxide (CO_2), the resulting product can be a waxy substance or a thick oil [98, 99]. Further supporting the fact that THC is an organic chemical, it is comprised of 21 carbon atoms, 30 hydrogen atoms, and 2 oxygen atoms and can be denoted as $C_{21}H_{30}O_2$ [100]. It should be further noted that cannabidiol (CBD) has the same chemical formula as THC because it is also comprised of 21 carbon atoms, 30 hydrogen atoms, and 2 oxygen atoms and can also be denoted as $C_{21}H_{30}O_2$ [101]. Since THC and CBD have the same chemical formulas, namely, $C_{21}H_{30}O_2$, they are known as isomers. This should not be surprising since both of these organic chemical compounds are extracted from the cannabis family of plants, namely, marijuana and hemp.

The previously mentioned solvent extraction process is also used to remove CBD from the hemp plant. The concern with this type of extraction process for both THC and CBD is the fact that the organic solvent used along with any residual insecticides, pesticides, and naturally occurring heavy metals can be concentrated in the resulting product. The heavy metals that can carry over to the resulting waxy or oil-like products is due to the fact that the cannabis plant is actually a "soil scrubber"; in fact, the cannabis plant is used in some areas in the world to clean up contaminated soil [102].

Cannabis plants also contain terpenes, which carry over with the THC and CBD extracts and give marijuana-based and hemp-based products their distinctive similar odors. Terpenes are also desirable additives because these compounds can either intensify or downplay the effects of both THC and CBD [103].

Vaping and Dabbing

There are two well-known methods to get THC quickly into the user's bloodstream, namely, by either vaping or dabbing. A "dab" is the product resulting from the solvent extraction of the THC from the marijuana plant. The extracted product is highly concentrated and therefore has a much greater potency (80%+ THC). Vaping and dabbing both require the use of heat in the form of an electrically energized coil (for vaping) or a manually heated "nail" composed of either ceramic, titanium, quartz, or glass (for dabbing) [104]. Vaping devices use a battery to heat/energize a metal or ceramic coil. When dabbing, a nail is normally heated to a very high temperature with a commercially available propane torch or other similar heating device [99]. On a YouTube video discussing how to clean a vape pen, the color of the coil appears to be a yellow in color, indicating a temperature of approximately 1,922°F (1,050°C)

[105]. Similarly, if dabbing, the glowing color of the nail indicates its approximate temperature.

As discussed previously, organic chemicals decompose into other compounds when they are exposed to an excessive amount of heat energy. Examples, previously discussed, were cooking oils heated to or above their "smoke point." THC and CBD will both therefore similarly decompose at elevated temperatures since they are lipids too and will similarly decompose.

Here are the recommended dab temperatures as documented on the "Torrch" website [106]:

- *32–310°F (0–154°C) – This range is generally too low to vaporize any type of cannabis concentrate. This will result in zero clouds and thus no flavor.*
- *315–450°F (157–232°C) – This is the range for your "low temp dabbing". In this range terpene profiles efficiently vaporize without burning. You will experience the maximum flavor and taste exactly the way the extractor meant for the extract to taste.*
- *450–600°F (232–315°C) – This is in range with a "medium temp dab" or a hybrid temperature. This range will deliver slightly lower flavor profiles while increasing cloud production.*
- *600–900°F (315–482°C) – This is the "high temp dab" range. You will start seeing rapid combustion and thick clouds. You lose terpene flavors as they lose their molecular structure at such high heats.*
- *900°F + (482°C+) – Anything above this temperature is generally frowned upon as certain carcinogens and toxins begin to release in vapor form. Hits will be cloudy, but extremely harsh with a distinct burnt taste.*

It should be noted that at 900°F (482°C), this vendor clearly states that "certain carcinogens and toxins begin to release in a vapor form." The vendor also states that at 600–900°F (315–482°C): "You will start seeing rapid combustion and thick clouds. You lose terpene flavors as they lose their molecular structure at such high heats." Also note that the target temperature for vaping is within the range of the smoke point of most cooking oils, which makes sense because both vaping and dabbing rely on the inhalation of smoke to achieve the desired effect(s) by the user. It can be concluded that if cooking oils release harmful compounds at or above their smoke point, and, since THC and CBD are both considered lipids, they too would release similar biologically harmful compounds when heated to or above their respective smoke points.

Additionally, researchers from the Portland State University Department of Chemistry, have found that multiple toxic compounds can be formed when dabbing [107]. The researchers state that "users posting online cite a preferred temperature around 710°F (378°C), but cite a range from 340°C to 482°C". The researchers further found that the following organic chemicals are likely formed when dabbing cannabis extracts because of their naturally occurring or augmented terpene content:

- 1, Methacrolein (MC)
- Methyl vinyl ketone
- Hydroxyacetone

- 4,3-Methylfuran
- 5,2-Methylnaphthalene
- 1,3-Butadiene
- Benzene
- 1-Methylcyclohexa-1
- 4-Diene
- 8, Benzene

The most concerning harmful chemical compounds identified were 1, methacrolein (*MC*), a noxious irritant and similar to acrolein; *benzene*, a known carcinogen; and *1,3-butadiene*, another known carcinogen [108].

Of particular note is this statement by the Oregon researchers, which is located in the "Conclusions" section of their research paper:

> The difficulty users find in controlling the nail temperature put users∗ at risk of exposing themselves to not only methacrolein but also benzene. Additionally, the heavy focus on terpenes as additives seen as of late in the cannabis industry is of great concern due to the oxidative liability (free-radical generation) of these compounds when heated.

∗Note: The researchers should have also considered the impairment that occurs when dabbing THC. This is another factor that could make manual temperature regulation when dabbing very difficult. Drug-induced impairment could also affect how well the temperature control of a vape pen is managed by the user.

Also, there is the distinct possibility of the generation of free radicals when dabbing and vaping THC or CBD, similar to what happens when overheating cooking oils, because both of these compounds have an O-H (oxygen-hydrogen) pair attached to its molecular structure, which can become a hydroxyl (O-H) radical or "free radical" upon decomposition. As discussed previously, free radicals are considered one of the causes of many diseases, such as atherosclerosis, cancer, and neurological disorders [109].

Terpene Hazards

The same researchers from the Portland State University Department of Chemistry listed the different terpenes that are associated with THC products and that are extracted from the marijuana plant or added to the product to augment the effects desired by user. They found that "myrcene was found to be the most abundant, followed by limonene, linalool, pinene, caryophyllene, and humulene; however, the plant can also contain up to 68 additional terpenic compounds in trace amounts." Additionally, they stated that "some consumers increase the terpenoid content by dipping butane hash oil in a vial of terpenes prior to use ("terp dipping")" [107].

These researchers focused on only the top three occurring terpenes, namely, myrcene, limonene, and linalool in their study. The hazards associated with these terpenes are easily found by referring to the respective Material Safety Data Sheet (MSDS) or newer Safety Data Sheet (SDS), which are required by the Occupational

Health and Safety Administration (OSHA) in workplaces where these chemical compounds are used. A summary of the hazards associated with these three terpenes in their natural (not decomposed) state are as follows:

- Myrcene [110]

  - Hazard statements

    Flammable liquid and vapor.
    Causes skin irritation.
    Causes serious eye irritation.
    May cause respiratory irritation.

  - Precautionary statements

    Avoid breathing dust/fume/gas/mist/vapors/spray.
    IF IN EYES: Rinse cautiously with water for several minutes. Remove contact lenses, if present and easy to do. Continue rinsing.

  - Potential health effects

    Inhalation may be harmful if inhaled. Causes respiratory tract irritation.
    May be harmful if absorbed through skin. Causes skin irritation.
    Causes eye irritation.
    Ingestion may be harmful if swallowed.

- Limonene [111]

  - Hazard statements

    Flammable liquid and vapor.
    May be harmful if swallowed.
    Causes skin irritation.
    May cause an allergic skin reaction.
    Very toxic to aquatic life.

  - Precautionary statements

    Avoid release to the environment.
    Wear protective gloves.

  - Potential health effects

    Inhalation may be harmful if inhaled. Causes respiratory tract irritation.
    May be harmful if absorbed through skin. Causes skin irritation.
    Causes eye irritation.
    Ingestion may be harmful if swallowed.

- Linalool [112]

  - Hazard statements

    Combustible liquid.
    May be harmful if swallowed.

Causes skin irritation.
Causes serious eye irritation.
May cause respiratory irritation.

– Precautionary statements

Avoid breathing dust/fume/gas/mist/vapors/spray.
IF IN EYES: Rinse cautiously with water for several minutes. Remove contact lenses, if present and easy to do. Continue rinsing.

– Potential health effects

Inhalation may be harmful if inhaled. Causes respiratory tract irritation. May be harmful if absorbed through skin. Causes skin irritation.
Causes eye irritation.
Ingestion may be harmful if swallowed.

Conclusions

The "vaping crisis" has been reported on numerous times by all of the major media outlets (radio, Internet, newsprint, radio, and television). Vaping is causing lung illnesses and lung damage to such a degree that hospital treatment is usually required, and in several notable cases, death occurs. What is always reported as possible causes are the additives in the vape cartridges and/or residual pesticides, herbicides, and even dangerous heavy metals because of lax regulation, which allowed the vape cartridge black market to grow ever larger.

The THC, CBD, and nicotine vape cartridges can have additives, which include flavorings, propylene glycol, vegetable glycerine, and vitamin E acetate (all organic chemicals). These additives along with the pesticides and herbicides can decompose into dangerous chemical compounds when heated to high temperatures, which is not surprising given the known behavior of organic chemicals during decomposition. What is important to consider is the fact that the majority (approximately 76%±) of those injured were vaping THC [113, 114].

What is not being reported is the fact that THC and CBD can also decompose when heated excessively and form chemical compounds that can also cause serious health issues, including lung ailments. Further, the naturally occurring or added terpenes themselves are lung irritants. For some reason though, THC and CBD and the associated terpenes are not being considered as part of the problem. Another concern is related to the proper temperature regulation by the user and/or control circuitry of the vaping device; this key detail is also not being discussed either.

Using chemistry and science as a basis, one can conclude that this crisis may simply be related to the decomposition of organic chemicals when heated at or above their respective smoke point, namely, the temperature at which decomposition begins to occur. Further, the organic chemical compounds of concern should also include THC and CBD. Even if the THC or CBD are not heated to or above their respective smoke points, the naturally occurring or added terpenes are known lung irritants. Also, investigators should also determine whether or not there is a dabbing component tied to the vaping crisis because both activities produce similar harmful by-products and also involve terpene inhalation, and those who vape THC and/or CBD may also dab THC and/or CBD. Simply stated, the vaping crisis may also be related to dabbing. Further, the Center for Disease Control (CDC) may also want to update its new acronym, EVALI, which stands for "electronic cigarette (e-cigarette), or vaping, product use associated lung injury," so that it includes dabbing.

Acknowledgments   Dr. Christine Miller, Dr. Kenneth Finn

Conflict of Interest   The author declares no competing financial interest.

References

Cannabinoids and the Respiratory System

1. Keyhani S, Steigerwald S, Ishida J, Vali M, Cerdá M, Hasin D, et al. Risks and benefits of marijuana use: a national survey of U.S. adults. Ann Intern Med. 2018;169(5):282–90.
2. Compton WM, Han B, Jones CM, Blanco C, Hughes A. Marijuana use and use disorders in adults in the USA, 2002–14: analysis of annual cross-sectional surveys. Lancet Psychiatry. 2016;3(10):954–64.
3. Malhotra J, Malvezzi M, Negri E, La Vecchia C, Boffetta P. Risk factors for lung cancer worldwide. Eur Respir J. 2016;48(3):889–902.
4. Zhang LR, Morgenstern H, Greenland S, Chang S-C, Lazarus P, Teare MD, et al. Cannabis smoking and lung cancer risk: pooled analysis in the International Lung Cancer Consortium. Int J Cancer. 2015;136(4):894–903.
5. Berthiller J, Straif K, Boniol M, Voirin N, Benhaïm-Luzon V, Ayoub WB, et al. Cannabis smoking and risk of lung cancer in men: a pooled analysis of three studies in Maghreb. J Thorac Oncol. 2008;3(12):1398–403.
6. Aldington S, Harwood M, Cox B, Weatherall M, Beckert L, Hansell A, et al. Cannabis use and risk of lung cancer: a case-control study. Eur Respir J. 2008;31(2):280–6.
7. Voirin N, Berthiller J, Benhaïm-Luzon V, Boniol M, Straif K, Ayoub WB, et al. Risk of lung cancer and past use of cannabis in Tunisia. J Thorac Oncol. 2006;1(6):577–9.
8. Park S, Myung S-K. Cannabis smoking and risk of cancer: a meta-analysis of observational studies. JGO. 2018;4(Supplement 2):196s.
9. Graef S, Choo CG, Warfield A, Cullen M, Woolhouse I. Small cell lung cancer in a 26-year-old man with significant cannabis exposure. J Thorac Oncol. 2011;6(1):218–9.
10. Huang Y-HJ, Zhang Z-F, Tashkin DP, Feng B, Straif K, Hashibe M. An epidemiologic review of marijuana and cancer: an update. Cancer Epidemiol Biomark Prev. 2015;24(1):15–31.
11. Tashkin DP, Shapiro BJ, Frank IM. Acute pulmonary physiologic effects of smoked marijuana and oral Δ9-tetrahydrocannabinol in healthy young men. N Engl J Med. 1973;289(7):336–41.
12. https://www.cnn.com/2016/10/21/health/colorado-marijuana-potency-above-national-average/index.html.
13. Hädener M, Vieten S, Weinmann W, Mahler H. A preliminary investigation of lung availability of cannabinoids by smoking marijuana or dabbing BHO and decarboxylation rate of THC- and CBD-acids. Forensic Sci Int. 2019;295:207–12.

14. Kempker JA, Honig EG, Martin GS. The effects of marijuana exposure on expiratory airflow. A study of adults who participated in the U.S. National Health and Nutrition Examination Study. Ann ATS. 2014;12(2):135–41.
15. Hancox RJ, Poulton R, Ely M, Welch D, Taylor DR, McLachlan CR, et al. Effects of cannabis on lung function: a population-based cohort study. Eur Respir J. 2010;35(1):42–7.
16. Pletcher MJ, Vittinghoff E, Kalhan R, Richman J, Safford M, Sidney S, et al. Association between marijuana exposure and pulmonary function over 20 years. JAMA. 2012;307(2):173–81.
17. Papatheodorou SI, Buettner H, Rice MB, Mittleman MA. Recent marijuana use and associations with exhaled nitric oxide and pulmonary function in adults in the United States. Chest. 2016;149(6):1428–35.
18. Tetrault JM, Crothers K, Moore BA, Mehra R, Concato J, Fiellin DA. Effects of marijuana smoking on pulmonary function and respiratory complications: a systematic review. Arch Intern Med. 2007;167(3):221–8.
19. https://www.thoracic.org/patients/patient-resources/resources/marijuana.pdf.
20. https://www.lung.org/get-involved/become-an-advocate/public-policy-position-lung-health.html.
21. Aldington S, Williams M, Nowitz M, Weatherall M, Pritchard A, McNaughton A, et al. Effects of cannabis on pulmonary structure, function and symptoms. Thorax. 2007;62(12):1058–63.
22. Hendriks L, Bootsma G, van Noord J. Cannabis use in patients with a primary spontaneous pneumothorax. Eur Respir J. 2011;38(Suppl 55):4693.
23. Johnson MK, Smith RP, Morrison D, Laszlo G, White RJ. Large lung bullae in marijuana smokers. Thorax. 2000;55(4):340–2.
24. Beshay M, Kaiser H, Niedhart D, Reymond MA, Schmid RA. Emphysema and secondary pneumothorax in young adults smoking cannabis. Eur J Cardiothorac Surg. 2007;32(6):834–8.
25. Weinberger AH, Delnevo CD, Wyka K, Gbedemah M, Lee J, Copeland J, et al. Cannabis use is associated with increased risk of cigarette smoking initiation, persistence, and relapse among adults in the United States. Nicotine Tob Res:ntz085.. [Internet]. 2019 May 21 [cited 29 Jul 2019]. Available from: https://doi.org/10.1093/ntr/ntz085.
26. Tan WC, Lo C, Jong A, Xing L, FitzGerald MJ, Vollmer WM, et al. Marijuana and chronic obstructive lung disease: a population-based study. CMAJ. 2009;180(8):814–20.
27. Macleod J, Robertson R, Copeland L, McKenzie J, Elton R, Reid P. Cannabis, tobacco smoking, and lung function: a cross-sectional observational study in a general practice population. Br J Gen Pract. 2015;65(631):e89–95.
28. Ghasemiesfe M, Ravi D, Vali M, Korenstein D, Arjomandi M, Frank J, et al. Marijuana use, respiratory symptoms, and pulmonary function: a systematic review and meta-analysis. Ann Intern Med. 2018;169(2):106–15.
29. McKenzie J, Copeland L, MacLeod J, Peter R. Respiratory symptoms associated with cannabis and tobacco use in a North Edinburgh primary care population. Eur Respir J. 2011;38(Suppl 55):4236.
30. McMillen RC, Gottlieb MA, Shaefer RMW, Winickoff JP, Klein JD. Trends in electronic cigarette use among U.S. adults: use is increasing in both smokers and nonsmokers. Nicotine Tob Res. 2014;17(10):1195–202.
31. Knapp AA, Lee DC, Borodovsky JT, Auty SG, Gabrielli J, Budney AJ. Emerging trends in cannabis administration among adolescent cannabis users. J Adolesc Health. 2019;64(4):487–93.
32. Schneider KE, Tormohlen KN, Brooks-Russell A, Johnson RM, Thrul J. Patterns of co-occurring modes of marijuana use among Colorado high school students. J Adolesc Health. 2019;64(6):807–9.
33. Giroud C, de Cesare M, Berthet A, Varlet V, Concha-Lozano N, Favrat B. E-cigarettes: a review of new trends in cannabis use. Int J Environ Res Public Health. 2015;12(8):9988–10008.
34. Spindle TR, Cone EJ, Schlienz NJ, Mitchell JM, Bigelow GE, Flegel R, et al. Acute effects of smoked and vaporized cannabis in healthy adults who infrequently use cannabis: a crossover Trial Acute effects of smoked vs vaporized cannabis use in infrequent cannabis Users Acute

effects of smoked vs vaporized cannabis use in infrequent cannabis users. JAMA Netw Open. 2018;1(7):–e184841.

35. Allen JG, Flanigan SS, Mallory LB, Jose V, Piers MN, Stewart James H, et al. Flavoring chemicals in E-cigarettes: diacetyl, 2,3-pentanedione, and acetoin in a sample of 51 products, including fruit-, candy-, and cocktail-flavored E-cigarettes. Environ Health Perspect. 2016;124(6):733–9.

36. https://www.fda.gov/news-events/press-announcements/statement-agencys-actions-tackle-epidemic-youth-vaping-and-court-ruling-application-submission.

37. Troutt WD, DiDonato MD. Carbonyl compounds produced by vaporizing cannabis oil thinning agents. J Altern Complement Med. 2017;23(11):879–84.

38. Lee M-S, Allen Joseph G, Christiani David C. Endotoxin and (1→3)-β-D-glucan contamination in electronic cigarette products sold in the United States. Environ Health Perspect. 127(4):047008.

39. Palazzolo DL, Crow AP, Nelson JM, Johnson RA. Trace metals derived from electronic cigarette (ECIG) generated aerosol: potential problem of ECIG devices that contain nickel. Front Physiol. 2017;7:663.

40. https://www.cnn.com/2019/08/03/health/vaping-hospitalizations-wisconsin-illinois/index.html.

41. https://www.nydailynews.com/life-style/health/ny-9-new-jersey-residents-in-hosp-after-vaping-20190820-mac5sqvppzdpxgnrdgenjxoyua-story.html.

42. https://www.star-telegram.com/news/local/article234184982.html.

43. https://www.foxnews.com/health/colorado-vaping-related-illness.

44. https://interactives.nejm.org/ile/cdc_vaping/index.html.

45. https://www.cdc.gov/tobacco/basic_information/e-cigarettes/severe-lung-disease.html.

46. Flower M, Nandakumar L, Singh M, Wyld D, Windsor M, Fielding D. Respiratory bronchiolitis-associated interstitial lung disease secondary to electronic nicotine delivery system use confirmed with open lung biopsy. Respirol Case Rep. 2017;5(3):e00230.

47. Agustin M, Yamamoto M, Cabrera F, Eusebio R. Diffuse alveolar hemorrhage induced by vaping. Case Rep Pulmonol. 2018;2018:9724530.

48. Thota D, Latham E. Case report of electronic cigarettes possibly associated with eosinophilic pneumonitis in a previously healthy active-duty sailor. J Emerg Med. 2014;47(1):15–7.

49. Modi S, Sangani R, Alhajhusain A. Acute lipoid pneumonia secondary to E-cigarettes use: an unlikely replacement for cigarettes. Chest. 2015;148(4):382A.

50. Blount BC, Karwowski MP, Morel-Espinosa M, et al. Evaluation of bronchoalveolar lavage fluid from patients in an outbreak of E-cigarette, or vaping, product use–associated lung injury — 10 states, August–October 2019. MMWR Morb Mortal Wkly Rep. 2019;68:1040–1.

51. Abdallah SJ, Smith BM, Ware MA, Moore M, Li PZ, Bourbeau J, et al. Effect of vaporized cannabis on exertional breathlessness and exercise endurance in advanced chronic obstructive pulmonary disease. A randomized controlled trial. Ann ATS. 2018;15(10):1146–58.

52. Huang J, Duan Z, Kwok J, Binns S, Vera LE, Kim Y, et al. Vaping versus JUULing: how the extraordinary growth and marketing of JUUL transformed the US retail e-cigarette market. Tob Control. 2019;28(2):146–51.

53. Hammond D, Wackowski OA, Reid JL, O'Connor RJ, International Tobacco Control Policy Evaluation Project (ITC) team. Use of JUUL E-cigarettes among youth in the United States. Nicotine Tob Res. . [Internet]. 27 Oct 2018 [cited 23 Aug 2019]. Available from: https://doi.org/10.1093/ntr/nty237.

54. Aleyan S, Cole A, Qian W, Leatherdale ST. Risky business: a longitudinal study examining cigarette smoking initiation among susceptible and non-susceptible e-cigarette users in Canada. BMJ Open. 2018;8(5):e021080.

55. Hammond D, Reid JL, Cole AG, Leatherdale ST. Electronic cigarette use and smoking initiation among youth: a longitudinal cohort study. CMAJ. 2017;189(43):E1328–36.

56. https://www.lung.org/stop-smoking/smoking-facts/e-cigarettes-and-lung-health.html.

57. Tashkin DP. Effects of marijuana smoking on the lung. Ann ATS. 2013;10(3):239–47.

58. Ribeiro LI, Ind PW. Effect of cannabis smoking on lung function and respiratory symptoms: a structured literature review. NPJ Prim Care Respir Med. 2016;26:16071.

59. Chatkin JM, Zabert G, Zabert I, Chatkin G, Jiménez-Ruiz CA, de Granda-Orive JI, et al. Lung disease associated with marijuana use. Archivos de Bronconeumología (English Edition). 2017;53(9):510–5.

60. Roth MD, Whittaker K, Salehi K, Tashkin DP, Baldwin GC. Mechanisms for impaired effector function in alveolar macrophages from marijuana and cocaine smokers. J Neuroimmunol. 2004;147(1):82–6.

61. Cescon DW, Page AV, Richardson S, Moore MJ, Boerner S, Gold WL. Invasive pulmonary aspergillosis associated with marijuana use in a man with colorectal cancer. JCO. 2008;26(13):2214–5.

62. Thu K, Hayes M, Miles S, Tierney L, Foy A. Marijuana "bong" smoking and tuberculosis. Intern Med J. 2013;43(4):456–8.

63. Oeltmann JE, Oren E, Haddad MB, Lake LK, Harrington TA, Ijaz K, et al. Tuberculosis outbreak in marijuana users, Seattle, Washington, 2004. Emerg Infect Dis. 2006;12(7):1156–9.

64. Morales I, Forseen C, Biddinger P, Keshavamurthy J, Thomson N, Fortson T. Marijuana: is it safe? A case of fatal marijuana-induced necrotizing bronchiolitis. Chest. 2016;150(4):401A.

65. Shams C, Dalal B. Cannabis-induced hemoptysis: a rare complication of a commonly used illicit substance. Chest. 2018;154(4):800A.

66. Weiss ZF, Gore S, Foderaro A. Pneumomediastinum in marijuana users: a retrospective review of 14 cases. BMJ Open Resp Res. 2019;6(1):e000391.

67. Anderson RP, Zechar K. Lung injury from inhaling butane hash oil mimics pneumonia. Respir Med Case Rep. 2019;26:171–3.

68. Sullivan N, Elzinga S, Raber JC. Determination of pesticide residues in cannabis smoke. J Toxicol. 2013;2013:378168.. 6 pages.

69. Raber JC, Elzinga S, Kaplan C. Understanding dabs: contamination concerns of cannabis concentrates and cannabinoid transfer during the act of dabbing. J Toxicol Sci. 2015;40(6):797–803.

70. Wei B, Alwis KU, Li Z, Wang L, Valentin-Blasini L, Sosnoff CS, et al. Urinary concentrations of PAH and VOC metabolites in marijuana users. Environ Int. 2016 Mar;88:1–8.

71. https://www.courthousenews.com/pot-smokers-warn-of-cyanide-from-pesticide/.

72. Wang C-T, Wiedinmyer C, Ashworth K, Harley PC, Ortega J, Vizuete W. Leaf enclosure measurements for determining volatile organic compound emission capacity from Cannabis spp. Atmos Environ. 2019;199:80–7.

73. Wang F, Li C, Liu W, Jin Y. Effect of exposure to volatile organic compounds (VOCs) on airway inflammatory response in mice. J Toxicol Sci. 2012;37(4):739–48.

74. Yoon HI, Hong Y-C, Cho S-H, Kim H, Kim YH, Sohn JR, et al. Exposure to volatile organic compounds and loss of pulmonary function in the elderly. Eur Respir J. 2010;36(6):1270–6.

75. Schober W, Szendrei K, Matzen W, Osiander-Fuchs H, Heitmann D, Schettgen T, et al. Use of electronic cigarettes (e-cigarettes) impairs indoor air quality and increases FeNO levels of e-cigarette consumers. Int J Hyg Environ Health. 2014;217(6):628–37.

76. Chen R, Aherrera A, Isichei C, Olmedo P, Jarmul S, Cohen JE, et al. Assessment of indoor air quality at an electronic cigarette (vaping) convention. J Expo Sci Environ Epidemiol. 2018;28(6):522–9.

77. https://no-smoke.org/wp-content/uploads/pdf/2018-Indoor-Air-Cannabis01-Schick.pdf.

78. Hoffman BC, Kuhl M, Harbeck RJ, Rabinovitch N. Cannabis allergy in a child with asthma chronically exposed to marijuana. J Allergy Clin Immunol Pract. 2020;8:422.. [Internet]. [cited 26 Aug 2019]. Available from: https://doi.org/10.1016/j.jaip.2019.06.042.

79. Decuyper II, Faber MA, Sabato V, Bridts CH, Hagendorens MM, Rihs H-P, et al. Where there's smoke, there's fire: cannabis allergy through passive exposure. J Allergy Clin Immunol Pract. 2017;5(3):864–5.

80. Silvers WS, Bernard T. Spectrum and prevalence of reactions to marijuana in a Colorado allergy practice. Ann Allergy Asthma Immunol. 2017;119(6):570–1.

81. Posis A, Bellettiere J, Liles S, Alcaraz J, Nguyen B, Berardi V, et al. Indoor cannabis smoke and children's health. Prev Med Rep. 2019;14:100853.
82. Wang X, Derakhshandeh R, Narayan S, Emmy L, Le S, Danforth Olivia M, et al. Abstract 19538: brief exposure to marijuana secondhand smoke impairs vascular endothelial function. Circulation. 2014;130(suppl_2):A19538.
83. Herrmann ES, Cone EJ, Mitchell JM, Bigelow GE, LoDico C, Flegel R, et al. Non-smoker exposure to secondhand cannabis smoke II: effect of room ventilation on the physiological, subjective, and behavioral/cognitive effects. Drug Alcohol Depend. 2015;151:194–202.
84. Cromar KR, Gladson LA, Perlmutt LD, Ghazipura M, Ewart GW. American Thoracic Society and Marron Institute report. Estimated excess morbidity and mortality caused by air pollution above American Thoracic Society–recommended standards, 2011–2013. Ann ATS. 2016;13(8):1195–201.
85. https://www.lung.org/stop-smoking/smoking-facts/marijuana-and-lung-health.html.

THC & CBD Decomposition and Terpene Hazards While Vaping or Dabbing

86. Life science: session 1. Annenberg Learners. https://www.learner.org/courses/essential/life/session1/closer2.html.
87. The difference between organic and inorganic. ThoughtCo, Anne Marie Helmenstine, Ph.D. 3 Jul 2019. https://www.thoughtco.com/difference-between-organic-and-inorganic-603912.
88. Thompson TE. Lipid biochemistry. Encyclopedia Britannica. https://www.britannica.com/science/lipid.
89. Alves E, Domingues MRM, Domingues P. Polar lipids from olives and olive oil: a review on their identification, significance and potential biotechnological applications. Foods. 2018;7:109.. Mass Spectrometry Centre, Department of Chemistry & QOPNA; University of Aveiro, Campus Universitário de Santiago; 10 July 2018: https://www.ncbi.nlm.nih.gov/pmc/articles/PMC6068626/.
90. Ruani A. Doctoral Researcher. Oils for cooking: which ones to avoid? The Health Sciences Academy. https://thehealthsciencesacademy.org/health-tips/oils-for-cooking/.
91. Achitoff-Gray N. What's a smoke point and why does it matter? 16 May 2014. https://www.seriouseats.com/2014/05/cooking-fats-101-whats-a-smoke-point-and-why-does-it-matter.html.
92. ATSDR. Public health statement for acrolein. Aug 2007. https://www.atsdr.cdc.gov/phs/phs.asp?id=554&tid=102.
93. Gavin J. Smoke point of cooking oils. 2 Feb 2018. https://www.jessicagavin.com/smoke-points-cooking-oils/.
94. Draper point. Wikipedia. https://en.wikipedia.org/wiki/Draper_point.
95. Forged in fire show. https://www.reddit.com/r/forgedinfireshow/comments/8tk6kt/temperature_color_chart/.
96. HeatersPlus.com. https://www.heatersplus.com/nichrome.html.
97. Kross B. Chief Detector Engineer. What's the melting point of steel? Jefferson Lab. https://education.jlab.org/qa/meltingpoint_01.html.
98. Sharma P, Murthy P, Bharath MMS. Chemistry, metabolism, and toxicology of cannabis: clinical implications. IJP. 2012;7(4):149–56: https://www.ncbi.nlm.nih.gov/pmc/articles/PMC3570572/.
99. King M. What's in that vape? cannabis & vaping. Public Health Insider. https://publichealth-insider.com/2019/07/12/whats-in-that-vape-cannabis-vaping/.
100. Dronabinol: PubChem; U.S. National Library of Medicine. https://pubchem.ncbi.nlm.nih.gov/compound/Dronabinol.
101. Cannabidiol: PubChem; U.S. National Library of Medicine. https://pubchem.ncbi.nlm.nih.gov/compound/Cannabidiol.

102. Doane S. Farmers in Italy fight soil contamination with cannabis. CBS Evening News. 12 Mar 2017. https://publichealthinsider.com/2019/07/12/whats-in-that-vape-cannabis-vaping/.
103. Jacobs M. The differences between cannabinoids and terpenes. Analytical Cannabis. 21 Feb 2019. https://www.analyticalcannabis.com/articles/the-difference-between-cannabinoids-and-terpenes-311502.
104. Nails D.. SmokeCartel.com, https://www.smokecartel.com/collections/titanium-ceramic-quartz-nails-and-dabber-tools.
105. Clean your atomizer – Protank EVOD MTE T3 Kanger. 19 Oct 2013. https://www.youtube.com/watch?v=g9FqlSikIpc.
106. Best temperature for dabs and concentrates. Torrch.com: https://torrchvapor.com/news/best-temperature-dabs-concentrates/.
107. Meehan-Atrash J, Luo W, Strongin RM. Toxicant formation in dabbing: the terpene story. Department of Chemistry, Portland University; ACS Omega 2017. https://pubs.acs.org/doi/pdf/10.1021/acsomega.7b01130.
108. 1,3 Butadiene; health effects. OSHA. https://www.osha.gov/SLTC/butadiene/healtheffects.html.
109. Lipinski B. Hydroxyl radical and its scavengers in health and disease: Joslin Diabetes Center, Harvard Medical School, Hindawi Publishing Co.; 11 June 2011. https://www.hindawi.com/journals/omcl/2011/809696/.
110. Myrcene material safety data sheet. Sigma-Aldrich. 13 Mar 2014. https://www.nwmissouri.edu/naturalsciences/sds/m/Myrcene.pdf.
111. Limonene material safety data sheet. Sigma-Aldrich. 13 Mar 2014. https://www.nwmissouri.edu/naturalsciences/sds/l/Limonene.pdf.
112. Linalool material safety data sheet. Sigma-Aldrich. 13 Mar 2014. https://www.nwmissouri.edu/naturalsciences/sds/l/Linalool.pdf.
113. Vaping: the good, the bad, and the popcorn lung. MPHonline.com: https://www.mphonline.org/vaping-public-health/.
114. O'Donnell J. Half of THC vape samples have risky Vitamin E acetate, but pesticides, heavy metals found too. USA Today. 11 Oct 2019. https://www.usatoday.com/story/news/health/2019/10/11/vaping-illness-thc-additives-include-vitamin-e-acetate-metals/3943427002/.

Chapter 9
Clinical Cardiovascular Effects of Cannabis Use

Cynthia Philip, Rebecca Seifried, Marcio Sommer Bittencourt, and Edward Hulten

Introduction

Cannabis is the most widely consumed illicit drug in the world today with an estimated 182.5 million users, which represents 3.8% of the global population. Cannabis is a complex mixture of several cannabinoids of which THC (Δ9-tetrahydrocannabinol) and cannabidiol (CBD) are the main active components. These components are present in variable amounts and proportions in each preparation. The activity of cannabis is likely influenced by terpenes and terpenoids, which vary in content and type [1]. Furthermore, the content of marijuana is not tightly regulated even in most legalized markets, which may lead to more intense concentrations of biologically active components as well as contamination with synthetic compounds or other illicit drugs.

The World Health Organization reports that marijuana use exceeds cocaine or opiates by an order of magnitude [2]. In North America, 15- to 64-year-olds abuse

---

Drs. Philip and Seifried were contributed equally to this work.

C. Philip · R. Seifried
Cardiology Service, Department of Medicine, Walter Reed National Military Medical Center and Uniformed Services University of Health Sciences, Bethesda, MD, USA

M. S. Bittencourt
Dalboni – DASA, São Paulo, Brazil

Hospital Israelita Albert Einstein & School of Medicine, Faculdade Israelita de Ciência da Saúde Albert Einstein, São Paulo, Brazil

Center for Clinical and Epidemiological Research, University Hospital & Sao Paulo State Cancer Institute, University of Sao Paulo, São Paulo, Brazil
e-mail: msbittencourt@mail.harvard.edu

E. Hulten (✉)
Fort Belvoir Community Hospital, Virginia, USA

© Springer Nature Switzerland AG 2020   209
K. Finn (ed.), *Cannabis in Medicine*,
https://doi.org/10.1007/978-3-030-45968-0_9

marijuana more than any other illicit substance with an estimated annual prevalence of 11.6% [2]. Despite its classification traditionally as an illicit substance in
many nations, in recent years in the United States, 33 states and the District of
Columbia have approved the clinical use of cannabis for various conditions and 10
states have legalized marijuana for recreational and medicinal purposes [3].
Medical use of marijuana focuses primarily upon its neurological and cognitive
effects to include management of chronic pain and fibromyalgia, relief of spasticity in multiple sclerosis, and as an anti-emetic in the treatment of chemotherapy-
induced nausea.

Until recent decades, the effects of cannabis on other organ systems beyond neurocognitive systems were not largely studied. However, a need for better understanding of cannabis effects upon the cardiovascular system has emerged with ever
more importance, given the rapid increase and spread in cannabis use and that cardiovascular disease remains the leading cause of mortality worldwide, with estimated global mortality of 17.9 million deaths in 2016 and 630,000 deaths within the
United States in 2015 [4]. A growing body of evidence has established that cannabis
has potential adverse biological and clinical effects on the cardiovascular system.
Cannabis consumption elicits numerous identified hormonal, adrenergic, vasospas-
tic, and atherogenic effects upon the vasculature. Furthermore, medical research has
demonstrated causal pathways for cannabis that cause arrhythmia, myocardial
infarction (MI), cerebrovascular accident, myocarditis, peripheral ischemia, pulmonary vascular disease, and sudden cardiac death.

With the recent increased legalization and use of cannabis in the United States as
well as worldwide, further research is needed to better understand the potential,
frequency, and severity of cardiovascular harm caused by this drug and to develop
public health educational programs about its adverse effects.

Biological Cardiovascular Effects of Cannabis

An important body of evidence has accumulated from basic science and observational studies regarding the biological and cardiovascular effects of cannabis on
human physiology. Despite this, the efforts of researchers in understanding the biological effects of cannabis are challenging due to confusions that arise as a result of
polysubstance use among cannabis subjects, which may or may not be fully disclosed to researchers, including tobacco, cocaine, alcohol, supplements, or illicit
drugs or other substances. Cannabis effects depend upon the affinity of cannabinoids for CBD receptors 1 and 2 (CB1, CB2). These receptors are present, to varying degrees, in different body tissues and are responsible for the subsequent central
and peripheral effects that we will further discuss in this section. CB1 receptors are
expressed predominantly in the brain, cardiac muscle, liver, gastrointestinal tract,
vascular endothelium, vascular smooth muscle cells, and kidney. CB2 receptors are
predominantly expressed in immune cells and on endothelial cells. Adipocytes,
platelets, and bronchial epithelium express both CB1 and CB2 receptors [5].

Marijuana use promulgates the formation of reactive oxygen species, decreases myocardial contractility, provokes a pro-inflammatory endothelial response, and promotes neointimal proliferation of vascular smooth muscle. It is, in part, because of these effects that marijuana use has been associated with adverse cardiovascular outcomes which include acute coronary syndromes, coronary artery dissection, coronary vasospasm, coronary thrombosis, arrhythmias, stroke, vasculitis, myocarditis, and cardiomyopathies [6].

Cannabis and Its Role in the Pathophysiology of Atherosclerosis

Cannabinoids affect atherogenesis via their effects on monocyte adhesion and cytokine expression. In atherogenesis, when vascular endothelium is injured, low-density lipoprotein cholesterol subsequently infiltrates the subendothelial layer. Concurrently, smooth muscle cells migrate to and infiltrate the intima of the vascular wall. Monocyte-derived macrophages accumulate oxidized low density lipoprotein resulting in the formation of foam cells, an early component of developing atherosclerotic plaque. Lipid uploading by macrophages is associated with the expression of inflammatory cytokines, which then activates type 1 T-helper cells (TH1). The TH1 cells then, in turn, stimulate the macrophages to continue to express inflammatory cytokines, which further contribute to the chronic atherosclerotic disease process [7].

In low doses, the main psychoactive component of marijuana, THC, decreases monocyte adhesion and infiltrates the vascular subendothelial layer via activation of CB2 receptors. Additionally, THC influences the macrophage's cytokine release, decreasing interferon-γ release, which in turn downregulates the type 1 T-helper cell (TH1) immune response. [5] Conversely, CB1 expression has been identified in macrophages of advanced atheroma, and a higher number of CB1 receptors exist in coronary atheroma patients with unstable angina compared to those with stable angina [8]. As monocytes differentiate into macrophages, there is increased expression of CB1 receptors. The increased CB1 receptors correlate with increased reactive oxygen species production and endothelial cell injury, and additionally, CB1 receptor agonism results in increased lipid accumulation in macrophages [9]. There have been several studies investigating the effect of CB1 receptor blockade, which resulted in decreased inflammatory cytokine production, and inhibition of monocyte recruitment. [5, 8, 10, 11] In a mouse study, a decreased atherosclerotic lesion development with CB1 receptor antagonism was observed, which the authors theorized was in part related to cholesterol inhibition and in part related to anti-inflammatory effects [11].

Cannabinoids also influence vascular smooth muscle cell growth and proliferation, which contribute to atherosclerosis and stent restenosis. CB2 agonism decreases the production of TNF-α, an inflammatory cytokine that signals smooth muscle cells to proliferate and infiltrate the intima. Conversely, CB1 antagonism

decreases platelet-derived growth factor production and agonism upregulates angio-
tensin 1 receptor leading to increased reactive oxygen species [5].

Although the relationship of CBD receptors to atherosclerosis is complex and
multifactorial, general studies have shown contrasting effects of CB1 and CB2
receptors on the development of atherosclerosis, with CB1 agonism promoting atherosclerosis while CB2 agonism preventing it.

Physiological Cardiovascular Effects of Cannabis

Marijuana exhibits dose-dependent increases upon the heart rate, cardiac output,
supine blood pressure, and postural hypotension [5, 12]. Heart rate can increase by
20–100%, with peak heart rate 10–30 minutes after inhaling marijuana smoke [13].
Smoking marijuana decreases time to maximum predicted heart rate with exertion
and decreases the maximum exercise capacity of even healthy individuals without
clinically significant coronary artery disease [5]. Increased activity of sympathetic
nervous system, stimulation of beta-adrenergic receptors with increased plasma
norepinephrine levels, inhibition of parasympathetic innervation of the heart, and
reflex tachycardia due to vasodilation are all proposed mechanisms for tachycardia
seen with cannabis use [14, 15].

Marijuana smoke exposure has been associated with the precipitation of angina
in people with existing coronary artery disease. In one study, the exercise time of
chronic stable angina patients decreased by an average of 48% after smoking one
marijuana cigarette versus 23% after smoking a nicotine cigarette [12, 16, 17]. One
proposed mechanism for the lower angina threshold is an increase in the levels of
carboxyhemoglobin with decreased oxygen-carrying capacity of red blood cells.
Additionally, catecholamine release increases heart rate and myocardial contractility, thereby resulting in oxygen demand [15]. These actions cause a net increase in
myocardial oxygen demand with a decrease in oxygen supply [17].

In one study of 147 patients with cannabis associated myocardial infarction (with
coronary imaging was available for 21 patients), 38% of patients had single-vessel
coronary thrombosis; another 38% had normal results [18]. While some myocardial
infarctions may be related to increased myocardial oxygen demand and decreased
oxygen supply, other patients have a culprit lesion which is proposed to be due to
disruption of vulnerable atherosclerotic plaque in response to hemodynamic effects
associated with cannabis use [19].

In a retrospective study of nearly 2.5 million hospitalized patients with history of
marijuana use, the burden of arrhythmia was evaluated and it occurred in about 2.7%
of patients with atrial fibrillation being the most common, followed by ventricular
tachycardia and atrial flutter [20]. Ventricular tachycardia with right bundle branch
block pattern and left axis deviation without significant atherosclerotic disease has
been described in the literature [21, 22] and it is hypothesized that it is triggered by
activity in Purkinje fibers or reentry in a small region of the inferior left ventricle
[22]. This form of ventricular tachycardia is responsive to verapamil therapy [22, 23].

In a case report of a 34-year-old male habitual marijuana user who developed ventricular tachycardia (VT), the VT was monomorphic with a right bundle branch block morphology and left axis deviation which responded to cardioversion [22]. He underwent coronary angiography and was found to have normal-appearing coronary arteries without stenosis, but had a marked reduction in coronary flow. After verapamil administration, he had normal coronary flow, and with repeat coronary angiography 3 days later, he again was found to have normal coronary flow. When initially undergoing electrophysiology testing, his VT was inducible, and after cessation of marijuana and treatment with verapamil, he no longer had inducible VT.

In addition to tachyarrhythmia, asystole has also been described in one case study [24], which showed that a 21-year-old male had recurrent episodes of presyncope and syncope while smoking marijuana. A Holter monitor demonstrated multiple symptomatic pauses, which corresponded to episodes where he was smoking marijuana. The proposed mechanism is thought to be due to a sudden increase in parasympathetic tone and parasympathetic activity, as demonstrated in mice [25]. CB1 receptor activation in the heart was found to have a triphasic response with initial vagally mediated fall in heart rate and blood pressure, then a brief non-sympathetically mediated pressor response, followed by a prolonged hypotensive effect due to decreased cardiac contractility and total peripheral resistance. Cannabinoids can elicit vasorelaxation, in part, by triggering the release of calcitonin gene-related peptide which induces vasorelaxation in isolated blood vessels [25].

The mechanisms of marijuana-induced myocardial infarction and ventricular arrhythmias are only partially understood, but these effects are thought to be due to the stimulation of the sympathetic nervous system and decrease in parasympathetic autonomic tone. This is demonstrated by slow or no flow in the coronary arteries, as TIMI grade coronary flow is a surrogate for blood flow in the microcirculation [22].

Sudden cardiac death or cardiomyopathy following cannabis use is rarer than myocardial infarction related to cannabis use; however, the exact incidence is difficult to determine as there may be underdiagnosis of marijuana as a causative agent for sudden death and myocardial infarction. For example, in the YOUNG MI registry, the adjusted hazard ratio for marijuana abuse was similar in effect size to cocaine for cardiovascular death, yet marijuana use may not be systematically tested for or reported as causal in MI or sudden death [6]. Bachs reviewed six cases of pathology review of likely acute cardiovascular cause of death and recent cannabis ingestion [15]. All subjects were young adults (17–43 years) whose sudden death appeared to be related solely to marijuana use. Toxicology studies revealed only presence of THC in the blood and urine, and all patients were healthy before sudden death.

There are a few case reports of stress cardiomyopathy due to cannabis use. One case report showed that a female with chronic cannabis use developed recurrent episodes of stress cardiomyopathy with reintroduction of cannabis [26]. The pathophysiology of stress cardiomyopathy in cannabis users is poorly defined, but it is thought to be associated with catecholamine surge. All studies investigating the role of cannabis in acute myocardial infarction and sudden death are observational which is hypothesis generating, but the infrequency of such reports prevents any certainty regarding the potential for direct effect of marijuana on left ventricle ejection fraction or sudden cardiac death.

There is likely a multifactorial etiology for some of the cardiovascular complications associated with cannabis use, and life style choices may play a significant role. The CARDIA study demonstrated that patients who use marijuana have a high caloric diet and were more likely to smoke tobacco and use other illicit drugs [27, 28].

Despite overall adverse cardiovascular physiologic and clinical effects of cannabis, paradoxically increasing reports of cannabis use among recreational and elite athletes have emerged. Although most competitive sports prohibit cannabis use during competition, no restriction may be required during training and some athletes report a perception of improved performance. However, as described above, cannabis would appear in sum to have deleterious effects on most athletic performance; thus, athletes' perceived performance enhancement may simply result from anxiolysis, pain mitigation, or placebo effect rather than a real cardiovascular performance enhancement [29].

Pulmonary Vascular Biological Effects of Cannabis

No ample literature is available regarding the biological effects of cannabis on the pulmonary vascular system, but cannabis has known associations with lung disease, resultant pulmonary vasoconstriction, and pulmonary hypertension. This is a problem that is understudied and underappreciated. Regular marijuana smokers complain of more chronic bronchitis symptoms of chronic productive cough and wheezing [30], but there has been mixed data regarding chronic marijuana smoking and the risk of developing emphysema and reduced lung function compared to that of nicotine cigarette smoking [31–33]. A mouse study evaluating the effects of marijuana smoke on lung tissue found that the mice developed severe pulmonary hyperresponsiveness, inflammation, and emphysema [34]. These effects are related to elevated concentrations of four inflammatory cytokines, MCP-1, IFN-y, TNF-α, and IL-12, which induce basophil and mast cell degranulation, induce nitric oxide synthase production, and enhance phagocytosis, IL-1 and PGE2 syntheses, and neutrophil accumulation. The activation of these cytokines leads to significant inflammation that eventually results in pulmonary tissue destruction [34].

The consequent severe lung disease results from parenchymal destruction as well as chronic pulmonary vascular disease including pulmonary hypertension.

Cerebrovascular Biological Effects of Cannabis

Cannabis-related cerebral infarction is an uncommon finding with less than 100 clinical cases reported in the literature. In a literature review examining 71 cannabis users with cerebral infarctions [18], a young (mean age 35.5 years) male predominance with a slight predilection for the posterior cerebral circulation was observed, with the majority being cerebellar and occipital infarctions. Most patients were regular users of marijuana and all had used marijuana within 24 hours of symptom onset. There is a temporal relationship between the use of cannabis and cannabis-associated cerebral infarct with studies demonstrating cerebral infarct or transient ischemic attacks (TIA) while actively smoking marijuana up to 30 minutes after cannabis inhalation [35]. There are several proposed mechanisms of cerebral infarcts and transient ischemic attacks after cannabis use, which include orthostatic hypotension with secondary impairment of autoregulation of cerebral blood flow or increased resistance in cerebral arteries, altered cerebral vasomotor function, supine hypertension and labile blood pressure, cardioembolism with atrial fibrillation or other arrhythmias, vasculopathy (toxic or with immune inflammatory), vasospasm, reversible cerebral vasoconstriction syndrome (RCVS) [36], and multifocal intra-cranial stenosis (MIS) [35]. Additionally, reduction in cerebral blood flow affects the cerebellum and causes cerebellar ischemia [37].

In a prospective cohort study of 48 patients admitted with acute ischemic stroke, of the patients who tested positive for cannabis (13 patients), there appeared to be a specific pattern of multifocal intracranial stenosis (MIS) in posterior cerebral arter-ies and superior cerebellar arteries appreciated on magnetic resonance angiography (MRA) and coronary angiography (CA), and upon follow-up, there was a partial or total reversibility of vasoconstriction within 3–6 months [38]. A study by Wolff et al. [35, 38] suggested reversible intracranial stenosis as a favored mechanism of action, but this contrasts with a subsequent literature review. Wolff et al. published a subsequent literature review of cannabis-associated acute cerebral infarct patients and a little more than half of those patients, 54% (n = 25), had abnormalities on cerebrovascular imaging [35].

Review of the literature highlights the difficulty in determining the mechanisms of stroke in cannabis users because in many of the cases reported, there was no adequate radiographic neurovascular evaluation during the acute phase of stroke and most patients did not have subsequent radiographic imaging upon follow-up. Furthermore, many of the patients may have reported or unreported polysubstance abuse [35, 39].

Peripheral Vascular Biological Effects of Cannabis

Numerous case reports have been published concerning cannabis or THC-associated arteritis, which may be one of the most frequent causes of peripheral arterial disease in adults under 50 years of age [40]. Cannabis use is associated with lower limb arteritis, which is mostly unilateral and has predominance in young males. Affected vessels often lack any evidence of conventional atherosclerotic disease. A literature review assessing 80 cannabis-associated arteritis patients [18] demonstrated that the average age of presentation was 28 years and 96% of these patients had involvement of their lower extremities. Most patients presented with painful distal necrosis of their limbs after several months of claudication, and vascular imaging revealed dis-tal arterial occlusions in 97% of patients and their occlusions were described as

Table 9.1 Summary of the major cardiovascular and cerebrovascular adverse effects related to cannabis inhalation

Cardiovascular	Peripheral	Cerebrovascular
Myocardial infarction	Arteritis	Reversible cerebral vasoconstriction
Coronary slow flow or	Vasculitis	syndrome
no-reflow	Ischemic ulcer	Transient ischemic attacks
Coronary vasospasm	Digital necrosis	Cerebral slow or no reflow
Coronary artery dissection	Raynaud's	Stroke
Coronary thrombosis	phenomenon	
Cardiac arrhythmia		
Worsened angina		
Tachycardia		
Hypertension and		
hypotension		
Myocarditis		

consistent with thromboangiitis obliterans (TAO) [18]. It is not clear whether cannabis-associated arteritis might be a subtype of TAO or whether it is an entirely different entity, as there is differing opinion in the literature [18, 40].

When compared with other TAO patients, patients with cannabis-associated limb arteritis are younger, more often male, have more frequent unilateral involvement of the lower limbs at clinical presentation, and have fewer occurrences of thrombophlebitis and Raynaud's phenomenon. In patients with cannabis arteritis, cannabis cessation was associated with arteritis remission, even during continued tobacco use. On the other hand, cannabis reintroduction after a period of cessation was associated with clinical arteritis recrudescence. Cannabis-associated arteritis has a poor prognosis with greater than 50% of patients requiring limb amputation without cannabis cessation [18].

Summary of Biological Effects of Cannabis (See Table 9.1)

The biological cardiovascular effects of cannabis are complicated with a dichotomy between the effects of CB1 versus CB2 agonism. Cannabis use has been associated with serious adverse cardiovascular outcomes, most of which are rare. The mechanisms for these adverse outcomes are not always well understood and confounding variables make a clear causal relationship difficult to establish. More research is required to better understand the biological cardiovascular effects of cannabis.

Cardiac Adverse Clinical Outcomes Caused by Cannabis Use

Angina

Studies have investigated the effect of inhaled cannabis on patients with exertional angina who were not regular users of cannabis. In one study, 10 male subjects of age

41–53 years exercised without smoking and then in a double-blind fashion smoked cannabis containing 18–20 mg THC; then the time taken to develop angina was investigated and considered as the primary endpoint. All patients had greater than 75% angiographically proven coronary stenosis in at least one major coronary artery [17]. In another study, 10 males 43–55 years of age underwent exercise after smoking marijuana versus placebo cigarette to evaluate time to development of angina [16]. Marijuana-containing cigarettes decreased exercise time to angina compared to the control by 48% whereas the placebo cigarette decreased exercise time to angina also, but by just 8.6% versus baseline [16, 17]. The authors hypothesized that the anginal effect of THC is attributable in part to the increased myocardial oxygen demands caused by faster increases in heart rate within minutes of inhalation.

Myocardial Infarction

Previously, cannabis users and the medical community underappreciated the risk of significant public health burden resulting from development of myocardial ischemia. However, over the past several years, there is a growing body of evidence that demonstrates the occurrence of acute coronary syndromes in otherwise young, healthy users of marijuana. Typically, they are young male patients without significant cardiovascular comorbidity who present with chest pain, ST segment elevation on ECG, and positive troponin after using marijuana. In many of the case reports, toxicology screening was negative for cocaine, opiates, and amphetamines while positive for marijuana, which suggests that marijuana use itself can be responsible for acute myocardial infarction [41].

A case–control study of patients after myocardial infarction has estimated that the risk of myocardial infarction in cannabis users is 4.8 times greater than the baseline in the first hour after cannabis use and is likely due to its short duration of action. In the second hour after smoking, the risk decreased to 1.7 times [12].

In 2017, Desai et al. published a retrospective analysis of over two million patients hospitalized with acute myocardial infarction between 2010 and 2014, and over 35,000 of those patients had a history of marijuana use. They found that the acute MI patients with history of marijuana use tended to be younger (average age 49 compared to 57 in the non-marijuana patients) and were more likely to be male and African American. Patients with a history of marijuana use had a 3–8% increase in lifetime odds of acute MI compared to patients without marijuana use. The length of stay and mortality rates were lower in the group with history of marijuana use; however, more patients were discharged against medical advice. The prevalence trends of dysrhythmias, respiratory failure, cardiogenic shock, and congestive heart failure complicating acute MI were higher in patients with cannabis use (Figs. 9.1 and 9.2) [42].

The YOUNG MI registry evaluated substance abuse among 2097 patients aged ≤50 years with first type 1 MI diagnosed at Brigham and Women's and Massachusetts General Hospital from 2000 and 2016. They noted a marijuana prevalence in 125

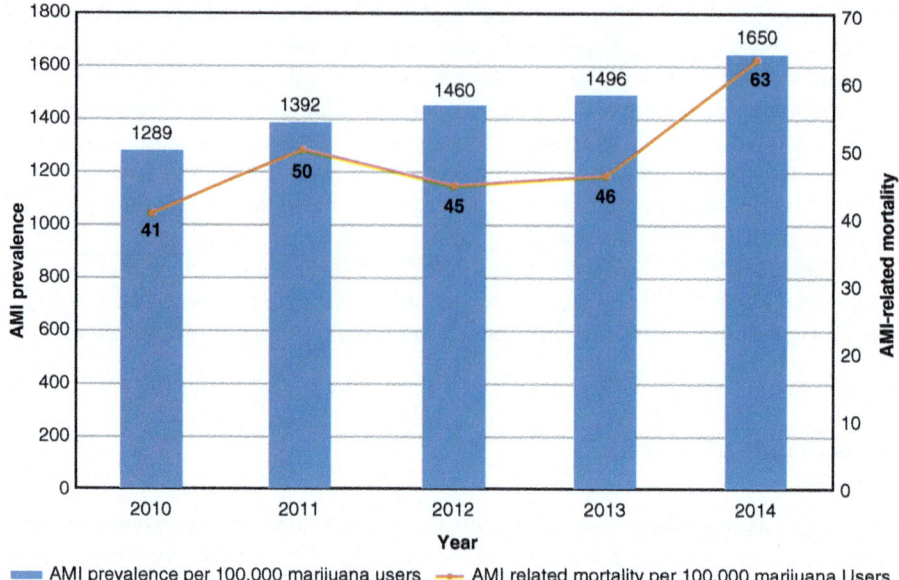

Fig. 9.1 Trends of acute myocardial infarction prevalence and mortality per 100,000 marijuana users in the United States [42]

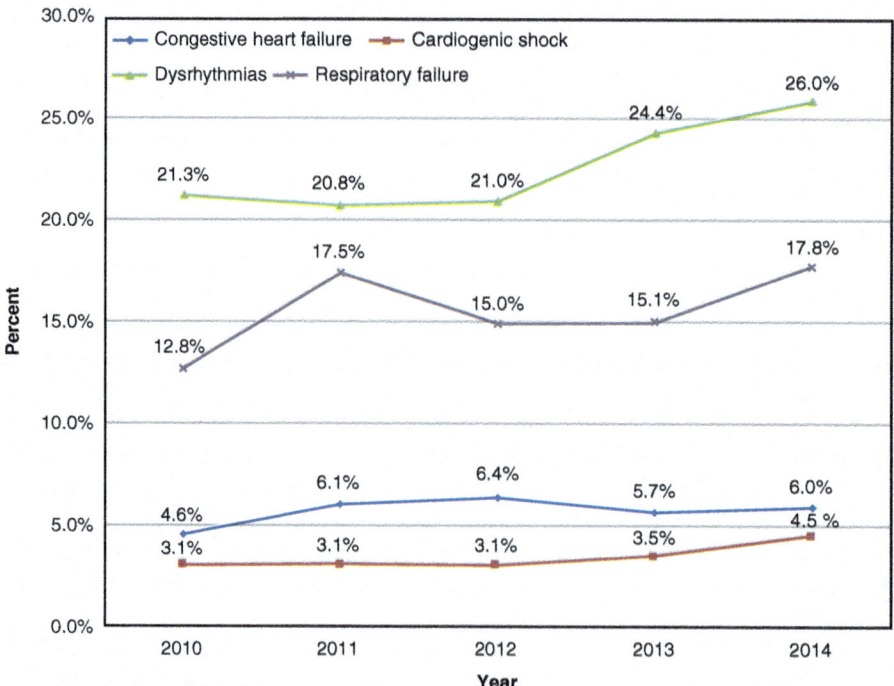

Fig. 9.2 Prevalence trends of congestive heart failure, cardiogenic shock, dysrhythmias, and respiratory failure in acute myocardial infarction patients with marijuana use (11–70 years) [42].

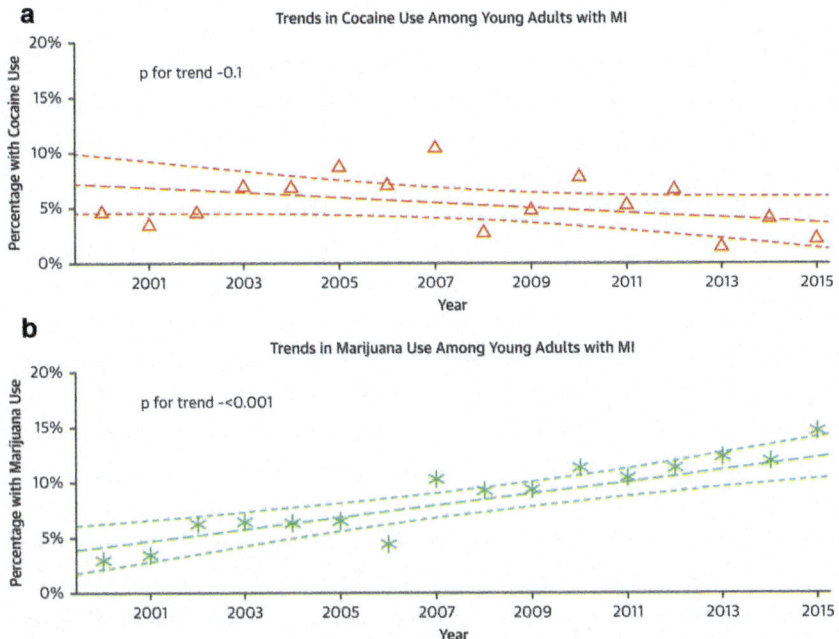

Fig. 9.3 Trends in substance use over time [6]. Trends in (**a**) cocaine and (**b**) marijuana use over the course of the study period, 2000–2016. The thick dashed line represented a fitted regression line and the thinner dashed line are confidence intervals. MI myocardial infarction. Triangles represents the percentage of patients with MI for the particular year who used cocaine. Asterisks represent the percentage of patients with MI for the particular year who used marijuana

(6.0%) young patients with MI, among whom 36 also tested positive for cocaine. This prevalence increased significantly over the 16-year study time, see Fig. 9.3 [6]. Initial presentation outside the hospital with cardiac arrest occurred in 4.0% of the patients, which was more common among those with substance abuse (8.0% vs. 3.5%; p . 0.003) and was associated more frequently with marijuana versus other substance abuse (8.8% vs. 3.5%; p . 0.007). After adjusting for age, presence of diabetes, hypertension, peripheral vascular disease, smoking, HDL-C, creatinine, medications at discharge, and length of stay, the authors noted that the hazard ratio for cardiovascular death due to marijuana was significant and similar in magnitude to cocaine – 2.13 (95% CI: 1.03–4.42; p . 0.042) for marijuana users versus 2.32 (95% CI: 1.11–4.85; p . 0.025) for cocaine (Fig. 9.4). [6].

Arrhythmia

Cardiac arrhythmias following recreational marijuana use have been described in case reports and case series. One observational study found that 2.7% of patients hospitalized with a history of marijuana use experienced arrhythmias. Males experienced more arrhythmias than females in this study (Fig. 9.7). The mean ages of

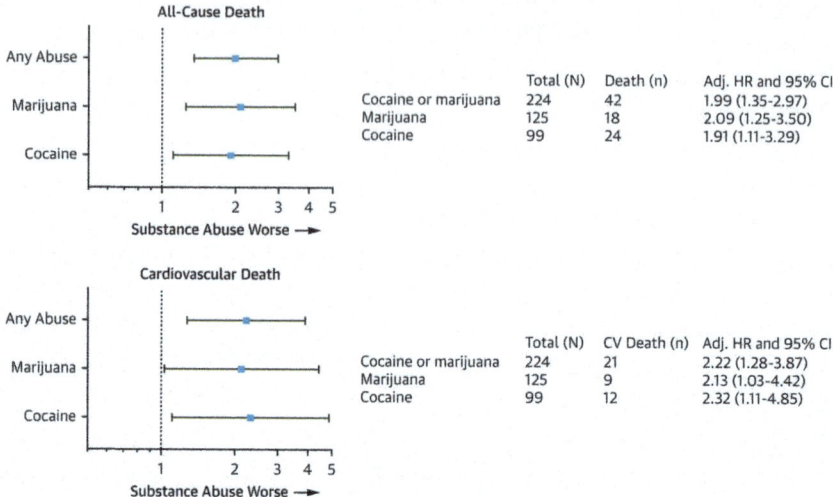

Fig. 9.4 Adjusted cardiovascular mortality and all-cause death [6]. Forest plots are shown for adjusted model of all-cause and cardiovascular (CV) death. All-cause death was adjusted for age, sex, presence of diabetes, hypertension, peripheral vascular diseases, smoking, high-density lipoprotein cholesterol, triglycerides, revascularization, creatinine, medications are discharge, and length of stay. CV death was adjusted for age, presence of diabetes, hypertension, peripheral vascular diseases, smoking, high-density lipoprotein cholesterol, creatinine, medications at discharge, and length of stay. Adj, HR adjusted hazard ratio; CI confidence interval

Fig. 9.5 Frequency of subtypes of arrhythmias per 100,000 hospitalized marijuana users [20]

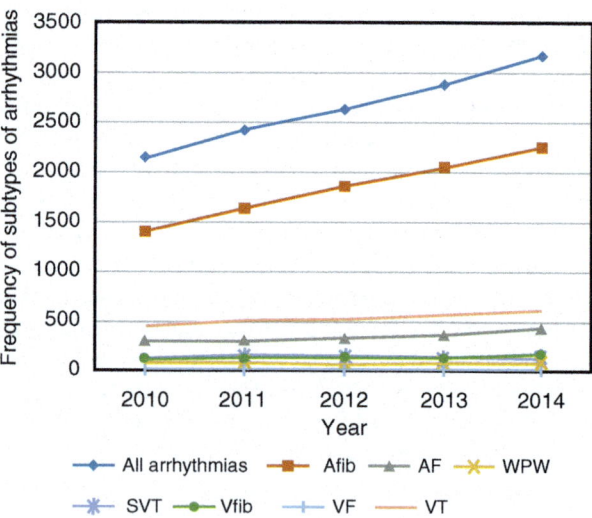

hospitalized marijuana users and marijuana users with arrhythmias were 36 and 51 years, respectively. Atrial fibrillation was the most common arrhythmia (1865/100,000 hospitalized patients) followed by ventricular tachycardia (532/100,000), atrial flutter (346/100,000), ventricular tachycardia (132/100,000),

Fig. 9.6 Frequency of all arrhythmias in hospitalized marijuana users by age [20]

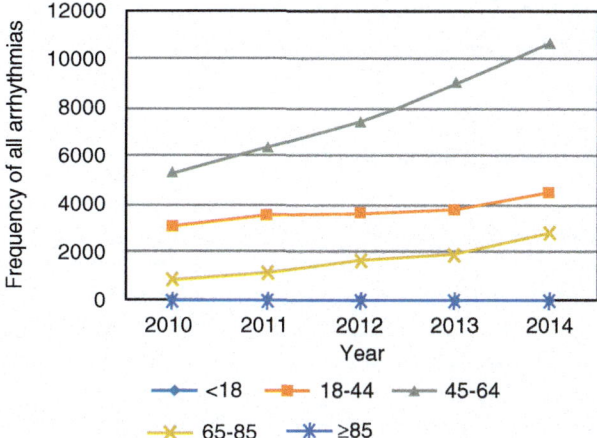

Fig. 9.7 Frequency of all arrhythmias in hospitalized marijuana users by sex [20]

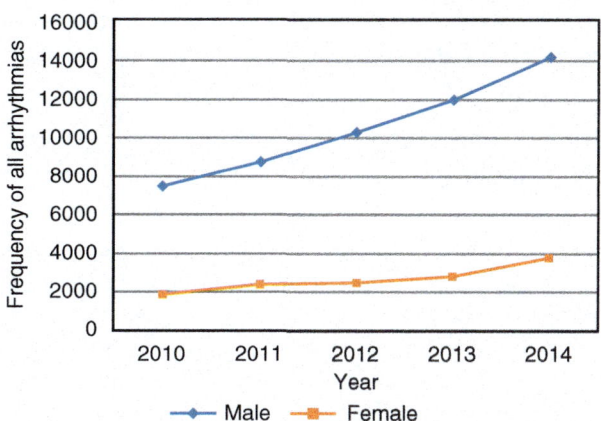

and ventricular fibrillation (136/100,000) (Figs. 9.5 and 9.6). Patients in the 45–65 age group showed highest incidence of arrhythmia [20]. Additionally, a case report identified marijuana as the only potentially causal factor in a 19-year-old man who presented with third-degree heart block requiring isopreteronol support in the intensive care unit. Heart block resolved after 1 day with cessation of marijuana in the hospital and evaluation revealed otherwise negative toxicology screen except for marijuana with unremarkable Borrelia and autoimmune titers, thyroid, electrolytes, chest X-ray, echocardiogram, coronary CT angiography, electrophysiologic study, and cardiac MRI. Five-day ambulatory ECG monitor after hospital discharge showed complete resolution of heart block with cessation of cannabis. The authors identified ten prior cases of symptomatic bradycardia attributed to cannabis in the published medical literature, ranging from sinus arrest to second- and third-degree heart blocks [43]..

Sudden Cardiac Death

Marijuana has traditionally been regarded as a relatively safe recreational drug, though some case reports link its use with sudden death. One comprehensive review showed that there were at least 35 reports of cases of significant cardiovascular emergencies and at least 13 deaths from a cardiovascular mechanism and there was likely to have been an underestimate of the true incidence of its contribution to sudden cardiac death. The age of the 13 people who died ranged from 17 to 52 years (median 37 years, all males). In eight of the cases, there was some degree of significant coronary atherosclerosis: three with superimposed thrombus, two with dilated cardiomyopathy, and at least three suffering from an acute myocardial infarction [1]. Five of the cases had little or obvious pathology, whose age ranged from 17 to 42 years (mean 31 years, all male). In all of these cases, the authors believed that cannabis significantly contributed to their deaths, possibly due to arrhythmia [1].

Myocarditis

There are at least five reports of pericarditis and myocarditis shortly after marijuana use in the literature. One of the cases was due to accidental exposure in an 11-month-old child which ultimately resulted in death [44]. Other published cases reported recovery with cannabis cessation and medical management [45–47].

Marijuana content, potential, and contiminants vary significantly; thus safety and regulation prove difficult even in legalized markets. The pathogenesis of pericarditis/myocarditis after marijuana use is unclear. Reports have shown fungi (*Aspergillus*, Penicillium), bacteria, microbial toxins such as aflatoxins, heavy metals (aluminum), and pesticides to contaminate marijuana. It is possible that contaminants may be the explanation, but further research is necessary to better explain the pathophysiology [48].

Pulmonary Vascular Adverse Clinical Outcomes

The inhalation of marijuana has been associated with adverse pulmonary outcomes such as chronic bronchitis and obstructive lung disease [49]. Studies have shown a dose-response relationship between cannabis and FEV1/FVC ratios, and it has been shown to increase total lung capacitance. This suggests that significant respiratory changes on spirometry occur in cannabis smokers, even at a young age [50, 51]. The incidence of cannabis-associated pulmonary hypertension is underreported and understudied. Because marijuana has been shown to promote lung disease, pulmonary hypertension may be an underappreciated public health burden of the legalization of marijuana.

Cerebrovascular Outcomes

Several case reports have been published in the literature implicating marijuana as the cause of ischemic cardiovascular accident (CVA) in young patients who smoke marijuana. One population-based study of hospitalized patients found an adjusted odds ratio of 1.76 for cannabis exposure associated with ischemic CVA [52]. One retrospective review of published cases linking marijuana use to stroke found that there was a majority of men versus women affected with a ratio of 4.9:1. Most of the strokes were ischemic strokes or transient ischemic attacks [35]. Hemorrhagic CVAs are less common, but have been associated with marijuana use as well. Similar to the elevated risk of myocardial infarction in the first hour after smoking marijuana, it appears that the risk of stroke is highest while smoking marijuana and up to half an hour after inhalation [39, 53–59]. The incidence of stroke-related

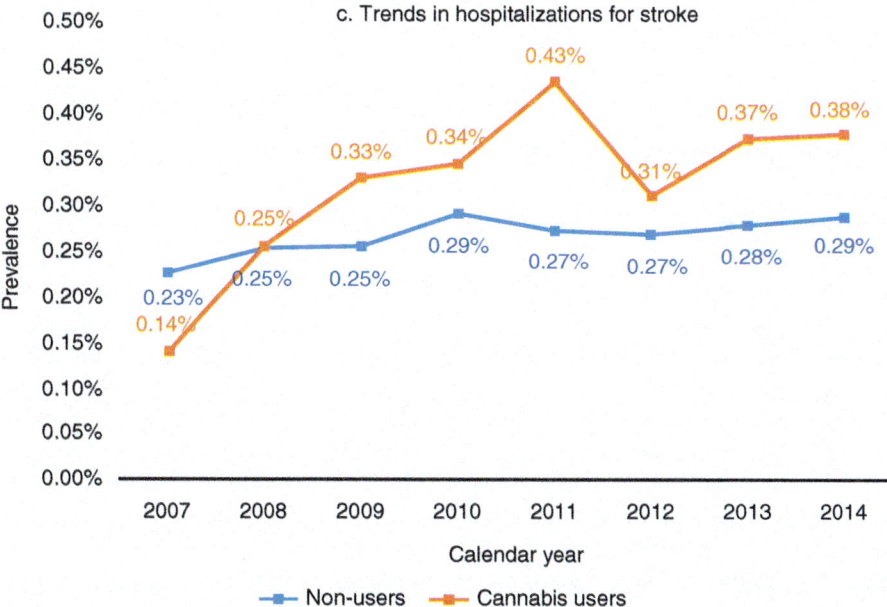

Fig. 9.8 The incidence of stroke-related admissions was higher among cannabis users vs. non-users (0.33% vs. 0.26%, $p < 0.001$) in a study of discharge records from the National Inpatient Sample (NIS) from 2007 to 2014 [60]

admissions among young patients aged 8–39 years was increased among cannabis users vs. non-users (0.33% vs. 0.26%, p <0.001) in a study of discharge records from the National Inpatient Sample (NIS) from 2007 to 2014 (Fig. 9.8) [60].

Reversible cerebral vasoconstriction syndrome (RCVS) is a neurological syndrome that affects young adults and is characterized by acute, severe headaches with or without neurological symptoms, and segmental cerebral artery vasoconstriction that appears as "beading" on neurovascular imaging. It tends to resolve within 12 weeks from the initial syndrome [61]. The majority of cases of RCVS can be attributed to a secondary factor that increases vascular tone, which includes vasoactive substances such as marijuana [62]. In one large prospective series, marijuana was the most common vasoactive substance to trigger RCVS in 30% of the patients (67 patients in total) [63]. Marijuana was found to be the definite triggering factor for RCVS in several of the reported cases [64–66]. The prognosis for all comers with RCVS is typically benign, but some patients experience permanent neurological deficits or death.

One retrospective cohort study from Denver, Colorado, looked at the demographics, suspected etiology, and outcomes in patients admitted with RCVS triggered by vasoactive substances with an interest in those triggered by marijuana. Marijuana was the identifiable trigger in four of the six cases and the two remaining cases used marijuana in combination with other drugs. Among the patients who used marijuana, there were five subarachnoid hemorrhages, one with ischemic stroke, and one death. The patients with RCVS attributable to marijuana tended to be younger (26.5 vs. 50.5 years old) and were less likely to be female (33% vs. 76%), but these associations were not statistically significant [67]..

Peripheral Vascular Adverse Clinical Outcomes

Cannabis Arteritis

Cannabis arteritis was first described in the 1960s and since then at least 70 cases have been published in the literature. The presentation of those who smoke marijuana is often very similar to that of young adults with thromboangitis obliterans who smoke tobacco products. In one large review, they found that the mean age of patients was estimated to be 28.5 years and there was a large male predominance (92.8%). The mean cannabis consumption was estimated at 3.8 joints per person per day with duration between 1 and 20 years. The cannabis is often mixed with tobacco, and thus it is difficult to attribute the effects to cannabis itself. However, cannabis may cause vasoconstriction and could have synergistic effects with tobacco [68]. One large retrospective review of patients who underwent lower extremity bypass surgery for peripheral vascular disease showed that patients who used drugs (38% marijuana) were more likely to present with clinically serious symptoms such as arterial embolism or thrombosis (Figs. 9.9 and 9.10), osteomyelitis, and cellulitis

Fig. 9.9 An exudative ulcerated lesion of the left hallux in a patient with cannabis arteritis [70]

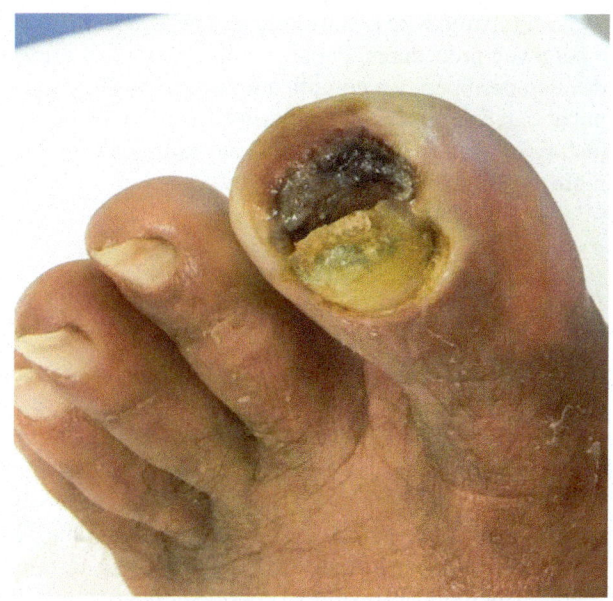

Fig. 9.10 Occlusion of the plantar arch of both feet in a patient with cannabis arteritis [70]

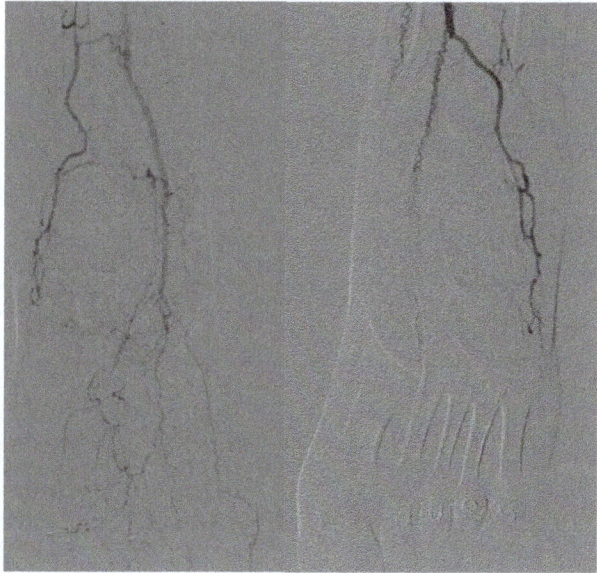

when compared with nondrug users. These patients were also more likely to undergo emergency procedures. Patients with a history of drug use were also more likely to develop perioperative complications such as kidney injury, CVA, respiratory complications, vascular and wound-related complications, and cellulitis. Patients with history of drug use had a higher rate of major amputations, along with longer and more expensive hospitalizations [69]..

Public Health Implications and Conclusion

Many states have legalized the medicinal and recreational use of marijuana due to potential beneficial effects. Our current evidence base lacks adequate scientific studies to provide thorough risk-benefit considerations for most marijuana use. There is an emerging body of evidence that suggests that patients exposed to marijuana are at risk for myocardial infarction, cerebrovascular disease, myocarditis, peripheral vascular complications, arrhythmias, and sudden cardiac death, and this should raise concerns about its safety and long-term effects. More evidence-based research including prospective cohort study on the effect of marijuana on the cardiovascular system will be necessary as legislative momentum leads to continued approval of marijuana in healthcare settings and recreational use.

Disclosures The authors report no financial conflicts of interest. The views expressed are those of the author and do not reflect any official policy of Fort Belvoir Community Hospital, Walter Reed National Military Medical Center, the Defense Health Agency, the Department of Defense, or the US government.

References

1. Drummer OH, Gerostamoulos D, Woodford NW. Cannabis as a cause of death: a review. Forensic Sci Int. 2019;298:298.
2. Crime UNOoDa. World drug report 2016 [October 06, 2019]. Available from: http://www.unodc.org/wdr2016/.
3. Procon.org. 33 Legal Medical Marijuana States and DC [October 06, 2019]. Available from: https://medicalmarijuana.procon.org/view.resource.php?resourceID=000881.
4. Benjamin EJ, Muntner P, Bittencourt MS. Heart disease and stroke statistics-2019 update: a report from the American Heart Association. Circulation. 2019;139(10):e56–e528.
5. Singla S, Sachdeva R, Mehta JL. Cannabinoids and atherosclerotic coronary heart disease. Clin Cardiol. 2012;35(6):329–35.
6. DeFilippis EM, Singh A, Divakaran S, Gupta A, Collins BL, Biery D, et al. Cocaine and marijuana use among young adults with myocardial infarction. J Am Coll Cardiol. 2018;71(22):2540–51.
7. Baidya SG, Zeng Q-T. Helper T cells and atherosclerosis: the cytokine web. Postgrad Med J. 2005;81(962):746–52.

8. Sugamura K, Sugiyama S, Nozaki T, Matsuzawa Y, Izumiya Y, Miyata K, et al. Activated endo-cannabinoid system in coronary artery disease and antiinflammatory effects of cannabinoid 1 receptor blockade on macrophages. Circulation. 2009;119(1):28–36.
9. Jiang LS, Pu J, Han ZH, Hu LH, He B. Role of activated endocannabinoid system in reg-ulation of cellular cholesterol metabolism in macrophages. Cardiovasc Res. 2008;81(4): 805–13.
10. Han KH, Lim S, Ryu J, Lee C-W, Kim Y, Kang J-H, et al. CB1 and CB2 cannabinoid receptors differentially regulate the production of reactive oxygen species by macrophages. Cardiovasc Res. 2009;84(3):378–86.
11. Dol-Gleizes F, Paumelle R, Visentin V, Marés A-M, Desitter P, Hennuyer N, et al. Rimonabant, a selective cannabinoid CB1 receptor antagonist, inhibits atherosclerosis in LDL receptor-deficient mice. Arterioscler Thromb Vasc Biol. 2009;29(1):12–8.
12. Mittleman MA, Lewis RA, Maclure M, Sherwood JB, Muller JE. Triggering myocardial infarction by marijuana. Circulation. 2001;103(23):2805–9.
13. Renault PF, Schuster CR, Heinrich R, Freeman DX. Marihuana: standardized smoke adminis-tration and dose effect curves on heart rate in humans. Science. 1971;174(4009):589–91.
14. Beaconsfield P, Ginsburg J, Rainsbury R. Marihuana Smoking. N Engl J Med. 1972;287(5):209–12.
15. Bachs L, Mørland H. Acute cardiovascular fatalities following cannabis use. Forensic Sci Int. 2001;124(2):200–3.
16. Aronow WS, Cassidy J. Effect of smoking marihuana and of a high-nicotine cigarette on angina pectoris. Clin Pharmacol Ther. 1975;17(5):549–54.
17. Aronow WS, Cassidy J. Effect of marihuana and placebo-marihuana smoking on angina pec-toris. N Engl J Med. 1974;291(2):65–7.
18. Desbois AC, Cacoub P. Cannabis-associated arterial disease. Ann Vasc Surg. 2013;27(7):996–1005.
19. Muller JE, Abela GS, Nesto RW, Tofler GH. Triggers, acute risk factors and vulnerable plaques: the lexicon of a new frontier. J Am Coll Cardiol. 1994;23(3):809–13.
20. Desai R, Patel U, Deshmukh A, Sachdeva R, Kumar G. Burden of arrhythmia in recreational marijuana users. Int J Cardiol. 2018;264:91–2.
21. Zipes DP, Foster PR, Troup PJ, Pedersen DH. Atrial induction of ventricular tachycardia: reentry versus triggered automaticity. Am J Cardiol. 1979;44(1):1–8.
22. Rezkalla SH, Sharma P, Kloner RA. Coronary no-flow and ventricular tachycardia associated with habitual marijuana use. Ann Emerg Med. 2003;42(3):365–9.
23. Belhassen B, Rotmensch HH, Laniado S. Response of recurrent sustained ventricular tachy-cardia to verapamil. Heart. 1981;46(6):679–82.
24. Menahem S. Cardiac asystole following cannabis (marijuana) usage–additional mechanism for sudden death? Forensic Sci Int. 2013;233(1–3):e3–5.
25. Pacher P, Batkai S, Kunos G. Blood pressure regulation by endocannabinoids and their recep-tors. Neuropharmacology. 2005;48(8):1130–8.
26. Kaushik M, Alla VM, Madan R, Arouni AJ, Mohiuddin SM. Recurrent stress cardiomyopathy with variable regional involvement: insights into etiopathogenetic mechanisms. Circulation. 2011;124(22):e556–e7.
27. Rodondi N, Pletcher MJ, Liu K, Hulley SB, Sidney S. Marijuana use, diet, body mass index, and cardiovascular risk factors (from the CARDIA study). Am J Cardiol. 2006;98(4):478–84.
28. Alshaarawy O, Sidney S, Auer R, Green D, Soliman EZ, Goff DC Jr, et al. Cannabis use and markers of systemic inflammation the coronary artery risk development in young adults study. Am J Med. 2019;132(11):1327.
29. Ware MA, Jensen D, Barrette A, Vernec A, Derman W. Cannabis and the health and perfor-mance of the elite athlete. Clin J Sport Med. 2018;28(5):480.
30. Tetrault JM, Crothers K, Moore BA, Mehra R, Concato J, Fiellin DA. Effects of marijuana smoking on pulmonary function and respiratory complications: a systematic review. Arch Intern Med. 2007;167(3):221–8.

31. Tashkin DP. Smoked marijuana as a cause of lung injury. Monaldi Arch Chest Dis. 2005;63(2):93.
32. Tashkin DP, Baldwin GC, Sarafian T, Dubinett S, Roth MD. Respiratory and immunologic consequences of marijuana smoking. J Clin Pharmacol. 2002;42(S1):71S–81S.
33. Taylor DR, Fergusson DM, Milne BJ, Horwood LJ, Moffitt TE, Sears MR, et al. A longitudinal study of the effects of tobacco and cannabis exposure on lung function in young adults. Addiction. 2002;97(8):1055–61.
34. Helyes Z, Kemény Á, Csekő K, Szőke É, Elekes K, Mester M, et al. Marijuana smoke induces severe pulmonary hyperresponsiveness, inflammation, and emphysema in a predictive mouse model not via CB1 receptor activation. Am J Phys Lung Cell Mol Phys. 2017;313(2):L267–L77.
35. Wolff V, Armspach J-P, Lauer V, Rouyer O, Bataillard M, Marescaux C, et al. Cannabis-related stroke: myth or reality? Stroke. 2013;44(2):558–63.
36. Uhegwu N, Bashir A, Hussain M, Dababneh H, Misthal S, Cohen-Gadol A. Marijuana induced reversible cerebral vasoconstriction syndrome. J Vasc Interv Neurol. 2015;8(1):36.
37. Inal T, Köse A, Köksal Ö, Armagan E, Aydın SA, Ozdemir F. Acute temporal lobe infarction in a young patient associated with marijuana abuse: an unusual cause of stroke. World J Emerg Med. 2014;5(1):72.
38. Wolff V, Lauer V, Rouyer O, Sellal F, Meyer N, Raul JS, et al. Cannabis use, ischemic stroke, and multifocal intracranial vasoconstriction: a prospective study in 48 consecutive young patients. Stroke. 2011;42(6):1778–80.
39. Singh NN, Pan Y, Muengtaweeponsa S, Geller TJ, Cruz-Flores S. Cannabis-related stroke: case series and review of literature. J Stroke Cerebrovasc Dis. 2012;21(7):555–60.
40. Grotenhermen F. Cannabis-associated arteritis. Vasa Suppl. 2010;39(1):43.
41. Franz CA, Frishman WH. Marijuana use and cardiovascular disease. Cardiol Rev. 2016;24(4):158–62.
42. Desai R, Patel U, Sharma S, Amin P, Bhuva R, Patel MS, et al. Recreational marijuana use and acute myocardial infarction: insights from nationwide inpatient sample in the United States. Cureus. 2017;9(11):e1816.
43. Van Keer JM. Cannabis-induced third-degree AV block. Case reports in emergency medicine. 2019;2019
44. Nappe TM, Hoyte CO. Pediatric death due to myocarditis after exposure to cannabis. Clin Pract Cases Emerg Med. 2017;1(3):166.
45. Leontiadis E, Morshuis M, Arusoglu L, Cobaugh D, Koerfer R, El-Banayosy A. Thoratec left ventricular assist device removal after toxic myocarditis. Ann Thorac Surg. 2008;86(6):1982–5.
46. Rodríguez-Castro CE, Haider Alkhateeb AE, Saifuddin F, Abbas A, Siddiqui T. Recurrent myopericarditis as a complication of marijuana use. Am J Case Rep. 2014;15:60.
47. Tournebize J, Gibaja V, Puskarczyk E, Popovic B, Kahn J-P. Myocarditis and cannabis: an unusual association. Toxicologie Analytique et Clinique. 2016;28(3):236.
48. Kariyanna PT, Jayarangaiah A, Singh N, Song T, Soroka S, Amarnani A, et al. Marijuana induced myocarditis: a new entity of toxic myocarditis. Am J Med Case Rep. 2018;6(9):169.
49. Gong H Jr, Fligiel S, Tashkin DP, Barbers RG. Tracheobronchial changes in habitual, heavy smokers of marijuana with and without tobacco. Am J Respir Crit Care Med. 1987;136(1):142–9.
50. Taylor DR, Poulton R, Moffitt TE, Ramankutty P, Sears MR. The respiratory effects of cannabis dependence in young adults. Addiction. 2000;95(11):1669–77.
51. Aldington S, Williams M, Nowitz M, Weatherall M, Pritchard A, McNaughton A, et al. Effects of cannabis on pulmonary structure, function and symptoms. Thorax. 2007;62(12):1058–63.
52. Westover AN, McBride S, Haley RW. Stroke in young adults who abuse amphetamines or cocaine: a population-based study of hospitalized patients. Arch Gen Psychiatry. 2007;64(4):495–502.
53. Barnes D, Palace J, O'Brien M. Stroke following marijuana smoking. Stroke. 1992;23(9):1381.
54. Mateo I, Pinedo A, Gomez-Beldarrain M, Basterretxea J, Garcia-Monco J. Recurrent stroke associated with cannabis use. J Neurol Neurosurg Psychiatry. 2005;76(3):435–7.

55. Lawson T, Rees A. Stroke and transient ischaemic attacks in association with substance abuse in a young man. Postgrad Med J. 1996;72(853):692–3.
56. Geller T, Loftis L, Brink DS. Cerebellar infarction in adolescent males associated with acute marijuana use. Pediatrics. 2004;113(4):e365–e70.
57. Zachariah SB. Stroke after heavy marijuana smoking. Stroke. 1991;22(3):406–9.
58. Álvaro LC, Iriondo I, Villaverde FJ. Sexual headache and stroke in a heavy cannabis smoker. Headache. 2002;42(3):224–6.
59. Finsterer J, Christian P, Wolfgang K. Occipital stroke shortly after cannabis consumption. Clin Neurol Neurosurg. 2004;106(4):305–8.
60. Desai R, Fong HK, Shah K, Kaur VP, Savani S, Gangani K, et al. Rising trends in hospitalizations for cardiovascular events among young cannabis users (18–39 years) without other substance abuse. Medicina. 2019;55(8):438.
61. Ducros A. Reversible cerebral vasoconstriction syndrome. Lancet Neurol. 2012;11(10): 906–17.
62. Sattar A, Manousakis G, Jensen MB. Systematic review of reversible cerebral vasoconstriction syndrome. Expert Rev Cardiovasc Ther. 2010;8(10):1417–21.
63. Ducros A, Boukobza M, Porcher R, Sarov M, Valade D, Bousser M-G. The clinical and radiological spectrum of reversible cerebral vasoconstriction syndrome. A prospective series of 67 patients. Brain. 2007;130(12):3091–101.
64. Koopman K, Teune L, Ter Laan M, Uyttenboogaart M, Vroomen P, De Keyser J, et al. An often unrecognized cause of thunderclap headache: reversible cerebral vasoconstriction syndrome. J Headache Pain. 2008;9(6):389.
65. Drazin D, Alexander MJ. Call-fleming syndrome (reversible cerebral artery vasoconstriction) and aneurysm associated with multiple recreational drug use. Case Rep Neurol Med. 2013;2013:729162.
66. Robert T, Marchini AK, Oumarou G, Uske A. Reversible cerebral vasoconstriction syndrome identification of prognostic factors. Clin Neurol Neurosurg. 2013;115(11):2351–7.
67. Jensen J, Leonard J, Salottolo K, McCarthy K, Wagner J, Bar-Or D. The epidemiology of reversible cerebral vasoconstriction syndrome in patients at a Colorado Comprehensive Stroke Center. J Vasc Interv Neurol. 2018;10(1):32.
68. Cottencin O, Karila L, Lambert M, Arveiller C, Benyamina A, Boissonas A, et al. Cannabis arteritis: review of the literature. J Addict Med. 2010;4(4):191–6.
69. Dakour-Aridi H, Arora M, Nejim B, Locham S, Malas MB. Association between drug use and in-hospital outcomes after infrainguinal bypass for peripheral arterial occlusive disease. Ann Vasc Surg. 2019;58:122.
70. Santos RP, Resende CIP, Vieira AP, Brito C. Cannabis arteritis: ever more important to consider. BMJ Case Rep. 2017;2017:bcr2016219111.

Chapter 10
Cannabinoids in Neurologic Conditions

Tyler E. Gaston, Jerzy P. Szaflarski, Allen C. Bowling, Ying Liu,
Tristan Seawalt, Maureen A. Leehey, E. Lee Nelson, Sharad Rajpal,
Alan T. Villavicencio, Andrew Bauer, and Sigita Burneikiene

Cannabis and Cannabinoids for the Treatment of Epilepsy

Tyler E. Gaston and Jerzy P. Szaflarski

Treatment of seizures and epilepsy with *cannabis* has been reported for millennia
[1–3]. However, the recent resurgence of the interest in *cannabis* and its derivatives
(e.g., cannabidiol (CBD) and d*elta (9)-tetrahydrocannabinol* (Δ^9-THC)) is the

T. E. Gaston (✉)
University of Alabama at Birmingham Epilepsy Center, Department of Neurology,
Birmingham, AL, USA
e-mail: tegaston@uabmc.edu

J. P. Szaflarski
University of Alabama at Birmingham Epilepsy Center, 312 Civitan International Research
Center, Birmingham, AL, USA
e-mail: jszaflarski@uabmc.edu

A. C. Bowling
NeuroHealth Institute, Englewood, CO, USA

Department of Neurology, University of Colorado, Aurora, CO, USA

Y. Liu · T. Seawalt · M. A. Leehey
Department of Neurology, University of Colorado School of Medicine, Aurora, CO, USA
e-mail: ying.3.liu@cuanschutz.edu; Tristan.seawalt@cuanschutz.edu; maureen.leehey@
cuanschutz.edu

E. L. Nelson · A. Bauer
Boulder Neurosurgical Associates, Boulder, CO, USA
e-mail: nelson@bnasurg.com; bauer@bnasurg.com

S. Rajpal · A. T. Villavicencio · S. Burneikiene
Boulder Neurosurgical Associates, Boulder, CO, USA

Justin Parker Neurological Institute, Boulder, CO, USA
e-mail: rajpal@bnasurg.com; atv@bnasurg.com; sigitab@bnasurg.com

© Springer Nature Switzerland AG 2020
K. Finn (ed.), *Cannabis in Medicine*,
https://doi.org/10.1007/978-3-030-45968-0_10

result of lay press popularization of the topic and the reports of such uses from parents of children suffering from treatment-resistant epilepsies (TREs) [3]. The societal pressures have resulted in gradual but perceptible changes in the legal environment and specific suggestions to reform it [4–6]. The initial lay press reports were followed by open-label, observational studies of artisanal *cannabis* products conducted concurrently to several randomized controlled trials (RCTs) of pharmaceutical-grade, highly purified CBD for the treatment of Lennox-Gastaut syndrome (LGS) and Dravet syndrome (DS) and for the treatment of seizures in patients with tuberous sclerosis complex (TSC) [7]. The impetus has been to predominantly study CBD as a non-euphoric cannabinoid. To date, several observational studies have also addressed the potential efficacy of artisanal products with variable phytocannabinoid content with a typically high proportion of CBD and low proportion of Δ^9-THC. Additionally, at least two studies of synthetic CBD have been completed, and some of their data have been reported [8, 9]. This chapter summarizes the known/hypothesized mechanisms of action (MOA) of Δ^9-THC and CBD, developments in artisanal *cannabis* products, reports of the expanded access programs (EAP), and, finally, results of RCTs for the treatment of seizures/epilepsy in patients with TREs, the adverse reactions to cannabinoids, and their interactions with other pharmaceuticals.

Mechanism of Action

In several recent studies, the involvement of the endocannabinoid system (ECS) has been postulated as one on the mainstays of seizure generation and maintenance. Therefore, modulating the ECS is thought to have a therapeutic potential in many human disorders, including epilepsy [10]. Basic science work has made great strides toward understanding the divergent roles of the ECS and the dynamics of its receptors (CB_1R and CB_2R) and neurotransmitters (anandamide (AEA) and 2-arachidonoylglycerol (2-AG)). The ECS is an "on-demand" system – the control of which depends on interplay between its neurotransmitters and their production, presence of distinct membrane transporters, and storage of AEA and 2AG and their delivery at a precisely defined moment [11]. Better understanding of the role of ECS in seizure generation and maintenance is particularly important in epilepsy where artisanal and FDA-approved treatments are now available [7, 12].

The mechanisms of action (MOA) of CBD and Δ^9-THC as they pertain to the treatment of seizures have been studied extensively but have been only partially elucidated [12]. In general, Δ^9-THC's agonist activity at CB_1R and CB_2R has demonstrated an anticonvulsant effect. CBD may exert some of its effects at the CB_1R and CB_2R level through an allosteric or indirect mechanism since it has overall low affinity for the endocannabinoid receptors. However, other MOAs likely underlie CBD's efficacy in treating seizures [13–16]. In fact, several studies indicate that CBD may also have antagonist activity at the CB_1Rs and CB_2Rs [17–19]. Further, Δ^9-THC, while predominantly anticonvulsant, has been reported to be also a proconvulsant in some studies [20]. In contrast to Δ^9-THC, proconvulsant properties of CBD have not been demonstrated to date [20]. CBD blocks AEA uptake and hydrolysis, effectively increasing AEA's availability to activate the CB_1Rs and CB_2Rs. Thus, while CBD appears to modulate the ECS, its entire anticonvulsant MOA continues to be somewhat unclear. However, there is increasing evidence for ECS' importance for the process of seizure generation and maintenance [10, 21].

To date, several primarily anticonvulsant MOAs of CBD have been proposed beyond ECS modulation. These include effects at the transient receptor potential (TRP) of vanilloid type 1 (TRPV1), G protein-coupled receptor 55 (GPR55), and inhibition of adenosine reuptake [22]. CBD activates TRPV1, which is also a receptor for AEA; action at TRPV1 may modulate calcium channels, leading to an increase in neuronal calcium influx and subsequent reduction in neural activity and glutamate release [12, 23–25]. In animals, CBD attenuated seizure and EEG activity, but these effects were reversed by CB_1R, CB_2R, and TRPV1 antagonists individually [24]. Interestingly, blockade of TRPV1 has also shown to abolish anticonvulsant activity, which essentially directly contradicts the postulation that CBD's agonist activity at TRPV1 results in anticonvulsant activity [25]. One possible explanation for this contradiction is that TRPV1 channels could possibly be "desensitized" in the presence of the binding of an agonist (i.e., CBD), and it is this desensitization that actually results in the anticonvulsant activity [24].

GPR55 is a "novel cannabinoid receptor" whose antagonism could have anticonvulsant effects, and CBD has antagonist action at this receptor [26]. These receptors are expressed in the hippocampus, pyramidal cells, and the interneurons in the pyramidal cell layer and can modulate hippocampal synaptic plasticity [27]. In an animal model, antagonism of GPR55 blocked CBD's actions on seizures and mimicked CBD's enhancement of inhibitory transmission in mouse dentate granule cells [28].

CBD also decreases neural excitability via inhibition of adenosine reuptake transporters (increasing adenosine availability at the receptor site) [29, 30]. Previously, adenosine levels have been shown to increase several fold in the epileptic hippocampus during a seizure to a level that is known to depress epileptiform activity *in vitro* and to remain elevated in the post-ictal period [29]. Adenosine is an endogenous purine neuromodulator with anticonvulsant and anti-inflammatory properties at the A_1 and A_2 receptors, respectively [30]. Finally, in a recent study, CBD has shown concentration-dependent ability to inhibit the equilibrative nucleoside transporter (ENT-1) and, thus, regulate extracellular adenosine levels [22].

There are many other actions of CBD that may contribute to its anticonvulsant properties, particularly in certain disease states or epilepsy syndromes. CBD preferentially targets mutant sodium channels, which would be of interest in certain epilepsy syndromes (e.g., Dravet Syndrome) where mutant sodium channels are the cause of seizures [31]. CBD blocks human T-type calcium channels – similar action is seen with other anti-seizure drugs (ASD); however, this activity in CBD is not felt to be extremely potent and thus is not considered a primary MOA [32]. Other possibilities include modulation of voltage-dependent anion selective channel protein (VDAC1) and tumor necrosis factor alpha release [29, 33, 34]. CBD also has anti-inflammatory properties by decreasing pro-inflammatory functions and signaling in astrocytes to prevent the increase in inflammatory cytokines (IL-6) in animal models of epilepsy [24, 35]. CBD does have affinity for the serotonin receptors $5-HT_{1A}$ and $5-HT_{2A}$, but this is considered to be a less plausible MOA as an animal study showed that pre-treatment with serotonin receptor antagonists did not block CBD's anticonvulsant effect [36].

An interesting area of study which could drive future directions of research is the "entourage effect." This is a proposed mechanism by which phytocannabinoids that are largely non-euphoric themselves (viz., CBD) appear to modulate the overall psychoactive effects of *cannabis* (primarily from Δ^9-THC) [37, 38]. Additionally, certain cannabinoids with less pharmacologic activity and terpenoids might contribute to a synergistic effect that might be lost with a highly purified product [39, 40].

Artisanal Cannabis *Product Use for the Treatment of Epilepsies*

In 2014, we reviewed the data regarding the treatment of epilepsy that were available at that time, and, based on those studies, we calculated that any improvement in seizures in response to *cannabis* products (defined as any decrease in seizure frequency) would be in the ~60% range [2]. Several studies, published since then, indicate such efficacy. These studies provide a relatively low level of evidence for artisanal product efficacy in this setting, and the reported efficacy needs to be viewed via the prism of open-label and frequently retrospective design, participants' and clinicians' expectation of efficacy, inconsistent response and adverse event monitoring, and lack of control groups [41–44]. Further, of importance is a recent meta-analysis that indicates there may be differences in response to artisanal *cannabis* products (extracts containing variable contents of all cannabinoids) when compared to purified CBD in that a much lower dose of artisanal *cannabis* products is needed vis-à-vis purified products (6.0 mg/kg/day vs. 25.3 mg/kg/day) indicating, in the opinion of the authors, the presence of the entourage effect [45].

One of the first large artisanal product studies described experiences from California, Maine, and Washington State [44]. In a retrospective data collection, the authors summarized the efficacy and adverse events in 272 patients with various clinical diagnoses including LGS, DS, and Rett syndrome, but the majority with unknown epilepsy etiology [44]. Overall, 37 (14%) found *cannabis* products ineffective, and 146/272 (54%) experienced >50% seizure reduction. However, since this was a retrospective study with data combined from several centers, the products utilized by patients (or suggested to patients by the providers) differed, and the specific CBD:Δ^9-THC content is unclear. In this study, California patients used predominantly high-CBD/low-Δ^9-THC products (ratio ranging from 15:1 to 27:1), Washington State patients used untested products with some of them self-medicating with home-made preparations, and Maine participants used tested/calibrated products that were tailored with a goal to achieve best possible response at doses of <0.1 mg/kg/day which, by some, could be considered homeopathic [44].

Of great importance are two studies that have not only evaluated the efficacy of artisanal products for seizure management but have also addressed the issue of expectation of efficacy [43, 46]. The first retrospective chart review in 75 children and adolescents focused on the response to oral *cannabis* extracts [43]. Fifty-seven percent reported improvement in seizure frequency with 33% of them reporting >50% seizure reduction with the response varying by residence status. The >50% improvement was noted in 47% of patients who relocated to Colorado to obtain *cannabis* extracts for the treatment of epilepsy (expectation of efficacy) compared to only 22% who were Colorado residents [43]. In this study, the seizure response varied by epilepsy syndrome with 88.9% of LGS patients and 23% of DS patients classified as responders. An expanded follow-up study reported that of the 119 patients, only 29% remained taking the *cannabis* product at the end of evaluation (±11.7 months; range 0.3–57 months) [46]. The relatively low retention rate in this study had two major drivers – lack of treatment response and cost of treatment – while the seizure benefit was the only factor associated with continued *cannabis* treatment. Again, relocation to Colorado was associated with 65% of users reporting benefit vs. 38% of users who were long-standing residents of the state [46].

Additional studies reported on the use of better characterized *cannabis* products for the treatment of epilepsy [47, 48]. The first study included 74 children and adolescents with epilepsy [48]. They used 20:1 CBD:Δ^9-THC ratio with the CBD dose titrated based on seizure response and adverse events up to 20 mg/kg/day [48]. The treatment resulted in 51% of participants reporting >50% improvement in seizures with 66/74 (89%) reporting some improvement. The second study also utilized artisanal 20:1 CBD:Δ^9-THC ratio plant-derived product in 46 children and adults with TRE [47]. The product obtained from a local dispensary was extensively tested for content and proportion of CBD:Δ^9-THC [47]. Participants who received doses of CBD higher than 11 mg/kg/day (and proportionally higher Δ^9-THC) reported more improvement compared to those received lower doses ($p = 0.043$), while lowering of concomitant ASDs did not affect the response. In 17 participants, addition of a vaporized form of *cannabis* to the treatment armamentarium resulted in additional improvements in some (6/17) [47]. This corresponds to anecdotal reports of patients utilizing vaporized *cannabis* products as abortive and oral products as preventive treatments. The improved seizure response with higher CBD dose in this study is in agreement with another study that tested the relationship between CBD dose, CBD serum level, and seizure response in one of the EAPs [49]. Finally, a medical record review indicated that "CBD-containing products" provided >50% improvement in seizure frequency in 39% of patients (predominantly children) with the effect being independent of the presence or absence of clobazam [50].

In addition to the CBD:Δ^9-THC studies described above, at least two studies have utilized artisanal preparation of pure CBD [51, 52]. In the first of the two studies, 66 children and young adults received crystalline preparation of 98–99% pure CBD in oily solution. Thirty-two of 66 (48.5%) reported >50% reduction in seizures, and 21.2% became seizure free [51]. In the second study, 29 children with developmental and epileptic encephalopathies received crystalline preparation of 98–99% pure CBD in medium-chain oil [52]. Of the participants, 37.9% had >50%

seizure reduction, and there was no difference in response reported between patients being treated (or not) with concomitant clobazam.

Several surveys have been conducted and reported to date. Perceived tolerability and efficacy of CBD-enriched *cannabis* products for the treatment of seizures were examined via an online survey of 117 parents of children with epileptic spasms and LGS [53]. The report indicates improvement in 85% of respondents and seizure freedom in 14% while utilizing median dose of CBD of 4.3 mg/kg/day. However, only a minority of patients were able to calculate the CBD/cannabinoid dose. Of parents who knew the CBD:Δ^9-THC content of their product, most indicated the ratio of 15:1 [53]. Two other surveys have been published recently [54, 55]. In the first survey of patient experiences with *cannabis* products, of the 976 responses that met the inclusion criteria, 15% adults and 13% of children with epilepsy were either currently using or had previously used various *cannabis* products to treat epilepsy [55]. Ninety percent of adults and 71% of children's parents reported that *cannabis* product use resulted in improved seizure frequency [55]. The number of previously tried ASDs was a significant predictor of medicinal *cannabis* use in both adults and children with epilepsy in uni- and multivariate analyses indicating that many had TRE. Another study by the same group conducted an in-person interview of 41 families that used one or more *cannabis* products for the treatment of epilepsy [54]. Of the 51 products tested, 38/51 were considered effective by their users. Of interest is that most of the tested *cannabis* products, contrary to the expectation, contained low CBD concentration while Δ^9-THC was present in almost all tested samples supporting the previous notion of low accuracy of the artisanal *cannabis* product labelling [56]. Finally, a survey of 43 Mexican children with various epilepsy diagnoses indicated that 81.3% had decrease in seizures in response to various cannabis products (majority utilized purified CBD approved by the Mexican equivalent of the US FDA) and 20.9% were able to decrease other seizure medications [57].

Open-Label Studies of Pharmaceutical-Grade CBD

The first published data on pharmaceutical-grade CBD's (Epidiolex®) efficacy for TREs come from an open-label study conducted at 11 epilepsy centers across the United States [58]. Participants were 137 children and adults who initiated therapy with CBD at a dose of 2–5 mg/kg/day. The dose could be titrated by 2–5 mg/kg a week until intolerance or a maximum dose of up to 50 mg/kg/day. The median decrease in total seizures was 34.6% with the responses varying between seizure types. Participants with focal seizures reported 55.0%, atonic seizures 54.3%, tonic seizures 36.5%, and tonic-clonic seizures 16.0% improvements [58]. Up to 37% of participants had an overall 50% or more reduction in seizures [58]. In a post hoc analysis, response rates were not different between patients with DS, LGS, and other participants. Long-term follow-up data from 25 EAPs were recently published [59]. Six hundred and seven participants with TRE ages 1–61 were enrolled with 580 included in the efficacy analysis. CBD was started at 2–10 mg/kg/day depending on the study site and was titrated up to a maximum dose of 50 mg/kg/day. After 12 weeks of treatment, participants observed a median monthly seizure reduction of 51% with the observed reductions not affected by dropouts. Responses remained stable over the duration of up to 96 weeks. Another study from the same population analyzed participants with the specific diagnosis of LGS and DS [60]. Overall, the results were similar to the ones reported in the larger dataset – while 28% of participants withdrew primarily because of lack of efficacy, the remaining patients reported 50% decrease in major motor seizures and 44% in seizures overall [60].

Single-center analyses reported similar results when compared to the overall EAP results [49, 61, 62]. The largest study included 132 adult and pediatric participants and showed the mean reduction at 12 weeks in all seizure types of 63.6% with the reductions sustained up to 48 weeks [49]. In this study, Chalfont Seizure Severity Scale (CSSS) showed improvement from a baseline score of 80.7 at enrollment to 39.3 at week 12 ($p < 0.0001$) with continued stable CSSS scores at 24 and 48 weeks. Another EAP study focused on longer-term follow-up [62]. In that study, of the 26 children ages 1–17, 15 (57%) discontinued treatment because of lack of efficacy. Only 35% continued treatment at 24 months with seven out of the remaining nine patients reporting >50% reduction in seizures [49]. Recently, another analysis was released – a correlation between CBD levels, CBD dose, and seizure response [63]. In an analysis of 100 participants from the same cohort, the authors were able to show a positive linear correlation between CBD dose in a 5–50 mg/kg/day range and CBD level ($r = 0.640$; $p < 0.001$). Further, the results of this study support the notion that higher CBD serum levels are associated with better seizure response after adjusting for age; in this study an increase in CBD serum level by 100 ng/mL was associated with approximately two counts reduction in seizure frequency per time period (1.87 96% confidence interval [CI] 0.34–3.39; $p = 0.018$). CBD seizure responses were not dependent on age group (pediatric vs. adult) [63].

Several other EAP studies have described CBD's effects on seizures in certain disease states. In addition to the mentioned above study of patients with LGS and DS [60], one study investigated the effects of CBD on 18 patients with TSC to show median 3-month seizure frequency reduction of 48.8% [61]. Patients taking concomitant CLB and CBD experienced 53.2% seizure reduction compared to 36.4% in patients who were treated with CBD alone indicating a potential interaction between these two ASDs in respect to improved seizure control with a combined approach. However, several other studies did not observe better seizure control in patients using CBD with CLB vs. CBD alone [50, 52, 64]. Seizure response to CBD in patients with various types of epileptic encephalopathies (CDKL5 deficiency disorder, Aicardi syndrome, Dup15q syndrome, and Doose syndrome) was also documented [65]. Mean 3-month seizure reduction was 51.4% and was sustained up to 48 weeks. A case series of seven children with refractory seizures due to febrile infection-related epilepsy syndrome (FIRES) received CBD in the acute ($n = 2$) or chronic ($n = 5$) phase of the illness [66]. In the two patients in the acute phase, one had cessation of status epilepticus, and the other patient (who died due to multiorgan failure thought to be due to prolonged isoflurane exposure) had only stimulus-induced seizures after CBD treatment. The five patients in the chronic phase had a mean seizure frequency reduction of 90.9% at 4 weeks and 65.3% at 48 weeks compared to baseline. A recently published study prospectively examined the efficacy of 50:1 CBD/THC pharmaceutical-grade product [67]. These authors were able to show 70.6% median motor seizure reduction in patients with DS with a RR of 63%. The dose of CBD and THC in this study ranged from 2 to 16 mg/kg/day and 0.14 to 0.32 mg/kg/day, respectively.

Finally, a report of an open-label synthetic CBD oral solution in a multicenter, open-label, flexible-dose study was recently reported in an abstract form [68]. In this study, patients who previously participated in a phase II multi-dose PK study were eligible to continue receiving 10, 20, or 40 mg/kg/day in two divided doses of CBD for up to 48 weeks, with dose changes at investigator discretion. Fifty-two patients were enrolled, and 45 (86.5%) completed the study with mean modal dose of CBD of 24.4 mg/kg/day. However, the abstract does not provide efficacy data and only reports on safety which does not appear to be different from other CBD products.

Randomized Controlled Trials of Pharmaceutical-Grade CBD

We were unable to identify any RCTs of artisanal *cannabis* products. Some of the initial studies included in the 2014 review were small randomized trials with CBD extracts from the *cannabis* plant with unclear purity that likely included some amounts of Δ^9-THC [2]. However, the results of these trials were inconclusive as to the efficacy of *cannabis* products for the treatment of epilepsy [42]. In the last few years, several phase II or III randomized controlled trials of pharmaceutical-grade (or synthetic) CBD have been completed (CBD for seizures in TSC data was reported to date only in an abstract form; NCT02544763).

The first study reported on the use of highly purified CBD (Epidiolex®) for the treatment of convulsive seizures in patients with DS (Table 10.1) [69]. In this double-blind, placebo-controlled study, patients were randomized to either receive CBD at 20 mg/kg/day or placebo in addition to the other ASDs they were taking prior to enrollment. The primary outcome measure was the change in convulsive seizures over a 14-week treatment period compared to a 4-week baseline. There was a significant decrease in monthly convulsive seizures from 12.4 to 5.9 in the CBD treatment group compared to 14.9–14.1 in the placebo group ($p = 0.01$ after adjusting for baseline differences between groups), and the responder rate for convulsive seizures was 43% for CBD vs. 27% for placebo ($p = 0.08$). The overall seizure frequency of all seizure types also improved in the CBD group ($p = 0.03$). However, there was no significant improvement in the non-convulsive seizures. Improvement in the Caregiver Global Impression of Change scale was seen in 62% in the CBD group vs. 34% of the patients treated with placebo ($p = 0.02$). There was a second DS study where participants received placebo or 5, 10, or 20 mg/kg/day of CBD, which is discussed in the "Interactions" section later in the chapter [70].

Table 10.1 Summary of references of *cannabis* studies in epilepsy

Reference	Number of participants	Age of participants	Diagnosis	Preparation	Dosage	Response
Artisanal (various or not tested ratios of CBD:Δ⁹-THC)						
Sulak et al. [44]	272	Adults and children	TRE, LGS, Dravet syndrome, Rett syndrome	Varied	Varied	61% reduction in seizures
Press et al. [43]	75	Children and adolescents	TRE	"Oral cannabis extracts"	Varied	57% reported improvement in seizure frequency
Treat et al. [46]	119	Children and adolescents	Varied syndromes/TRE	"Oral cannabis extracts"	Varied	65% vs. 38%, $p = 0.01$ (moved to Colorado vs. residents)
Tzadok et al. [48]	74	Children	TRE	20:1 CBD:THC	1–20 mg/kg/day	89% reported decrease in seizures
Hausman-Kedem et al. [47]	46	Adults and children	TRE	20:1 CBD:THC	11.4 mg/kg/day (avg dose)	80% reduction in patients taking >11 mg/kg/day, 50% reduction <11 mg/kg/day
Porcari et al. [50]	108	Children	TRE	"CBD oil"	Varied	39% RR
Neubauer et al. [51]	66	Children and adolescents	TRE	Crystalline CBD in oily solution	1–3 mg/kg/day starting dose up to 16 mg/kg/day maximum	48.5% RR; 21.2% became seizure free
Pietrafusa et al. [52]	29	Children	Developmental and epileptic encephalopathies	Crystalline CBD in medium-chain oil	2–5 mg/kg/day starting dose up to 25 mg/kg/day maximum	37.9% RR

(continued)

Table 10.1 (continued)

Reference	Number of participants	Age of participants	Diagnosis	Preparation	Dosage	Response
Hussain et al. [53]	117	Children	TRE, LGS, epileptic spasms	Unknown, if reported 15:1 CBD:THC	Median dose 4.3 mg/kg/day	85% reported improvement in seizure frequency (survey)
Suraev et al. [54]	976	Adults and children	TRE	Varied	Varied	90% adults and 71% children reported seizure improvement (survey)
Suraev et al. [55]	41	Children	Mostly TRE	Varied	Varied	38/51 products were considered efficacious by the users; survey
Aguirre-Velazquez [57]	43	Children	Varied syndromes/TRE	Varied cannabis products	Varied	81.3% had decrease in seizures (survey)
Open label studies of pharmaceutical-grade Cannabidiol (Epidiolex®)						
Devinsky et al. [58]	162 (137 in efficacy analysis)	Adults and children	TRE	Highly purified CBD oral solution	2–50 mg/kg/day	34.6% median seizure reduction
Szaflarski et al. [59]	580	Adults and children	TRE	Highly purified CBD oral solution	2–50 mg/kg/day	51% median seizure reduction
Laux et al. [60]	58 (sub-cohort of study in [59])	Adults and children	LGS and DS	Highly purified CBD oral solution	2–50 mg/kg/day	44% total seizure reduction
Szaflarski et al. [49]	132	Adults and children	TRE	Highly purified CBD oral solution	5–50 mg/kg/day	63.6% mean seizure reduction at 12 weeks
Hess et at [61]	18	Adults and children	Tuberous sclerosis	Highly purified CBD oral solution	5–50 mg/kg/day	48.8% median seizure reduction at 12 weeks

Table 10.1 (continued)

Reference	Number of participants	Age of participants	Diagnosis	Preparation	Dosage	Response
Devinsky et al. [65]	55	Adults and children	Epileptic encephalopathies	Highly purified CBD oral solution	5–50 mg/kg/day	51.4% mean seizure reduction at 12 weeks
Gofshteyn et al. [66]	7	Children	FIRES	Highly purified CBD oral solution	5–25 mg/kg/day	6/7 had improved seizure frequency
McCoy et al. [67]	20	Children	DS	50:1 CBD/THC	2–16 mg/kg/day CBD; 0.14–0.23 mg/kg/day THC	63% RR; 70.6% median motor seizure reduction
Randomized control trials of pharmaceutical-grade cannabidiol (Epidiolex®)						
Devinsky et al. [69]	120	Children	Dravet syndrome	Highly purified CBD oral solution	20 mg/kg/day	43% RR (vs. 27% in placebo group)
Devinsky et al. [71]	171	Adults and children	LGS	Highly purified CBD oral solution	20 mg/kg/day	43.9% RR (vs. 21.8% in placebo group)
Thiele et al. [73]	225	Adults and children	LGS	Highly purified CBD oral solution	10 or 20 mg/kg/day	41.9% (20 mg/kg), 37.2% (10 mg/kg), 17.2% (placebo)
Thiele et al. [see below]	201	Adults and children	TSC	Highly purified CBD oral solution	25 or 50 mg/kg/day	48.6% (25 mg/kg), 47.5% (50 mg/kg), 26.5% (placebo) RR

Abbreviations: *LGS* Lennox-Gastaut syndrome, *TRE* treatment-resistant epilepsy, *TSC* tuberous sclerosis complex, *RR* responder >50% reduction in seizures, TSC trial reference: http://ir.gwpharm.com/news-releases/news-release-details/gw-pharmaceuticals-reports-positive-phase-3-pivotal-trial

The first LGS study consisted of 171 participants who reported drop seizures and were randomized to receive placebo or 20 mg/kg/day of CBD, with the primary endpoint being change from baseline in drop seizure frequency. With a 4-week baseline period and a 14-week treatment period, the median percentage reduction in drop seizure frequency per month from baseline was 43.9% in the CBD group vs. 21.8% in the placebo group ($p = 0.0135$). Responder rate for drop seizure reduction was 44% during the treatment phase and 46% in the maintenance phase in the CBD group. The second RCT for LGS had the same primary endpoint of reduction of drop seizure frequency [71]. In this dose-ranging study, patients were randomized to placebo and 10 or 20 mg/kg/day of CBD with response measured at 14 weeks when compared to 4-week baseline. Of the 225 enrolled patients, median percent reduction in drop seizures was 41.9% in the 20 mg/kg/day CBD group, 37.2% in the 10 mg/kg/day CBD group, and 17.2% in the placebo group, with comparisons between treatment and placebo groups being significant. Responder rates for drop seizures were 39%, 36%, and 14% in the 20 mg/kg/day, 10 mg/kg/day, and placebo groups, respectively.

A recently completed NCT02544763 trial of CBD for the treatment of seizures in patient with TSC was also positive (http://ir.gwpharm.com/news-releases/news-release-details/gw-pharmaceuticals-reports-positive-phase-3-pivotal-trial). The data from this trial were presented at the 2019 International TSC Research Conference. Two hundred twenty-four patients were randomized to receive placebo or CBD at 25 or 50 mg/kg/day – seizure reduction was significant when compared to placebo in both active treatment groups, but there was no difference in seizure response between the 25 and 50 mg/kg/day groups (48.6% vs. 47.5%, respectively).

There are two recently completed randomized controlled trials that failed to show efficacy of synthetic CBD for the treatment of epilepsy. In a study by Zynerba Pharmaceuticals (zynerba.com), a transdermal delivery of CBD did not produce statistically significant reduction of seizures in patients with refractory epilepsy with focal seizures [8]. This trial was conducted in 188 patients who were randomized to receive either 195 mg of ZYN002 4.2% gel every 12 hours, 97.5 mg of ZYN002 4.2% gel every 12 hours, or placebo. Overall, patients on the low dose of ZYN002 had 18.4% seizure reduction vs. 14% on high dose vs. 8.7% seizure reduction for placebo. The final report of this RCT is not available at this time. Further, Insys Therapeutics, Inc. recently reported completion of a phase II RCT of synthetic CBD for the treatment of infantile spasms [72]. In this study, patients received synthetic CBD product orally up to a maximum dose of 20 mg/kg/day, and response was monitored via overnight video/EEG to determine the presence or absence of hypsarrhythmia and the seizure burden (before and after 14 days of CBD treatment). Of the nine enrolled patients, one was classified as responder after 14 days of treatment with CBD but was reported to relapse later. No additional data are available at this time.

Another recently completed RCT showed lack of efficacy of CBDV vs. placebo for the treatment of focal onset epilepsy in 162 adults; both the placebo and active arms showed ~40% seizure reduction from baseline (GW Pharmaceuticals; gwpharm.com).

Adverse Effects

Adverse effects of artisanal products have been reported. In one study, in addition to typical adverse events of increased seizures and fatigue/somnolence, the authors reported positive effects of improved behavior/alertness (33%), improved language

(10%), and improved motor skills (10%) [43]. Another study reported increased appetite, while positive adverse effects including improved sleep, alertness, and mood were reported in >50% of participants [53]. One of the studies from Israel reported aggressive behavior and worsening of seizures; some patients had somnolence, fatigue, gastrointestinal disturbances, and irritability [48]. Finally, 46% of participants reported adverse events including somnolence in 14% in the second study from Israel [47].

Reported side effects in both the open-label EAPs and the RCTs of highly purified CBD (Epidiolex®) have been similar. In the EAPs [59], diarrhea (29.2%) and somnolence (22.4%) were the most common AEs, with other AEs including upper respiratory infection (12.4%), decreased appetite (12.4%), convulsion (16.8%), vomiting (11.4%), fatigue (10.7%), pyrexia (10.4%), status epilepticus (7.4%), and pneumonia (6.8%). Somnolence and diarrhea appear to be dose-related. Further, the AE of somnolence appears to be related to concomitant clobazam use, as somnolence was much more common in patients taking clobazam (38% of those taking clobazam vs. 14% not taking clobazam). Abnormal liver function tests (LFTs; alanine aminotransferase/aspartate aminotransferase elevations >3 times the upper limit of normal) were seen in 10% of patients, but the majority (75%) of these abnormalities were found in patients taking concomitant valproate. In this study, 5.2% (n = 31/607) of patients discontinued CBD due to AEs.

No dose-related effects were reported in the first published RCT in DS [69] because patients in the CBD treatment group only received one dose (20 mg/kg/day). In this study, AEs were similar to the EAP data, with diarrhea (31% in treatment group vs. 10% in placebo) and somnolence (36% in treatment group vs. 10% in placebo) being the most common side effects, again with most participants (18/22) reporting sedation also taking clobazam. LFT abnormalities were also seen in this study, and they led to withdrawal of three patients in the treatment group and one patient in the placebo group, all of which were also taking valproate. There were nine other patients who had LFT elevations but continued in the trial; the LFTs returned to normal even though they continued CBD treatment. In the safety trial in DS [70], rash was more frequently reported (five in CBD group vs. one in placebo group), with a diffuse maculopapular rash, localized rash, papular rash, viral rash, and concomitant rash and hives seen in the CBD group and diaper rash seen in one patient in the placebo group.

In the LGS trial [73], reported side effects in patients receiving CBD were the same and included diarrhea, somnolence, decreased appetite, and vomiting. Of the patients who had adverse events, the events resolved by the end of the trial in 45 (61%) of patients receiving CBD and 38 (64%) of patients in the placebo group. Three patients had to withdraw from the study due to LFT elevations. AEs led to withdrawal from the study for one patient due to each: diarrhea, vomiting, acute hepatic failure, viral infection, increased concentration of another ASD, convulsion, lethargy, restlessness, acute respiratory distress syndrome, hypercapnia, hypoxia, pneumonia aspiration, and rash. All patients who had respiratory distress were all taking concomitant clobazam.

Drug-Drug Interactions

We were unable to identify studies that directly address the drug-drug interactions of artisanal Δ^9-THC. However, studies of synthetic Δ^9-THC or its analogues indicate potential interactions with other pharmaceuticals [74]. For example, WIN55,212-2 mesylate (WIN), a non-selective CB_1R/CB_2R agonist, has been shown to enhance anticonvulsant effects of several ASDs including phenytoin, phenobarbital, carbamazepine, ethosuximide, and valproate in animal seizure models in a dose-dependent manner; however, such effect was not observed for clonazepam. Whether similar effects of naturally occurring Δ^9-THC can be expected will need to be determined.

However, there are now a few studies that address the drug-drug interactions of/ with CBD, and these are described here. A recent open-label, fixed-sequence study in healthy volunteers assessed the effect of CBD on steady-state pharmacokinetics of CLB and N-desmethyl-clobazam (N-CLB), stiripentol, and valproate (VPA) and the reciprocal effect of CLB, stiripentol, and valproate on CBD and its metabolites 7-OH-CBD and 7-COOH-CBD [75]. Overall, the concomitant use of CBD had little effect on CLB and VPA exposure, but it resulted in increased exposure to N-CLB and stiripentol. Further, analysis of the interaction between CLB and CBD revealed that it has resulted in increased 7-OH-CBD and that stiripentol decreased 7-OH-CBD exposure by 29% and 7-COOH-CBD exposure by 13% [75]. A recent compilation of several CBD interaction studies in healthy and epilepsy participants confirmed a bidirectional drug-drug interaction between CBD and CLB/N-CLB, lack of interaction with VPA, and lack of effect on 4-ene-VPA (4-ene-VPA is a putative hepatotoxin) [76]. Further, it documented that CBD had no effect on CYP3A4 and, thus, that it is unlikely to cause clinically significant drug-drug interactions with other medicines metabolized by this enzyme, e.g., midazolam [76].

Of particular importance for the epilepsy community are the studies of interactions with other ASDs. In addition to the studies mentioned above (CLB/N-CLB, VPA, stiripentol, and midazolam), several other studies have identified a PK interaction with CLB. In a study of 13 children taking concomitantly CLB and CBD, the mean CLB and N-CLB plasma levels were increased after treatment with CBD compared to pre-treatment baseline, though the CLB level increases were not significant [77]. Increased N-CLB levels were associated with sedation and resulted in reduction of CLB dose; this interaction is likely a result of CBD's inhibition of CYP2C19, the enzyme responsible for metabolizing N-CLB [76, 78]. One issue that has been under debate and not completely resolved is whether CBD's efficacy in epilepsy can be mostly accounted for by the presence of concomitant CLB. In one open-label study of TRE and another in TSC, there were significant differences in the responder rates, with significantly higher response rates in patients who were taking concomitant CLB [58, 61]. In a different open-label study in TRE, there were no sustained differences in seizure frequency and severity reduction at 12 weeks between patients taking clobazam with CBD vs. those not taking CLB [64]. However, no study has been designed to specifically answer this question, and all published data are from exploratory analyses.

In a dose-ranging RCT in DS, changes in ASD levels with CBD treatment were reported [70]. The authors measured levels of CLB/N-CLB, VPA, stiripentol, topiramate (TPM), and levetiracetam (LEV). While there was a significant increase in N-CLB levels in all CBD groups, levels of the other ASDs remained unchanged. However, into account needs to be taken the relatively small number of participants in each arm [79]. Further, the focus of this study was on PK rather than efficacy and on testing of serum levels of CBD and its metabolites 6-OH-CBD, 7-OH-CBD, and 7-COOH-CBD [70]. Of note is that of the 6/22 patients receiving valproate developed elevated transaminases – this is similar to another recently reported study [59]. However, none of these elevations met criteria for drug-induced liver injury, and all patients' LFTs ultimately returned to normal. Another recent study focused on the interaction between brivaracetam (BRV) and CBD to show 95–280% increases in BRV level in response to CBD co-administration [80]. Out of two patients enrolled in this study, two had minor adverse events leading to BRV decreases in one of them.

In an open-label study, levels of all standard ASDs with the exception of BRV were measured in 39 adult and 42 pediatric patients [79]. With CBD co-administration, there were significant increases in levels of CLB, N-CLB, rufinamide, and TPM in all patients; in adults only, there were also increases seen in the serum levels of eslicarbazepine and zonisamide levels. However, the mean changes in levels exceeded normal therapeutic range for CBZ and N-CLB only. Additionally, patients taking concomitant VPA had significant changes in mean ALT and AST levels compared to patients not taking VPA, though VPA levels did not change significantly from baseline. One study reported an interaction between CBD and warfarin and another on an interaction between *cannabis* and warfarin, with the presence of CBD increasing the international normalized ratio (INR) and thus necessitating adjustments in warfarin dosing [81, 82]. Finally, there is one case report from another open-label CBD study that demonstrates an interaction between CBD and tacrolimus, with a threefold increase in tacrolimus levels seen with initiation of CBD; this led to the patient demonstrating symptoms of tacrolimus toxicity [83]. Ultimately, this patient required holding of the tacrolimus for a period of time and subsequent tacrolimus dose adjustments as CBD treatment continued.

Effects of Food on CBD

It is important to recognize that the relationship between the CBD dose (including synthetic CBD) and CBD plasma levels is linear (dose proportional) [9, 63, 71]. However, a substantial variability of the CBD levels possibly relates to other factors, e.g., food intake status/fatty meals, high first-pass metabolism, or individual absorption rates [84]. For example, there is a relationship between delivery method (e.g., liquid vs. capsule) and serum level [85]. Another reason for the observed variability in the relationship between CBD dose and level may be the fact that oral bioavailability of CBD is overall low in humans (<10%), highly variable, and much lower than for other administration routes such as intranasal or transdermal, where higher exposure to CBD is typically observed [86]. A recent single ascending and multiple-dose pharmacokinetic (PK) trial of CBD in healthy controls examined the effect of food on CBD PK parameters [87]. Overall, CBD T_{max} was 4–5 hours with the major metabolites being 7-carboxy-CBD, 7-hydroxy-CBD, and 6-hydroxy-CBD. Plasma exposure to CBD increased in a less than dose-proportional manner. CBD reached steady state after approximately 2 days. A high-fat meal increased CBD plasma exposure (T_{max} and AUC) by 4.85- and 4.2-fold, respectively; there was no effect of food on T_{max} or terminal half-life [87].

Conclusions

Understanding of the efficacy and safety of *cannabis* products in the treatment of TRE has expanded significantly in the last few years, with high-quality data emerging in the form of RCTs for pharmaceutical-grade CBD. The results of these RCTs have led to FDA approval of one highly purified formulation of CBD. It appears CBD has a novel MOA compared to the vast majority of other ASDs, which makes it a desirable adjunctive option for patients with TRE. There are potential AEs and drug-drug interactions, but overall studies indicate that CBD is well tolerated with only LFT and certain ASD level monitoring recommended. While these data are promising, it is important to note that these data cannot be generalized to all available CBD and *cannabis* products. Future controlled studies of various ratios of CBD and Δ^9-THC are needed as there could be further therapeutic potential of these compounds for patients with epilepsy.

Multiple Sclerosis and Cannabis – Benefits, Risks, and Special Considerations

Allen C. Bowling

History and Demographics of Use

There is a long history of cannabis use in MS. The first published account of the potential benefit of cannabis in MS, reported in *Journal of the American Medical Association* in 1979, described the effects of tetrahydrocannabinol (THC) on nine people with MS-associated spasticity [88].

Since that publication, there have been dozens of clinical studies of variable quality that have examined potential symptom-alleviating as well as disease-modifying effects of cannabis in MS [89–93]. The majority of these studies have focused on MS-associated pain and spasticity. Some of these studies included nabiximols, a pharmaceutical-grade cannabis product, which was first approved for use in MS in the United Kingdom in 2010 and subsequently in more than two dozen other countries [93].

For thousands of years before these published studies in MS, cannabis was claimed to be beneficial for pain and spasticity in other conditions [94]. In several ancient cultures, cannabis was used for pain and "neuralgia." In ancient Greece, Galen claimed that cannabis could be used for spasms and pain. In the mid-1800s, O'Shaughnessy, an Irish physician, described the use of cannabis for pain as well as severe spasms associated with tetanus and rabies. More recently, from 1851 to 1942, in the United States, multiple editions of the *US Pharmacopeia* included cannabis and listed analgesia as one of its potential therapeutic uses [94].

The legal acceptance of cannabis in the United States has vacillated significantly over the past century. Since the late 1990s, there has been a growing trend for legalization of cannabis for medical as well as recreational use. The vast majority of states have now legalized some form of medical marijuana, and, in these states, commonly approved conditions include MS, pain, or spasticity [89, 95].

In the United States, cannabis use appears to be greater in those with MS than in the general population. In the general population, 8.3% are "current" users; men use more often (10.6%) than women (6.2%) [89]. Studies in MS indicate that 9–38% are current users and that, as in the general population, cannabis use is more common in men than women [96, 97].

Fund of Knowledge – Health Professionals, Dispensary Staff

Health professionals and dispensary staff are critical points of contact for educating and providing informed decision-making about cannabis to those with MS. Multiple studies have found that health professionals and dispensary staff lack cannabis education and training and may thereby provide misinformation, be unable to provide appropriate information, and ultimately be unable to provide optimal care and facilitate informed decision-making in this area [98].

Several North American studies indicate that health professionals do not have an adequate fund of knowledge about cannabis. In one US study of physician residents and fellows, 89.5% stated that they were not at all prepared to recommend cannabis and 38.5% were not at all prepared to answer questions [99]. In a Colorado survey of physicians, nurse practitioners, physician assistants, and medical assistants, 1–2% reported being completely trained about the health risks of cannabis [100]. The majority of US states do not require training for physicians who provide cannabis recommendations [98]. Canadian studies of physicians and nurse practitioners found that there is a large gap between current and desired cannabis knowledge [101, 102].

There are significant limitations with the information, as well as products, that are recommended and sold by staff at US cannabis dispensaries. Most states do not require cannabis training for dispensary staff [98]. One study of dispensary staff found that 80% do not have any medical or scientific training, 94% provide advice about specific products, 78% provide recommendations for products that have not been shown to be effective or could exacerbate conditions, and 21% recommend products in order to move them out of inventory [98].

Pharmacology

Components of cannabinoid (CB) pharmacology are theoretically intriguing for their relevance to MS. The cannabinoid 1 receptor (CB1R), the most abundant G-coupled receptor in the central nervous system (CNS), acts as a "synaptic circuit breaker" to maintain homeostasis by suppressing excessive activity in neurons that are excitatory (such as glutamatergic) as well as inhibitory (such as gamma amino-butyric acid (GABA)-ergic). The circuit breaker action in inhibitory and excitatory pathways is referred to as depolarization-induced suppression of excitation (DSE) and depolarization-induced suppression of inhibition (DSI), respectively. The CBR1 is present in regions and pathways that are critical for pain and spasticity. CB-induced DSE and DSI in these areas may thereby alleviate pain and spasticity [103].

CBs have many non-CB1R-mediated pharmacological actions, some of which may be relevant to symptomatic as well as disease-modifying effects in MS. For example, in terms of symptoms, some CBs, including cannabidiol (CBD), may produce pain-relieving effects through actions on the transient receptor potential channels [104]. Anti-spasticity effects may be mediated by CB actions on big-conductance calcium-activated potassium channels [105]. Possible disease-modifying effects could be produced by immune-modulating effects of cannabinoid 2 receptors (CB2Rs), which are present on lymphocytes, or CB actions that could be neuroprotective, including effects on oxidative damage, excitotoxicity, and calcium flux [106, 107].

Efficacy in MS

Among all medical conditions that have undergone formal clinical trial testing with cannabis, MS is one of the most extensively studied. There are 17 randomized controlled trials (RCTs) that have studied cannabis effects on MS symptoms, and many of these have reported beneficial effects with pharmaceutical-grade preparations for spasticity, pain, and bladder dysfunction. These studies have overall included more 3000 patients [89–93]. RCTs of cannabis as an MS disease-modifying therapy are more limited and have not reported therapeutic effects [108].

RCTs have evaluated multiple MS symptoms. The largest number of high-quality RCTs has evaluated spasticity, pain, and bladder dysfunction. Individual trials and meta-analyses of these trials have generally reported therapeutic effects for subjective or self-reported outcome measures. The RCTs for these three MS symptoms have been placebo-controlled; there are not any RCTs that have used conventional symptomatic medications as active comparators. For spasticity, therapeutic effects have been observed with subjective outcome measures but not with objective outcome measures, such as the Ashworth and Modified Ashworth scales. There are fewer RCTs of bladder dysfunction than pain or spasticity, but these studies have also generally reported beneficial effects. RCTs for MS symptoms have not been entirely consistent. For example, the largest and longest RCT found that placebo was favored over cannabis with the outcomes of subjective spasticity, pain, and bladder dysfunction. Cannabis has not shown therapeutic effects in multiple RCTs of MS-associated tremor [89–93].

In the most rigorous study of RCTs in this area, a systematic review and meta-analysis that followed international standards were conducted on clinical trial data for spasticity, pain, and bladder dysfunction [92]. Unlike previous similar studies, this analysis was able to determine pooled estimates of outcomes by standardizing outcome measures in different trials. With this approach, it was found that there were statistically significant differences that favored cannabis relative to placebo in outcome measures for pain, spasticity, and bladder dysfunction. The standardized mean difference (SMD), which is a measure of the magnitude of the treatment effect, was modest for all three symptoms. Most of the therapeutic effects had absolute SMDs that were between 0.09 and 0.25, which is generally indicative of a mild effect size [109] and is less than the SMDs of 0.58–2.41 for several conventional MS symptomatic therapies, such as lioresal for spasticity and solifenacin and oxybutynin for bladder dysfunction. This meta-analysis also found that, for unclear reasons, the treatment effect was less when industry-funded studies were excluded. Finally, the analysis was limited by the heterogeneity of the analyzed trials, including differences in study designs, study populations, treatment duration, cannabis preparations, and outcome measures. This meta-analysis concluded that the MS trials "suggest a limited efficacy" of cannabis for spasticity, pain, and bladder dysfunction [92].

Unfortunately, it is not possible to use the results of the RCTs in MS to guide clinical practice with products from US cannabis dispensaries. This is because, as noted, the cannabis products in the high-quality RCTs were pharmaceutical-grade cannabis preparations and these preparations are not available in US dispensaries.

Dosing and Formulations

The majority of the MS RCTs have used nabiximols, an oromucosal spray, and Cannador, an oral cannabis extract. These preparations are high-quality, pharmaceutical-grade products with mixtures of THC and cannabidiol (CBD) with THC:CBD ratios of approximately 1:1 for nabiximols and 2:1 for Cannador. There are not any RCTs of pure CBD in MS [93].

MS clinical trial protocols have used various doses and frequency schedules [93]. The frequency for oral administration has generally been twice daily, while that for oromucosal administration has been extremely variable with dosing up to 48 times daily. Starting doses have been 5–15 milligrams (mg) for THC and 2.5 mg for CBD. Average and maximal final daily doses for THC have been 20–40 mg and approximately 120 mg, respectively, while those for CBD have be approximately 10 mg and 120 mg, respectively. Titration times have been 3–5 weeks.

For discontinuation of cannabis, formal recommendations generally do not exist. In the case of pharmaceutical-grade CBD, which is approved by the Food and Drug Administration (FDA) for some forms of pediatric epilepsy, precautions are given in the Prescribing Information (PI) to slowly taper the dose since rapid discontinuation of this product, like any other anticonvulsant, could provoke seizures, especially in those with underlying seizure disorders [110]. For patients who are using products that are predominantly THC, clinicians should be aware that discontinuation may be difficult in those who are addicted to THC.

Safety

In spite of cannabis use by humans for thousands of years, rigorous understanding of its safety in recreational and medical use, including MS, is still poorly understood. This is probably due to multiple factors that have hindered safety studies, including limited formal clinical trials, diverse cannabis preparations, self-report data, illegality, and widespread but poorly studied and monitored recreational use. Cannabis safety data for smoking, which is the most common mode of administration, is especially limited. While some safety information is available from clinical trials, much of the higher-quality data is derived from large databases, including emergency room visits and hospitalizations. Case reports also provide safety information, but this is often of limited and variable quality [89].

In clinical trials for MS and other neurological and non-neurological conditions, cannabis is generally well tolerated. Common side effects reported in cannabis clinical trials, listed in descending order of frequency, are dizziness, dry mouth, nausea, fatigue, somnolence, euphoria, vomiting, disorientation, drowsiness, confusion, loss of balance, and hallucinations [111]. In MS RCTs specifically, meta-analysis found that cannabis treatment was more likely than placebo to cause dizziness or vertigo, dry mouth, fatigue, feeling drunk, impaired balance or ataxia, memory impairment, and somnolence [92].

In MS, a possible adverse effect of cannabis that is of significant concern is stroke due reversible cerebral vasoconstriction syndrome (RCVS) [112–114]. RCVS is characterized by segmental cerebral vasoconstriction and specific vasoactive triggers, including cannabis. One study of 40 RCVS patients in Colorado found that cannabis was involved in 33% of those who had vasoactive triggers and that those with cannabis-associated RCVS were more likely to be younger and male than those with other forms of RCVS [115]. RCVS is often, but not always, associated with thunderclap headache [116]. Neurological deficits due to RCVS may mimic an MS attack. Importantly, steroids, which are used to treat MS attacks, may worsen neurological deficits or even cause death in those with RCVS [117, 118]. Therefore, clinicians caring for those with MS should be aware that RCVS may mimic an MS attack and should use caution with steroid use in patients who use cannabis and have symptoms that are consistent with an MS attack but could also be consistent with RCVS. Also, RCVS risk could be greater in those with MS who use cannabis in combination with sphingosine-1-phosphate inhibitors (fingolimod and siponimod) since fingolimod has been associated with RCVS [119].

There are other potential neurological side effects that are relevant to MS. THC, in contrast with CBD, has been associated with proconvulsant effects [120]. Visual difficulties and weakness have been reported with cannabis [121]. In those under age 25, cannabis may impair brain development [89]. Neuropsychological deficits and impaired cerebral compensatory mechanisms have been associated with cannabis use in MS [122]. Some of these deficits, including memory, processing speed, and executive function, have been found to improve after 28 days of abstinence in people with MS who are frequent, long-term cannabis users [123]. In the general population, cannabis use is associated with impaired memory, attention, and learning [124]. Driving a motor vehicle may be impaired by cannabis-associated cognitive dysfunction, including slowed reaction time, increased lane weaving, and decreased critical tracking and attention [125]. Psychiatric risks that have been associated with cannabis include addiction, worsening of anxiety and depression, increased suicidality (ideation, attempt, death), and development of schizophrenia and other psychoses [89].

Multiple possible non-neurological side effects of cannabis, which should be incorporated into the decision-making process about cannabis use in MS, are summarized below:

- *Carcinogenesis:* possible non-seminoma testicular cancer [89]
- *Cardiovascular:* triggering of myocardial infarction [89], orthostatic hypotension [126]
- *Driving and operating machinery:* approximate twofold increased risk of motor vehicle accidents [89]
- *Gastrointestinal:* cannabis hyperemesis syndrome [2], hepatocellular injury (especially with CBD) [110], decreased gut motility [127]
- *Infection:* increased infection risk with CBD [110]
- *Mutagenesis, fertility:* for women, lower birth weight, increased pregnancy complications, increased risk of infant admission to ICU [89]; for men, lower sperm concentration and sperm counts [128]

There are also unknown side effects of cannabis. Products from US dispensaries may contain unknown amounts of contaminants that have established and unstudied side effects in humans (see "Special Considerations for Dispensary Products"). Also, formal safety studies of specific cannabinoids are limited, especially with long-term use and use of highly concentrated THC products that have recently become available.

Comorbidities, MS Symptoms, and Cannabis

Due to its safety profile, cannabis should be used with caution or avoided in those with MS who have specific comorbid conditions or MS symptoms. The most common comorbid conditions in MS, depression and anxiety [129], may be worsened by cannabis [89]. Also, the increased suicide risk of MS [130] may be increased further by cannabis use [89]. Those with seizure disorders should avoid THC-containing products [120]. MS-associated constipation could be worsened with cannabis due to its inhibitory effect on gut motility [127]. Other cannabis-relevant conditions include personal and family history of addiction and psychosis, stroke, coronary artery disease, pulmonary disease, liver disease, and testicular cancer.

Drug Interactions

Drug interactions of cannabis, especially US dispensary products, are not well understood. This is due to the possible presence in a single cannabis product of more than 100 different cannabinoids, each of which may have different drug interactions that are poorly understood [131–133]. Limited studies at this time indicate that CBD may actually have more drug interactions than THC [131].

There are general considerations about cannabis interactions. Cannabis may increase the sedating effects of alcohol and medications [131–133]. Many MS medications have potential sedating effects, especially those used for spasticity, such as lioresal, tizanidine, and benzodiazepines [105]. Also, cannabis may interact with anticonvulsants that may be used in those with MS, including topiramate, rufinamide, clobazam, zonisamide, eslicarbazepine, and valproic acid [131].

There are potential specific interactions of cannabis with MS DMTs. CBD may be hepatotoxic. The PI for pharmaceutical-grade CBD states that liver function tests should be obtained before starting CBD and also 1, 3, and 6 months after starting CBD and periodically thereafter [110]. In those with MS, hepatotoxicity may be increased by concomitant administration of CBD with DMTs that are also potentially hepatotoxic, including interferons, teriflunomide, fingolimod, siponimod, cladribine, natalizumab, and alemtuzumab [134]. Teriflunomide toxicity may also be increased through the breast cancer resistance protein (BCRP) since teriflunomide is a substrate for BCRP [135] and CBs inhibit this transporter system [131]. Cladribine effectiveness may be decreased, and levels and toxicity may be increased because cladribine is a substrate for two transporters that are inhibited by CBs, equilibrative nucleoside transporter 1 (ENT1) [136] and BCRP [131]. Finally, siponimod levels and toxicity may be increased by CB inhibition of two cytochrome P450 isoforms, 2C9 and 3A4 [132, 137].

Special Considerations for Dispensary Products

There are special considerations that need to be taken into account for cannabis products that are sold in US dispensaries. These considerations do not apply to conventional prescription medications because, in contrast to dispensary products, the manufacture and labelling of conventional medications are strictly regulated and these products are prescribed and dispensed by trained, licensed professionals (physicians and pharmacists). Since these considerations are unique to cannabis dispensary products, many clinicians may not be familiar with them.

Labelling

There are multiple studies that have reported potentially dangerous inaccuracies in the labelling of cannabis dispensary products. For example, a study of 75 cannabis products from California and Washington found that 83% of the products were inaccurately labelled and concluded that the labelling failed to meet the basic label accuracy standards for pharmaceuticals [138].

Toxic and Infectious Risks

Dispensary products may contain contaminants, some of which are associated with neurotoxicity and infection risk. Neurotoxicity may be of particular concern to those with MS because MS-associated neurological disability may increase vulnerability to neurotoxicity and may also make it difficult to diagnose neurotoxic syndromes. Cannabis-associated infection risks may be increased by DMT-induced immunosuppression.

Multiple contaminants have been found in US dispensary products. Pesticides and solvents, some of which have significant health risks, including neurotoxicity, have been reported in up to 70–80% of dispensary products [138–140]. Since the cannabis plant avidly absorbs heavy metals from the soil in which it is grown, cannabis products may be contaminated with heavy metals, some of which are neurotoxic [138]. Finally, vaporizing and smoking produce potentially harmful compounds. Vaporizing has been associated with significant lung injury that may be fatal [141]. Smoking produces ammonia, heavy metals, carbon monoxide, mutagens, carcinogens, and polycyclic hydrocarbons [140].

There are potential infection risks with cannabis. In the clinical trials of pharmaceutical-grade CBD, the overall infection risk was higher with CBD than placebo [110]. This risk could be higher in those with MS who are immunocompromised due to MS DMTs. There is limited evidence that cannabis use is a risk factor for tuberculosis (TB) [142]. Multiple MS DMTs should not be used in those with active or latent TB, including teriflunomide, cladribine, and alemtuzumab [134]. The cannabis microbiome includes many microbes, especially gram-negative bacilli and fungi, that may be pathogenic to humans, especially those who are immunocompromised [143–145]. There are particular fungi in the cannabis microbiome [143–145] that have been associated with infections with the use of specific MS DMTs including *Aspergillus* [146] with alemtuzumab and *Cryptococcus* with fingolimod [147] and natalizumab [148].

Some *Penicillium* species in the cannabis microbiome produce compounds that may be toxic to humans. For example, paxilline, which is produced by *Penicillium paxilli*, is a tremorgenic mycotoxin, and citrinin, produced by *Penicillium citrinum*, is a nephrotoxin [144, 145].

Dispensary Staff There are significant limitations of dispensary staff. As discussed elsewhere in this chapter (see "Fund of Knowledge—Health Professionals, Dispensary Staff"), the majority of US dispensary staff do not have any medical or scientific training and are not required to obtain cannabis training [98]. One study found that dispensary staff make recommendations for products that have not been shown to be effective or could worsen patients' conditions, some of which are relevant to MS or MS comorbidities. For example, 78% of staff recommend high THC or high CBD preparations for MS, 33% recommend THC for depression, 13% recommend THC for anxiety, and 7% recommend THC for epilepsy [98]. A study of workers in the Colorado cannabis industry, including dispensary staff, found that 33% use cannabis while driving to work, 18% use while at work, and 27% use while driving home from work [149]. This raises the concern that staff are cognitively impaired while interacting with, and making recommendations to, customers.

Conclusion

Health professionals may play a critical role in addressing cannabis use in MS. The majority of people with MS may not understand the complexity of cannabis use in MS and may not have access to objective lay information on this topic. Health professionals who are educated on the MS-relevant aspects of cannabis may thus provide education, facilitate informed cannabis decision-making, and optimize safe and appropriate cannabis use in those patients who choose to use it.

Key Takeaways

1. Many people with MS are interested in and use cannabis, and many health professionals are not well educated about cannabis.
2. Cannabis has potential therapeutic symptomatic effects in MS, including alleviation of pain, spasticity, and bladder dysfunction.
3. Cannabis has potential side effects and drug interactions, and, in the case of US dispensary products, there are "special considerations," including possible contaminants, incorrect labelling, and limitations of dispensary staff services.
4. Health professionals who are educated about the MS-relevant benefits, risks, and "special considerations" of cannabis may play an important role in facilitating informed decision-making about cannabis as well as optimizing the safe and appropriate use of cannabis in their patients.
5. For people with MS, efforts should be made to develop and provide access to cannabis products that have been shown to be effective, do not have contaminant and labelling issues, and are dispensed by staff who are educated and trained.

The Evidence for Cannabis Use in Movement Disorders

Ying Liu, Tristan Seawalt, and Maureen A. Leehey

The Evidence for Cannabis Use in Movement Disorders

The US Food and Drug Administration (FDA) has not approved any forms of cannabis as an indication for Parkinson disease or any other movement disorder. The American Academy of Neurology (AAN) states that presently the benefits of cannabis to treat neurological disorders are not substantiated by enough non-anecdotal evidence. The AAN is also concerned about long-term safety as well as the effects of the innumerous unstudied cannabinoids in cannabis [150].

In the 33 states with Medical Marijuana Programs (MMPs), persons with debilitating medical conditions are allowed to use cannabis products as an alternative treatment. Depending on jurisdiction, there are over 50 distinct qualifying debilitating medical conditions. Some movement disorders, e.g., Tourette syndrome, Huntington's disease, Parkinson disease, and dystonia, are on many state's lists of qualifying medical marijuana conditions, with Parkinson disease being the most common movement disorder. Other movement disorders that may benefit from cannabis, such as essential tremor, restless legs syndrome, and rapid eye movement (REM) sleep behavior disorder, have not been listed as qualifying conditions. Despite MMP implication of cannabis as an effective alternative treatment, according to the National Academies of Sciences, only limited evidence can be found for its use in Tourette syndrome, and insufficient evidence supports its use in Parkinson disease, Huntington's disease, and dystonia regarding efficacy and safety [151].

Due to the limited research on this Schedule I Controlled Substance (Comprehensive Drug Abuse Prevention and Control Act, 1970), physicians are left without evidence-based resources when answering questions from their clinic patients, many of whom expect definitive answers regarding their use of cannabis to treat their specific condition. This review presents the preclinical and clinical evidence of the effects of cannabis in movement disorders (Tables 10.2, 10.3, 10.4, and 10.5) and the quality of this evidence (Table 10.6). Since cannabis is a plant consisting of hundreds of chemicals with complex interactions with the human endocannabinoid system, this review emphasizes the type of cannabinoid-related drug used in each study, as well as its dose, whenever this information is available. The major cannabis extracts and synthetic compounds used in these studies are presented in Table 10.5. Delta-9-tetrahydrocannabinol (Δ9-THC) and cannabidiol (CBD) are the most frequently studied compounds found in cannabis plants. Both THC and CBD interact with human endocannabinoid system: THC binds with the cannabinoid 1 (CB_1) receptors in the brain, while CBD binds weakly, and CBD can interfere with the binding of THC to CB_1 receptors.

Parkinson Disease

Parkinson disease (PD) is the second most common neurodegenerative disease and is clinically characterized by progressive disabling tremor, slowness, stiffness, balance impairment, as well as many non-motor symptoms such as cognitive deficits, psychiatric symptoms, autonomic dysfunction, pain, fatigue, insomnia, and rapid eye movement (REM) sleep behavior disorder. In 2016, PD affected approximately 6.1 million people globally, compared to 2.5 million in 1990 [152]. The economic burden of PD in the United States is documented as at least $14.4 billion a year [153]. The cause of PD remains largely unknown. Treatments, including medications and surgery, cannot cure PD but can help control symptoms. Because the pathogenesis of PD results in low levels of dopamine in the brain, current medications function to increase or substitute for dopamine in its role as a neurotransmitter. However, these treatments sometimes produce unsatisfactory results and often

Table 10.2 Efficacy and tolerability of cannabis products in movement disorders

Reference	Class	Design	Group size	Study drug	Treatment dose and duration	Outcomes	Tolerability AEs	Withdrawals
Parkinson disease (÷)								
Carroll et al. 2004 [178]	I	R-DB-PC, crossover	19 (17 completed)	Cannador, THC 2.5 mg, CBD 1.25 mg, oral	THC 0.146 mg/kg/day (0.032–0.25 mg/kg/day) or placebo; 4 weeks. (THC blood level 0.25–5.4 ng/mL)	No objective or subjective improvement in dyskinesias or parkinsonism	18 types of AEs reported; similar types of AEs in both groups; more frequency in cannabis group	None
Chagas et al. 2014 [176]	II	R-DB-PC	21 (7 per group)	99.9% CBD, oral	CBD 75 mg/day, 300 mg/day or placebo; 6 weeks	Objective assessment: no effects on UPDRS. Subjective assessments: only 300 mg/day improved PDQ-39 ($p = 0.05$)	No AEs reported	None
Sieradzan et al. 2001 [179]	III	R-DB-PC, crossover	7	Nabilone (synthetic THC), oral	0.03 mg/kg/day	Objective assessments: reduced total Rush Dyskinesia Disability Scale scores ($p < 0.05$)	8 types of AEs reported. (§)	Two withdrawals, one due to vertigo and one to postural hypotension
Mesnage et al. 2004 [177]	III	R-DB-PC	24 (4 neurokinin B, 4 neurotensin, 4 SR 141713, 12 placebo)	Rimonabant, CB₁ antagonist, oral	20 mg/day, 16 days	Objective assessments: not change in UPDRS part III and IV	No AEs reported	None

Study	Level	Study type	N	Intervention	Dose	Results	AEs	Withdrawals
Chagas et al. 2014 [180]	IV	Case report	4	99.9% CBD, oral	75 mg/day, or 300 mg/day, 6 weeks	Subjective assessments: prompt and substantial reduction in the frequency of RBD-related events	No AEs reported	None
Zuardi et al. 2009 [175]	IV	Open-label study	6	99.9% CBD, oral	CBD, up to 400 mg/day, 4 weeks	Objective assessments: BPRS total score decreased ($p < 0.001$). No change on UPDRS sub-scores and MMSE. Subjective assessments: PPQ decreased, $p = 0.001$	No AEs observed	None
Lotan et al. 2014 [172]	IV	Open-label observational study	28 (22 completed)	Cannabis*, smoke	Single dose, 0.5 g	Objective assessments: UPDRS total score ($p < 0.001$) and tremor ($p = 0.000$), rigidity ($p = 0.004$) and bradykinesia ($p = 0.000$) sub-scores improved. Subjective: Visual analog scale score ($p < 0.001$) and present pain intensity scale ($p < 0.001$) improved	6 types of AEs reported	Six withdrawals, due to inability to smoke, vomiting, dizziness, and psychosis

(continued)

Table 10.2 (continued)

Reference	Class	Design	Group size	Study drug	Treatment dose and duration	Outcomes	Tolerability AEs	Withdrawals
Frankel et al. 1990 [174]	IV	Case series report	5	Marijuana leaf (2.9% THC by weight), smoke	1 g	No improvement in tremor	2 types of AEs reported	N/A
Shohet et al. 2017 [173]	IV	Open-label observational study	20	Cannabis*, smoke or inhale	1 g of cannabis single dose, smoking or inhalation, for motor symptoms assessment. 1 g of cannabis daily, smoking or inhalation, for at least 10 weeks for sensory testing	Objective assessment: motor UPDRS scores ($p < 0.0001$), cold pain threshold ($p = 0.02$), and mean heat pain threshold ($p = 0.05$) improved Subjective assessment: PRI ($p = 0.001$) and VAS ($p = 0.0005$) improved	No AEs reported	N/A
Venderova et al. 2004 [154]	IV	Anonymous questionnaire survey	85	Fresh or dried leaves*, Oral	Half a teaspoon, mostly. (Urine level of 11-nor-δ-THCOOH ranging 43.10 ng/mL to 147.43 ng/mL in 7 participants)	Subjective reports: 39 participants reported improvement in general, 26 in rest tremor, 38 in bradykinesia, 32 in muscle rigidity, 12 in L-dopa-induced dyskinesia, 4 reported worse symptoms	Three discontinued due to unspecified AEs	N/A

Study	Level	Design	N	Intervention	Dose	Outcomes	AEs	
Finseth et al. 2015 [155]	IV	Self-administered survey	9	Cannabis*	No data available	Subjective reports: 5 reported "great improvement" in motor, sleep, motor symptoms or quality of life	No AEs reported	N/A
Balash et al. 2017 [156]	IV	Retrospective telephone survey	47	Cannabis sativa flowers and leaves, smoking or oil ingestion* (38/47)	Average 0.9 g/day (0.2–2.25)	Subjective reports: reduction in complaints of falling, stiffness, tremor, pain, mood, and sleep	Six discontinued medical cannabis due to loss of consciousness, hallucinations, fatigue, or postural instability 9 types of AEs reported	N/A
HD (€)								
Lopez-Sendon Moreno et al. 2016 [198]	I	R-DB-PC, crossover	24	Sativex® (2.7 mg THC/2.5 mg CBD per spray), Oral spray	Up to 12 sprays/day, 12 weeks (treatment compliance, assessed checking the returned packages and urine test, reached 95.8%)	Sativex® was safe and well tolerated in persons with HD Objective assessments: no differences on motor, cognitive, behavioral, and functional scores	13 types of AEs reported Dizziness or disturbance in attention in Sativex® more than placebo ($p = 0.045$). The frequency of rest of AEs similar in both periods	None

(continued)

Table 10.2 (continued)

Reference	Class	Design	Group size	Study drug	Treatment dose and duration	Outcomes	Tolerability AEs	Withdrawals
Consroe et al. 1991 [197]	III	R-DB-PC, crossover	15	Oral CBD* from US National Institute on Drug Abuse (NIDA)	10 mg/kg/day, 6 weeks (plasma levels of CBD ranging 5.9–11.2 ng/mL)	Objective assessments: no change in chorea severity, disability score, HD staging scheme, tongue extension, finger tapping, screw-and-nut test, Hopkins SCL-90R, recall, physician's assessment. Subjective assessments: no change in subjective assessment	No AEs reported	None
Curtis et al. 2009 [196]	II	R-DB-PC, crossover	44 (37 completed)	Nabilone, synthetic THC, oral	1 or 2 mg/day, 5 weeks	Objective assessments: no change in the UHDRS motor score. Improved chorea sub-score ($p = 0.009$)	4 types of AEs reported. (§)	One withdrawal due to sedation
Curtis et al. 2006 [195]	IV	Single case report	1	Nabilone, synthetic THC, oral	1 mg/day, 5 years	Subjective report: behavior and chorea improved	No AEs reported	N/A

	Level	Study type	N	Drug, route	Dose	Assessments/outcomes	AEs	Withdrawals
Muller-Vahl et al. 1999 [194]	IV	Single case report	1	Nabilone, synthetic THC, oral	1.5 mg, single dose	Objective assessments: chorea and motor impairment scale scores increased	1 type of AE reported	N/A
Dystonia (¥)								
Zadikoff et al. 2011 [208]	III	R-DB-PC, crossover	9 (7 completed)	Dronabinol tablet, Marinol®, 2.5 mg THC/tablet, oral	Up to 15 mg/day, 3 weeks	Objective assessments: no effects on TWSTRS part A Subjective assessments: no effects on TSWTRS part B and C, GIS, or VAP	7 types of AEs reported. (§)	One withdrawal due to insomnia and heart racing
Fox et al. 2002 [207]	III	R-DB-PC, crossover	15 (13 completed)	Nabilone, synthetic THC, oral	0.03 mg/kg, single dose	Objective assessments: no reduction in dystonia movement scale portion of the Burke-Fahn-Marsden dystonia scale	2 types of AEs reported. No difference in postural fall in blood pressure between placebo and nabilone ($p > 0.05$)	Two withdrawals due to postural hypotension or sedation
Consroe et al. 1986 [209]	IV	Open-label study	5	CBD*, oral	600 mg/day, 6 weeks	Subjective reports: dystonia improved	7 types of AEs reported	No withdrawals
Sandyk et al. 1986 [241]	IV	Case report	2	CBD*, oral	200 mg, single dose	Objective assessments: spasmodic torticollis and generalized torsion dystonia improved	No AEs reported	N/A

(continued)

Table 10.2 (continued)

Reference	Class	Design	Group size	Study drug	Treatment dose and duration	Outcomes	Tolerability AEs	Withdrawals
Chatterjee et al. 2002 [210]	IV	Single case report	1	Herbal cannabis*, smoked	Smoke one "joint," 3 weeks	Subjective report: pain and dystonia relieved.	2 types of AEs reported	N/A
Uribe Roca et al. 2005 [211]	IV	Single case report	1	Smoked marijuana*	3 or 4 g, single dose	Objective assessments: Burke-Fähn-Marsden dystonia rating scale scores improved	2 types of AEs reported	N/A
Tourette syndrome (£)								
Muller-Vahl et al. 2002 [227]	II	R-DB-PC, crossover	12	THC, oral	5.0, 7.5 or 10.0 mg, single dose, (significant correlation between tic improvement and maximum plasma 11-OH-THC)	Objective assessments: improved sub-scores, CMT (TSGS) improved ($p = 0.015$) Subjective assessments: TSSL improved ($p = 0.015$)	11 types of AEs reported in THC period only	None
Muller-Vahl et al. 2003 [228, 242]	III	R-DB-PC	24 (17 completed)	THC, oral	Up to 10 mg/day, 6 weeks (urine and serum test of THC and its metabolites excluded additional marijuana use)	Objective assessments: TS-CGI ($p = 0.008$), STSSS ($p = 0.033$), YGTSS ($p = 0.061$) improved Subjective assessment: TSSL improved ($p < 0.05$)	3 types of AEs reported in TCH and placebo groups	One withdrawal due to anxiety and restlessness

Thaler et al. 2019 [225]	IV	Telephone survey	42	Medical cannabis*	No data available	Subjective reports: high subjective satisfaction by most participants	8 types of AEs reported	N/A
Muller-Vahl et al. 1998 [224]	IV	Interview survey	64 interviewed, 17 reported prior use of marijuana	Smoked marijuana*	No data available	Subjective reports: 82% experienced a reduction or complete remission of motor and vocal tics and an amelioration of premonitory urges and obsessive-compulsive symptoms	No AEs reported	N/A
Abi-Jaoude et al. 2017 [226]	IV	Retrospective study (chart review and interview)	19	Cannabis*	No data available	Objective assessments: YGTSS ($p < 0.001$) and CGI ($p < 0.001$) improved Subjective assessments: Y-BOCS ($p = 0.001$), PUTS ($p < 0.001$) and ASRS ($p < 0.001$) improved	13 types of AEs reported	N/A
Jakubovski et al. 2017 [243]	IV	Case report	1	Vaporized Bedrocan® 22% THC and 1% CBD	0.6 g/day of vaporized medical cannabis, 8 months	Subjective report: vocal blocking tics improved	1 AE reported	N/A

(continued)

Table 10.2 (continued)

Reference	Class	Design	Group size	Study drug	Treatment dose and duration	Outcomes	Tolerability	
							AEs	Withdrawals
Jakubovski et al. 2017 [243]	IV	Case report	1	Vaporized dronabinol	Up to 16.8 mg dronabinol/day, 8 months	Subjective report: vocal blocking tics improved	No AEs reported	N/A
Muller-Vahl et al. 2002 [221]	IV	Single case report	1	THC, oral	10 mg/day	Objective assessments: GCIS (5 → 4), STSS (5 → 4), and YGTSS (81 → 46) improved Subjective reports: TSSL (46 → 16) and PE (23 → 9) improved	2 types of AEs reported	N/A
Szejko et al. 2018 [222]	IV	Single case report	1	THC, oral	Up to 29.4 mg THC/day, 4 months	Objective assessments: YGTSS-TSS (percentage improvement from baseline, −28.9%), rush video-based tic rating scale (−8.4%), YGTSS-GS (−60.3%), and CGI-I (−40%) improved Subjective assessments: PE (−72.7%), GTS-QOL (−83.3%) improved	No AEs reported	N/A

Muller-Vahl et al. 1999 [244]	IV	Single case report	1	THC, oral	10 mg THC, single dose	Objective assessment: Tourette syndrome global scale (41 → 7) improved Subjective report: motor and vocal tics improved about 70%	No AEs reported	N/A
Szejko et la. 2019 [223]	IV	Single case report	1	Vaporized medicinal cannabis* and oral pure THC	Vaporization of 0.15 g cannabis (equivalent to 33 mg THC), and 7 mg oral THC	Objective assessment: YGTSS (29 → 19), rush video-based tic rating scale (17 → 13), impairment score of the YGTSS (30 → 10), YGTSS-GS (59 → 29), CGI-SS (3 → 2) improved Subjective assessment: improved in Parent Tic Questionnaire (56 → 4), PE (23 → 15), GTW-QOL (42 → 2)	No AEs reported	N/A
Hasan et al. 2010 [220]	IV	Single case report	1	THC, oral	15 mg/day, 9 weeks (plasma level of Δ9-THC 0.8 ng/mL, 11-OH-THC 1.5 ng/mL, THC-COOH 25 ng/mL)	Objective assessments: YGTSS improved (97 → 54) Subjective assessment: GTS-QOL improved (54 → 21)	1 AE reported	N/A

(continued)

Table 10.2 (continued)

Reference	Class	Design	Group size	Study drug	Treatment dose and duration	Outcomes	Tolerability AEs	Withdrawals
Brunnauer et al. 2011 [217]	IV	Single case report	1	THC, oral	Up to 15 mg/day, 2 weeks	Objective assessment: YGTSS (89 → 22), concentration (from percentage 39 to 58), and visual perception (from percentage 44 to 72) improved	No AEs reported	N/A
Hemming et al. 1993 [218]	IV	Single case report	1	Cannabis leaf*, smoked	No data available	Subjective report: Tourette symptoms resolved completely	No AEs reported	N/A
Kanaan et al. 2017 [214]	IV	Single case report	1	Sativex® 2.7 mg THC/2.5 mg CBD per spray, oral spray	Up to 3 * 3 puff/day (= 24.3 mg THC and 22.5 mg CBD), 2 weeks	Objective assessments: YGTSS-TTS (45 → 35), MRVS (17 → 7), YGTSS-GS (85 → 55) improved Subjective assessments: TSSL (89 → 33), PUTS (34 → 22), GCI for PU (65 → 40), GTS-QOL (51 → 11), GTS-QOL-VAS (50 → 85) improved	No AEs reported	N/A

| Pichler et al. 2019 [215] | IV | Single case report | Dronabinol and oral CBD | 10 mg dronabinol plus 20 mg CBD/day, 1 year | Objective assessment: YGTSS improved (73 → 44) | No AEs reported | N/A |
| Trainor et al. 2016 [216] | IV | Single case report | Sativex® 2.7 mg THC/2.5 mg CBD per spray, oral spray | 10.8 mg THC/10 mg CBD/day, 4 weeks | Objective assessments: ORVRS (176 → 27) and YGTSS (71 → 36) improved | No AEs reported | N/A |

R randomized, *DB* double-blind, *PC* placebo-controlled, *CBD* cannabidiol, *THC* tetrahydrocannabinol, *AE* adverse event, *UPDRS* Unified Parkinson Disease Rating Scale, *PDQ-39* Parkinson Disease Questionnaire-39, *BPRS* Brief Psychiatric Rating Scale, *PPQ* Parkinson Psychosis Questionnaire, *MMSE* Mini-Mental State Examination, *PRI* Pain Rating Index, *VAS* Visual Analogue Scale, *UHDRS* Unified Huntington's Disease Rating Scale, *TWSTRS* Toronto Western Hospital Spasmodic Torticollis Rating Scale, *GIS* Global Impression Scale, *VAP* visual analog pain, *TS-CGI* Tourette Syndrome Clinical Global Impression Scale, *STSSS* Shapiro Tourette Syndrome Severity Scale, *YGTSS* Yale Global Tic Severity Scale, *TSSL* Tourette Syndrome Symptom List, *YGTSS-ITS* Total Tic Score of the Yale Global Tic Severity Scale, *PUTS* Premonitory Urges for Tics Scale, *Y-BOCS* Yale-Brown Obsessive-Compulsive Scale, *ASRS* Adult ADHD Self-Report Scale, version 1.1, *CGI-S* Clinical Global Impression Severity, *GCIS* Global Clinical Impression Scales, *PE* premonitory experiences, *MRVS* Modified Rush Video-Based Tic Scale, *GCI for PU* Global Clinical Impairment for premonitory urges, *GTS-QOL* GTS-Quality of Life, *GTS-QoL-VAS* Visual Analogue Scale for satisfaction of the GTS-QOL, *ORVRS* Original Rush Videotape Rating Scale, *11-OH-THC* 11-hydroxy-Δ9-tetrahydrocannabinol, *THC-COOH* 11-nor-Δ9-tetrahydrocannabinol-9-carboxylic-acid, *UTI* urinary tract infection

*Asterisk means the percent of THC in the plant material was not provided, so the exact dose taken is not known. (÷) means AEs reported in PD studies. (€) means AEs reported in dystonia studies. (£) means AEs reported in HD studies. (¥) means AEs reported in Tourette syndrome studies. (§) means that the authors didn't state the difference of frequency or types of AEs between treatment and placebo

Table 10.3 AEs reported in movement disorders

Movement disorders	AEs (common)	AEs
Parkinson disease (PD) (‡)	Dizziness, sedation	Altered taste, anxiety, cognitive decline, confusion, constipation, cough, decreased concentration, detached, diarrhea, disorientation, dyspnea, dry mouth, euphoria, hallucination, hyperacusis, hypoglycemia, muscular pain, nausea, nightmares, palpitations, paranoia, postural hypotension, psychosis, somnolence, unsteadiness, UTI, vertigo, vivid dreams
Huntington's disease (HD) (€)	Dizziness, sedation	Anxiety, behavioral changes, cognitive decline, diarrhea, disturbance in attention, euphoria, fever, headache, increased choreatic movements, insomnia, local infection, muscular pain, somnolence, upper respiratory infection, vomiting
Dystonia (¥)	Dizziness, sedation	Bitter taste, blurred vision, dry mouth, exacerbated hypokinesia, exacerbated resting tremor, postural hypotension, psychomotor slowing, somnolence, vertigo
Tourette syndrome (£)	Dizziness, sedation	Anxiety, ataxia, cognitive decline, confusion, decreased concentration, decreased motivation, dry eyes, dry mouth, euphoria, fatigue, feeling of a "high," galactorrhea, hallucination, headache, hot flush, increased appetite, increased tics, irritability, nausea, psychosis, sensitivity to noise or light, tremble, wheezing

(‡) means AEs reported in PD studies. (€) means AEs reported in HD studies. (¥) means AEs reported in dystonia studies. (£) means AEs reported in Tourette syndrome studies

Table 10.4 Cannabis products and related adverse events reported in movement disorder studies

Cannabis type	Class I (N/n)	Class II (N/n)	Class III (N/n)	Class IV (N/n)
Cannabis smoking	0	0	0	14(9)
THC, oral	0	1(1)	1(1)	6(2)
Dronabinol, oral	0	0	1(1)	2(0)
Nabilone, oral	0	1(1)	2(2)	2(1)
CBD, oral	0	1(0)	1(0)	5(1)
Cannador, oral	1(1)	0	0	0
Sativex®, oral spray	1(1)	0	0	2(0)
Rimonabant, oral	0	0	1(0)	0

Class I–IV are grades of the studies according to the American Academy of Neurology classification scheme for therapeutic articles (Appendix)
N the number of studies, n the number of studies that reported AEs in cannabis treatment group or period, *CBD* cannabidiol, *THC* tetrahydrocannabinol

cause adverse effects. In many states, PD is one of the MMP qualifying conditions. Some persons with PD recall using cannabis to treat motor symptoms and non-motor symptoms [154–156].

Preclinical Research

Animal studies have shown evidence of therapeutic efficacy of cannabinoids in PD, alleviating motor symptoms and reducing levodopa-induced involuntary movements, i.e., dyskinesia. Interestingly, these effects were found when animal models

Table 10.5 AEs reported in cannabis product studies

Adverse events	Cannabis smoked	THC, oral	Dronabinol, oral	Nabilone, oral	CBD, oral	Cannador oral	Sativex® oral spray	Rimonabant, oral	Total
Cannabis type	Percentage of THC not provided	Δ9-THC	Synthetic THC	Synthetic THC	99.9% purity of CBD	THC 2.5 mg/ CBD 1.25 mg	A botanical extract with equimolecular combinations of Δ9-THC and CBD (2.7 mg THC/2.5 mg CBD per spray)	SR141716, CB$_1$ antagonist, first approved in Europe in 2006, withdrawn worldwide in 2008 due to serious psychiatric side effects	
Dizziness	✓	✓	✓	✓	✓	✓	✓		7
Dry mouth	✓	✓	✓		✓	✓			5
Decreased concentration	✓	✓				✓	✓		4
Somnolence	✓			✓		✓	✓		4
Altered taste	✓		✓			✓			3
Anxiety	✓	✓				✓			3
Cognitive decline	✓			✓			✓		3
Euphoria	✓	✓		✓					3
Postural hypotension			✓	✓	✓				3
Sedation	✓			✓		✓			3
Confusion	✓					✓			2
Diarrhea						✓	✓		2
Fatigue	✓	✓							2
Feeling of a "high"	✓	✓							2
Hallucination	✓			✓					2
Headache	✓	✓					✓		2

(continued)

Table 10.5 (continued)

Adverse events	Cannabis smoked	THC, oral	Dronabinol, oral	Nabilone, oral	CBD, oral	Cannador oral	Sativex® oral spray	Rimonabant, oral	Total
Musculoskeletal pain						√	√		2
Nausea		√				√			2
Sensitivity to noise or light	√			√					2
Unsteadiness			√	√					2
Vertigo		√		√					2
Ataxia		√							1
Behavioral changes							√		1
Blurred vision			√						1
Constipation						√			1
Cough	√								1
Decreased motivation	√								1
Detached						√			1
Disorientation				√					1
Dry eyes	√								1
Dyspnea	√								1
Exacerbated hypokinesia					√				1
Exacerbated resting tremor					√				1
Fever							√		1
Galactorrhea		√							1
Hot flush		√							1
Hypoglycemia	√								1
Increased appetite	√								1
Increased choreatic movements				√					1

Increased tics	✓								1
Insomnia							✓		1
Irritability	✓								1
Local infection							✓		1
Nightmares						✓			1
Palpitation	✓					✓			1
Paranoia									1
Psychomotor slowing					✓				1
Psychosis	✓								1
Tremble		✓							1
Upper respiratory infection									1
UTI						✓			1
Vivid dreams						✓			1
Vomiting							✓		1
Wheezing	✓								1
Subtotal	25	14	6	12	7	16	13	0	

Table 10.6 Class and number of the cannabis studies in movement disorders

Disease	Class I study	Class II study	Class III study	Class IV study
Parkinson disease	1	1	2	6
Huntington's disease	1	1	1	2
Dystonia	0	0	2	4
Tourette syndrome	0	1	1	14

were treated with both cannabinoid receptor type 1 (CB_1) agonists and antagonists. Moreover, there is a dose-dependent effect; both CB_1 agonists and antagonists have no effects or impair normal motor function at higher doses. Low doses of CB_1 antagonists have been reported to improve locomotor activities and reduce levodopa-induced dyskinesia more consistently than CB_1 agonists [157–166].

CB_1 antagonists that have been used in animal studies include rimonabant (SR141716, first approved in Europe in 2006 but was withdrawn worldwide in 2008 due to serious psychiatric adverse effects), AM251, Δ^9-THCV, and cannabis extract [157–166]. Most studies exhibited a positive therapeutic effect of CB_1 antagonists, especially rimonabant, in PD. Intraperitoneal injection of 0.05 and 0.1 mg/kg of rimonabant, alone or with levodopa, enhanced ambulation and attenuated motor inhibition in 6-hydroxydopamine-lesioned rat models without influencing brain dopamine levels, indicating a dopamine-independent mechanism [158–161, 164]. The effects of cannabinoid antagonists can be eliminated indirectly by a CB_1 agonist, confirming the existence of CB_1-mediated modulation of the nigrostriatal dopaminergic tone. Higher doses, 0.5–1.0 mg/kg, of intraperitoneal injections of rimonabant tended to aggravate bradykinesia [164].

Administering lower dosages is critical when using CB_1 antagonists in PD due to its dose-dependent effects. Oral administration of 1 mg/kg of rimonabant in rat models and 1–3 mg/kg in cynomolgus monkeys, along with co-administration of levodopa, significantly decreased levodopa-induced dyskinesia without significantly affecting the antiparkinsonian action of levodopa [158, 160]. These animal studies also showed less loss of dopaminergic cells and a less denervated striatum in comparison with levodopa treatment alone in 6-hydroxydopamine (6-OHDA)-lesioned animals [158]. Some researchers point out that long-term co-administration of levodopa with cannabinoid-antagonist-based therapy may not only alleviate motor symptoms but also delay or even arrest the degeneration of dopaminergic cells in the substantia nigra.

Paradoxically, cannabinoid agonists such as WIN55,212-2, nabilone, and HU-210 also have positive effects on levodopa-induced dyskinesia, or increase antiparkinsonian action of levodopa, but with a very narrow therapeutic window at low doses [162, 165–169]. Other studies have reported conflicting results. Some cannabinoid agonists, like THC and levonantradol, were not effective and sometimes increased hypokinesia induced by reserpine in a dose- and time-dependent manner, producing no therapeutic effects [170, 171].

It is speculated that cannabinoid agonists and antagonists might be effective only in specific phases of the disease and under certain circumstances [159, 163, 164].

The dosage of cannabinoid agonists/antagonists and the severity of PD conditions may be critical for future consideration of cannabis use in the PD population.

Clinical Research

Motor Symptoms A questionnaire surveying 85 persons with PD found that many reported cannabis alleviated their PD motor symptoms; based on subjective experience reports, 45% of the participants had improvement in bradykinesia, 37% in muscle rigidity, and 31% in rest tremor [154]. In another standardized telephone survey among 47 persons with PD who used medical cannabis for at least 3 months, 73% reported moderate improvements in tremor and stiffness [156]. In these two surveys, participants preferred different types of delivery of cannabis, usually a teaspoon of fresh or dried leaves orally with a meal in the former survey while smoking cannabis flowers and leaves, average daily dose of 0.9 g in the latter. Neither of the surveys provided the percentage of THC in products used.

In an open-label study, a single administration of smoking cannabis (0.5 g cannabis, percentage of THC not provided) was found to significantly improve the motor Unified PD Rating Scale (UPDRS) scores as well as the tremor, rigidity, and bradykinesia subscale scores; a trend, but not significant, was also found for improvement of posture in the 22 participants that had an average of 7.3 years (range 2–18) since their diagnosis of PD. The effects after the single dose lasted 2–3 hours [172]. Benefit was also found in a similar study in which 20 persons with PD improved their UPDRS motor scores 30 minutes after smoking or vaporizing 1 g of cannabis (percentage of THC not provided) [173]. However, a case series study of five persons with PD with severe tremor did not exhibit similar results: none reported alleviation of tremor after a single dose of smoking cannabis (1 g cannabis, 2.9% THC by weight, about 29 mg of THC) [174].

Several other cannabis products, such as oral cannabidiol (CBD), CB_1 receptor antagonist, and cannabis extract (THC and CBD), were used in clinical trials but failed to find a significant beneficial effect on motor symptoms. An open-label study reported that oral CBD (powder form, approximately 99.9% pure, dissolved in corn oil), 400 mg/day for 4 weeks in six persons with PD and psychosis, did not improve their UPDRS motor scores [175]. In a randomized, double-blind, placebo-controlled study, using the same CBD product, the study team found similar results in UPDRS scores. Twenty-one PD participants received a placebo or CBD (75 or 300 mg/day) for 6 weeks. No improvement was noted in their UPDRS motor scores [176]. In these studies of CBD, the small sample size and the mild motor symptoms most of the participants exhibited may have decreased the power to detect significant change. Another randomized, double-blind, placebo-controlled study used a CB_1 receptor antagonist, rimonabant, at 20 mg/day for 16 days in four persons with a mean of 13 years of PD. Rimonabant has shown benefit in motor symptoms in animal models at low doses. However, in this clinical trial, rimonabant did not improve the UPDRS motor scores significantly [177]. The number of participants in this study was again small, diminishing the study's power to detect significant change. A Class I randomized, double-blind, placebo-controlled crossover study to provide high-quality evidence regarding the effects of a cannabis extract (Cannador, with capsules of 2.5 mg THC and 1.25 mg CBD) in PD was performed [178]. Seventeen persons with 14 years of PD received oral cannabis extract followed by a placebo, or vice versa, with each treatment phase lasting for 4 weeks. Though there was a slight trend for participants to feel that their tremor improved while on active treatment, the difference was not significant. The lack of treatment effect in this study may have been because of the low dosage of cannabis product. Based on body weight, the mean dose was 0.146 mg/kg/day of THC. For example, if a participant weighed 84 kg, he took 12.26 mg of THC and 6.13 mg of CBD per day. This dosage may have been too low to have an effect. The authors checked blood levels, which showed that most participants had a peak level of THC (within 2 hours of cannabis extract ingestion) ranging from 0.25 to 5.4 ng/ml. THC level of 5 ng/ml is considered to be enough to charge someone with driving under the influence (DUI) in Colorado. The wide variability in blood level was even present between participants taking the same dose of cannabis.

Besides the classic PD motor symptoms of tremor, slowness, stiffness, and balance impairment, many persons with PD develop disabling involuntary movements after taking levodopa, i.e., dyskinesia. Many animal studies have provided evidence of the therapeutic effects of cannabinoid agonists and antagonists on levodopa-induced dyskinesia. However, evidence from clinical trials is too minimal to verify these therapeutic effects. Only one randomized, controlled, crossover study has shown that the orally consumed synthetic CB_1 agonist, nabilone (0.03 mg/kg/day), significantly reduced dyskinesia, assessed using the Rush Dyskinesia Disability Scale in seven participants [179]. In this study, the percentage reduction in the total levodopa-induced dyskinesia with nabilone compared with placebo ranged from 3.8% to 62%, with two of the seven participants having improvements of 62% and 42% and the remaining five persons having less improvement (between 3.8% and 17.4%). This result is not sufficient to prove a benefit of nabilone on levodopa-induced dyskinesia. Two other randomized, controlled studies exhibited negative results, one using Cannador (2.5 mg THC and 1.25 mg CBD per capsule, up to 0.146 mg/kg/day of THC) [178] and the other using rimonabant, 20 mg/day [177], which was found to be effective on levodopa-induced dyskinesia in animal studies [158, 160, 165]. Persons in the rimonabant study were mid-stage PD and had a good response to levodopa. Further studies are needed to evaluate the effects of cannabis on levodopa-induced dyskinesia in a more diverse PD population and at different dosages.

Non-motor Symptoms In clinic and telephone surveys, participants reported using cannabis to treat their PD symptoms and found benefit in mood, sleep, pain, and quality of life [155, 156]. Similar findings were reported in clinical trials. A 4-week open-label study of oral CBD (powder form, approximately 99.9% pure, dissolved in corn oil) in six persons with PD and psychosis showed that psychosis significantly decreased with CBD (up to 400 mg/day) [175]. The same CBD product given orally at a dose of 75 or 300 mg/day reduced the frequency of REM sleep behavior disorder events among four persons with PD [180] and improved the Parkinson Disease Questionnaire-39 (PDQ-39) at 300 mg/day [176] in seven participants. Thirty-eight persons with PD had significant reduction of subjective pain scales (Visual Analog Scale and Present Pain Intensity Scale or Pain Rating Index) after a single dose of cannabis smoking (0.5 or 1 g of cannabis, percentage of THC not provided), eight had mild pain relief, and 12 reported greatly improved quality of sleep [172, 173]. Further, 14 participants had a significant decrease in their Visual Analog Scale scores and had a trend, but not significant reduction, in their Pain Rating Index after 10–40 weeks (median 14 weeks) of smoking or vaporizing 1 g of cannabis (percentage of THC also not provided) [173]. However, a randomized, controlled, crossover study produced a negative result: none of the scores (PDQ-39, McGill Pain score, and Visual Analogue Sleep Scale) showed a significant change after 4 weeks of cannabis (Cannador, 2.5 mg THC and 1.25 mg CBD per capsule, up to 0.146 mg/kg/day of THC) [178]. In this latter study, the low dose likely contributed to the lack of treatment effect.

These studies are summarized in Table 10.2, which also shows the effects of cannabis in other movement disorders. Tables 10.3, 10.4, and 10.5 show the cannabis products and/or related adverse events in movement disorder and cannabis studies. Table 10.6 shows the quality of these studies. The studies were graded according to the American Academy of Neurology classification scheme for therapeutic articles (Appendix).

Safety and Tolerability

Given the different forms of cannabis studied, it was generally well-tolerated but less so for those with THC or THC-related products. Dizziness, dry mouth, decreased concentration, somnolence, and cognitive complaints were the most common adverse events. Though no adverse events were reported, two participants withdrew when treated with nabilone, one due to vertigo and one due to postural hypotension. The grades of the adverse events were not reported. In the open-label observational study, six participants discontinued smoking cannabis (percentage of THC not provided) due to intolerability of severe adverse effects, including vomiting, dizziness, and psychosis. The survey studies also reported participants discontinued cannabis treatment due to adverse events, such as loss of consciousness, hallucinations, and postural instability. There were no serious adverse events attributed to cannabis. There were no adverse events reported in CBD-treated participants.

Huntington's Disease

Huntington's disease (HD) is a neurodegenerative disease, characterized by progressive motor, behavioral, and cognitive decline with a clinical course of 15–20 years. The prevalence of HD ranges from 1 to 7/1,000,000 in Asian populations and 10.6

to 13.7/100,000 in Western populations. Decreased quality of life is reported among persons with HD as well as by adults and children at risk of developing the disorder, and this may start as early as the time of diagnosis of the parent. There are currently no disease-modifying treatments, and symptomatic management is limited. Symptoms, such as bradykinesia, dystonia, rigidity, ataxia, gait disturbance, and cognitive impairment, do not respond well to current treatments.

HD is caused by an autosomal dominantly inherited CAG trinucleotide repeat expansion in the huntingtin (HTT) gene, resulting in a protein, huntingtin, containing an excess number of glutamine units. The huntingtin protein is toxic to brain cells, especially medium-sized spiny GABAergic neurons in striatum [181–183]. GABAergic striatal efferent neurons degenerate progressively in HD [184–187]. GABAergic neurons contain the major population of CB_1 receptors in the basal ganglia structures. CB_1 receptor binding was found decreased at all stages and in all regions of basal ganglia in HD [184].

HD is one of the MMP qualifying conditions in many states, but there is not sufficient evidence to show that cannabis or cannabinoids are effective for symptoms such as chorea and neuropsychiatric disorders [151]. Preclinical studies have validated the findings in postmortem HD human tissue [184] as well as in HD animal models that there is a progressive loss of CB_1 receptors in the substantia nigra, lateral globus pallidus, and putamen [188]. These findings support the theory that enhancing endocannabinoid activity might be a promising treatment, especially in the early or intermediate hyperkinetic phase of HD, before CB_1 receptors decrease significantly. Many drugs, such as CB_1 receptor agonists, endocannabinoid reuptake inhibitors, and metabolism inhibitors (also called indirect cannabinoid agonists, like fatty acid amide hydrolysis (FAAH)), have been used in HD animal and human studies; however, these studies exhibit inconsistent results.

Preclinical Research

Endocannabinoid reuptake inhibitors were suggested to be effective in reducing the hyperkinetic activity and attenuating the decreased inactivity in some 3-nitropropionic acid (3-NP)-lesioned HD rat models but failed to exhibit anti-hyperkinetic activity in other 3-NP-lesioned HD models and failed to protect against the death of GABAergic neurons in malonate-lesioned HD models [189–191]. The effects of anti-hyperkinesia sometimes were reversed when models were pre-treated with capsaicin, a vanilloid receptor (VR1) agonist, indicating a role for these receptors in the anti-hyperkinetic effects of endocannabinoid reuptake inhibitors [190]. VR1 agonists also displayed anti-hyperkinetic activity alone or combined with a CB_1 agonist [190, 192]. The CB_1 agonist alone only produced modest anti-hyperkinetic effects [190] or showed no effect on motor testing but significantly increased seizure events [193], indicating possible imbalances in excitatory/inhibitory neurotransmitter tone occurring in HD. Inhibiting the enzyme fatty acid amide hydrolase (FAAH) showed no efficacy in reducing hyperkinesia or altering the progressive deterioration of motor performance [190, 193].

Clinical Research

The effect of nabilone, a synthetic CB_1 receptor agonist that mimics THC, in two single persons with HD yielded contradictory results. One had marked increase in choreatic movement after taking a single dose, 1.5 mg [194], whereas the other had a significant reduction in chorea and irritability when taking 1 mg/day for 5 years [195]. A positive effect of oral nabilone on chorea was further confirmed in a randomized, double-blind, placebo-controlled, crossover study [196]. In this study, 1 or 2 mg/day for 5 weeks, there were significantly improved Unified Huntington's Disease Rating Scale (UHDRS) sub-scores for chorea, among the 37 persons with HD ($p = 0.009$), while there was no change in total motor score of the UHDRS ($p = 0.5$). However, two other randomized, controlled trials did not find therapeutic effects of CBD or Sativex® in HD. In the CBD study, which was a crossover design, 15 persons took 10 mg/kg/day (mean dose of 700 mg day) oral CBD (obtained from the US National Institute on Drug Abuse) for 6 weeks. There were no beneficial effects on chorea or other motor and cognitive tests [197]. However, while on CBD, plasma levels of CBD were in low nanogram concentrations, 11.2 ng/ml at week 6, so an insufficient CBD dose may have contributed to the negative results. In the other randomized, controlled study, Sativex® mouth spray solution (2.7 mg THC/2.5 mg CBD per spray), up to 12 spray/day, for 12 weeks, was tested in 25 persons with HD, with mean time from disease onset of 6.6 years [198]. No differences on motor, cognitive, behavioral, and functional scores were detected. Given the findings of progressive loss of CB_1 receptors in persons with HD and animal models and the hypothesis that cannabinoids have therapeutic potential in the earlier phases of the disease, it may be that the absence of clinical changes in this study was related to the use of the drug in too advanced state of the disease progression [198] but could also be due to the dose being too low.

Safety and Tolerability

CBD, which may have been a very low dose given the mg/ml plasma levels, had no associated adverse events. Nabilone was well tolerated, except one treatment-related serious adverse event: one person taking concomitant temazepam experienced severe sedation and withdrew from the study. Drowsiness and forgetfulness were the most frequently reported adverse events during the nabilone administration period. Common adverse events for Sativex® included dizziness, disturbance in attention, anxiety, and sleepiness.

Dystonia

Dystonia is a relatively common movement disorder that may be primary (idiopathic) or occur as part of another disorder and is characterized by sustained or intermittent muscle contractions causing abnormal, often repetitive, movements, postures, or both [199]. The disorder may involve one or multiple body regions, resulting in disability and decreased quality of life [200]. There is no satisfying medication. Neuroimaging and electrophysiologic studies suggested that dystonia is associated with abnormal activity in the basal ganglia, especially the globus pallidus [201–204], where CB_1 receptors are highly expressed. This indicates potential anti-dystonic effects of CB_1 receptor agonists and antagonists.

Preclinical Research

Higher doses of CB_1 receptor agonists, like (+)-WIN55.212-2 at 5 or 10 mg/kg, significantly reduced dystonia; however, these agonists also induced severe central adverse events, including the reduction of spontaneous motor activity, catalepsy, jumping, and hypothermia, in mutant dystonic hamsters [205, 206]. Co-administration of individually ineffective doses of CB_1 receptor agonists and diazepam resulted in reduced dystonia without causing catalepsy or depression of spontaneous locomotion. The anti-dystonic and cataleptic effects of (+)-WIN55,212-2 were completely blocked by pre-treatment with rimonabant (CB_1 receptor antagonist). The authors also found that CBD, which has low affinity to cannabinoid receptors, did not exert any beneficial effects on dystonia at doses of 50, 100, and 150 mg/kg. These findings indicate the beneficial effects of (+)-WIN55,212-2 might be selectively mediated by the activation of CB_1 receptors. It was hypothesized that CB_1 receptor agonists, which are located presynaptically on GABA terminals within the internal globus pallidus (GPi), reduce GABA reuptake, enhance the responsiveness of GABA receptors, or modulate GABA release, thereby managing dystonic symptoms [206–208].

Clinical Research

Interestingly, though CBD was not effective on dystonia in animal models, anecdotal reports and small uncontrolled clinical trials have reported that oral CBD (in capsules, 100–600 mg/day) had beneficial effects [209]. Some persons with coexisting parkinsonian features experienced exacerbated hypokinesia and resting tremor [209]. Isolated cases also have shown improvements in dystonia through self-medicated smoking or inhaling 3–4 g/day of cannabis [210, 211]. However, this was not confirmed in two small double-blind, randomized, placebo-controlled, cross-over studies [207, 208]. Unlike the CB_1 receptor agonist in animal studies, nabilone, another synthetic cannabinoid receptor agonist, was not beneficial in dystonia when administered at a single dose of 0.03 mg/kg among 15 persons with primary dystonia. Two persons were withdrawn from the study, one due to postural hypotension the other to marked sedation [207]. Nabilone was also used in 0.03 mg/kg doses in both PD animal studies and clinical trials, but in those studies was found to significantly reduce levodopa-induced dyskinesia [169, 179]. It was postulated that stimulation of the CB_1 receptors with a higher dose of nabilone or a different CB_1 receptor agonist might have significant beneficial effects in dystonia. Adverse events did occur at high doses of (+)-WIN55,212-2 in animal studies, and the adverse effects induced by CBD and nabilone in clinical trials limit their therapeutic use.

Without finding significant effects of nabilone among primary dystonia persons, the same author with a different study team in Toronto Western Hospital movement disorders center conducted another double-blind, randomized, placebo-controlled, crossover study using dronabinol (Marinol®, synthetic THC). Doses of dronabinol consist of 2.5 mg of THC, and the new study sought to determine the efficacy of synthetic THC in cervical dystonia. Nine participants were randomized to dronabinol (15 mg/day of THC) and a placebo in an 8-week crossover trial with 3 weeks for each treatment period. Two participants withdrew from the study: one due to adverse effects and the other was lost to follow-up. Dronabinol was ineffective in reducing cervical dystonia symptoms [208]. The dose used in the dronabinol study, 15 mg/day of THC, which was 0.2 mg/kg/day if a person weighed 75 kg, was about five times higher than that in the nabilone study (0.03 mg/kg) but still lower than that used in animal studies (5 or 10 mg/kg) [205, 206]. These two well-designed studies indicated that synthetic THC, at low dose, may not be useful in the treatment of dystonia.

Safety and Tolerability

In animal studies, high doses of CB_1 receptor agonists induced severe central adverse events, such as reduction of spontaneous motor activity, catalepsy, jumping, and hypothermia in mutant dystonic hamsters. Thus caution is needed for human studies. In clinical trials, adverse events were reported in most of the participants using smoked cannabis (THC concentration not provided), oral CBD at 600 mg/day, or synthetic THC. The common adverse events, including postural hypotension, sedation, dry mouth, somnolence, lightheadedness, blurred vision, bitter taste, dizziness, and palpitations, were mild and resolved on discontinuing or decreasing the drug. There were no serious adverse events, but a few persons withdrew due to intolerability, i.e., insomnia, a feeling of heart racing, postural hypotension, and sedation.

Tics and Tourette Syndrome

Tourette syndrome (TS) is a developmental neuropsychiatric disorder characterized by chronic motor and phonic tics with a universal prevalence of 0.52% [212]. Tics are the hallmark of TS; are typically preceded by an urge to move, i.e., "premonitory urge"; and tend to develop between 2 and 15 years of age, peak during adolescence, and diminish greatly or resolve in the early 20s. TS also has comorbid features such as attention-deficit hyperactivity disorder, obsessive-compulsive disorder, and other behavioral, mood, and sleep disorders. An interaction between social and environmental factors and multiple genetic factors is thought to be the cause. The only FDA-approved drugs for TS are dopamine receptor blockers. These medications reduce tics, but often not the other symptoms, and are poorly tolerated [213].

There is no direct preclinical evidence showing the role of the endocannabinoid system in the pathology or treatment of TS. Results from preclinical and clinical studies on other movement disorders indicate the possible involvement of the CB_1 receptor system in the pathophysiology of TS through the modulation of dopaminergic neurotransmission. This involvement indicates a potential beneficial effect of CB_1 receptor agonists in TS. Based on shared symptoms in these movement disorder studies, smoking marijuana and orally consuming THC have been tried by persons with TS and researchers.

Case reports have shown the successful administration of cannabis (smoked or vaporized cannabis, oral THC, Sativex®) and a synthetic cannabinoid (Dronabinol) in reducing motor and verbal tics as well as associated behavioral disorders among minor and adult persons with TS [214–223]. Two surveys [224, 225] and one retrospective study [226] also suggested beneficial effects of cannabis. One survey of 64 persons with TS reported that 17 (27%) had used cannabis (percentage of THC not provided) and 14 (82%) experienced a reduction or complete remission of tics. Of these 14, 9 had moderate or marked reduction, 4 had complete remission of tics, and 1 only had improvement of premonitory urges. The other survey was done via a telephone interview consisting of 42 persons with TS who had at least 1 year of medical cannabis treatment. Participants reported reduction in tic severity, better sleep, and improved mood as positive effects of medical cannabis (also no percentage of THC provided). Only four (9.5%) had no improvements with their symptoms.

In the retrospective study [226], with the addition of clinical chart review, 19 persons with TS who used cannabis regularly for at least 2 years were interviewed by psychiatrists using standardized questionnaires regarding their cannabis use (no data available on ratio of THC to CBD). There was an average of 60% reduction in the Yale Global Tic Severity Scale – total tic scores and 18 of the 19 participants (94.7%) were rated as "very much improved" or "much improved" on the Clinical Global Impression Improvement scale by clinicians.

Beneficial effects of oral THC were also suggested in two small randomized, double-blind, placebo-controlled trials [227, 228]. One was a crossover study with 12 persons treated with a single dose of 5.0, 7.5, or 10.0 mg of THC. Three to four hours after administration, participants had statistically significantly improvement in tics on the self-rating scale (Tourette syndrome symptom list) with significant or trending-toward-significant improvement in the examiner rating scale, the Tourette's Syndrome Global Scale. The other randomized, controlled trial was a 6-week parallel study in which seven participants took up to 10 mg/day of oral THC and ten received placebo. The examiner and patient ratings as well as the videotape-based rating scale showed a significant or a trending-toward-significant reduction in tics. These results support reports of benefit of THC from surveys and case reports. However, given the limitations of these studies, such as small sample size, selection bias, short-term treatment, and large number of items tested, the AAN evidence-based systematic review, Cochrane review, and National Academy of Sciences have determined that there is limited to insufficient evidence to support or refute the use of THC in TS [91, 151, 229].

Over the past few years, CBD has been mixed with THC in medications, such as nabiximols (Sativex®, oromucosal spray, 2.7 mg of THC, and 2.5 mg of CBD), in treating TS, but all results thus far come from anecdotal reports. Larger, well-designed, and controlled studies are needed to verify the effects of THC, CBD, and mixtures of THC and CBD in TS.

Safety and Tolerability

The studies in TS mainly involved THC and THC-related compounds; only very low doses of CBD were given in the Sativex® product; thus the adverse events were likely due to THC. Adverse events, mostly mild, occurred in many participants; no serious adverse events were reported. One person stopped oral THC due to anxiety and restlessness. One person in the retrospective study discontinued cannabis due to experiencing severe irritability. Common adverse events included anxiety, ataxia, cognitive decline, confusion, decreased concentration, decreased motivation, dry eyes, dry mouth, euphoria, fatigue, feeling of a "high," galactorrhea, hallucination, headache, hot flush, increased appetite, increased tics, irritability, nausea, psychosis, sensitivity to noise or light, trembling, and wheezing. Most of the adverse events were transient and resolved after stopping the drug.

Only a few persons under the age of 18, with TS, have reported using cannabis, so the safety and tolerability of cannabis have not been established among minors with TS. The effects of medical cannabis on brain structure or function among adolescents are not clear. The endocannabinoid system plays an important role in neurodevelopment, by being involved in synaptic pruning and white matter development during prenatal, post-natal, and adolescence periods and even into early adulthood. Adolescence is a period of vulnerability to cannabis exposure which might disrupt the endocannabinoid system, alter the trajectory of brain development, and cause persistent, long-term alterations in brain structure and brain function. Clinical studies have found that in adolescents, chronic or heavy recreational cannabis use can impair memory, attention, decision-making, and inhibitory control in brain functions and caused abnormalities in hippocampal volume and gray matter density in brain structure [230–232].

Other Movement Disorders

Some persons with other movement disorders, such as essential tremor, restless legs syndrome, and rapid eye movement (REM) sleep behavior disorder, also used medical cannabis to treat their symptoms. However, these disorders have not been listed as qualifying medical marijuana conditions. There have been no data reported from controlled clinical trials. One case report suggested handwriting in essential tremor might be improved with the administration of oral THC [233]. A randomized, double-blind, placebo-controlled crossover trial is currently being conducted at the University of California, San Diego, to evaluate the safety and efficacy of a combined oral formulation of THC and CBD in essential tremor (https://clinicaltrials.gov/ct2/show/NCT03805750?term=cannabis&cond=Essential+Tremor&rank=1). The effects of cannabis on restless legs syndrome was reported in six persons, who reported total relief as well as improvements of sleep quality after smoking cannabis or sublingual administration of CBD [234]. A case series reported four persons with PD and REM sleep behavior disorder who were treated with oral CBD for 6 weeks. Three of them, 75 mg/day, had total relief of REM sleep behavior disorder during the treatment period. One participant on 300 mg/day reported a reduction of episodes from two to four times to once a week [180]. Lacking evidences from controlled clinical trials, the safety and efficacy of cannabis in these movement disorders are unclear.

Discussion

This review presents the current preclinical and clinical evidence for the effects of cannabis and cannabis-related products in movement disorders. To date, there is a paucity of high-quality studies and a large amount of anecdotal reports. While there are some randomized, controlled trials, there are methodological issues, for example, the total number of participants is small. Efficacy has not been established in any movement disorder, and the studies bring up concerns regarding tolerability and safety.

The PD literature describes persons discontinuing study drugs, mainly THC, due to adverse effects such as loss of consciousness, dizziness, vomiting, psychosis, hallucinations, postural instability, and sedation. Some studies focused on reports from those who completed the study but not on those who dropped out due to adverse events. Dizziness was one of the most common adverse effects of cannabinoids. Dizziness, falls, and cognition are common concerns posed by the elderly. The AAN reports a potential adverse effect of taking cannabis products to be lightheadedness associated with loss of balance and falls in healthy controls (https://www.aan.com/Guidelines/home/GetGuidelineContent/650). Further, postural instability, as an adverse event, was reported in some persons with PD or HD. Also of concern, cognitive function, such as forgetfulness, poor concentration, or short-term amnesia, was subjectively reported to decline among persons with PD, HD, and Tourette syndrome when using cannabis.

Liver function is another safety issue to consider. Epidiolex®, a highly purified form of CBD, has been associated with liver enzyme changes in severe forms of epilepsy, mostly in pediatric populations [235]. Researchers from the University of Arkansas for Medical Sciences reported that CBD may be harmful to the liver: mice given relatively high doses showed signs of liver damage, possibly of a cholestatic nature, within 24 hours of administration [236]. The data from the University of Alabama at Birmingham (UAB) CBD open-label compassionate-use study showed a higher, but still within normal range level of aspartate aminotransferase (AST) and alanine aminotransferase (ALT) in participants taking concomitant Epidiolex® and valproate compared to those not taking valproate ($p = 0.026$ for ALT, $p = 0.003$ for AST). This indicated a potential effect of the combination of valproate and CBD on liver function or an increased effect of CBD on the negative effects of valproate on liver functions [237]. More research in humans on the effects of cannabis, especially CBD and especially in vulnerable populations, on liver function is needed.

There are a number of reasons that, as yet, there is not definitive information regarding the efficacy and safety of cannabis use in movement disorders despite the large amount of research that has been accomplished. These include the complexity of cannabis, different modes of administration, potency variability, and host factors. Further, there are considerable barriers to research, at least in the United States.

A major issue is that cannabis is not one drug – it is a plant that is composed of hundreds of chemicals. Studies report effects of cannabis plant material, extracted mixtures of major and minor components of cannabis plants, and synthetic products that mimic cannabis components, e.g., THC or CBD, or target endocannabinoid receptors. For example, in HD all the reports studied THC or a THC-related study drug; only one included CBD but at very low dose. Further, the modes of administration, e.g., smoked vs. oral, vary in studies and can cause persons to have immediate, intense (smoked) or gradual, and subtle or no (oral) effects. In addition, there are a number of host factors to consider.

Host factors that play a role in study outcomes include the participants' stage and characteristics of the disease, age, renal and liver function, concomitant medications, and comorbidities [238]. For example, specific cannabis-related products may have benefits in persons with early-stage but not late-stage disease and perhaps benefits in anxiety but not tremor. Also, the aged brain is more vulnerable to psychoactive drugs, i.e., THC, so the same dose may be beneficial in young persons but toxic in the elderly [239]. Any time there are comorbidities being treated with multiple medicines, there is a higher risk of drug interactions. Cannabis has been found to inhibit hepatic drug metabolism and decrease activities of p-glycoprotein and other drug transporters [240]. For example, CBD is metabolized via the CYP450 enzymes 2C19 and 3A4 and is an inhibitor of these isoenzymes. As such, efficacy of medications metabolized in similar pathways could be affected. Cannabis products are documented to interact with alcohol, anticoagulants, antiplatelet drugs, CNS depressants, protease inhibitors, and selective serotonin reuptake inhibitors [131, 239]. It is therefore important to inform people of possible interactions their current medications may have when taken with cannabis.

Another important issue to consider is the difficulty of accomplishing relevant research. Much of cannabis research to date has been done outside of the United States. While the National Institutes of Health funds cannabis research, US investigators face tough regulatory barriers, especially regarding obtaining relevant study drugs. While many good quality cannabis products are available in the US retail market, at the present time, investigators are limited to using products approved by agencies of the federal government. The results of research using cannabis products produced locally would be more reflective of the experience persons with movement disorders would have from products they are actually using.

CBD products, including CBD cannabis extract and hemp CBD, are becoming more popular in the United States, Canada, and European countries. Hemp CBD products, defined in the United States as having less than 0.3% THC, can be found easily online and at local markets, while cannabis products with CBD concentrations higher than THC are obtained at dispensaries. Hemp products are not FDA regulated, may have inaccurate labelling of CBD or THC contents, and may contain significant levels of THC. While these studies in movement disorders have not produced definitive guidelines for clinicians, they and others have started to provide information regarding tolerability and dosing. Given the popularity of CBD, this information is useful.

Conclusions

While the recreational and medical legalization of cannabis and cannabis products spreads globally, it is important for clinicians to understand the benefits and safety of using cannabis. Unfortunately, research to date has not provided adequate information to guide clinicians. There are not enough good quality data to determine that any forms of cannabis are effective in movement disorders. The strongest evidence of therapeutic benefit is that THC may reduce tics, but this evidence is relatively weak given that studies had small numbers of participants, short duration, and product integrity questions. Further, the majority of persons with problematic tics are minors with Tourette syndrome, and the effects of cannabis on the developing brain are not adequately studied.

The research data does suggest that THC may be poorly tolerated among persons with PD, especially when smoked, and that overall CBD has less adverse effects in the populations studied. More toxicity from cannabis products may occur with increasing dosage as well as host factors such as older age, stage and symptoms of their disease, relevant concomitant medications, and others.

There are a variety of cannabis products on the market. Patients with movement disorders should talk with their doctors before using cannabis since it interacts with many other medications and supplements. Smoking dispensary cannabis or using vape cartridges is not a good health choice, particularly in light of recent pulmonary illnesses, including deaths, that have been reported to be related to dispensary marijuana products. As of August 27, 2019, 215 possible cases of severe pulmonary diseases associated with the use of e-cigarettes containing cannabinoid products such as THC or CBD have been reported from 25 states, according to the federal Centers for Disease Control and Prevention (CDC). The detailed information and recommendations for clinicians, public health officials, and the public can be found on the website of CDC (https://emergency.cdc.gov/han/han00421.asp?fbclid=

IwAR2m9K_c211LVjp54MO-fs1bAJls-GJqK96lfso-ghyFoH-HjepnFBezrrU) and two other resources (https://www.washingtonpost.com/health/2019/09/05/contaminant-found-vaping-products-linked-deadly-lung-illnesses-state-federal-labs-show/; https://abcnews.go.com/Health/wireStory/oregon-vape-death-patient-thc-device-dispensary-65394889?fbclid=IwAR0FcmdT9bdey8EcfMqMWwf-tZzkZQuu-DEXQHw-7e1Xrx3yBnC2-8-WKKXw). Patients also need to discuss the routes of cannabis administration and dosing with their doctors. Providers may consult recommendations and evidence-based resources from AAN [91] and National Academies of Sciences [151].

Cannabinoids in Neurosurgery

E. Lee Nelson, Sharad Rajpal, Alan T. Villavicencio, Andrew Bauer, and Sigita Burneikiene

It has been almost 50 years since marijuana has been classified by the Department of Health and Human Services as a schedule 1 substance in the United States based on "a considerable void in our knowledge." Five decades later, the same void remains pertaining to its use in neurosurgery patients. Recently, research into cannabinoids expanded exponentially, with basic science advancing more rapidly than clinical applications.

There is some evidence suggesting that cannabis or cannabinoids may be effective as an adjunctive treatment for conditions including refractory epilepsy [245], controlling pain and spasticity symptoms of multiple sclerosis [91, 246, 247], or treatment of chronic non-cancer pain [111, 248]. Nevertheless, the list of cannabinoids' negative consequences [249, 250], particularly recreational marijuana, is long, and an abbreviated list as it relates to the central nervous system is shown in Table 10.7.

Table 10.7 Neurological consequences of recreational marijuana

Impaired short-term memory
Impaired motor coordination
Cognitive impairment
Structural changes in the brain including white matter degradation and demyelination
Reductions in left frontal fractional anisotropy (FA)
Increased apparent diffusion coefficients in the right genu of the corpus callosum
Impaired axonal connectivity of the right fornix, splenium, and commissural fibers
Impaired prefrontal cortical activity in adolescents and reduced processing efficiency during novel working memory tasks
Increased risk of motor vehicle accidents

As we review the published literature for the treatment of neurosurgical conditions, we must keep in mind that marijuana itself already has such a long list of health-related warnings; we should not underestimate its power to harm as we look for its ability to heal. We plan to look at cannabinoids for the treatment of chronic low back and radicular pain, malignant gliomas, traumatic spinal cord and brain injury, and cerebrovascular disease.

Chronic Low Back and Radicular Pain

Chronic pain is one of the primary indications reported by medical cannabis users [248, 251, 252]. Cannabinoids act through CB1- and CB2-specific mechanisms to suppress pain on spinal, central, and peripheral levels [253, 254] along with anti-inflammatory effects [255]. Although chronic pain is one of the conditions that have substantial [248] and sometimes conflicting evidence of efficacy [256], according to the National Academies of Sciences Engineering and Medicine report, the conclusive evidence was mostly for neuropathic and cancer-related pain [257].

In an extensive systematic review and meta-analysis, Whiting et al. [111] identified a total of 28 randomized and placebo-controlled trials that evaluated different types of synthetic and plant-derived cannabinoids for the treatment of chronic pain. The authors concluded that moderate-quality evidence is available to support the use of cannabinoids in chronic pain for a modest reduction in pain (37% vs. 31%; OR 1.41, 95% CI 0.99–2.00) and a modest average reduction in pain scores (−0.46, 95% CI −0.80 to −0.11) compared with placebo. Although there were no apparent differences for pain reduction between the reported conditions, the majority of these studies evaluated neuropathic and cancer pain (central, peripheral, or not specified), but none of them included studies looking at pain associated with degenerative spine disease. Cannabinoids were associated with an increased risk of adverse events.

A more recent systematic review published in 2018 by Stockings et al. examined the effectiveness of cannabinoids in chronic non-cancer pain patients and reached a similar conclusion [258]. This study included a total of 47 randomized controlled trials and 57 observational studies and analyzed them independently. Again, the authors noted that the majority of the studies enrolled patients with neuropathic and multiple sclerosis-related pain and only a very few studies included patients with neck and low back pain conditions. The authors reported a modest impact on pain outcomes for cannabinoids, with 29% of patients reporting a 30% reduction in pain compared with 25.9% in the placebo group. The authors noted that in this review, the number of patients required to treat to benefit was high at 24, while the number of patients needed to harm was 6 and they felt like cannabinoids were unlikely to be a highly effective medication for the treatment of chronic non-cancer pain. The most significant reduction in pain intensity was reported for short-term follow-up studies with a smaller or non-significant reduction noted in longer-term studies.

A prospective, open-label study included 39 (23.8%) patients suffering from radicular low back pain among a mixed group of patients ($n = 206$) with various chronic pain conditions and symptoms lasting for longer than 3 months who had a proper trial with two first- and second-line analgesic drugs [259]. The majority of the patients smoked cannabis cigarettes, and the mean monthly dose was 43.2 (±17) g. At the mean follow-up time of 7 months, the pain symptom score improved in 65.9% and worsened in 26.1% of all participants. There was also a statistically significant improvement in various quality of life domains, including sleep. Forty-four percent of patients on opioid therapy discontinued opioid treatment, or the median dose decreased from 60 to 45 mg for those who continued using opioids, but this reduction was not statistically significant. The upper and lower body physical disability scores did not change significantly, which may have suggested that the perception of pain was affected rather than objectively assessed clinical outcomes. There were no differences in the pain symptom score improvement between neuropathic and non-neuropathic pain patients. Eleven of 206 (5.3%) patients discontinued treatment due to side effects. This study was limited by the lack of a control group and its open-label design. We cannot draw any conclusions about smoking cannabis for the radicular low back pain patient from this study because they comprised a small subset of the cohort and the subgroup analysis was not available.

Yassin et al. [260] reported a total of 46 patients who were diagnosed with sciatica due to spinal stenosis, disc herniation, or failed back surgery syndrome underwent at least 12 months of treatment and failed at least two narcotic drugs. The patients were offered treatment with medical cannabis (MCT) at 20 g per month and four dosages per day, but the exact content of tetrahydrocannabinol (THC) was not controlled. After 12 months, the patients reported statistically significant improvement on the Brief Pain Inventory, VAS, and SF-12 scales, along with an active range of motion improvement. A total of 27 out of 46 (59%) patients stopped opiate therapy, and 20 out of 34 (59%) returned to work. These were remarkable results, and one strong point of this study was a longer-term follow-up compared with the median follow-up of 8 weeks reported for the majority of the studies investigating the effectiveness of cannabinoids for chronic pain patients. There is also no data on the actual dosage of THC delivered to these patients. The study, however, is limited by the fact that it was not randomized and not controlled, and therefore, it is difficult to draw conclusions about the effectiveness of MCT.

Mondello et al. [261] reported a total of 11 patients with refractory failed back surgery syndrome who were prescribed a daily mean dose of 68.5 (range, 50–100) mg consisting of THC (oleic suspension 19%) and CBD (<1%) without discontinuing spinal cord stimulation therapy. All other oral analgesic therapies were discontinued 2 months prior to the enrollment. At the baseline, the mean pain rating score was 8.15 ± 0.98, which was reduced to 4.72 ± 0.9 at the 12-month follow-up. The patients also reported a statistically significant improvement in all Brief Pain Inventory items, including general activities, mood, walking abilities, normal work, sleep and enjoyment of life, and relations with other people. There were no reports of serious adverse events or the need to discontinue therapy. The study lacked a control group and the sample size was small.

A single-center, placebo-controlled, double-blind pilot study enrolled a total of 30 patients with chronic and therapy-resistant pain related to a pathologic status of the skeletal and locomotor system [262]. The crossover design was employed, and the subjects received either nabilone (oral daily dose of 0.25–1.0 mg) or placebo for 4 weeks with a 5-week washout period followed by 16 weeks with free choice of study drugs. The authors reported significantly lower current and average spinal pain intensity and the quality of life improvement with nabilone. The number of participants who favored nabilone was four times higher than those who preferred the placebo.

Although clinical evidence of cannabis efficacy for chronic radicular pain management is lacking, so does the evidence that opioids are effective for this indication. Opioids are the most frequently prescribed medication, but the effectiveness for chronic low back pain management is based on short-term, uncontrolled, or population-based studies [263–266].

Cannabinoid Use and Its Impact on Perioperative or Trauma Pain

Cannabinoids may offer some benefit in the treatment of pain, but preoperative cannabinoid use can result in sleep disturbance and higher postoperative pain scores in patients undergoing surgery. In Liu et al. study of 3793 patients undergoing major orthopedic surgery, including spinal fusion surgery, 155 patients were found to be on cannabinoids prior to surgery. They were younger, tended to be male, were more likely to need spine surgery, and were more likely to be on opioids preoperatively. After propensity matching the cannabinoid users against the non-cannabinoid users, they achieved a well-matched cohort (age, type of surgery, gender, preoperative opioid use, depression, anxiety, administration of regional analgesia). They found cannabinoid users had a higher intensity of pain postoperatively and more sleep disturbance postoperatively [267]. This data appears consistent with the report by Salottolo et al. (2018) that looked at pain scores following traumatic injuries in marijuana users and found that they had statistically significant higher pain scores than non-marijuana users. In addition, they found that chronic marijuana use in these patients resulted in a much higher opioid consumption following injury than in the episodic or non-marijuana user [268].

In addition to these studies that demonstrate some of the challenges in pain management that might be seen in marijuana users, Twardowski et al. reports that marijuana users require significant more sedation for endoscopic procedures than non-users [269]. This is something that has been at least anecdotally reported by many anesthesiologists.

In summary, while there is evidence that cannabinoids may offer some reduction of pain for those who are suffering from chronic neuropathic and cancer-related pain, there is also evidence of increased adverse events when using cannabinoids, and understanding the true "costs" of cannabinoids in achieving this benefit will require more studies. In addition, this reduction of pain intensity appears to be more apparent over a short term rather than a sustained benefit. There are few clinical trials evaluating back pain, and these suffer from major methodological limitations, including variations in the substances and doses administered, routes of administration, schedules, and inclusion of various pain conditions. None of the studies published so far used phenotypic profiling that differentiates the underlying pathophysiological mechanisms and identifies personalized treatment approaches. In addition, there has not yet been a study looking at the effectiveness of cannabinoids in the treatment of acute back or radicular pain. It is important to point out that these studies were done with products that generally are unavailable in the United States or with synthetic cannabinoids. These findings do not apply to dispensary cannabis.

Alternative to Opioids

Since the implementation of marijuana laws in the United States, there may have been a reduction in the prescription of conventional pain medications, including opioids [270–272]. Initially, it was also thought that the introduction of medical cannabis laws in 1999 was associated with a reduction in opioid overdose mortality [273]; however, a more recent paper presented contradictory results documenting a 23% increase in mortality rates [274].

Acting through different pharmacological mechanisms, cannabinoids synergistically interact with the opioid system, so it may be possible to reduce the doses of each agent, potentially resulting in reduced side effects [275]. As rates of opioid addiction have risen to alarming levels, this could be a reasonable alternative worth considering. Still, the clinical studies investigating the risk and benefits of cannabinoids as a replacement or partial substitution therapy are currently lacking. Besides the study that was previously described [259], we were able to locate another retrospective survey study of 244 subjects who used medical cannabis for chronic pain [272]. Sixty-four percent of patients reported a decrease in opioid use, and 45% of patients reported improved quality of life. A significant correlation (R − 0.37; $p = 0.002$) between the reduction of side effects and opioid use decrease was also noted. Unfortunately, this was a cross-sectional study that simply asked medical cannabis users about their habits and is subject to selection bias that likely undermines any significant conclusions from this study.

Of note, European Pain Federation, based on the panel expert opinion, cautions against prescribing cannabis with high doses of opioids and benzodiazepines [276], and the College of Family Physicians of Canada recommends pharmaceutically developed products instead of sold at dispensaries for neuropathic and cancer pain, but not as first- and second-line therapy [277].

No clinical trials have looked at using cannabis as a treatment for opioid addiction. Two studies have been published that suggest the opposite. In the *Journal of Addiction Medicine* 2018 study [278], "medical cannabis use was positively associated with greater use and misuse of prescription opioids." Another study in the *American Journal of Psychiatry* found that cannabis use increased the risk of developing nonmedical prescription opioid use and opioid use disorder [279]. There is, therefore, no high-quality data to suggest that cannabinoids are truly an alternative to opioids, and further controlled studies are needed.

Malignant Gliomas

In 2014, Rocha et al. [280] performed a systematic review of the cannabinoid therapy for gliomas and its antitumor effects. Reduction in tumor size and antiangiogenic and antimetastatic effects along with apoptotic death and cell cycle arrest through cannabinoid system were the most frequently described mechanisms in vivo and/or in vitro studies. Among the potential treatment strategies, such substances as ajulemic acid, CBD, JWH-133, endogenous cannabinoid anandamide, ceramide, and especially CBD/THC combinations were listed.

Despite the reported increasing evidence of cannabinoids' anticancer properties in preclinical research, clinical studies have yet to demonstrate any effect on survival rates. Some cancer patients may benefit from cannabis as a palliative treatment to relieve pain, lack of appetite, nausea symptoms, or sleep problems [281]. Among a total of 2970 cancer patients that were studied, 126 patients were diagnosed with CNS cancer, and once the patients who died or discontinued the treatment were excluded, 59 (67.8%) remaining patients reported at least moderate or significant improvement in their condition without serious side effects.

The first human pilot study was performed by Guzman et al. [282] and enrolled nine patients diagnosed with glioblastoma multiforme who failed standard therapy (surgery, external beam radiotherapy] and had clear tumor progression. These patients received THC (>96.5%), which was administered intracranially into the recurrent tumor resection cavity. The age of patients varied from 35 to 69 years and all had Karnofsky scores $\geq$70. There was no control group for this study and patients received diverse doses of THC. Although a temporary reduction of tumor proliferation was observed in three of the five patients who received more than one treatment cycle, the median survival time from the resection of tumor relapse was 24 weeks (range, 15–33), which is comparable to the survival rates using standard treatment strategies for recurrent glioblastoma [283].

A few other pilot studies were performed in patients with recurrent glioblastoma [284]. An open-label phase I study (safety and tolerability) enrolled a total of six patients who received temozolomide (TMZ) and a combination of THC and CBD (2.5:2.7 mg/mL per 100 μL oromucosal spray). This was followed by the phase II study (efficacy, safety, pharmacokinetics), which enrolled 21 patients who were treated with TMZ and randomized to receive either THC/CBD oromucosal spray ($n = 12$) or placebo ($n = 9$). Overall median survival and survival at 1 year was 662 and 369 days compared with 83% and 44% ($p = 0.042$) for the investigational and placebo arms, respectively. Severe treatment-emergent adverse events were reported in 50% of the investigational group patients compared with 44% mostly moderate events in the placebo group. Of note, the reported effective THC and CBD doses were several times higher and often supraphysiological (up to 25 mg/kg THC) in the preclinical studies [280]. This is a small pilot study sponsored by the company providing the THC/CBD drug (Sativex, GW Pharmaceuticals, Cambridge, UK), and while the results are very promising, they need to be confirmed with a more extensive study, preferably with genotypically classified tumors.

Furthermore, the putative antitumor effects seem to fall short of preventing brain tumor development [285]. A longitudinal managed-care cohort study enrolled 133,881 participants and followed them for up to 21 (mean 13.2 ± 6.7) years. A total of 130 (0.1%) subjects developed primary adult-onset gliomas. Individuals who smoked marijuana at least once per month had a modestly increased risk (2.8-fold; 95% CI 1.3–6.2) to develop gliomas compared to non-users. A marginal statistical significance (OR = 2.8; $p = 0.07$) to develop astrocytoma was also found in children who had gestational exposure to marijuana [286].

Cannabinoids may have anticancer properties for the tumors themselves, but they are also being promoted as having anti-inflammatory, immune-modulating abilities that could work counter to their anticancer properties. Further studies will be needed to determine whether they will become useful in the treatment of gliomas or other cancers of the nervous system. In the case of gliomas specifically, we would need to know whether they can shift the Kaplan-Meier curve to the right, change its slope, or even more importantly extend the area under the tail of the curve indefinitely.

Spinal Cord Injury

The endocannabinoid system is substantially upregulated in the spinal cord after injury by overproduction of anandamide and 2-arachidonoylglycerol, which are thought to be related protective mechanisms limiting secondary damage and improving functional outcomes. Prevention of the progressive demyelination, normalization of astrocyte reactivity and inhibition of glial scar formation, or controlling lymphocyte infiltration and chronic inflammation were attempted in experimental studies [287].

As alternative therapies are being sought to alleviate symptoms related to spinal cord injury (SCI), there are a limited number of publications on clinical applications for pain and spasticity. Wilsey et al. [288] performed a double-blind crossover study which enrolled a total of 42 patients with injury ($n = 29$) (90% of whom were either previous or current cannabis users) or disease of the spinal cord and randomized to the placebo, 2.9% THC, or 6.7% THC arms. The authors reported a better risk-benefit ratio of the lower dose, although the effectiveness of the two active treatments did not significantly differ ($p = 0.06$). After controlling for psychoactive and subjective effects, a significant pain reduction was reported ($p < 0.0004$) in 45%, 70%, and 88% of patients in the placebo, 2.9% THC, and 6.7% THC arms, respectively, reported at least 30% reduction in pain intensity. One of the major limitations of this study was that it was an 8-hour human laboratory experiment lasting 120 days.

A small randomized, double-blind, crossover pilot study ($n = 5$) was published by Rintala et al. [289]. The authors compared dronabinol with diphenhydramine as an active control and did not find that dronabinol was more effective in relieving chronic neuropathic pain below the injury level.

Cardenas and Jensen [290] surveyed a total of 117 SCI patients suffering from chronic pain. The pain relief provided by opioids (mean 6.27 ± 3.05 on the 0–10 pain relief scale) was comparable to pain relief provided by marijuana (6.62 ± 2.54). The authors also noted that the patients were less likely to continue the treatment with opioids.

Spasticity is another common side effect of SCI that cannot always be managed effectively with the currently available drugs. Although the application of cannabinoids was extensively studied in patients with multiple sclerosis [111, 247], the origin of spasticity differs, and these results cannot be directly applied to SCI patients. Hagenbach et al. [291] enrolled a total of 25 patients with traumatic SCI in an open-label, dose-ranging study and administered oral or rectal synthetic THC with mean daily doses of 31 and 43 mg, respectively. The authors reported a significant improvement of spasticity symptoms and noted that at least 15–20 mg of THC was needed to achieve a therapeutic effect. Of note, five (23%) patients reported pain increase, four (18%) of them dropped out, while another four patients (18%) reported pain relief. A total of eight (36%) patients reported sleepiness and seven (32%) anxiety symptoms.

A small double-blind, placebo-controlled, crossover study was performed by Pooyania et al. [292], which enrolled 12 SCI patients with spasticity and administered 0.5–1.0 mg of nabilone. There was a significant decrease in spasticity in the most involved muscle (0.909 ± 0.85, $p = 0.003$) and in muscle groups ($p = 0.001$) reported.

The endocannabinoid system and its role in modulating spinal cord injury and the sequela of SCI are areas deserving further study. There is yet no apparent or proven benefit of cannabinoids in improving outcome after SCI, and they join a long list of previous and current substances under investigation for this purpose, the most prominent of which recently was methylprednisolone. Despite years of clinical enthusiasm for steroids, their benefit in SCI is even less clear today. Cannabinoids show somewhat more promise in treating the sequela of SCI, and while this benefit might appear modest, the morbidity of SCI is so significant that patients would welcome even a modest benefit. It is important though to recognize that this benefit comes with risks that are not to be understated.

Traumatic Brain Injury

Various mechanisms involved in neuroprotection provided by cannabinoids were demonstrated in preclinical studies, including reduced inflammatory response, glutamate excitotoxicity, free radical damage, and decreased vasospasm [293–295]. However, only a few published reports are available documenting the attempts to use cannabinoids as a therapeutic modality involving these neuroprotective mechanisms in traumatic brain injury (TBI).

Although consumption of marijuana was related to higher adjusted odds (2.8; 95% CI 1.79–4.39) of TBI history compared to adult non-users [296], some researchers claim that a positive THC screen may also be associated with decreased mortality in adult patients sustaining TBI [297]. This retrospective review included 446 subjects, 18.4% of which had a positive THC screen. Overall mortality was significantly lower: 2.4% and 9.9% in THC-positive vs. THC-negative patients, respectively. These results contradicted a study on a synthetic cannabinoid analog in severe TBI patients who were randomized to receive either 150 mg of dexanabinol ($n = 432$) or placebo ($n = 429$) within 6 hours of injury [298]. There were no differences in outcomes (extended Glasgow scale) between the groups at the 6-month follow-up: 215 (50%) patients in the active treatment group had unfavorable outcomes compared with 214 (51%) patients in the placebo group.

Therapeutic benefits of cannabinoids in the treatment of TBI deserve further investigation, but it is clear that any possible therapeutic benefit administered after a TBI is not to be confused with a secondary "benefit" of recreational use of cannabis. The data is clear that using cannabis increases your risk of TBI, and this data is borne out by what we have at least observed empirically in the emergency rooms of our trauma centers.

Cerebrovascular

Similar to TBI, a hypothesis was raised that THC may protect against cerebrovascular damage associated with stroke [299] or CBD may have a preventative effect against stroke [300]. However, there is a growing body of clinical evidence supporting the notion that cannabis consumption is associated with cerebrovascular risk. Besides several case reports [301–305], there have been prospective studies [306, 307] and retrospective reviews [308, 309] published documenting associations between cannabis use and ischemic or hemorrhagic stroke. This contradicts preclinical studies, which demonstrated neuroprotective effects through macrophage/microglial downregulation and anti-inflammatory mechanisms [310] or antioxidative properties [311]. On the contrary, orthostatic hypotension, impairment of cerebral circulation, vasculitis, vasospasm, cerebral mitochondrial dysfunction, atrial fibrillation, and inhibition of warfarin metabolism may play an adverse role according to clinical studies [81, 305, 312–315].

In 2003, 14.4% of hemorrhagic strokes among young adults (18–44 years old) in Texas were explained by illicit drug abuse, including marijuana [309]. Controlling for all other risk factors, the cannabis users had a slightly higher risk (OR 1.36, 95% CI 0.90–2.06) for hemorrhagic stroke. Likewise, Behrouz et al. [316] included 108 patients with aneurysmal subarachnoid hemorrhage in a retrospective study, which compared cannabinoid-positive patients (25.9%) to patients with a negative urine drug screen. The cannabis use was associated with more severe symptoms (OR 1.48; 95% CI 1.08–2.03; $p = 0.02$), delayed cerebral ischemia (OR 2.68; 95% CI 1.03–6.99; $p = 0.01$), and possibly worse outcome, and the patients had higher hospital mortality (14.3% vs. 3.8%; $p = 0.052$).

A more recent study by Malhotra et al. [317] reported on clinical outcomes and severity of intracranial hemorrhage (ICH). The authors studied cannabis as an independent predictor of ICH and utilized the Nationwide Inpatient Sample comparing 2,496,165 patients who used cannabis to 116,163,454 non-users. The prevalence of ICH was higher in users (relative risk 1.11, 95% CI 1.07–1.16) and especially in younger adults (relative risk 2.45, 95% CI 2.22–2.69), but other factors, including illicit drug use, could not be ruled out. The cannabis users had higher in-hospital mortality (OR 1.26, 95% CI 1.12–1.41) despite fewer adverse discharge dispositions (OR 0.78, 95% CI 0.72–0.86) and reduced length of hospitalization (OR 0.54, 95% CI 0.48–0.61). They also had fewer complications, including sepsis, deep venous thrombosis, blood transfusions, prolonged mechanical ventilation, tracheostomy, gastrostomy, and feeding tube (all $p < 0.0001$). The same database was also used to analyze associations of cannabis use with hospitalizations for aneurysmal subarachnoid hemorrhage (aSAH), which included 2104 cannabis users and 91,948 non-users [318]. The cannabis use was an independent predictor of aSAH (OR 1.18, 95% CI 1.12–1.24), but it was not associated with symptomatic vasospasm, inpatient mortality, or adverse discharge disposition.

There was one study that at least partially contradicted the previously described findings. Napoli et al. [319] utilized an international, multicenter, observational registry to determine associations with cannabis use. Out of 725 intracerebral hemorrhage patients who had urine toxicology screens, 8.6% were cannabinoid-positive. Clinical, radiological, or mortality rates did not differ, but it was noted that cannabinoid-positive patients had significantly lower ICH scores (0 vs. 2, $p = 0.017$). Although the effect was small (OR 0.544, 95% CI 0.330–0.895, $p = 0.017$), cannabinoid-positive patients had better functional outcomes as measured on the modified Rankin Scale at discharge.

Marijuana also appears to be a vasoactive trigger in the reversible cerebral vasoconstriction syndrome (RCVS) [114, 115, 320]. Typically, RCVS afflicts young adults, predominantly women, who present with headache and many with neurological signs and symptoms that may or may not be reversible. They can suffer ischemic strokes or intracerebral hemorrhages. Vasoactive substances are usually to blame for RCVS, and 1/3 of the time marijuana is the trigger. RCVS secondary to marijuana appears in a younger cohort (26.5 vs. 51 years) and afflicts males more than females (67% male vs. 33% female) [115].

Cannabinoids, therefore, appear to be implicated in a number of adverse cerebrovascular disorders, including stroke, aneurysmal subarachnoid hemorrhage, RCVS, and intracerebral hemorrhage (ICH).

Conclusions

Maroon et al. [321] in a review of neurological conditions recognized a powerful therapeutic potential of phytocannabinoids, especially the benefits of neuroprotection, but also acknowledged the lack of human trials and evidence needed for clinical applications. Summarizing the results of clinical evidence for neurosurgical conditions, we have concluded that there is limited evidence to support or deny any benefits of the cannabinoid effectiveness for neurosurgery patients. Further epidemiological and clinical studies with rigorous study designs overcoming methodological limitations are needed to clarify contradictory findings. It should be noted that performing clinical trials involving cannabinoids is associated with immense regulatory barriers, logistic challenges, and restricted access due to the cannabis Schedule I classification. At least partially, these challenges are responsible for methodological shortcomings: a lack of uniformity for concentrations and even the substance studied in these clinical trials as different strains may have different THC concentrations and CBD content resulting in different ratios. Dispensary cannabis lacks the product integrity needed to conduct scientific studies as it is poorly tested, poorly regulated, and frequently contaminated. It will be difficult to use these products in scientific studies, and we would, therefore, support the efforts of the FDA in approving and developing pharmaceutical cannabinoids.

While there is some data to suggest the efficacy of the cannabinoids in the treatment of chronic cancer-related and neuropathic pain, there is not yet the evidence for benefit in acute spine-related pain. We have also seen that it increases your risk of trauma, traumatic brain injury, stroke, ICH, and aneurysmal subarachnoid hemorrhage and can increase your chance of developing cancer, including a glioma. This list goes on and on, but this does not mean that cannabinoids will not be proven to have medical utility. They have been shown to have some effect on modulating pain, but can they be used to help treat a spinal cord injury, a brain injury, and a stroke patient? Can they help patients with malignant gliomas survive longer? These are all questions that should be asked, and we owe it to the public to be able to answer them with evidence. Until we have this conclusive scientific validation on short- and long-term safety and efficacy, and the health risks of cannabinoids, we should be the reason to limit their use of cannabinoids at the present time.

Appendix. American Academy of Neurology Classification of Evidence

Therapeutic

Class I A randomized, controlled clinical trial of the intervention of interest with masked or objective outcome assessment, in a representative population. Relevant baseline characteristics are presented and substantially equivalent among treatment groups, or there is appropriate statistical adjustment for differences.

The following are also required:

(a) Concealed allocation
(b) Primary outcome(s) clearly defined
(c) Exclusion/inclusion criteria clearly defined

(d) Adequate accounting for dropouts (with at least 80% of enrolled subjects completing the study) and crossovers with numbers sufficiently low to have minimal potential for bias

(e) For non-inferiority or equivalence trials claiming to prove efficacy for one or both drugs, the following are also required∗:

1. The authors explicitly state the clinically meaningful difference to be excluded by defining the threshold for equivalence or non-inferiority.
2. The standard treatment used in the study is substantially similar to that used in previous studies establishing efficacy of the standard treatment (e.g., for a drug, the mode of administration, dose, and dosage adjustments are similar to those previously shown to be effective).
3. The inclusion and exclusion criteria for patient selection and the outcomes of patients on the standard treatment are comparable to those of previous studies establishing efficacy of the standard treatment.
4. The interpretation of the results of the study is based upon a per protocol analysis that takes into account dropouts or crossovers.

Class II A randomized controlled clinical trial of the intervention of interest in a representative population with masked or objective outcome assessment that lacks one criteria a–e above or a prospective matched cohort study with masked or objective outcome assessment in a representative population that meets b–e above. Relevant baseline characteristics are presented and substantially equivalent among treatment groups, or there is appropriate statistical adjustment for differences.

Class III All other controlled trials (including well-defined natural history controls or patients serving as own controls) in a representative population, where outcome is independently assessed or independently derived by objective outcome measurement.∗∗

Class IV Studies not meeting Class I, II, or III criteria including consensus or expert opinion.

∗Note that numbers 1–3 in Class Ie are required for Class II in equivalence trials. If any one of the three is missing, the class is automatically downgraded to Class III.

∗∗Objective outcome measurement: an outcome measure that is unlikely to be affected by an observer's (patient, treating physician, investigator) expectation or bias (e.g., blood tests, administrative outcome data).

References

Cannabis and Cannabinoids for the Treatment of Epilepsy

1. Russo EB. Cannabis and epilepsy: an ancient treatment returns to the fore. Epilepsy Behav. 2017;70:292–7.
2. Szaflarski JP, Bebin EM. Cannabis, cannabidiol, and epilepsy--from receptors to clinical response. Epilepsy Behav. 2014;41:277–82.

3. Maa E, Figi P. The case for medical marijuana in epilepsy. Epilepsia. 2014;55:783–6.
4. Cohen PA, Sharfstein J. The opportunity of CBD - reforming the law. N Engl J Med. 2019;381:297.
5. Mead A. The legal status of cannabis (marijuana) and cannabidiol (CBD) under U.S. law. Epilepsy Behav. 2017;70:288–91.
6. Yang YT, Szaflarski JP. The US Food and Drug Administration's Authorization of the first cannabis-derived pharmaceutical: are we out of the haze? JAMA Neurol. 2018;76:135.
7. Gaston TE, Szaflarski JP. Cannabis for the treatment of epilepsy: an update. Curr Neurol Neurosci Rep. 2018;18:73.
8. O'Brien TJ, Berkovic SF, French JA, Messenheimer J, Gutterman D. Transdermal cannabidiol (CBD) gel for the treatment of focal epilepsy in adults. Annual Meeting of the American Epilepsy Society; 2018.
9. Wheless JW, Dlugos D, Miller I, et al. Pharmacokinetics and tolerability of multiple doses of pharmaceutical-grade synthetic cannabidiol in pediatric patients with treatment-resistant epilepsy. CNS Drugs. 2019;33:593–604.
10. Szaflarski JP. The highs and lows of the endocannabinoid system-another piece to the epilepsy puzzle? Epilepsy Curr. 2018;18:315–7.
11. Pacher P, Kunos G. Modulating the endocannabinoid system in human health and disease--successes and failures. FEBS J. 2013;280:1918–43.
12. Gaston TE, Friedman D. Pharmacology of cannabinoids in the treatment of epilepsy. Epilepsy Behav. 2017;70:313–8.
13. Pertwee RG. The diverse CB1 and CB2 receptor pharmacology of three plant cannabinoids: delta9-tetrahydrocannabinol, cannabidiol and delta9-tetrahydrocannabivarin. Br J Pharmacol. 2008;153:199–215.
14. Wallace MJ, Blair RE, Falenski KW, Martin BR, DeLorenzo RJ. The endogenous cannabinoid system regulates seizure frequency and duration in a model of temporal lobe epilepsy. J Pharmacol Exp Ther. 2003;307:129–37.
15. Wallace MJ, Martin BR, DeLorenzo RJ. Evidence for a physiological role of endocannabinoids in the modulation of seizure threshold and severity. Eur J Pharmacol. 2002;452:295–301.
16. Wallace MJ, Wiley JL, Martin BR, DeLorenzo RJ. Assessment of the role of CB1 receptors in cannabinoid anticonvulsant effects. Eur J Pharmacol. 2001;428:51–7.
17. McPartland JM, Duncan M, Di Marzo V, Pertwee RG. Are cannabidiol and Delta(9)-tetrahydrocannabivarin negative modulators of the endocannabinoid system? A systematic review. Br J Pharmacol. 2015;172:737–53.
18. Perucca E. Cannabinoids in the treatment of epilepsy: hard evidence at last? J Epilepsy Res. 2017;7:61–76.
19. Thomas A, Baillie GL, Phillips AM, Razdan RK, Ross RA, Pertwee RG. Cannabidiol displays unexpectedly high potency as an antagonist of CB1 and CB2 receptor agonists in vitro. Br J Pharmacol. 2007;150:613–23.
20. Rosenberg EC, Patra PH, Whalley BJ. Therapeutic effects of cannabinoids in animal models of seizures, epilepsy, epileptogenesis, and epilepsy-related neuroprotection. Epilepsy Behav. 2017;70:319–27.
21. Cleeren E, Casteels C, Goffin K, et al. Positron emission tomography imaging of cerebral glucose metabolism and type 1 cannabinoid receptor availability during temporal lobe epileptogenesis in the amygdala kindling model in rhesus monkeys. Epilepsia. 2018;59:959–70.
22. Nichol K, Stott C, Jones N, Gray R, Bazelot M, Whalley BJ. The proposed multimodal mechanism of action of cannabidiol (CBD) in epilepsy: modulation of intracellular calcium and adenosine signalling. In: Annual meeting of the American Epilepsy Society. Philadelphia; 2018.
23. Bisogno T, Hanus L, De Petrocellis L, et al. Molecular targets for cannabidiol and its synthetic analogues: effect on vanilloid VR1 receptors and on the cellular uptake and enzymatic hydrolysis of anandamide. Br J Pharmacol. 2001;134:845–52.
24. Vilela LR, Lima IV, Kunsch EB, et al. Anticonvulsant effect of cannabidiol in the pentylenetetrazole model: pharmacological mechanisms, electroencephalographic profile, and brain cytokine levels. Epilepsy Behav. 2017;75:29–35.

25. Naziroglu M. TRPV1 channel: a potential drug target for treating epilepsy. Curr Neuropharmacol. 2015;13:239–47.
26. Ryberg E, Larsson N, Sjogren S, et al. The orphan receptor GPR55 is a novel cannabinoid receptor. Br J Pharmacol. 2007;152:1092–101.
27. Hurst K, Badgley C, Ellsworth T, et al. A putative lysophosphatidylinositol receptor GPR55 modulates hippocampal synaptic plasticity. Hippocampus. 2017;27:985–98.
28. Kaplan JS, Stella N, Catterall WA, Westenbroek RE. Cannabidiol attenuates seizures and social deficits in a mouse model of Dravet syndrome. Proc Natl Acad Sci U S A. 2017;114:11229–34.
29. During MJ, Spencer DD. Adenosine: a potential mediator of seizure arrest and postictal refractoriness. Ann Neurol. 1992;32:618–24.
30. Sebastiao AM, Ribeiro JA. Fine-tuning neuromodulation by adenosine. Trends Pharmacol Sci. 2000;21:341–6.
31. Patel RR, Barbosa C, Brustovetsky T, Brustovetsky N, Cummins TR. Aberrant epilepsy-associated mutant Nav1.6 sodium channel activity can be targeted with cannabidiol. Brain. 2016;139:2164–81.
32. Ross HR, Napier I, Connor M. Inhibition of recombinant human T-type calcium channels by Delta9-tetrahydrocannabinol and cannabidiol. J Biol Chem. 2008;283:16124–34.
33. Devinsky O, Cilio MR, Cross H, et al. Cannabidiol: pharmacology and potential therapeutic role in epilepsy and other neuropsychiatric disorders. Epilepsia. 2014;55:791–802.
34. Rimmerman N, Ben-Hail D, Porat Z, et al. Direct modulation of the outer mitochondrial membrane channel, voltage-dependent anion channel 1 (VDAC1) by cannabidiol: a novel mechanism for cannabinoid-induced cell death. Cell Death Dis. 2013;4:e949.
35. Kozela E, Juknat A, Vogel Z. Modulation of astrocyte activity by cannabidiol, a nonpsycho-active cannabinoid. Int J Mol Sci. 2017;18:E1669.
36. Pelz MC, Schoolcraft KD, Larson C, Spring MG, Lopez HH. Assessing the role of serotoner-gic receptors in cannabidiol's anticonvulsant efficacy. Epilepsy Behav. 2017;73:111–8.
37. Ben-Shabat S, Fride E, Sheskin T, et al. An entourage effect: inactive endogenous fatty acid glycerol esters enhance 2-arachidonoyl-glycerol cannabinoid activity. Eur J Pharmacol. 1998;353:23–31.
38. Russo EB. The case for the entourage effect and conventional breeding of clinical cannabis: no "strain" no gain. Front Plant Sci. 2018;9:1969.
39. McPartland JM, Russo EB. Cannabis and cannabis extracts. J Cannabis Ther. 2001;1:103–32.
40. Russo EB. Taming THC: potential cannabis synergy and phytocannabinoid-terpenoid entourage effects. Br J Pharmacol. 2011;163:1344–64.
41. Espay AJ, Norris MM, Eliassen JC, et al. Placebo effect of medication cost in Parkinson disease: a randomized double-blind study. Neurology. 2015;84:794–802.
42. Gloss D, Vickrey B. Cannabinoids for epilepsy. Cochrane Database Syst Rev. 2014;3:CD009270.
43. Press CA, Knupp KG, Chapman KE. Parental reporting of response to oral cannabis extracts for treatment of refractory epilepsy. Epilepsy Behav. 2015;45:49–52.
44. Sulak D, Saneto R, Goldstein B. The current status of artisanal cannabis for the treatment of epilepsy in the United States. Epilepsy Behav. 2017;70:328–33.
45. Pamplona FA, da Silva LR, Coan AC. Potential clinical benefits of CBD-rich cannabis extracts over purified CBD in treatment-resistant epilepsy: observational data meta-analysis. Front Neurol. 2018;9:759.
46. Treat L, Chapman KE, Colborn KL, Knupp KG. Duration of use of oral cannabis extract in a cohort of pediatric epilepsy patients. Epilepsia. 2017;58:123–7.
47. Hausman-Kedem M, Menascu S, Kramer U. Efficacy of CBD-enriched medical cannabis for treatment of refractory epilepsy in children and adolescents - an observational, longitudinal study. Brain and Development. 2018;40:544–51.
48. Tzadok M, Uliel-Siboni S, Linder I, et al. CBD-enriched medical cannabis for intractable pediatric epilepsy: the current Israeli experience. Seizure. 2016;35:41–4.
49. Szaflarski JP, Bebin EM, Cutter G, et al. Cannabidiol improves frequency and severity of sei-zures and reduces adverse events in an open-label add-on prospective study. Epilepsy Behav. 2018;87:131.

50. Porcari GS, Fu C, Doll ED, Carter EG, Carson RP. Efficacy of artisanal preparations of cannabidiol for the treatment of epilepsy: practical experiences in a tertiary medical center. Epilepsy Behav. 2018;80:240–6.
51. Neubauer D, Perkovic Benedik M, Osredkar D. Cannabidiol for treatment of refractory childhood epilepsies: experience from a single tertiary epilepsy center in Slovenia. Epilepsy Behav. 2018;81:79–85.
52. Pietrafusa N, Ferretti A, Trivisano M, et al. Purified cannabidiol for treatment of refractory epilepsies in pediatric patients with developmental and epileptic encephalopathy. Paediatr Drugs. 2019;21:283.
53. Hussain SA, Zhou R, Jacobson C, et al. Perceived efficacy of cannabidiol-enriched cannabis extracts for treatment of pediatric epilepsy: a potential role for infantile spasms and Lennox-Gastaut syndrome. Epilepsy Behav. 2015;47:138–41.
54. Suraev A, Lintzeris N, Stuart J, et al. Composition and use of cannabis extracts for childhood epilepsy in the Australian community. Sci Rep. 2018;8:10154.
55. Suraev AS, Todd L, Bowen MT, et al. An Australian nationwide survey on medicinal cannabis use for epilepsy: history of antiepileptic drug treatment predicts medicinal cannabis use. Epilepsy Behav. 2017;70:334–40.
56. Vandrey R, Raber JC, Raber ME, Douglass B, Miller C, Bonn-Miller MO. Cannabinoid dose and label accuracy in edible medical cannabis products. JAMA. 2015;313:2491–3.
57. Aguirre-Velazquez CG. Report from a survey of parents regarding the use of cannabidiol (medicinal cannabis) in Mexican children with refractory epilepsy. Neurol Res Int. 2017;2017:2985729.
58. Devinsky O, Marsh E, Friedman D, et al. Cannabidiol in patients with treatment-resistant epilepsy: an open-label interventional trial. Lancet Neurol. 2016;15:270–8.
59. Szaflarski JP, Bebin EM, Comi AM, et al. Long-term safety and treatment effects of cannabidiol in children and adults with treatment-resistant epilepsies: expanded access program results. Epilepsia. 2018;59:1540–8.
60. Laux LC, Bebin EM, Checketts D, et al. Long-term safety and efficacy of cannabidiol in children and adults with treatment resistant Lennox-Gastaut syndrome or Dravet syndrome: expanded access program results. Epilepsy Res. 2019;154:13–20.
61. Hess EJ, Moody KA, Geffrey AL, et al. Cannabidiol as a new treatment for drug-resistant epilepsy in tuberous sclerosis complex. Epilepsia. 2016;57:1617–24.
62. Sands TT, Rahdari S, Oldham MS, Caminha Nunes E, Tilton N, Cilio MR. Long-term safety, tolerability, and efficacy of cannabidiol in children with refractory epilepsy: results from an expanded access program in the US. CNS Drugs. 2019;33:47–60.
63. Szaflarski JP, Hernando K, Bebin EM, et al. Higher cannabidiol plasma levels are associated with better seizure response following treatment with a pharmaceutical grade cannabidiol. Epilepsy Behav. 2019;95:131–6.
64. Gaston TE, Bebin EM, Cutter G, et al. Drug–drug interactions with cannabidiol (CBD) appear to have no effect on treatment response in an open-label expanded access Program. Epilepsy Behav. 2019;98:201–6.
65. Devinsky O, Verducci C, Thiele EA, et al. Open-label use of highly purified CBD (Epidiolex(R)) in patients with CDKL5 deficiency disorder and Aicardi, Dup15q, and Doose syndromes. Epilepsy Behav. 2018;86:131–7.
66. Gofshteyn JS, Wilfong A, Devinsky O, et al. Cannabidiol as a potential treatment for febrile infection-related epilepsy syndrome (fires) in the acute and chronic phases. J Child Neurol. 2017;32:35–40.
67. McCoy B, Wang L, Zak M, et al. A prospective open-label trial of CBD/THC cannabis oil in Dravet syndrome. Ann Clin Transl Neurol. 2018;5:1077.
68. Cilio MR, Wheless JW, Parikh N, Miller I. Long-term safety of pharmaceutical cannabidiol oral solution as adjunctive treatment for pediatric patients with treatment-resistant epilepsy. AES Annual Meeting; 2018.
69. Devinsky O, Cross JH, Laux L, et al. Trial of cannabidiol for drug-resistant seizures in the Dravet syndrome. N Engl J Med. 2017;376:2011–20.

70. Devinsky O, Patel AD, Thiele EA, et al. Randomized, dose-ranging safety trial of cannabidiol in Dravet syndrome. Neurology. 2018;90:e1204–11.
71. Devinsky O, Patel AD, Cross JH, et al. Effect of cannabidiol on drop seizures in the Lennox-Gastaut syndrome. N Engl J Med. 2018;378:1888–97.
72. Hussain SA, et al. Synthetic pharmaceutical grade cannabidiol for treatment of refractory infantile spasms: a multicenter phase-2 study. Epilepsy Behav. 2020;102:106826.
73. Thiele EA, Marsh ED, French JA, et al. Cannabidiol in patients with seizures associated with Lennox-Gastaut syndrome (GWPCARE4): a randomised, double-blind, placebo-controlled phase 3 trial. London: Lancet; 2018.
74. Miziak B, Walczak A, Szponar J, Pluta R, Czuczwar SJ. Drug-drug interactions between antiepileptics and cannabinoids. Expert Opin Drug Metab Toxicol. 2019;15:407–15.
75. Morrison G, Crockett J, Blakey G, Sommerville K. A phase 1, open-label, pharmacokinetic trial to investigate possible drug-drug interactions between clobazam, stiripentol, or valproate and cannabidiol in healthy subjects. Clin Pharmacol Drug Dev. 2019;8:1009.
76. Szaflarski JP, Gidal G, Patsalos P, VanLandingham K, Critchley D, Morrison G. Drug-drug interaction studies with coadministration of cannabidiol and clobazam, valproate, stiripentol, or midazolam in healthy volunteers and adults with epilepsy. In: Annual meeting of the American Academy of Neurology. Philadelphia; 2019.
77. Geffrey AL, Pollack SF, Bruno PL, Thiele EA. Drug-drug interaction between clobazam and cannabidiol in children with refractory epilepsy. Epilepsia. 2015;56:1246–51.
78. Jiang R, Yamaori S, Okamoto Y, Yamamoto I, Watanabe K. Cannabidiol is a potent inhibitor of the catalytic activity of cytochrome P450 2C19. Drug Metab Pharmacokinet. 2013;28:332–8.
79. Gaston TE, Bebin EM, Cutter GR, Liu Y, Szaflarski JP, Program UC. Interactions between cannabidiol and commonly used antiepileptic drugs. Epilepsia. 2017;58:1586–92.
80. Klotz KA, Hirsch M, Heers M, Schulze-Bonhage A, Jacobs J. Effects of cannabidiol on brivaracetam plasma levels. Epilepsia. 2019;60:e74–7.
81. Damkier P, Lassen D, Christensen MMH, Madsen KG, Hellfritzsch M, Pottegard A. Interaction between warfarin and cannabis. Basic Clin Pharmacol Toxicol. 2019;124:28–31.
82. Grayson L, Vines B, Nichol K, Szaflarski JP, Program UC. An interaction between warfarin and cannabidiol, a case report. Epilepsy Behav Case Rep. 2018;9:10–1.
83. Leino AD, Emoto C, Fukuda T, Privitera M, Vinks AA, Alloway RR. Evidence of a clinically significant drug-drug interaction between cannabidiol and tacrolimus. Am J Transplant. 2019;19:2944.
84. Moghimipour E, Ameri A, Handali S. Absorption-enhancing effects of bile salts. Molecules. 2015;20:14451–73.
85. Birnbaum AK, Karanam A, Marino SE, et al. Food effect on pharmacokinetics of cannabidiol oral capsules in adult patients with refractory epilepsy. Epilepsia. 2019;60:1586.
86. Paudel KS, Hammell DC, Agu RU, Valiveti S, Stinchcomb AL. Cannabidiol bioavailability after nasal and transdermal application: effect of permeation enhancers. Drug Dev Ind Pharm. 2010;36:1088–97.
87. Taylor L, Gidal B, Blakey G, Tayo B, Morrison G. A phase I, randomized, double-blind, placebo-controlled, single ascending dose, multiple dose, and food effect trial of the safety, tolerability and pharmacokinetics of highly purified cannabidiol in healthy subjects. CNS Drugs. 2018;32:1053–67.

Multiple Sclerosis and Cannabis – Benefits, Risks, and Special Considerations

88. Check WA. Marijuana may lessen spasticity of MS. JAMA. 1979;241(23):2476.
89. National Academies of Sciences, Engineering, and Medicine. The health effects of cannabis and cannabinoids: current state of evidence and recommendations for research. Washington, D.C.: The National Academies Press; 2017.

90. Yadav V, Bever C, Bowen J, Bowling A, Weinstock-Guttman B, Cameron M, et al. Summary of evidence-based guideline: complementary and alternative medicine in multiple sclerosis: report of the guideline development subcommittee of the American Academy of Neurology. Neurology. 2014;82(12):1083–92.

91. Koppel BS, Brust JC, Fife T, Bronstein J, Youssof S, Gronseth G, et al. Systematic review: efficacy and safety of medical marijuana in selected neurologic disorders: report of the guideline development Subcommittee of the American Academy of neurology. Neurology. 2014;82(17):1556–63.

92. Torres-Moreno MC, Papaseit E, Torrens M, Farré M. Assessment of efficacy and tolerability of medicinal cannabinoids in patients with multiple sclerosis: a systematic review and meta-analysis. JAMA Netw Open. 2018;1(6):e183485.

93. Rice J, Cameron M. Cannabinoids for treatment of MS symptoms: state of the evidence. Curr Neurol Neurosci Rep. 2018;18(8):50.

94. Russo EB. History of cannabis and its preparations in saga, science, and sobriquet. Chem Biodivers. 2007;4(8):1614–48.

95. Anon. 33 legal medical marijuana states and DC. Available from: https://medicalmarijuana.procon.org/view.resource.php?resourceID=000881&gclid=EAIaIQobChMI-aSByov-l4wIV3__jBx3DtQXnEAAYASAAEgJIAfD_BwE. Accessed 2 Aug 2019.

96. Gupta S, Fellows K, Weinstock-Guttman B, Hagemeier J, Zivadinov R, Ramanathan M. Marijuana use by patients with multiple sclerosis. Int J MS Care. 2019;21(2):57–62.

97. Weinkle L, Domen CH, Shelton I, Sillau S, Nair K, Alvarez E. Exploring cannabis use by patients with multiple sclerosis in a state where cannabis is legal. Mult Scler Relat Disord. 2019;27:383–90.

98. Haug NA, Kieschnick D, Sottile JE, Babson KA, Vandrey R, Bonn-Miller MO. Training and practices of cannabis dispensary staff. Cannabis Cannabinoid Res. 2016;1(1):244–51.

99. Evanoff AB, Quan T, Dufault C, Awad M, Bierut LJ. Physicians-in-training are not prepared to prescribe medical marijuana. Drug Alcohol Depend. 2017;180:151–5.

100. Brooks E, Gundersen DC, Flynn E, Brooks-Russell A, Bull S. The clinical implications of legalizing marijuana: are physician and non-physician providers prepared? Addict Behav. 2017;72:1–7.

101. Ziemianski D, Capler R, Tekanoff R, Lacasse A, Luconi F, Ware MA. Cannabis in medicine: a national educational needs assessment among Canadian physicians. BMC Med Educ. 2015;15:52.

102. Balneaves LG, Alraja A, Ziemianski D, McCuaig F, Ware M. A national needs assessment of Canadian nurse practitioners regarding cannabis for therapeutic purposes. Cannabis Cannabinoid Res. 2018;3(1):66–73.

103. Benarroch EE. Synaptic effects of cannabinoids: complexity, behavioral effects, and potential clinical implications. Neurology. 2014;83(21):1958–67.

104. Muller C, Morales P, Reggio PH. Cannabinoid ligands targeting TRP channels. Front Mol Neurosci. 2018;11:487.

105. Baker D, Pryce G, Visintin C, Sisay S, Bondarenko AI, Vanessa Ho WS, et al. Big conductance calcium-activated potassium channel openers control spasticity without sedation. Br J Pharmacol. 2017;174(16):2662–81.

106. Giacoppo S, Mazzon E. Can cannabinoids be a potential therapeutic tool in amyotrophic lateral sclerosis. Neural Regen Res. 2016;11(12):1896–9.

107. Pryce G, Baker D. Potential control of multiple sclerosis by cannabis and the endocannabinoid system. CNS Neurol Disord Drug Targets. 2012;11(5):624–41.

108. Ball S, Vickery J, Hobart J, Wright D, Green C, Shearer J, et al. The cannabinoid use in progressive inflammatory brain disease (CUPID) trial: a randomised double-blind placebo-controlled parallel-group multicentre trial and economic evaluation of cannabinoids to slow progression in multiple sclerosis. Health Technol Assess. 2015;19(12).:vii-viii, xxv-xxxi,:1–187.

109. Faraone SV. Interpreting estimates of treatment effects: implications for managed care. P T. 2008;33(12):700–11.

110. Food and Drug Administration (FDA). Epidiolex full prescribing information. Available from: www.accessdata.fda.gov/drugsatfda_docs/label/2018/210365lbl.pdf. Accessed 12 Aug 2019.
111. Whiting PF, Wolff RF, Deshpande S, Di Nisio M, Duffy S, Hernandez AV, et al. Cannabinoids for medical use: a systematic review and meta-analysis. JAMA. 2015;313(24):2456–73.
112. Singhal AB, Hajj-Ali RA, Topcuoglu MA, Fok J, Bena J, Yang D, et al. Reversible cerebral vasoconstriction syndromes: analysis of 139 cases. Arch Neurol. 2011;68(8):1005–12.
113. Wolff V, Jouanjus E. Strokes are possible complications of cannabinoids use. Epil Behav. 2017;70(Pt B):355–63.
114. Ducros A. Reversible cerebral vasoconstriction syndrome. Lancet Neurol. 2012;11(10):906–17.
115. Jensen J, Leonard J, Salottolo K, McCarthy K, Wagner J, Bar-Or D. The epidemiology of reversible cerebral vasoconstriction syndrome in patients at a Colorado comprehensive stroke Center. J Vasc Interv Neurol. 2018;10(1):32–8.
116. Wolff V, Ducros A. Reversible cerebral vasoconstriction syndrome without typical thunderclap headache. Headache. 2016;56(4):674–87.
117. Mawet J. Avoidance of steroids in the reversible cerebral vasoconstriction syndrome. Neurology. 2017;88(3):224–5.
118. Kunchok A, Castley HC, Aldous L, Hawke SH, Torzillo E, Parker GD, et al. Fatal reversible cerebral vasoconstriction syndrome. J Neurol Sci. 2018;385:146–50.
119. Belliston S, Sundararajan J, Hammond N, Newell K, Lynch S. Reversible cerebral vasoconstriction syndrome in association with fingolimod use. Int J Neurosci. 2017;127(9):831–4.
120. Devinsky O, Cilio MR, Cross H, Fernandez-Ruiz J, French J, Hill C, et al. Cannabidiol: pharmacology and potential therapeutic role in epilepsy and other neuropsychiatric disorders. Epilepsia. 2014;55(6):791–802.
121. Benbadis SR, Sanchez-Ramos J, Bozorg A, Giarratano M, Kalidas K, Katzin L, et al. Medical marijuana in neurology. Expert Rev Neurother. 2014;14(12):1453–65.
122. Pavisian B, MacIntosh BJ, Szilagyi G, Staines RW, O'Connor P, Feinstein A. Effects of cannabis on cognition in patients with MS: a psychometric and MRI study. Neurology. 2014;82(21):1879–87.
123. Feinstein A, Meza C, Stefan C, Staines RW. Coming off cannabis: a cognitive and magnetic resonance imaging study in patients with multiple sclerosis. Brain. 2019;142(9):2800–12.
124. Bosker WM, Karschner EL, Lee D, Goodwin RS, Hirvonen J, Innis RB, et al. Psychomotor function in chronic daily cannabis smokers during sustained abstinence. PLoS One. 2013;8(1):e53127.
125. Busardò FP, Pellegrini M, Klein J, di Luca NM. Neurocognitive correlates in driving under the influence of cannabis. CNS Neurol Disord Drug Targets. 2017;16(5):534–40.
126. Goyal H, Awad HH, Ghali JK. Role of cannabis in cardiovascular disorders. J Thorac Dis. 2017;9(7):2079–92.
127. Camilleri M. Cannabinoids and gastrointestinal motility: pharmacology, clinical effects, and potential therapeutics in humans. Neurogastroenterol Motil. 2018;30(9):e13370.
128. Gundersen TD, Jørgensen N, Andersson AM, Bang AK, Nordkap L, Skakkebæk NE, et al. Association between use of marijuana and male reproductive hormones and semen quality: a study among 1,215 healthy young men. Am J Epidemiol. 2015;182(6):473–81.
129. Marrie RA, Miller A, Sormani MP, Thompson A, Waubant E, Trojano M, et al. Recommendations for observational studies of comorbidity in multiple sclerosis. Neurology. 2016;86(15):1446–53.
130. Feinstein A, Pavisian B. Multiple sclerosis and suicide. Mult Scler. 2017;23(7):923–7.
131. Brown JD, Winterstein AG. Potential adverse drug events and drug-drug interactions with medical and consumer cannabidiol (CBD) use. J Clin Med. 2019;8(7):E989.
132. Alsherbiny MA, Li CG. Medicinal cannabis-potential drug interactions. Medicines (Basel). 2018;6(1):E3.
133. Bouquié R, Deslandes G, Mazaré H, Cogné M, Mahé J, Grégoire M, et al. Cannabis and anticancer drugs: societal usage and expected pharmacological interactions - a review. Fundam Clin Pharmacol. 2018;32(5):462–84.

134. Rae-Grant A, Day GS, Marrie RA, Rabinstein A, Cree BAC, Gronseth GS, et al. Practice guideline recommendations summary: disease-modifying therapies for adults with multiple sclerosis: report of the guideline development, dissemination, and implementation Subcommittee of the American Academy of neurology. Neurology. 2018;90(17):777–88.
135. Kis E, Nagy T, Jani M, Molnár E, Jánossy J, Ujhellyi O, et al. Leflunomide and its metabolite A771726 are high affinity substrates of BCRP: implications for drug resistance. Ann Rheum Dis. 2009;68(7):1201–7.
136. Carrier EJ, Auchampach JA, Hillard CJ. Inhibition of an equilibrative nucleoside transporter by cannabidiol: a mechanism of cannabinoid immunosuppression. Proc Natl Acad Sci U S A. 2006;103(20):7895–900.
137. Food and Drug Administration (FDA). Siponimod full prescribing information. Available from: https://www.accessdata.fda.gov/drugsatfda_docs/label/2019/209884s000lbl.pdf. Accessed 20 Aug 19.
138. Russo EB. Current therapeutic cannabis controversies and clinical trial design issues. Front Pharmacol. 2016;7:309.
139. Raber JC, Elzinga S, Kaplan C. Understanding dabs: contamination concerns of cannabis concentrates and cannabinoid transfer during the act of dabbing. J Toxicol Sci. 2015;40(6):797–803.
140. Pizzorno J. What should we tell our patients about marijuana. Integr Med (Encinitas). 2016;15(6):8–12.
141. Perrine CG, Pickens CM, Boehmer TK, King BA, Jones CM, DeSisto CL, et al. Characteristics of a multistate outbreak of lung injury associated with E-cigarette use, or vaping - United States, 2019. MMWR Morb Mortal Wkly Rep. 2019;68(39):860–4.
142. French CE, Coope CM, McGuinness LA, Beck CR, Newitt S, Ahyow L, et al. Cannabis use and the risk of tuberculosis: a systematic review. BMC Public Health. 2019;19(1):1006.
143. Thompson GR, Tuscano JM, Dennis M, Singapuri A, Libertini S, Gaudino R, et al. A microbiome assessment of medical marijuana. Clin Microbiol Infect. 2017;23(4):269–70.
144. McKernan K, Spangler J, Zhang L, Tadigotla V, Helbert Y, Foss T, et al. Cannabis microbiome sequencing reveals several mycotoxic fungi native to dispensary grade cannabis flowers. F1000Res. 2015;4:1422.
145. McKernan K, Spangler J, Helbert Y, Lynch RC, Devitt-Lee A, Zhang L, et al. Metagenomic analysis of medicinal cannabis samples. F1000Res. 2016;5:2471.
146. Russo CV, Saccà F, Paternoster M, Buonomo AR, Gentile I, Scotto R, et al. Post-mortem diagnosis of invasive pulmonary aspergillosis after alemtuzumab treatment for multiple sclerosis. Mult Scler. 2020;26:123. https://doi.org/10.1177/1352458518813110.
147. Chong I, Wang KY, Lincoln CM. Cryptococcal meningitis in a multiple sclerosis patient treated with Fingolimod: a case report and review of imaging findings. Clin Imaging. 2019;54:53–6.
148. Gundacker ND, Jordan SJ, Jones BA, Drwiega JC, Pappas PG. Acute cryptococcal immune reconstitution inflammatory syndrome in a patient on natalizumab. Open Forum Infect Dis. 2016;3(1):ofw038.
149. Walters KM, Fisher GG, Tenney L. An overview of health and safety in the Colorado cannabis industry. Am J Ind Med. 2018;61(6):451–61.

The Evidence for Cannabis Use in Movement Disorders

150. John CM, Brust DF, Narayanaswami P, Patel A, Song S, Youssof S, Stock A. AAN position: use of medical marijuana for neurologic disorders. 2018.
151. National Academies of Sciences E, Medicine, Health, Medicine D, Board on Population H, Public Health P, et al. The National Academies Collection: reports funded by National Institutes of Health. The health effects of cannabis and cannabinoids: the current state of evidence and recommendations for research. Washington, D.C.: National Academies Press. (US) Copyright 2017 by the National Academy of Sciences. All rights reserved; 2017.

152. GBD 2016 Neurology Collaborators. Global, regional, and national burden of Parkinson's disease, 1990-2016: a systematic analysis for the global burden of disease study 2016. Lancet Neurol. 2018;17(11):939–53.
153. Kowal SL, Dall TM, Chakrabarti R, Storm MV, Jain A. The current and projected economic burden of Parkinson's disease in the United States. Mov Disord. 2013;28(3):311–8.
154. Venderova K, Ruzicka E, Vorisek V, Visnovsky P. Survey on cannabis use in Parkinson's disease: subjective improvement of motor symptoms. Mov Dis. 2004;19(9):1102–6.
155. Finseth TA, Hedeman JL, Brown RP 2nd, Johnson KI, Binder MS, Kluger BM. Self-reported efficacy of cannabis and other complementary medicine modalities by Parkinson's disease patients in Colorado. Evid Based Complement Alternat Med. 2015;2015:874849.
156. Balash Y, Bar-Lev Schleider L, Korczyn AD, Shabtai H, Knaani J, Rosenberg A, et al. Medical cannabis in Parkinson disease: real-life patients' experience. Clin Neuropharmacol. 2017;40(6):268–72.
157. Garcia C, Palomo-Garo C, Garcia-Arencibia M, Ramos J, Pertwee R, Fernandez-Ruiz J. Symptom-relieving and neuroprotective effects of the phytocannabinoid Delta(9)-THCV in animal models of Parkinson's disease. Br J Pharmacol. 2011;163(7):1495–506.
158. Gutierrez-Valdez AL, Garcia-Ruiz R, Anaya-Martinez V, Torres-Esquivel C, Espinosa-Villanueva J, Reynoso-Erazo L, et al. The combination of oral L-DOPA/rimonabant for effective dyskinesia treatment and cytological preservation in a rat model of Parkinson's disease and L-DOPA-induced dyskinesia. Behav Pharmacol. 2013;24(8):640–52.
159. Gonzalez S, Scorticati C, Garcia-Arencibia M, de Miguel R, Ramos JA, Fernandez-Ruiz J. Effects of rimonabant, a selective cannabinoid CB1 receptor antagonist, in a rat model of Parkinson's disease. Brain Res. 2006;1073–4:209–19.
160. van der Stelt M, Fox SH, Hill M, Crossman AR, Petrosino S, Di Marzo V, et al. A role for endocannabinoids in the generation of parkinsonism and levodopa-induced dyskinesia in MPTP-lesioned non-human primate models of Parkinson's disease. FASEB J. 2005;19(9):1140–2.
161. Kelsey JE, Harris O, Cassin J. The CB(1) antagonist rimonabant is adjunctively therapeutic as well as monotherapeutic in an animal model of Parkinson's disease. Behav Brain Res. 2009;203(2):304–7.
162. Walsh S, Gorman AM, Finn DP, Dowd E. The effects of cannabinoid drugs on abnormal involuntary movements in dyskinetic and non-dyskinetic 6-hydroxydopamine lesioned rats. Brain Res. 2010;1363:40–8.
163. Cao X, Liang L, Hadcock JR, Iredale PA, Griffith DA, Menniti FS, et al. Blockade of cannabinoid type 1 receptors augments the antiparkinsonian action of levodopa without affecting dyskinesias in 1-methyl-4-phenyl-1,2,3,6-tetrahydropyridine-treated rhesus monkeys. J Pharmacol Exp Ther. 2007;323(1):318–26.
164. Fernandez-Espejo E, Caraballo I, de Fonseca FR, El Banoua F, Ferrer B, Flores JA, et al. Cannabinoid CB1 antagonists possess antiparkinsonian efficacy only in rats with very severe nigral lesion in experimental parkinsonism. Neurobiol Dis. 2005;18(3):591–601.
165. Segovia G, Mora F, Crossman AR, Brotchie JM. Effects of CB1 cannabinoid receptor modulating compounds on the hyperkinesia induced by high-dose levodopa in the reserpine-treated rat model of Parkinson's disease. Mov Disord. 2003;18(2):138–49.
166. Morgese MG, Cassano T, Cuomo V, Giuffrida A. Anti-dyskinetic effects of cannabinoids in a rat model of Parkinson's disease: role of CB(1) and TRPV1 receptors. Exp Neurol. 2007;208(1):110–9.
167. Martinez A, Macheda T, Morgese MG, Trabace L, Giuffrida A. The cannabinoid agonist WIN55212-2 decreases L-DOPA-induced PKA activation and dyskinetic behavior in 6-OHDA-treated rats. Neurosci Res. 2012;72(3):236–42.
168. Gilgun-Sherki Y, Melamed E, Mechoulam R, Offen D. The CB1 cannabinoid receptor agonist, HU-210, reduces levodopa-induced rotations in 6-hydroxydopamine-lesioned rats. Pharmacol Toxicol. 2003;93(2):66–70.
169. Fox SH, Henry B, Hill M, Crossman A, Brotchie J. Stimulation of cannabinoid receptors reduces levodopa-induced dyskinesia in the MPTP-lesioned nonhuman primate model of Parkinson's disease. Mov Disord. 2002;17(6):1180–7.

170. Meschler JP, Howlett AC, Madras BK. Cannabinoid receptor agonist and antagonist effects on motor function in normal and 1-methyl-4-phenyl-1,2,5,6-tetrahydropyridine (MPTP)-treated non-human primates. Psychopharmacology. 2001;156(1):79–85.
171. Moss DE, McMaster SB, Rogers J. Tetrahydrocannabinol potentiates reserpine-induced hypokinesia. Pharmacol Biochem Behav. 1981;15(5):779–83.
172. Lotan I, Treves TA, Roditi Y, Djaldetti R. Cannabis (medical marijuana) treatment for motor and non-motor symptoms of Parkinson disease: an open-label observational study. Clin Neuropharmacol. 2014;37(2):41–4.
173. Shohet A, Khlebtovsky A, Roizen N, Roditi Y, Djaldetti R. Effect of medical cannabis on thermal quantitative measurements of pain in patients with Parkinson's disease. Eur J Pain (London). 2017;21(3):486–93.
174. Frankel JP, Hughes A, Lees AJ, Stern GM. Marijuana for parkinsonian tremor. J Neurol Neurosurg Psychiatry. 1990;53(5):436.
175. Zuardi AW, Crippa JA, Hallak JE, Pinto JP, Chagas MH, Rodrigues GG, et al. Cannabidiol for the treatment of psychosis in Parkinson's disease. J Psychopharmacol. 2009;23(8):979–83.
176. Chagas MH, Zuardi AW, Tumas V, Pena-Pereira MA, Sobreira ET, Bergamaschi MM, et al. Effects of cannabidiol in the treatment of patients with Parkinson's disease: an exploratory double-blind trial. J Psychopharmacol. 2014;28(11):1088–98.
177. Mesnage V, Houeto JL, Bonnet AM, Clavier I, Arnulf I, Cattelin F, et al. Neurokinin B, neurotensin, and cannabinoid receptor antagonists and Parkinson disease. Clin Neuropharmacol. 2004;27(3):108–10.
178. Carroll CB, Bain PG, Teare L, Liu X, Joint C, Wroath C, et al. Cannabis for dyskinesia in Parkinson disease: a randomized double-blind crossover study. Neurology. 2004;63(7):1245–50.
179. Sieradzan KA, Fox SH, Hill M, Dick JP, Crossman AR, Brotchie JM. Cannabinoids reduce levodopa-induced dyskinesia in Parkinson's disease: a pilot study. Neurology. 2001;57(11):2108–11.
180. Chagas MH, Eckeli AL, Zuardi AW, Pena-Pereira MA, Sobreira-Neto MA, Sobreira ET, et al. Cannabidiol can improve complex sleep-related behaviours associated with rapid eye movement sleep behaviour disorder in Parkinson's disease patients: a case series. J Clin Pharm Ther. 2014;39(5):564–6.
181. McColgan P, Tabrizi SJ. Huntington's disease: a clinical review. Eur J Neurol. 2018;25(1):24–34.
182. Wyant KJ, Ridder AJ, Dayalu P. Huntington's disease-update on treatments. Curr Neurol Neurosci Rep. 2017;17(4):33.
183. Deng YP, Albin RL, Penney JB, Young AB, Anderson KD, Reiner A. Differential loss of striatal projection systems in Huntington's disease: a quantitative immunohistochemical study. J Chem Neuroanat. 2004;27(3):143–64.
184. Glass M, Dragunow M, Faull RL. The pattern of neurodegeneration in Huntington's disease: a comparative study of cannabinoid, dopamine, adenosine and GABA(a) receptor alterations in the human basal ganglia in Huntington's disease. Neuroscience. 2000;97(3):505–19.
185. Albin RL, Reiner A, Anderson KD, Dure LS, Handelin B, Balfour R, et al. Preferential loss of striato-external pallidal projection neurons in presymptomatic Huntington's disease. Ann Neurol. 1992;31(4):425–30.
186. Faull RL, Waldvogel HJ, Nicholson LF, Synek BJ. The distribution of GABAA-benzodiazepine receptors in the basal ganglia in Huntington's disease and in the quinolinic acid-lesioned rat. Prog Brain Res. 1993;99:105–23.
187. Reiner A, Albin RL, Anderson KD, D'Amato CJ, Penney JB, Young AB. Differential loss of striatal projection neurons in Huntington disease. Proc Natl Acad Sci U S A. 1988;85(15):5733–7.
188. Lastres-Becker I, De Miguel R, Fernandez-Ruiz JJ. The endocannabinoid system and Huntington's disease. Curr Drug Targets CNS Neurol Disord. 2003;2(5):335–47.

189. de Lago E, Fernandez-Ruiz J, Ortega-Gutierrez S, Cabranes A, Pryce G, Baker D, et al. UCM707, an inhibitor of the anandamide uptake, behaves as a symptom control agent in models of Huntington's disease and multiple sclerosis, but fails to delay/arrest the progression of different motor-related disorders. Eur Neuropsychopharmacol. 2006;16(1):7–18.

190. Lastres-Becker I, de Miguel R, De Petrocellis L, Makriyannis A, Di Marzo V, Fernandez-Ruiz J. Compounds acting at the endocannabinoid and/or endovanilloid systems reduce hyperkinesia in a rat model of Huntington's disease. J Neurochem. 2003;84(5):1097–109.

191. Lastres-Becker I, Hansen HH, Berrendero F, De Miguel R, Perez-Rosado A, Manzanares J, et al. Alleviation of motor hyperactivity and neurochemical deficits by endocannabinoid uptake inhibition in a rat model of Huntington's disease. Synapse (N Y). 2002;44(1):23–35.

192. de Lago E, Urbani P, Ramos JA, Di Marzo V, Fernandez-Ruiz J. Arvanil, a hybrid endocannabinoid and vanilloid compound, behaves as an antihyperkinetic agent in a rat model of Huntington's disease. Brain Res. 2005;1050(1–2):210–6.

193. Dowie MJ, Howard ML, Nicholson LF, Faull RL, Hannan AJ, Glass M. Behavioural and molecular consequences of chronic cannabinoid treatment in Huntington's disease transgenic mice. Neuroscience. 2010;170(1):324–36.

194. Muller-Vahl KR, Schneider U, Emrich HM. Nabilone increases choreatic movements in Huntington's disease. Mov Disord. 1999;14(6):1038–40.

195. Curtis A, Rickards H. Nabilone could treat chorea and irritability in Huntington's disease. J Neuropsychiatry Clin Neurosci. 2006;18(4):553–4.

196. Curtis A, Mitchell I, Patel S, Ives N, Rickards H. A pilot study using nabilone for symptomatic treatment in Huntington's disease. Mov Disord. 2009;24(15):2254–9.

197. Consroe P, Laguna J, Allender J, Snider S, Stern L, Sandyk R, et al. Controlled clinical trial of cannabidiol in Huntington's disease. Pharmacol Biochem Behav. 1991;40(3):701–8.

198. Lopez-Sendon Moreno JL, Garcia Caldentey J, Trigo Cubillo P, Ruiz Romero C, Garcia Ribas G, Alonso Arias MA, et al. A double-blind, randomized, cross-over, placebo-controlled, pilot trial with Sativex in Huntington's disease. J Neurol. 2016;263(7):1390–400.

199. Albanese A, Bhatia K, Bressman SB, Delong MR, Fahn S, Fung VS, et al. Phenomenology and classification of dystonia: a consensus update. Mov Disord. 2013;28(7):863–73.

200. Page D, Butler A, Jahanshahi M. Quality of life in focal, segmental, and generalized dystonia. Mov Disord. 2007;22(3):341–7.

201. Vitek JL. Pathophysiology of dystonia: a neuronal model. Mov Disord. 2002;17(Suppl 3):S49–62.

202. Moro E, LeReun C, Krauss JK, Albanese A, Lin JP, Walleser Autiero S, et al. Efficacy of pallidal stimulation in isolated dystonia: a systematic review and meta-analysis. Eur J Neurol. 2017;24(4):552–60.

203. Brecl Jakob G, Pelykh O, Kosutzka Z, Pirtosek Z, Trost M, Ilmberger J, et al. Postural stability under globus pallidus internus stimulation for dystonia. Clin Neurophysiol. 2015;126(12):2299–305.

204. Sharma N. Neuropathology of dystonia. Tremor Other Hyperkinet Mov (N Y). 2019;9:569.

205. Richter A, Loscher W. (+)-WIN 55,212-2, a novel cannabinoid receptor agonist, exerts antidystonic effects in mutant dystonic hamsters. Eur J Pharmacol. 1994;264(3):371–7.

206. Richter A, Loscher W. Effects of pharmacological manipulations of cannabinoid receptors on severity of dystonia in a genetic model of paroxysmal dyskinesia. Eur J Pharmacol. 2002;454(2–3):145–51.

207. Fox SH, Kellett M, Moore AP, Crossman AR, Brotchie JM. Randomised, double-blind, placebo-controlled trial to assess the potential of cannabinoid receptor stimulation in the treatment of dystonia. Mov Disord. 2002;17(1):145–9.

208. Zadikoff C, Wadia PM, Miyasaki J, Chen R, Lang AE, So J, Fox SH. Cannabinoid, CB1 agonists in cervical dystonia: failure in a phase IIa randomized controlled trial. Basal Ganglia. 2011;1:91–5.

209. Consroe P, Sandyk R, Snider SR. Open label evaluation of cannabidiol in dystonic movement disorders. Int J Neurosci. 1986;30(4):277–82.

210. Chatterjee A, Almahrezi A, Ware M, Fitzcharles MA. A dramatic response to inhaled cannabis in a woman with central thalamic pain and dystonia. J Pain Symptom Manag. 2002;24(1):4–6.
211. Uribe Roca MC, Micheli F, Viotti R. Cannabis sativa and dystonia secondary to Wilson's disease. Mov Disord. 2005;20(1):113–5.
212. Scharf JM, Miller LL, Gauvin CA, Alabiso J, Mathews CA, Ben-Shlomo Y. Population prevalence of Tourette syndrome: a systematic review and meta-analysis. Mov Disord. 2015;30(2):221–8.
213. Jankovic J. Therapeutic developments for tics and myoclonus. Mov Disord. 2015;30(11):1566–73.
214. Kanaan AS, Jakubovski E, Muller-Vahl K. Significant tic reduction in an otherwise treatment-resistant patient with Gilles de la Tourette syndrome following treatment with nabiximols. Brain Sci. 2017;7(5):E47.
215. Pichler EM, Kawohl W, Seifritz E, Roser P. Pure delta-9-tetrahydrocannabinol and its combination with cannabidiol in treatment-resistant Tourette syndrome: a case report. Int J Psychiatry Med. 2019;54(2):150–6.
216. Trainor D, Evans L, Bird R. Severe motor and vocal tics controlled with Sativex(R). Australas Psychiatry. 2016;24(6):541–4.
217. Brunnauer A, Segmiller FM, Volkamer T, Laux G, Muller N, Dehning S. Cannabinoids improve driving ability in a Tourette's patient. Psychiatry Res. 2011;190(2–3):382.
218. Hemming M, Yellowlees PM. Effective treatment of Tourette's syndrome with marijuana. J Psychopharmacol. 1993;7(4):389–91.
219. Sandyk R, Awerbuch G. Marijuana and Tourette's syndrome. J Clin Psychopharmacol. 1988;8(6):444–5.
220. Hasan A, Rothenberger A, Munchau A, Wobrock T, Falkai P, Roessner V. Oral delta 9-tetrahydrocannabinol improved refractory Gilles de la Tourette syndrome in an adolescent by increasing intracortical inhibition: a case report. J Clin Psychopharmacol. 2010;30(2):190–2.
221. Emrich KRM-VUSHM. Combined treatment of Tourette syndrome with Δ9-THC and dopamine receptor antagonists. J Cannabis Ther. 2002;2(3–4):10.
222. Szejko N, Ewgeni J, Fremer C, Kunert K, Müller-Vahl K. Delta-9-tetrahydrocannabinol for the treatment of a child with Tourette syndrome: case report. EJMCR. 2018;2(2):3.
223. Szejko N, Jakubovski E, Fremer C, Müller-Vahl KR. Vaporized cannabis is effective and well-tolerated in an adolescent with Tourette syndrome. Med Cannabis Cannabinoid. 2019;2:4.
224. Muller-Vahl KR, Kolbe H, Schneider U, Emrich HM. Cannabinoids: possible role in patho-physiology and therapy of Gilles de la Tourette syndrome. Acta Psychiatr Scand. 1998;98(6):502–6.
225. Thaler A, Arad S, Schleider LB, Knaani J, Taichman T, Giladi N, et al. Single center experience with medical cannabis in Gilles de la Tourette syndrome. Parkinsonism Relat Disord. 2019;61:211–3.
226. Abi-Jaoude E, Chen L, Cheung P, Bhikram T, Sandor P. Preliminary evidence on cannabis effectiveness and tolerability for adults with Tourette syndrome. J Neuropsychiatry Clin Neurosci. 2017;29(4):391–400.
227. Muller-Vahl KR, Schneider U, Koblenz A, Jobges M, Kolbe H, Daldrup T, et al. Treatment of Tourette's syndrome with delta 9-tetrahydrocannabinol (THC): a randomized crossover trial. Pharmacopsychiatry. 2002;35(2):57–61.
228. Muller-Vahl KR, Schneider U, Prevedel H, Theloe K, Kolbe H, Daldrup T, et al. Delta 9-tetrahydrocannabinol (THC) is effective in the treatment of tics in Tourette syndrome: a 6-week randomized trial. J Clin Psychiatry. 2003;64(4):459–65.
229. Curtis A, Clarke CE, Rickards HE. Cannabinoids for Tourette's syndrome. Cochrane Database Syst Rev. 2009;(4):Cd006565.
230. Burggren AC, Shirazi A, Ginder N, London ED. Cannabis effects on brain structure, function, and cognition: considerations for medical uses of cannabis and its derivatives. Am J Drug Alcohol Abuse. 2019;45:1–17.

231. Lubman DI, Cheetham A, Yucel M. Cannabis and adolescent brain development. Pharmacol Ther. 2015;148:1–16.
232. Meruelo AD, Castro N, Cota CI, Tapert SF. Cannabis and alcohol use, and the developing brain. Behav Brain Res. 2017;325(Pt A):44–50.
233. Sutherland DP. Effect of marijuana on essential tremor: a case report [abstract]. Mov Disord. 2016;31(suppl 2). https://www.mdsabstracts.org/abstract/effect-of-marijuana-on-essential-tremor-a-case-report/.
234. Megelin T, Ghorayeb I. Cannabis for restless legs syndrome: a report of six patients. Sleep Med. 2017;36:182–3.
235. Sekar K, Pack A. Epidiolex as adjunct therapy for treatment of refractory epilepsy: a comprehensive review with a focus on adverse effects. F1000Res. 2019;8:F1000 Faculty Rev-234.
236. Ewing LE, Skinner CM, Quick CM, Kennon-McGill S, McGill MR, Walker LA, et al. Hepatotoxicity of a cannabidiol-rich cannabis extract in the mouse model. Molecules. 2019;24(9):E1694.
237. Gaston TE, Bebin EM, Cutter GR, Liu Y, Szaflarski JP. Interactions between cannabidiol and commonly used antiepileptic drugs. Epilepsia. 2017;58(9):1586–92.
238. Shah RR. Drug development and use in the elderly: search for the right dose and dosing regimen (parts I and II). Br J Clin Pharmacol. 2004;58(5):452–69.
239. Ujvary I, Hanus L. Human metabolites of cannabidiol: a review on their formation, biological activity, and relevance in therapy. Cannabis Cannabinoid Res. 2016;1(1):90–101.
240. Bergamaschi MM, Queiroz RH, Zuardi AW, Crippa JA. Safety and side effects of cannabidiol, a Cannabis sativa constituent. Curr Drug Saf. 2011;6(4):237–49.
241. Sandyk R, Snider SR, Consroe P, Elias SM. Cannabidiol in dystonic movement disorders. Psychiatry Res. 1986;18(3):291.
242. Muller-Vahl KR, Prevedel H, Theloe K, Kolbe H, Emrich HM, Schneider U. Treatment of Tourette syndrome with delta-9-tetrahydrocannabinol (delta 9-THC): no influence on neuropsychological performance. Neuropsychopharmacology. 2003;28(2):384–8.
243. Jakubovski E, Muller-Vahl K. Speechlessness in Gilles de la Tourette syndrome: cannabis-based medicines improve severe vocal blocking tics in two patients. Int J Mol Sci. 2017;18(8):E1739.
244. Muller-Vahl KR, Schneider U, Kolbe H, Emrich HM. Treatment of Tourette's syndrome with delta-9-tetrahydrocannabinol. Am J Psychiatry. 1999;156(3):495.

Cannabinoids in Neurosurgery

245. Stockings E, Zagic D, Campbell G, Weier M, Hall WD, Nielsen S, et al. Evidence for cannabis and cannabinoids for epilepsy: a systematic review of controlled and observational evidence. J Neurol Neurosurg Psychiatry. 2018;89(7):741–53.
246. Collin C, Ehler E, Waberzinek G, Alsindi Z, Davies P, Powell K, et al. A double-blind, randomized, placebo-controlled, parallel-group study of Sativex, in subjects with symptoms of spasticity due to multiple sclerosis. Neurol Res. 2010;32(5):451–9.
247. Zajicek J, Fox P, Sanders H, Wright D, Vickery J, Nunn A, et al. Cannabinoids for treatment of spasticity and other symptoms related to multiple sclerosis (CAMS study): multicentre randomised placebo-controlled trial. Lancet. 2003;362(9395):1517–26.
248. Boehnke KF, Gangopadhyay S, Clauw DJ, Haffajee RL. Qualifying conditions of medical cannabis license holders in the United States. Health Aff (Millwood). 2019;38(2):295–302.
249. Volkow ND, Baler RD, Compton WM, Weiss SR. Adverse health effects of marijuana use. N Engl J Med. 2014;370(23):2219–27.
250. Mandelbaum DE, de la Monte SM. Adverse structural and functional effects of marijuana on the brain: evidence reviewed. Pediatr Neurol. 2017;66:12–20.
251. Ilgen MA, Bohnert K, Kleinberg F, Jannausch M, Bohnert AS, Walton M, et al. Characteristics of adults seeking medical marijuana certification. Drug Alcohol Depend. 2013;132(3):654–9.

252. Light MK, Orens A, Lewandowski B, Pickton T. Market size and demand for marijuana in Colorado. http://www.cannabisconsumer.org/uploads/9/7/9/6/97962014/market_size_and_demand_study_july_9_2014[1].pdf.
253. Castillo PE, Younts TJ, Chavez AE, Hashimotodani Y. Endocannabinoid signaling and synaptic function. Neuron. 2012;76(1):70–81.
254. Mackie K. Distribution of cannabinoid receptors in the central and peripheral nervous system. Handb Exp Pharmacol. 2005;168:299–325.
255. Klein TW, Newton CA. Therapeutic potential of cannabinoid-based drugs. Adv Exp Med Biol. 2007;601:395–413.
256. Hauser W, Welsch P, Klose P, Radbruch L, Fitzcharles MA. Efficacy, tolerability and safety of cannabis-based medicines for cancer pain: a systematic review with meta-analysis of randomised controlled trials. Schmerz. 2019;33:424.
257. Medicine TNAoSa. The health effects on cannabis and cannabinoids. Washington, D.C.: National Academies Press; 2017. ISBN: 978-0-309-45304-2.
258. Stockings E, Campbell G, Hall WD, Nielsen S, Zagic D, Rahman R, et al. Cannabis and cannabinoids for the treatment of people with chronic noncancer pain conditions: a systematic review and meta-analysis of controlled and observational studies. Pain. 2018;159(10):1932–54.
259. Haroutounian S, Ratz Y, Ginosar Y, Furmanov K, Saifi F, Meidan R, et al. The effect of medicinal cannabis on pain and quality-of-life outcomes in chronic pain: a prospective open-label study. Clin J Pain. 2016;32(12):1036–43.
260. Yassin M, Robinson D. Effect of medicinal cannabis therapy (MCT) on severity of chronic low back pain, sciatica and lumbar range of motion. Int J Anesth Pain Med. 2016;2(1:5)1–4.
261. Mondello E, Quattrone D, Cardia L, Bova G, Mallamace R, Barbagallo AA, et al. Cannabinoids and spinal cord stimulation for the treatment of failed back surgery syndrome refractory pain. J Pain Res. 2018;11:1761–7.
262. Pinsger M, Schimetta W, Volc D, Hiermann E, Riederer F, Polz W. Benefits of an add-on treatment with the synthetic cannabinomimetic nabilone on patients with chronic pain--a randomized controlled trial. Wien Klin Wochenschr. 2006;118(11–12):327–35.
263. Buynak R, Shapiro DY, Okamoto A, Van Hove I, Rauschkolb C, Steup A, et al. Efficacy and safety of tapentadol extended release for the management of chronic low back pain: results of a prospective, randomized, double-blind, placebo- and active-controlled phase III study. Expert Opin Pharmacother. 2010;11(11):1787–804.
264. Eriksen J, Jensen MK, Sjogren P, Ekholm O, Rasmussen NK. Epidemiology of chronic nonmalignant pain in Denmark. Pain. 2003;106(3):221–8.
265. Jamison RN, Raymond SA, Slawsby EA, Nedeljkovic SS, Katz NP. Opioid therapy for chronic noncancer back pain. A randomized prospective study. Spine. 1998;23(23):2591–600.
266. Vorsanger GJ, Xiang J, Gana TJ, Pascual ML, Fleming RR. Extended-release tramadol (tramadol ER) in the treatment of chronic low back pain. J Opioid Manag. 2008;4(2):87–97.
267. Liu CW, Bhatia A, Buzon-Tan A, Walker S, Ilangomaran D, Kara J, et al. Weeding out the problem: the impact of preoperative cannabinoid use on pain in the perioperative period. Anesth Analg. 2019;129(3):874–81.
268. Salottolo K, Peck L, Tanner Ii A, Carrick MM, Madayag R, McGuire E, et al. The grass is not always greener: a multi-institutional pilot study of marijuana use and acute pain management following traumatic injury. Patient Saf Surg. 2018;12:16.
269. Twardowski MA, Link MM, Twardowski NM. Effects of cannabis use on sedation requirements for endoscopic procedures. J Am Osteopath Assoc. 2019;119:307–11.
270. Bradford AC, Bradford WD. Medical marijuana laws reduce prescription medication use in medicare part D. Health Aff (Millwood). 2016;35(7):1230–6.
271. Boehnke KF, Scott JR, Litinas E, Sisley S, Williams DA, Clauw DJ. Pills to pot: observational analyses of cannabis substitution among medical cannabis users with chronic pain. J Pain. 2019;20:830.

272. Boehnke KF, Litinas E, Clauw DJ. Medical cannabis use is associated with decreased opiate medication use in a retrospective cross-sectional survey of patients with chronic pain. J Pain. 2016;17(6):739–44.

273. Bachhuber MA, Saloner B, Cunningham CO, Barry CL. Medical cannabis laws and opioid analgesic overdose mortality in the United States, 1999-2010. JAMA Intern Med. 2014;174(10):1668–73.

274. Shover CL, Davis CS, Gordon SC, Humphreys K. Association between medical cannabis laws and opioid overdose mortality has reversed over time. Proc Natl Acad Sci U S A. 2019;116(26):12624–6.

275. Corchero J, Manzanares J, Fuentes JA. Cannabinoid/opioid crosstalk in the central nervous system. Crit Rev Neurobiol. 2004;16(1–2):159–72.

276. Hauser W, Finn DP, Kalso E, Krcevski-Skvarc N, Kress HG, Morlion B, et al. European pain federation (EFIC) position paper on appropriate use of cannabis-based medicines and medical cannabis for chronic pain management. Eur J Pain. 2018;22(9):1547–64.

277. Allan GM, Ramji J, Perry D, Ton J, Beahm NP, Crisp N, et al. Simplified guideline for prescribing medical cannabinoids in primary care. Can Fam Physician. 2018;64(2):111–20.

278. Bachhuber MA, Arnsten JH, Cunningham CO, Sohler N. Does medical cannabis use increase or decrease the use of opioid analgesics and other prescription drugs? J Addict Med. 2018;12(4):259–61.

279. Olfson M, Wall MM, Liu SM, Blanco C. Cannabis use and risk of prescription opioid use disorder in the United States. Am J Psychiatry. 2018;175(1):47–53.

280. Rocha FC, Dos Santos Junior JG, Stefano SC, da Silveira DX. Systematic review of the literature on clinical and experimental trials on the antitumor effects of cannabinoids in gliomas. J Neuro-Oncol. 2014;116(1):11–24.

281. Bar-Lev Schleider L, Mechoulam R, Lederman V, Hilou M, Lencovsky O, Betzalel O, et al. Prospective analysis of safety and efficacy of medical cannabis in large unselected population of patients with cancer. Eur J Intern Med. 2018;49:37–43.

282. Guzman M, Duarte MJ, Blazquez C, Ravina J, Rosa MC, Galve-Roperh I, et al. A pilot clinical study of Delta9-tetrahydrocannabinol in patients with recurrent glioblastoma multiforme. Br J Cancer. 2006;95(2):197–203.

283. van Linde ME, Brahm CG, de Witt Hamer PC, Reijneveld JC, Bruynzeel AME, Vandertop WP, et al. Treatment outcome of patients with recurrent glioblastoma multiforme: a retrospective multicenter analysis. J Neuro-Oncol. 2017;135(1):183–92.

284. Short SC, Little C. A 2-part safety and exploratory efficacy randomized double-blind, placebo-controlled study of a 1:1 ratio of the cannabinoids cannabidiol and delta-9-tetrahydrocannabinol (CBD;THC) plus dose-intense temozolomide (TMZ) in patients with recurrent glioblastoma multiforme (GBM). Society for Neuro-Oncology 22nd Annual Scientific Meeting, 16–19 November 2017, San Francisco, USA, 2017.

285. Efird JT, Friedman GD, Sidney S, Klatsky A, Habel LA, Udaltsova NV, et al. The risk for malignant primary adult-onset glioma in a large, multiethnic, managed-care cohort: cigarette smoking and other lifestyle behaviors. J Neuro-Oncol. 2004;68(1):57–69.

286. Kuijten RR, Bunin GR, Nass CC, Meadows AT. Gestational and familial risk factors for childhood astrocytoma: results of a case-control study. Cancer Res. 1990;50(9):2608–12.

287. Arevalo-Martin A, Molina-Holgado E, Garcia-Ovejero D. Cannabinoids to treat spinal cord injury. Prog Neuro-Psychopharmacol Biol Psychiatry. 2016;64:190–9.

288. Wilsey BL, Deutsch R, Samara E, Marcotte TD, Barnes AJ, Huestis MA, et al. A preliminary evaluation of the relationship of cannabinoid blood concentrations with the analgesic response to vaporized cannabis. J Pain Res. 2016;9:587–98.

289. Rintala DH, Fiess RN, Tan G, Holmes SA, Bruel BM. Effect of dronabinol on central neuropathic pain after spinal cord injury: a pilot study. Am J Phys Med Rehabil. 2010;89(10):840–8.

290. Cardenas DD, Jensen MP. Treatments for chronic pain in persons with spinal cord injury: a survey study. J Spinal Cord Med. 2006;29(2):109–17.

291. Hagenbach U, Luz S, Ghafoor N, Berger JM, Grotenhermen F, Brenneisen R, et al. The treatment of spasticity with Delta9-tetrahydrocannabinol in persons with spinal cord injury. Spinal Cord. 2007;45(8):551–62.

292. Pooyania S, Ethans K, Szturm T, Casey A, Perry D. A randomized, double-blinded, crossover pilot study assessing the effect of nabilone on spasticity in persons with spinal cord injury. Arch Phys Med Rehabil. 2010;91(5):703–7.

293. Fernandez-Ruiz J, Moro MA, Martinez-Orgado J. Cannabinoids in neurodegenerative disorders and stroke/brain trauma: from preclinical models to clinical applications. Neurotherapeutics. 2015;12(4):793–806.

294. Castillo A, Tolon MR, Fernandez-Ruiz J, Romero J, Martinez-Orgado J. The neuroprotective effect of cannabidiol in an in vitro model of newborn hypoxic-ischemic brain damage in mice is mediated by CB(2) and adenosine receptors. Neurobiol Dis. 2010;37(2):434–40.

295. Shohami E, Cohen-Yeshurun A, Magid L, Algali M, Mechoulam R. Endocannabinoids and traumatic brain injury. Br J Pharmacol. 2011;163(7):1402–10.

296. Ilie G, Adlaf EM, Mann RE, Ialomiteanu A, Hamilton H, Rehm J, et al. Associations between a history of traumatic brain injuries and current cigarette smoking, substance use, and elevated psychological distress in a population sample of Canadian adults. J Neurotrauma. 2015;32(14):1130–4.

297. Nguyen BM, Kim D, Bricker S, Bongard F, Neville A, Putnam B, et al. Effect of marijuana use on outcomes in traumatic brain injury. Am Surg. 2014;80(10):979–83.

298. Maas AI, Murray G, Henney H 3rd, Kassem N, Legrand V, Mangelus M, et al. Efficacy and safety of dexanabinol in severe traumatic brain injury: results of a phase III randomised, placebo-controlled, clinical trial. Lancet Neurol. 2006;5(1):38–45.

299. Hillard CJ. Endocannabinoids and vascular function. J Pharmacol Exp Ther. 2000;294(1):27–32.

300. Scharf EL. Translating endocannabinoid biology into clinical practice: cannabidiol for stroke prevention. Cannabis Cannabinoid Res. 2017;2(1):259–64.

301. Zachariah SB. Stroke after heavy marijuana smoking. Stroke. 1991;22(3):406–9.

302. Mateo I, Pinedo A, Gomez-Beldarrain M, Basterretxea JM, Garcia-Monco JC. Recurrent stroke associated with cannabis use. J Neurol Neurosurg Psychiatry. 2005;76(3):435–7.

303. Duchene C, Olindo S, Chausson N, Jeannin S, Cohen-Tenoudji P, Smadja D. Cannabis-induced cerebral and myocardial infarction in a young woman. Rev Neurol (Paris). 2010;166(4):438–42.

304. Bal S, Khurana D, Lal V, Prabhakar S. Posterior circulation stroke in a cannabis abuser. Neurol India. 2009;57(1):91–2.

305. Singh NN, Pan Y, Muengtaweeponsa S, Geller TJ, Cruz-Flores S. Cannabis-related stroke: case series and review of literature. J Stroke Cerebrovasc Dis. 2012;21(7):555–60.

306. Wolff V, Lauer V, Rouyer O, Sellal F, Meyer N, Raul JS, et al. Cannabis use, ischemic stroke, and multifocal intracranial vasoconstriction: a prospective study in 48 consecutive young patients. Stroke. 2011;42(6):1778–80.

307. Barber PA, Pridmore HM, Krishnamurthy V, Roberts S, Spriggs DA, Carter KN, et al. Cannabis, ischemic stroke, and transient ischemic attack: a case-control study. Stroke. 2013;44(8):2327–9.

308. Rumalla K, Reddy AY, Mittal MK. Recreational marijuana use and acute ischemic stroke: a population-based analysis of hospitalized patients in the United States. J Neurol Sci. 2016;364:191–6.

309. Westover AN, McBride S, Haley RW. Stroke in young adults who abuse amphetamines or cocaine: a population-based study of hospitalized patients. Arch Gen Psychiatry. 2007;64(4):495–502.

310. Zarruk JG, Fernandez-Lopez D, Garcia-Yebenes I, Garcia-Gutierrez MS, Vivancos J, Nombela F, et al. Cannabinoid type 2 receptor activation downregulates stroke-induced classic and alternative brain macrophage/microglial activation concomitant to neuroprotection. Stroke. 2012;43(1):211–9.

311. Hampson AJ, Grimaldi M, Axelrod J, Wink D. Cannabidiol and (−)Delta9-tetrahydrocannabinol are neuroprotective antioxidants. Proc Natl Acad Sci U S A. 1998;95(14):8268–73.
312. Ducros A, Boukobza M, Porcher R, Sarov M, Valade D, Bousser MG. The clinical and radiological spectrum of reversible cerebral vasoconstriction syndrome. A prospective series of 67 patients. Brain. 2007;130(Pt 12):3091–101.
313. Wolff V, Schlagowski AI, Rouyer O, Charles AL, Singh F, Auger C, et al. Tetrahydrocannabinol induces brain mitochondrial respiratory chain dysfunction and increases oxidative stress: a potential mechanism involved in cannabis-related stroke. Biomed Res Int. 2015;2015:323706.
314. Wolff V, Armspach JP, Beaujeux R, Manisor M, Rouyer O, Lauer V, et al. High frequency of intracranial arterial stenosis and cannabis use in ischaemic stroke in the young. Cerebrovasc Dis. 2014;37(6):438–43.
315. Herning RI, Better WE, Tate K, Cadet JL. Cerebrovascular perfusion in marijuana users during a month of monitored abstinence. Neurology. 2005;64(3):488–93.
316. Behrouz R, Birnbaum L, Grandhi R, Johnson J, Misra V, Palacio S, et al. Cannabis use and outcomes in patients with aneurysmal subarachnoid hemorrhage. Stroke. 2016;47(5):1371–3.
317. Malhotra K, Rumalla K, Mittal MK. Association and clinical outcomes of marijuana in patients with intracerebral hemorrhage. J Stroke Cerebrovasc Dis. 2018;27(12):3479–86.
318. Rumalla K, Reddy AY, Mittal MK. Association of recreational marijuana use with aneurysmal subarachnoid hemorrhage. J Stroke Cerebrovasc Dis. 2016;25(2):452–60.
319. Di Napoli M, Zha AM, Godoy DA, Masotti L, Schreuder FH, Popa-Wagner A, et al. Prior cannabis use is associated with outcome after intracerebral hemorrhage. Cerebrovasc Dis. 2016;41(5–6):248–55.
320. Uhegwu N, Bashir A, Hussain M, Dababneh H, Misthal S, Cohen-Gadol A. Marijuana induced reversible cerebral vasoconstriction syndrome. J Vasc Interv Neurol. 2015;8(1):36–8.
321. Maroon J, Bost J. Review of the neurological benefits of phytocannabinoids. Surg Neurol Int. 2018;9:91.

Chapter 11
Ocular Conditions and the Endocannabinoid System

Finny T. John and Jean R. Hausheer

Patients commonly ask about the use of marijuana for treatment of glaucoma, especially in the setting of increasing legalization across the United States and Canada. Currently in the United States, there are 33 states in addition to the District of Columbia, Guam, and Puerto Rico that have legalized either medical, recreational, or both uses of marijuana, while Canada has federally legalized the use of this substance.

The ocular endocannabinoid system has become a point of active research for its involvement in three separate functions within the ocular system: intraocular pressure (IOP) control, visual processing, and inflammatory regulation. Marijuana clinical trials in the United States remain limited in large part because of current Schedule I classification, defined as "no medical indication but high abuse potential," but also because of its relatively short duration of action, high cost, ocular irritation with topical (eye drop) routes of administration, and general health risks and side effects [1]. Scientific references to the effect of marijuana on the ocular system have stemmed from 1971 and extend to present day.

Glaucoma describes a complex disease that is characterized by progressive damage of the optic nerve over time, constriction of peripheral visual fields, and irreversible blindness if left untreated (Figs. 11.1 and 11.2).

Glaucoma affects approximately 3 million Americans and more than 60 million people worldwide. Its most common form is primary open-angle glaucoma (POAG), which is a slowly progressive disorder that destroys cells in the nerve fiber layer of the retina and results in an enlarged cup-to-disc ratio of the optic nerve (Figs. 11.3 and 11.4).

F. T. John
Department of Ophthalmology, University of Oklahoma Health Sciences Center,
Dean McGee Eye Institute, Oklahoma City, OK, USA

J. R. Hausheer (✉)
Department of Ophthalmology, University of Oklahoma Health Sciences Center,
Dean McGee Eye Institute, Lawton, OK, USA

© Springer Nature Switzerland AG 2020
K. Finn (ed.), *Cannabis in Medicine*,
https://doi.org/10.1007/978-3-030-45968-0_11

Less common forms of glaucoma include narrow or closed-angle, normal tension, pigmentary, pseudoexfoliative, traumatic, uveitic, neovascular, congenital, and other secondary forms. Gonioscopy using a contact lens with a reflecting mirror or prism during slit lamp examination can provide some information about the anatomical angle between the cornea and iris, which can help narrow the potential causes of a patient's glaucoma (Fig. 11.5).

The loss of nerve fiber layer cells is manifested initially as diminished or absent peripheral vision but can ultimately result in complete loss of central vision. Researchers have not yet identified all of the triggers linked with POAG but have

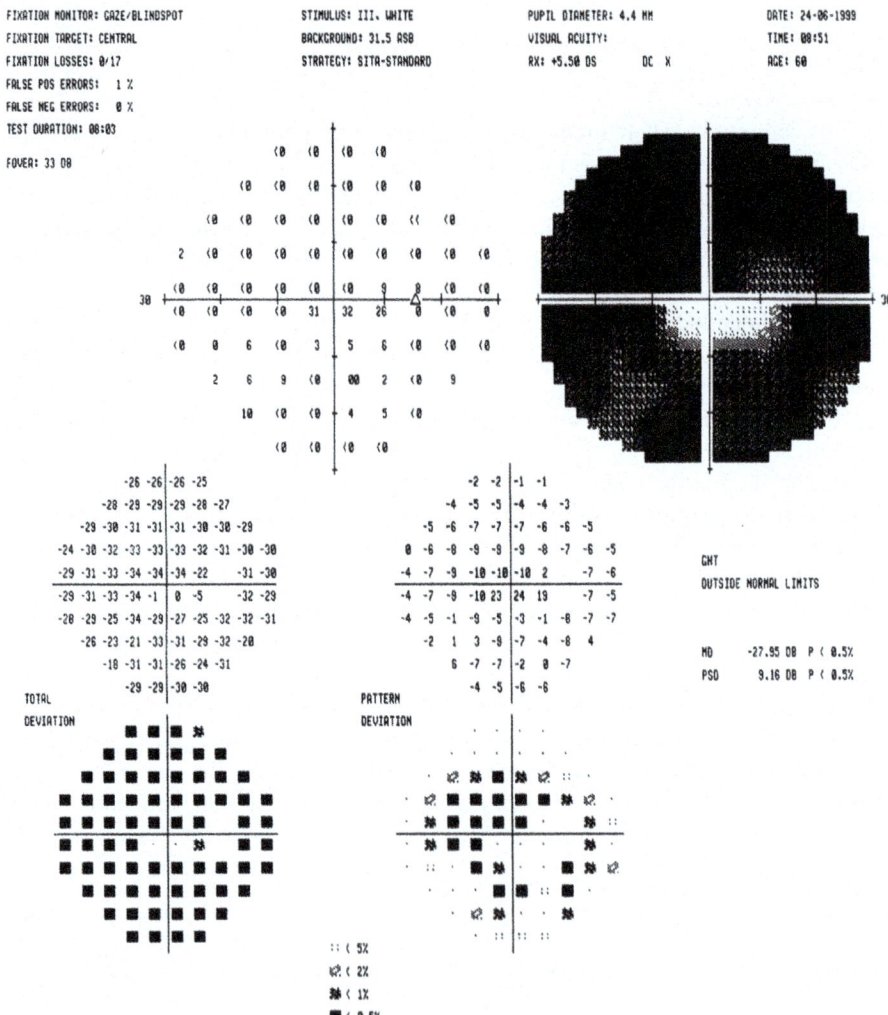

Figs. 11.1 and 11.2 Humphrey visual field 24-2 testing in a patient with severe glaucoma, with dense peripheral constriction and defects approaching central fixation point [2]

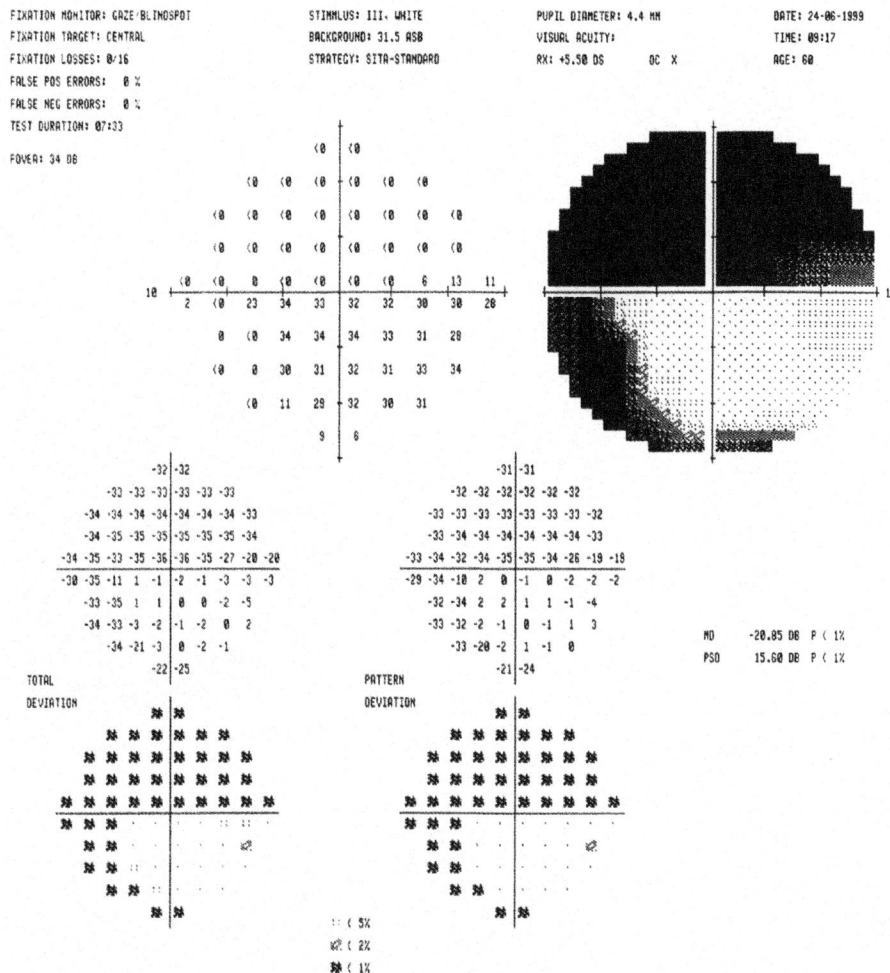

Fig. 11.1 and 11.2   (continued)

found multiple factors that put individuals at risk for development of the disease. These factors include older age, African American race, positive family history, decreased central corneal thickness, increased vertical cup-to-disc ratios of the optic nerve, and elevated IOP. Of these, the only modifiable risk factor is IOP, which is the target of modern-day glaucoma therapy.

Intraocular pressure is a function of the production and drainage of aqueous humor within the ocular system. Aqueous humor is produced by the ciliary body, a highly metabolically active structure that sits posterior to the iris, and it is formed primarily by active secretion but also through diffusion and ultrafiltration. This fluid travels through the posterior chamber, moves anteriorly through the pupil, and exits the eye via trabecular meshwork or uveoscleral outflow pathways (Fig. 11.6).

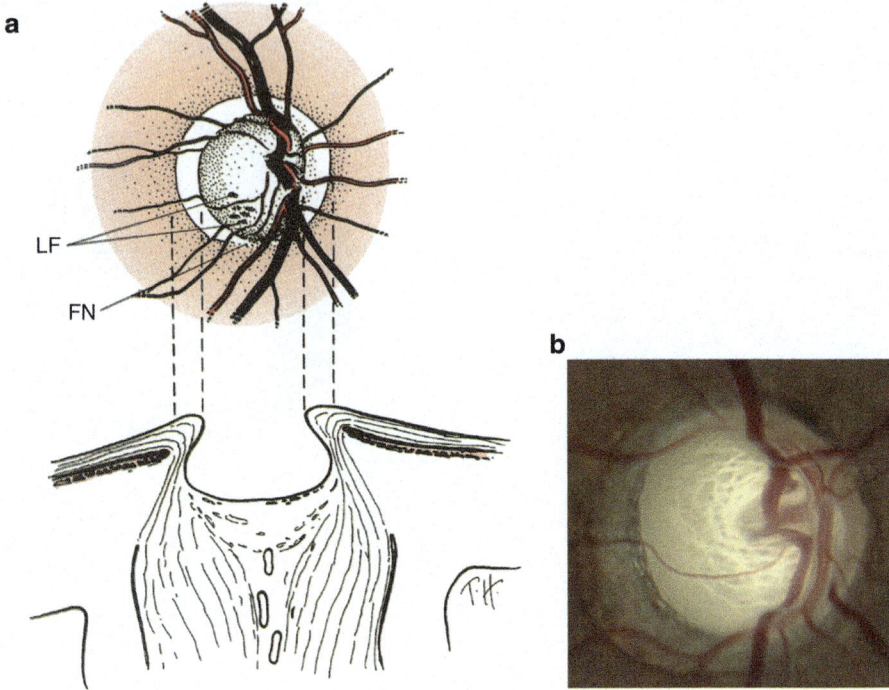

Fig. 11.3 (**a**) Representative diagram of the thinning of the nerve fiber layer and deepening of the optic nerve cup. (**b**) Glaucoma-related enlarged cup-to-disc ratio of the nerve, with nasalization of central vasculature [3]

Fig. 11.4 Enlarged cup-to-disc ratio of the optic nerve secondary to long-standing glaucoma. Note significant thinning of upper and lower aspects of optic nerve [4]

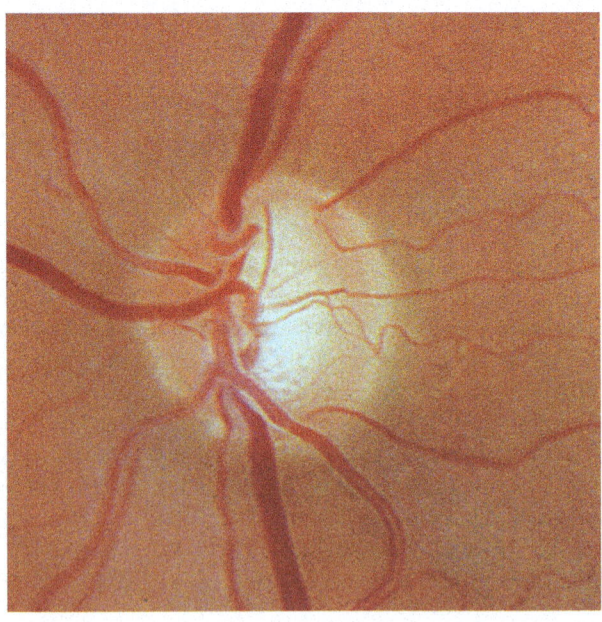

Fig. 11.5 Gonioscopic evaluation reveals angle structures, which is helpful in identifying etiology or classifying type of glaucoma [5]

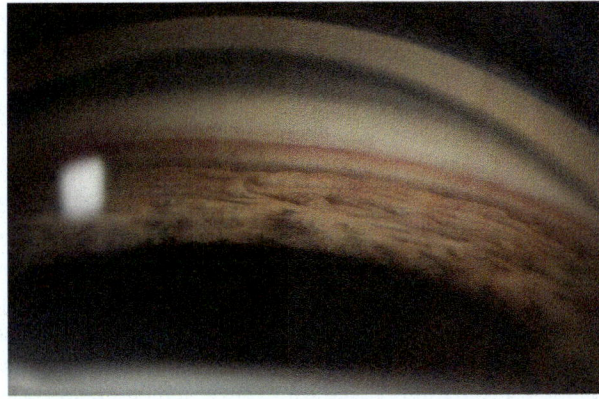

Fig. 11.6 Schematic diagram of aqueous production and outflow pathways within the human eye. Red arrow denotes the trabecular meshwork outflow pathway, while green arrow denotes the uveoscleral outflow pathway [6]

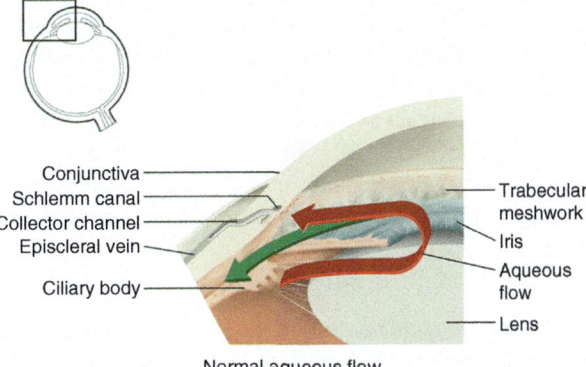

When there is excessive aqueous humor production or insufficient drainage, the IOP will rise. While the relationship between elevated IOP and glaucomatous optic nerve damage is well-supported by research, the exact causative mechanism is unclear.

Effective treatment of glaucoma, achieved with oral medication or topical eye drops, laser, or surgery, classically translates to sustained, continuous control of IOP. Oral carbonic anhydrase inhibitors or topical ocular antihypertensive drops are affordable solutions that are dosed once or twice a day and alter IOP by acting at different sites of the aqueous humor formation and drainage pathways. The mechanisms are well-described in other resources and are beyond the scope of this chapter. If IOP remains uncontrolled or if the patient does not tolerate oral or topical therapy because of systemic side effects, an ophthalmologist may offer laser therapy targeting the trabecular meshwork to increase aqueous humor outflow. Alternatively, there are surgical options for controlling elevated eye pressure, which include the use of drainage tube implants, scleral flaps, or, more recently, implantation of devices made of heparin-coated titanium and other materials to safely shunt fluid away from the anterior chamber toward other regions of the eye. If none of the above achieves sufficient IOP control and there is evidence of disease progression, the ciliary body epithelium can be destroyed with laser or cryotherapy to reduce aqueous humor production.

Despite these efficacious treatment options, there has been increasing public interest to find alternative, natural remedies to treat glaucoma, as well as other ocular diseases. The plant *Cannabis sativa*, from which marijuana is derived, has long been recognized to have medicinal properties [7]. In 1964, the active component of marijuana, delta 9-tetrahydrocannabinol (THC), was isolated and defined structurally [8]. The cannabis plant contains more than 100 unique chemical components classified as cannabinoids. These ingredients actively bind to specific endocannabinoid receptors in the brain and many other organs of the body, including the eye. Of note, the two most prevalent components of the cannabis plant are delta-9-tetrahydrocannabinol (THC), which creates a psychotropic effect in users, and cannabidiol (CBD), which has minimal psychotropic influence.

There are numerous ongoing studies to evaluate the efficacy of endocannabinoid (ECB)-based therapeutics for treatment of glaucoma, as well as other ophthalmic diseases including uveitis, ischemic retinal disease, diabetic retinopathy, and age-related macular degeneration. At a molecular level, endocannabinoids are endogenous lipids that act as neuromodulators targeting the same receptors within the body that bind THC and CBD. Endocannabinoids are different than other neuromodulators in that they are not synthesized in advance and stored in vesicles, but rather exist in cell membranes and are cleaved by specific enzymes on an as-needed basis [9].

The human ECB system has three major components:

- ECB *molecules* such as 2-arachidonoylglycerol (2-AG), anandamide (N-arachidonoyl ethanolamine) (AEA), and N-palmitylethanolamide (PEA)
- Classical and nonclassical *receptors* such as CB1 and CB2, GPR18, GPR55, TRPV1, and PPAR alpha/beta/gamma
- *Enzymes* that synthesize and degrade ECBs such as diacylglycerol lipase (DGL), fatty acid amide hydrolase (FAAH), and many others [10]

The concentration of ECB receptors varies by the specific structure of the eye. For example, the retina and trabecular meshwork each contain many more receptors than the crystalline lens [11].

A recent study published by a group at Indiana University looked specifically at two cannabinoids found in marijuana, CBD and THC (materials supplied by the National Institute on Drug Abuse drug supply program, dissolved in Tocrisolve™ solvent), and their effects on IOP [12]. The researchers found that a single topical CBD (5 mM) eye drop in mice *increased* IOP by 18 percent for at least 4 hours after administration compared to mice treated with the vehicle in the contralateral eye. This effect disappeared if the CB1 receptor was knocked out prior to drop use. This finding implicates the CB1 receptor as a key target for these molecules. On the contrary, the group also found that a single topical THC (5 mM) eye drop *decreased* eye pressure by up to 30 percent within 8 hours. Interestingly, THC drops affected IOP differently in male and female rats, with males having a much larger decline in pressures secondary to THC compared to females. These results highlight that the IOP effects of THC and CBD may counteract one another in a complex mechanism, with a biologic variable potentially involved as well. Ultimately, this study shows that additional research is necessary to further understand the effects of these compounds on IOP (including translational research in human beings, using well-tolerated formulations) and that marijuana cannot be safely or reliably used as monotherapy for diseases like glaucoma.

A review of current literature reveals that many synthetic cannabinoids, which bind to CB1 receptors similar to THC or CBD, are being studied for their effects on various aspects of the ocular system. Specifically, IOP can be reduced by synthetic aminoalkylindoles (e.g., WIN 55212-2) via a mechanism similar to topical beta blockers that are used for glaucoma, but without a sustained effect [10, 13]. Additionally, studies have shown that CB1 agonists appear to have a neuroprotective effect on retinal ganglion cells in ischemia-reperfusion settings, with the co-administration of CB1 antagonists blunting this beneficial effect. Nevertheless, the potency or duration of effect remains unspecified [10].

Recent studies have also shown CB2 receptor agonists temper inflammation within the eye, as is commonly seen with disease states like anterior, intermediate, and posterior uveitis. Specifically, studies have shown that these molecules decrease inflammatory cell infiltration in the retina, reducing overall cellular infiltrates and granulomas in a dose-dependent manner [14]. Toguri et al. (2014) similarly demonstrated that the topical CB2 receptor synthetic agonist, HU-308 (dissolved in Tocrisolve solvent for topical application at 1.5%), reduces leukocyte-endothelial adhesions within iridal microcirculation of rats, dampening inflammation more significantly than comparable treatments (e.g., topical steroids or nonsteroidal anti-inflammatory medications) [15]. This effect was dampened with the co-administration of CB2 receptor antagonist, AM630, administered by intravenous route. These findings suggest a role for the CB2 receptor pathway in moderating intraocular inflammation.

Studies have also demonstrated potential therapeutic benefits of CB1 and CB2 receptor agonists on corneal nociceptors causing pain in acute corneal pathology, such as alkali burns. Yang et al. showed that receptor activation by synthetic cannabinoids like WIN 55212-2 appears to stimulate corneal wound healing and stromal thickening at a more rapid rate [16]. Furthermore, the study showed that CB1 −/− mice had more significant CD11b staining, consistent with upregulated monocyte and neutrophil stromal infiltration associated with increased corneal fibrosis compared to WT mice, suggesting the necessity of the ECB system for this healing process without overactivation of the innate immune response. On an unrelated note, disease states like diabetic retinopathy and age-related macular degeneration are associated with lower levels of ECB-degrading enzymes, suggesting a role for the ECB system in the pathophysiology of these blinding conditions [10].

Finally, in 2007, the oral synthetic cannabinoid, dronabinol (7.5 mg Marinol, Unimed Pharmaceuticals, Chicago, IL, USA), was studied in its effects on lowering IOP as well as influencing retinal hemodynamics [17]. Eight healthy medical doctors underwent IOP testing, blood pressure measurement, and fluorescein angiography with scanning laser ophthalmoscopy before and 2 hours after ingestion of the substance. There was a statistically significant decrease in IOP (13.2 to 11.8 mmHg, $p = 0.038$) as well as a reduction in retinal arteriovenous passage time (on average, 1.77–1.57 seconds, $p = 0.028$), without a significant effect on blood pressure or heart rate. The researchers concluded that dronabinol could be potentially useful in ocular circulatory disorders including glaucoma, where decreased retinal circulation is often noted. On the contrary, in a study published in 1978, researchers found that this same substance increased blood flow through the iris, ciliary body, and choroid, but not the retina in rabbits [18].

While these may be interesting discoveries in various animal models, there remains a large gap between our understanding of the ocular endocannabinoid system and the implementation of ECB-based therapy to successfully treat human ophthalmic disease. Furthermore, there is a large difference between the purified, synthetic agonists used in these studies and dispensary cannabis ingested by patients who are intending to self-treat ophthalmic disease, the latter of which often contains over 480 chemicals including at least 66 cannabinoids that can vary greatly in concentrations and safety profiles depending on the source [19]. The lack of consistency counters the requirements of regulatory bodies like the FDA with regard to standardized and accepted treatment options for human disease. Future research will likely be directed toward identifying biased agonists or allosteric modulators with increased receptor affinity that can decrease the required drug dose necessary to treat disease, as well as isolating inhibitors of ECB-degrading enzymes. This could potentially increase duration of drug effect while reducing behavioral and systemic side effects associated with marijuana use. Future research must also transform from animal models into more reliable human clinical trials before any ECB-based therapies could be safely recommended for patients with glaucoma and other ocular disease.

Proponents of marijuana use for glaucoma treatment cite a study from the early 1970s, where Hepler and Frank showed both marijuana and one of its ingredients, THC, could reduce IOP [20]. Over the years, other studies have confirmed the IOP-lowering effect of THC by various modes of administration including inhalational [21], oral [22], intravenous [23], sublingual [24], and topical routes [25].

However, in order to achieve therapeutic levels of marijuana in the bloodstream to treat glaucoma, an individual would need to smoke approximately six to eight times a day [26]. At this frequency, an individual would likely be physically and mentally unable to perform tasks requiring attention and focus (e.g., studying, working, driving). This dosing frequency could be even higher with the pharmacologic tolerance that a patient would develop with chronic use of this substance [27, 28]. Studies also indicate a direct relationship between drug concentration and decrease in IOP from baseline; higher concentrations result in greater reductions in pressure. This would translate to reliance on extremely potent forms of marijuana for adequate treatment of disease. These studies did not find a relationship between potency and duration of effect, so one may still need to smoke every 3–4 hours around the clock, regardless of the substance potency, to achieve any purported therapeutic effect [19].

Oral and sublingual consumption is associated with variable systemic absorption as well as poorly tolerated global side effects [22, 26]. Given this, the topical eye drop approach would appear to be an optimal route of administration. However, delta-9-tetrahydrocannabinol (THC) has been investigated in the form of topical application, and these forms were found to be less effective compared to inhalational, oral, or intravenous marijuana [29]. This is may be because ocular penetration with THC compounds is poor due to the highly lipophilic and poorly hydrophilic nature of the cannabinoid extracts. Furthermore, these substances commonly create intolerable ocular irritation, conjunctival hyperemia, decreased lacrimation, and corneal damage [29]. Overall, several studies have failed to demonstrate a substantial hypotensive effect of topical THC within the eye [29, 30].

The American Glaucoma Society position statement in 2010 declared that there is no scientific basis for the use of marijuana in the treatment of glaucoma "unless a well-tolerated formulation…with a much longer duration of action is shown in rigorous clinical testing to reduce damage to the optic nerve and preserve vision." In addition to marijuana failing to achieve sustained IOP-lowering effects, the organization notes that the drug is associated with tachycardia and systemic hypotension, a potentially devastating effect on a glaucomatous optic nerve that may already have inadequate blood supply [26, 31]. While the organization expresses optimism that a locally administered, well-tolerated drug targeting the ocular ECB system can potentially augment IOP control, it expressly disavows the use of marijuana in any form as a primary or sole treatment for glaucoma.

The American Academy of Ophthalmology issued statements in 2009 and 2014, from their Complementary Therapy Task Force, stating that "no scientific evidence has been found that [marijuana] demonstrates increased benefit or diminished risk in the treatment of glaucoma compared with the wide variety of pharmaceutical agents now available" [32]. Similarly, in 2010, the Canadian Ophthalmological Society of Eye Physicians and Surgeons stated it "does not support the medical use of marijuana for the treatment of glaucoma due to the short duration of action, the incidence of undesirable psychotropic and other systemic side effects and the absence of scientific evidence showing a beneficial effect on the course of the disease. This is in contrast to other more effective and less harmful medical, laser, and surgical modalities for the treatment of glaucoma" [33]. In November 2018, the Canadian Ophthalmological Society issued another position statement discouraging medical use of cannabis for dry eye disease, "due to its undesirable side-effects, including dry eye symptoms if smoked, and the absence of scientific evidence showing any beneficial effect at this time" [34].

Navigating the complex and intricate web of factors that influence public perception with respect to glaucoma and medical marijuana will require an equally intricate patient-centered approach if physicians who treat glaucoma patients are to effectively address false perceptions and transcend the clash between scientific evidence and truth versus popular culture [35]. This undeniable clash places unprecedented importance on considering the patient perspective. It is not enough to simply detect patient misconceptions on the topic of marijuana and glaucoma. We must mold our practices to correct these errors in understanding using a patient-centered compassionate and evidence-based approach.

In 2015, Belyea and colleagues published a study that investigated the attitudes of glaucoma patients in Washington, DC toward the legality of marijuana and its use as a potential treatment agent [36]. This study was performed in the context of legalization of the drug in the city as well as 21 other states for medicinal purposes. Approximately 59.8% of study participants (122 of 204) reported awareness about the potential use of marijuana to treat glaucoma. The authors identified that the following factors contribute to patient intention to use marijuana for treatment of their glaucoma: younger age, lower level of education, and prior marijuana use. Newer factors contributing to this decision now include increasing legalization of marijuana, false beliefs regarding marijuana's efficacy in glaucoma treatment, and disregard for the associated costs to purchase and use the drug. The authors stressed that the best way to alter these perspectives is to place greater emphasis on evidence-based reasoning and to offer a thorough explanation of FDA-approved glaucoma therapies.

Interestingly, Belyea et al. found that patient satisfaction with current glaucoma management options was dependent on a combination of personal, cultural, socioeconomic, and health-related factors that were all superimposed on past experiences with healthcare services. In their study, the physician's ability to convey respect and empathy for patient needs and values, engagement of family members, and capacity to provide emotional support alongside high-quality, easy-to-comprehend educational materials were the key ingredients to improved patient-centered care and outcomes.

Perhaps this is a reminder for physicians to sit down and spend greater time with each of our patients and their family members in our clinics, listen more attentively, and care more deeply about their concerns regarding their ocular health. This will establish a greater degree of trust in the physician-patient relationship as we move forward together toward newer treatment options and scientific discoveries.

Key Points
- The clinical utility of marijuana for the treatment of glaucoma and other ocular diseases is limited by the short duration of effect on intraocular pressures, propensity for tolerance, and inability to separate reproducible therapeutic action and benefit from the undesirable physical, neuropsychological, and behavioral effects of the drug.
- Delta-9-tetrahydrocannabinol (THC) appears to lower intraocular pressure, but recent studies show cannabidiol (CBD) may increase intraocular pressure; both are found in marijuana and can cause tachycardia and systemic hypotension, which can compromise vascular flow to an otherwise unhealthy optic nerve in glaucoma.
- Patients should be counseled regarding the lack of reputable scientific evidence demonstrating superiority of cannabinoid-containing products over FDA-approved and currently used medications, laser, and surgical interventions to treat glaucoma and other ocular disease.

References

1. Drug scheduling. (2012, Sept 4). Retrieved 24 June 2019, from https://www.dea.gov/drug-scheduling.
2. American Academy of Ophthalmology. 2018-2019 BCSC: basic and clinical science course - glaucoma. San Francisco: American Academy of Ophthalmology; 2018. Figure 3-23, 81.
3. American Academy of Ophthalmology. 2018-2019 BCSC: basic and clinical science course - glaucoma. San Francisco: American Academy of Ophthalmology; 2018. Figure 3-13, 65.
4. American Academy of Ophthalmology. 2018-2019 BCSC: basic and clinical science course - glaucoma. San Francisco: American Academy of Ophthalmology; 2018. Figure 3-15, 68.
5. American Academy of Ophthalmology. 2018-2019 BCSC: basic and clinical science course - glaucoma. San Francisco: American Academy of Ophthalmology; 2018. Figure 3-5, 52.
6. American Academy of Ophthalmology. 2018-2019 BCSC: basic and clinical science course - glaucoma. San Francisco: American Academy of Ophthalmology; 2018. Figure 1-2, 20.
7. Zlas J, Stark H, Seligman J, Levy R, Werker E, Breuer A, Mechoulam R. Early medical use of cannabis. Nature. 1993;363(6426):215.
8. Gaoni Y, Mechoulam R. Isolation, structure, and partial synthesis of an active constituent of hashish. J Am Chem Soc. 1964;86(8):1646–7. https://doi.org/10.1021/ja01062a046.
9. Iancu R, Coman I, Barac C, Hammoud MA, Cherecheanu AP. Endocannabinoid system and ocular vascularization. Nepal J Ophthalmol. 2018;10(2):168–75. https://doi.org/10.3126/nepjoph.v10i2.20464.
10. Cairns, E. A., Toguri, J. T., Porter, R. F., Szczesniak, A., & Kelly, M. E. (2016). Seeing over the horizon – targeting the endocannabinoid system for the treatment of ocular disease. J Basic Clin Physiol Pharmacol, 27(3). doi:https://doi.org/10.1515/jbcpp-2015-0065.
11. Toguri JT, Caldwell M, Kelly ME. Turning down the thermostat: modulating the endocannabinoid system in ocular inflammation and pain. Front Pharmacol. 2016;7 https://doi.org/10.3389/fphar.2016.00304.
12. Miller S, Daily L, Leishman E, Bradshaw H, Straiker A. Δ9-tetrahydrocannabinol and cannabidiol differentially regulate intraocular pressure. Invest Ophthalmol Vis Sci. 2018;59(15):5904. https://doi.org/10.1167/iovs.18-24838.
13. Chien FY. Effect of WIN 55212-2, a cannabinoid receptor agonist, on aqueous humor dynamics in monkeys. Arch Ophthalmol. 2003;121(1):87. https://doi.org/10.1001/archopht.121.1.87.
14. Xu H, Cheng CL, Chen M, Manivannan A, Cabay L, Pertwee RG, et al. Anti-inflammatory property of the cannabinoid receptor-2-selective agonist JWH-133 in a rodent model of autoimmune uveoretinitis. J Leukoc Biol. 2007;82(3):532–41. https://doi.org/10.1189/jlb.0307159.
15. Toguri JT, Lehmann C, Laprairie RB, Szczesniak AM, Zhou J, Denovan-Wright EM, Kelly ME. Anti-inflammatory effects of cannabinoid CB2receptor activation in endotoxin-induced uveitis. Br J Pharmacol. 2014;171(6):1448–61. https://doi.org/10.1111/bph.12545.
16. Yang Y, Yang H, Wang Z, Varadaraj K, Kumari S, Mergler S, et al. Cannabinoid receptor 1 suppresses transient receptor potential vanilloid 1-induced inflammatory responses to corneal injury. Cell Signal. 2013;25(2):501–11. https://doi.org/10.1016/j.cellsig.2012.10.015.
17. Plange N, Arend KO, Kaup M, Doehmen B, Adams H, Hendricks S, et al. Dronabinol and retinal Hemodynamics in humans. Am J Ophthalmol. 2007;143(1):173–4. https://doi.org/10.1016/j.ajo.2006.07.053.
18. Green K, Wynn H, Padgett D. Effects of Δ9-tetrahydrocannabinol on ocular blood flow and aqueous humor formation. Exp Eye Res. 1978;26(1):65–9. https://doi.org/10.1016/0014-4835(78)90152-5.
19. Green K. Marijuana smoking vs cannabinoids for glaucoma therapy. Arch Ophthalmol. 1998;116(11):1433. https://doi.org/10.1001/archopht.116.11.1433.
20. Hepler RS. Marihuana smoking and intraocular pressure. JAMA. 1971;217(10):1392. https://doi.org/10.1001/jama.1971.03190100074024.
21. Merritt JC, Crawford WJ, Alexander PC, Anduze AL, Gelbart SS. Effect of marihuana on intraocular and blood pressure in glaucoma. Ophthalmology. 1980;87(3):222–8. https://doi.org/10.1016/s0161-6420(80)35258-5.

22. Merritt JC, McKinnon S, Armstrong JR, et al. Oral delta 9-tetrahydrocannabinol in heterogeneous glaucomas. Ann Ophthalmol. 1980;12:947–50.
23. Purnell WD, Gregg JM. Delta(9)-tetrahydrocannabinol, euphoria and intraocular pressure in man. Ann Ophthalmol. 1975;7(7):921–3.
24. Tomida I, Azuara-Blanco A, House H, Flint M, Pertewee RG, Robson PJ. Effect of sublingual application of cannabinoids on intraocular pressure: a pilot study. J Glaucoma. 2006;15(5):349–53. https://doi.org/10.1097/01.ijg.0000212260.04488.60.
25. Merritt JC, Olsen JL, Armstrong JR, Mckinnon SM. Topical Δ9-tetrahydrocannabinol in hypertensive glaucomas. J Pharm Pharmacol. 1981;33(1):40–1. https://doi.org/10.1111/j.2042-7158.1981.tb13699.x.
26. Jampel H. American Glaucoma Society position statement: marijuana and the treatment of glaucoma. J Glaucoma. 2010;19(2):75–6. https://doi.org/10.1097/ijg.0b013e3181d12e39.
27. Ramaekers JG, Wel JH, Spronk DB, Toennes SW, Kuypers KP, Theunissen EL, Verkes RJ. Erratum: Cannabis and tolerance: acute drug impairment as a function of cannabis use history. Sci Rep. 2016;6(1) https://doi.org/10.1038/srep31939.
28. Colizzi M, Bhattacharyya S. Cannabis use and the development of tolerance: a systematic review of human evidence. Neurosci Biobehav Rev. 2018;93:1–25. https://doi.org/10.1016/j.neubiorev.2018.07.014.
29. Jay WM, Green K. Multiple-drop study of topically applied 1% 9-tetrahydrocannabinol in human eyes. Arch Ophthalmol. 1983;101(4):591–3. https://doi.org/10.1001/archopht.1983.01040010591012.
30. Green K, Roth M. Ocular effects of topical administration of 9-tetrahydrocannabinol in man. Arch Ophthalmol. 1982;100(2):265–7. https://doi.org/10.1001/archopht.1982.01030030260 7006.
31. Jadoon KA, Tan GD, O'Sullivan SE. A single dose of cannabidiol reduces blood pressure in healthy volunteers in a randomized crossover study. JCI Insight. 2017;2(12) https://doi.org/10.1172/jci.insight.93760.
32. Marijuana in the treatment of glaucoma CTA – 2014. (2017, Oct 30). Retrieved 24 June 2019, from https://www.aao.org/complimentary-therapy-assessment/marijuana-in-treatment-of-glaucoma-cta%2D%2Dmay-2003.
33. Buys YM, Rafuse P. (2010, Apr). Medical use of marijuana for glaucoma. Retrieved 24 June 2019, from https://www.cos-sco.ca/advocacy-news/position-policy-statements/medical-use-of-marijuana-for-glaucoma/.
34. Mostofian F, Baig K. (2018, Nov). Medical use of cannabis for dry eye disease. Retrieved 24 June 2019, from https://www.cos-sco.ca/wp-content/uploads/2019/04/MedUseCannabisDryEye-COS_CCEDRSS_e.pdf.
35. Higginbotham EJ, Higginbotham LA. Shaping patients' perspective of medical marijuana for glaucoma treatment. JAMA Ophthalmol. 2016;134(3):265. https://doi.org/10.1001/Jamaophthalmol.2015.5290.
36. Belyea DA, Alhabshan R, Rio-Gonzalez AM, Chadha N, Lamba T, Golshani C, et al. Marijuana use among patients with glaucoma in a city with legalized medical marijuana use. JAMA Ophthalmol. 2016;134(3):259. https://doi.org/10.1001/jamaophthalmol.2015.5209.

Chapter 12
Cannabis in Oncology and Symptom Management

Matthew Chung and Salahadin Abdi

Cannabis and Cancer Care

Growing popularity of alternative medicine and cannabis has raised numerous questions regarding the potential of cannabis use beyond palliative and symptomatic treatment in cancer care. Due to increasing interest in the natural benefits of cannabis, in an era of legalized cannabis and readily accessible mainstream media, inaccurate claims regarding cannabis and its role in the treatment of cancer have become rampant [46, 87]. In effort to prevent patients from foregoing conventional cancer therapy as a result of this misinformation, it is the responsibility of the medical community to ensure that these patients are well informed to avoid consequences including avoidable deaths.

Laboratory Studies

THC exerts a variety of biological effects by mimicking endogenous substances, including the endocannabinoids anandamide and 2-arachidonylglyercol (2-AG) that of which bind and activate specific cannabinoid receptors. Thus far, there have been two G protein coupled, cannabinoid-specific receptors that have been cloned and characterized from animal studies in the form of CB1 and CB2. CB1 receptor is predominantly found in the central nervous system with a minority in the peripheral nervous system and various extraneural sites (including vascular endothelium, spleen, eye, and testis) [34]. The CB2 receptor is primarily expressed in the immune system at the cellular and tissue level of lymphocytes to lymph nodes, respectively [34]. An

M. Chung (✉) · S. Abdi
Department of Pain Medicine, Division of Anesthesia, Critical Care and Pain Medicine, The University of Texas MD Anderson Cancer Center, Houston, TX, USA
e-mail: mchung1@mdanderson.org; sabdi@mdanderson.org

© Springer Nature Switzerland AG 2020
K. Finn (ed.), *Cannabis in Medicine*,
https://doi.org/10.1007/978-3-030-45968-0_12

exciting area of research includes the applicability of these two receptors as potential targets for anticancer agents.

Mechanisms of cannabinoid antitumor action are still unclear and inconsistent; however, the current leading proposals include the induction of apoptosis [29, 31, 83], cell cycle arrest [20, 62, 63], and the inhibition of angiogenesis and metastasis [8, 14, 76].

Additionally, it has been proposed that cannabinoids have utility as adjuvant therapies for cancer treatment, but the true usefulness still remains unclear. Thus far only two studies have been carried out involving gamma radiation and tamoxifen.

Although the large majority of studies pertaining to cannabinoid use in cancer have been for their palliative effects, the utility of cannabinoids as anticancer therapies still has room to develop. As stated, there have been proposed mechanisms of how cannabinoids may have antitumorigenic potential in culture and animal models; however, these have not successfully translated to in vivo studies as they have been disappointingly ineffective and/or toxic when tested.

Clinical Studies

To date, there are no active clinical trials involving the use of cannabis or its derivatives in the treatment of cancer. The only trial that has been published includes a phase 1 cohort of nine terminal patients with known recurrent glioblastoma, involving the use if intratumoral injection of delta-9-THC that demonstrated no significant clinical benefit with fair safety profile [35, 95].

Several trials have previously been reported to be completed without any finalized published data. These trials included a phase 2 pilot study of 21 participants with recurrent glioblastoma multiforme involving the use of nabiximol alongside temozolomide compared to a placebo arm of temozolomide. A report by GW Pharmaceuticals reported an 83% 1-year survival compared to the 53% in the placebo arm ($p = 0.042$) [85], prompting a flurry of media including one politician and his family to use this as a platform for the legalization of cannabis for treatment of cancer. Another trial including 60 solid tumor cancer patients used oral CBD as a single salvage treatment without any published results at this time (NCT 02255292).

In a phase II trial, Yeshurun et al. demonstrated the potential immunosuppressive and anti-inflammatory effects CBD may have as prophylactic treatment for patients undergoing stem cell transplantation. In their study, they had 48 participants with acute leukemia or myelodysplastic syndrome received CBD 300 mg/day alongside their conventional prophylaxis treatment. After comparing these patients from 101 historical controls, they demonstrated a lower incidence of grade 2 to grade 4 graft versus host disease, necessitating the need for randomize control studies [101].

In so far as the pediatric population, there are no clinical trials to date for the use of cannabis as treatment for cancer. Published reports thus far in this population have been limited to case reports suggesting cannabis as a promising anticancer treatment [27, 88].

Cannabis and Symptom Management in Cancer Care

Cannabis has been long used as an avenue for pain relief [82] and often perceived by clinicians with negative connotation due to their association with illegal substances [10], often excluding individuals from candidacy from traditional (albeit limited) pain relief in the form of opiates. Medical cannabis refers to the use of cannabis or cannabinoids (derivatives of the former) as medical therapy to treat and alleviate symptoms. Beyond these notions, cannabis is commonly used by cancer patients during therapy, frequently without the oncologist's knowledge [16]. This poses increasing concern due the influence of cannabis, cancer therapy, and cancer.

In a study that allowed 17,000 patients to enroll for the use of cannabis for cancer symptoms, the most common causes for use of cannabis were pain, well-being, appetite, and nausea [97]. Surprisingly, only 42% listed their oncologist as providing information regarding the use of cannabis to address their symptoms. To further elaborate on prescription practices and the attitudes of the physician regarding the use of cannabinoids as part of their management, a survey involving 166 physicians from a region of Canada found that cannabinoid prescription was at a rate of only 27% (for any indication). Among those who prescribed cannabinoids did so for fewer or equal to five patients in the last year, which was explained due in large part from lack of comfort with prescription of cannabinoids. Factors of improving degree of comfort included need for guidance and education including guidelines (i.e., dosing) and need for robust evidence. Limitations to this report included prescribing practice for only cannabinoids and not medical marijuana added, concern that the reported prescription rate was an overestimate as nonresponders may have not decided to complete the survey because they did not prescribe or were not comfortable with prescribing cannabinoids. The authors and the surveys conducted concluded that guidelines and education were needed [91].

A cross-sectional survey of 937 cancer patients conducted at a cancer center in the state of Washington (where medical and recreational use of cannabis is legalized) included 24% reported regular cannabis users. Additionally, reported non-mutually exclusive reasons for cannabis use among these patients were physical symptoms (75%), neuropsychiatric symptoms, recreational use/enjoyment, and treatment of cancer. Among the physical symptoms that were reported included pain, nausea, and loss of appetite. Interestingly, the majority of patients preferred to obtain information regarding cannabis from their care team, but less than 15% of patients reported receiving information from their cancer physician or nurse [71].

Cancer Pain

Animal Studies

Although proposals in the effectiveness of cannabinoids in cancer pain has often been discussed since the 1970s, it was not until the mode of action was further elucidated by peripheral action and at both CB1 and CB2 receptors [12, 23, 33, 84] that cannabinoids had affirmed an avenue for analgesia in multiple types of cancer pain.

Primary treatment for cancer pain has previously surrounded the use of opioids; however, due to ineffective relief, side effects, as well as the development of tolerance, there are increasing popularity of patients switching from opiate use to cannabinoid use.

Cannabinoids have demonstrated ability to potentiate analgesic effects of morphine [4] and curtail the incidence of tolerance [15]. Analgesia has been achieved through the activation of the two cannabinoid receptor types (CB1 and CB2). While CB1 is localized to the spinal dorsal horn, periaqueductal grey, and dorsal root ganglia, the CB2 receptors are found in immune cells and keratinocytes [96].

In a model involving the inoculation of osteolytic cells into the humerus of mice, a nonselective CB1/CB2 agonist (WIN55,212) was intraperitoneally administered, effectively creating time and dose-related systemic antihyperalgesia [47]. Given the known side effect of loss of coordination and catalepsy in the induction of CB1 receptors, this effect was confirmed secondary to behavior via the cannabinoid receptor rather than the former. In a fibrosarcoma mouse model, the CB1 receptor was isolated and identified as having antihyperalgesic effect through the following use of various combinations of nonselective agonists (CP 55,940), selective antagonists (SR 141716A), and a selective CB2 antagonist (SR 144528) [37].

To address the role of peripheral cannabinoid receptors in carcinoma pain, Guerrero examined allodynia in an oral squamous cell cancer mouse model with intratumor administration of WIN55,212 or selective CB2 agonist (AM1241) attenuated mechanical hyperalgesia without any temporal association to a tumor growth effect. Interestingly, Guerrero also demonstrated increased CB1 receptor expression in the dorsal root ganglia ipsilateral to the inflicting cancer.

The disparity seen between this model and the previous fibrosarcoma model may have been from different profiles emanating from their respective primary cancers as well as well as the route of cannabinoid administration (local vs systemic).

In three separate studies involving the implementation of vincristine, cisplatin, and paclitaxel, cannabinoids were demonstrated to be effective in relieving the induced chemotherapy-induced peripheral neuropathy (CIPN). These studies demonstrated that spinal sites of action were implicated both CB1 and CB2; receptor-mediated processes were involved in the suppression of CIPN [48–50, 78, 98].

Human Studies

Cancer pain is secondary to cancer-related growth of tissue or secondary to treatments implemented to address it in the form of bone, neuropathic, visceral, or somatic pain. When cancer pain is severe and persistent, this is often resistant to conventional therapy including opiates. The control of pain is a cornerstone of cancer treatment promoting enhanced quality of life, improved functioning, improved compliance, and a way for patients to have an improved outlook on life.

Oral delta-9-THC effects were measured for cancer pain in a double-blind, placebo-controlled study involving 10 patients using domains of intensity of pain and relief of pain [68]. Among various dosages, there was substantial analgesic effects with 15 and 20 mg doses of cannabinoid delta-9-THC. In a follow up study involving 36 patients with the use of 10 mg of delta-9-THC, there was comparable analgesic relief as to 60 mg doses of codeine. In this same study, 20 mg doses of delta-9-THC demonstrated analgesic equivalence to 120 mg of codeine, however was mired with intolerable side effects including somnolence, ataxia and blurred vision [68].

In a multicenter, double-blind, placebo-controlled study including 177 patients with advanced cancer with moderate-to-severe cancer-related pain over a 2-week time frame, THC:CBD nabiximols extract and THC extract were compared for their analgesic management [44]. After these patients were randomized to a THC/CBD extract, THC extract, or placebo extract group, they determined that the combination nabiximol extract was efficacious for pain relief as an adjunctive treatment for those that did not achieve an analgesic response to opioids [44]. In an open-label extension study from the previous study, involving 43 patients found that some patients continued to find relief with prolonged and long-term use of the THC/CBD oromucosal spray without need for increasing dose of spray or dose of other analgesics [45].

In a randomized, placebo-controlled, graded-dose trial involving 268 advanced cancer patients with poorly controlled pain refractory to opioid therapy, improved pain control and sleep were seen with nabiximol sprays at lower to medium doses (1–4 and 6–10 sprays/day) compared to placebo [77]. Adverse effects were demonstrated with the higher-dose group compared to placebo. This study was in contrast to one by Lichtman et al. involving 397 treatment refractory advanced cancer patients in a similar randomized, placebo-controlled setting that demonstrated nabiximol was not superior to placebo [55].

Chemotherapy-induced peripheral neuropathy (CIPN) is a dose-limiting side effect associated with several regularly used chemotherapeutic agents including taxanes, platinum-based agents, and vinca alkaloids. In a randomized, placebo-controlled crossover study involving 16 patients with chemotherapy-induced neuropathic pain, nabiximol was administered with no significant difference between the treatment and placebo group. In the same study, among those who responded (five patients), an average reported decrease of 2.6 points on an 11-point numerical scale was made, calling for a larger scale study [57].

A prospective observational study assessed the effectiveness of adjuvant nabilone therapy in advanced cancer patients undergoing pain and other associated symptoms (including nausea, anxiety, and depression). Following 30 days of follow-up patients who were treated with nabilone found improvement in pain, nausea, anxiety, distress, and pain compared to untreated patients. Additionally, there was an associated decreased use or greater tendency to discontinue adjuvant pain therapies including opiates, non-steroidal anti-inflammatories, tricyclic antidepressants, and gabapentin to name a few [58].

Preclinical observations that cannabis augments analgesic effects of opiates in a synergistic effect were further elaborated in a pharmacokinetic study involving 21 chronic pain patients. This study group was given vaporized cannabis in addition to either sustained release morphine or oxycodone for 5 days. The morphine arm had associated decrease in mean pain score while the oxycodone did not [4]. Several limitations including size of participant pool, duration of study, and lack of a placebo-control calls for further studies to explain the relationship of how cannabis affects the metabolism of opiates before translating these findings into regular practice.

The use of nabiximols, a combination cannabis extract comprising of THC and CBD in a 1:1 ratio is currently approved for use by Canada, New Zealand, and various countries in Europe for treatment of spasticity in multiple sclerosis. Added, Canada additionally has an indicated use of nabiximols for advanced cancer pain. Fallon et al. reported the results of two phase 3, double-blinded, randomized, placebo-controlled, multicenter trials involving the use of nabiximols in advanced cancer patients for treatment of chronic pain that were optimized on opiate therapy. On the basis of a primary endpoint using a numerical rating scale score (NRS), there was no difference in the use treatment group compared to placebo. Interestingly, a pooled analysis of these trials conducted in the United States (reported as 30% of the trial population) demonstrated improvement for nabiximols compared to the placebo in a subset of patients that were less than 65 years of age [24].

Appetite Stimulation

Animal Studies

The appetite stimulating action of the cannabis plant has largely been attributed to the effect of delta9-tetrahydrocannabinol (THC) properties. Since the 1970s THC has been demonstrated to stimulate feeding in a variety of animal models following systemic or central administrations. Studies have demonstrated the belief that endocannabinoid activity upon CB1 receptor, particularly in associated areas of the hypothalamic nuclei and nucleus accumbens, has associated effects on eating motivation and nutrition behavior. The hyperphagic actions of THC have been replicated with CB1 cannabinoid receptors, largely with agonist endocannabinoid use including anandamide and 2-arachidonoylglycerol (2-AG).

Supporting evidence for endocannabinoid involvement in appetite regulation was demonstrated in a mouse model involving CB1 receptor knockout mice (Cb1−/−) where these animals were fed either standard chow or a high-fat diet. CB1(−/−) mice did not display hyperphagia characteristic of wild-type mice (CB1+/+) and did not develop obesity. Additionally, the Cb1 knockout mice demonstrated a reduced hyperphagic response to fasting, eating less than wild-type mice.

Previous identification of two cannabinoid receptor subtypes of CB1 and CB2 receptors that are predominantly expressed in the central nervous system with some expression in gastrointestinal, adipose, and hepatic tissues, linking endocannabinoids to processes related to energy storage and metabolism that may affect appetite.

Human Studies

Appetite and weight loss are common side-effects of cancer and its associated treatments. In practice, appetite loss, involuntary weight loss, and nutritional deficiencies can be indicators of cancer severity and quality of life, physical functionality, and survival timeline.

In advanced cancer, the cause of appetite loss is believed in part to be caused by catabolism driven by pro-inflammatory cytokines, tumor products as a host reaction to tumor, and neurohormonal alterations (including hypoanabolism) [103]. Appetite loss can also have contributing secondary factors such as depression/psychosocial stress, nausea, constipation, taste alterations, or pain.

In so far as the clinical use of marijuana for appetite, significant evidence resides in the treatment of HIV wasting syndrome as advanced stages of cancer or HIV infection, and there are similar findings of progressive weight loss and loss of appetite. In placebo-controlled studies of HIV patients, smoking marijuana led to an increase in food intake which may be mediated through elevation in ghrelin and leptin as well as decreased levels of peptide tyrosine that of which regulates appetite.

Two controlled studies have demonstrated dronabinol (oral THC) that stimulates appetite and helps slow chronic weight loss in adults suffering from advanced cancers. The first was seen in a study in 1976 by Regeleson in a pool of 54 patients with advanced cancer. These patients were given dronabinol at 0.1 mg/kg three times a day. Secondly, a study by Jatoi et al. involved 469 patients with advanced cancer that had previously demonstrated weight loss. These patients were divided into treatment arms of dronabinol at a 2.5 mg BID dose, an oral megesterol at an 800 mg/day dose arm, alongside a combined treatment pool. They found that megesterol had greater efficacy over dronabinol with appetite (75% versus 11%) and weight gain (11% versus 3%), without any significant differences with the combination therapy [41].

Three additional controlled studies involving HIV-AIDS-related patients (with associated weight loss) and the use of THC (in the use of dronabinol or smoked THC) demonstrated marked, statistically significant stimulation of appetite and weight maintenance, or gain compared to placebo controls [3, 6, 92].

An additional randomized, placebo-controlled trial involving 46 cancer patients, and the use of dronabinol demonstrated improved and enhanced chemosensory perception with dronabinol use. More specifically, the dronabinol treatment arm demonstrated altered preference, appeal for foods, increased appetite, and increased intake of protein [11].

Currently, oral synthetic TCH or dronabinol is used as an appetite stimulant for the treatment of anorexia and weight loss associated with AIDS and not for advanced cancer. Dronabinol is available for use in 2.5, 5, and 10 mg capsules that can be taken up to a maximum dosage of 10 mg twice a day. Added, there are no published studies to date that have explored the effect of inhaled cannabis involving cancer patients and any impact on appetite to date.

Nausea and Vomiting Due to Chemotherapy

Development of chemotherapy treatment has been very useful in oncology practice as this has helped prolonged the lives of many patients. The use of these drugs, however, pose very difficult challenges to patients and their clinicians as they often have many associated side effects, most notably nausea and vomiting.

The emetic reflex has included vomiting, retching, and a sensation of nausea. Vomiting is a protective reflex to remove ingested toxins from the upper gastrointestinal tract. The sense of nausea serves as a warning and typically results in the cessation of ingestion and an associated aversion to repeat ingestion of the said toxin. Uniquely to cancer patients, the protective vomiting reflex does not apply as this does not remove the toxin.

Three types of emetic episodes have been described: (1) acute nausea and/or vomiting with temporal association of chemotherapy, (2) delayed nauseas and/or vomiting that proceeds after 24 hours of chemotherapy, and (3) anticipatory nausea and/or vomiting (ANV) with re-exposure to associations of the toxin [1]. ANV is potentiated with increased intensity of initial acute emetic episode. ANV has been demonstrated in at least half of patients treated, occurring in later cycles of chemotherapy.

Animal Studies

Animal models developed to assess the potential antiemetic properties of cannabinoids have been developed with the use of cats, pigeons, ferrets, least shrews, *Cryptotis parva*, and the house musk shrew *(Suncus murinus)* [70]. Rats and mice were largely excluded in these studies because they do not vomit in response to a toxin challenge [59].

The isolation of the cannabinoid receptors (CB1 and CB2) alongside the discovery of their respective endogenous ligands of anandamide and 2-aracidonoyl glycerol (2-AG) paved the way to further elucidate the findings we now have regarding the antiemetic effects of cannabinoids [25, 26].

It was in a shrew and ferret model (Van Sickle and Darmani) that the site of emesis was localized to the brainstem within the dorsal vagal complex.

The CB1 receptors have been demonstrated in the GI tract and enteric nervous system as well as in the dorsal vagal complex including the area postrema, nucleus tractus of the solitary tract, and dorsal motor nucleus in these animal models [72, 73, 93, 94], wherein cannabinoid agonists act mainly to decrease motility and act centrally to attenuate emesis.

Through various shrew models by Darmani, the endogenous cannabinoid system demonstrated a role in the both the regulation of emesis (by blocking CB1 receptors to block the antiemetic activity of cannabinoids as well as inducing emesis with higher doses of CB1 receptor antagonists) while also demonstrating a potential for promotion of emesis (with demonstration of 2-AG as a potent emetogenic agent and anandamide as a weak antiemetic) [19].

In studies involving lithium-induced emesis, THC and non-psychoactive CBD were used in shrew models demonstrating a dose-dependent suppression of lithium-induced vomiting with THC. CBD in this model produced a biphasic effect with lower doses demonstrating suppression while higher doses (20–40 mg/kg) demonstrating enhancement of lithium-induced vomiting. In these same lithium-induced vomiting models, CBD was confirmed to not act at the CB1 receptor (via reversal agent of SR-141716 that of which reversed the THC suppression but not the CBD), thereby raising further questions of alternative routes for controlling nausea and vomiting [60].

The dorsal vagal complex is densely populated with CB1 and 5HT3 receptors. In a shrew model involving combined treatment of ondansetron and Delta9-THC demonstrated complete suppression of cisplatin-induced vomiting and retching, wherein independent administrations at a similar dose was ineffective [17, 18]. Notably, the effective independent THC dose was measurably higher than the administered THC dose in the combined treatment, suggesting potential for fewer side effects at higher doses [53]. Studies have demonstrated the interaction of the cannabinoid system with the serotonergic system in the control of emesis [51].

The use of cannabis in the successful treatment of anticipatory nausea and vomiting is limited as the model of nausea was largely founded on a conditioned gaping model in rats (rats do not have a physiologic equivalent to humans as they are unable to vomit). However, the use of shrews has suggested the role of attenuating properties of cannabis through THC in re-exposure to lithium toxin models [56, 69, 70].

Human Studies

Nausea and vomiting, largely in the form of chemotherapy-induced nausea and vomiting (CINV), are the most common complaint as it is seen in up to 75% of those undergoing chemotherapy [86]. As common as these complaints arise by patients, 40% of cancer patients often fail to achieve adequate control of these symptoms [22]. The psychological impact that these symptoms convey contribute toward the development of anticipatory nausea and vomiting. Unfortunately, these symptoms contribute to reduced quality of life and feelings of helplessness and may additionally affect adherence to chemotherapy [89, 104, 105] and impaired survival as a consequence.

Several risk factors that have been identified as contributing to CINV include use of the degree of emetogenic potential of an antineoplastic therapy (i.e., platinum or anthracycline-based), previous experience of poorly controlled emesis, age, gender, history of hyperemesis gravidarum, duration of sleep the night prior to chemotherapy, anticipatory nausea/vomiting, and first cycle of chemotherapy.

Although cannabis has been used for centuries for various therapeutic applications including nausea and vomiting, cannabinoids and their antiemetic properties were investigated prior to the discovery of 5-HT3 antagonists. Nabilone (Cesamet) was the first cannabinoid agonist introduced in the 1980s for suppression of nausea and vomiting by chemotherapy [66] followed by Delta9-THC [28], dronabinol as an antiemetic and as an appetite stimulant [74].

Among all the studies conducted thus far (28 studies), the large majority of studies have surrounded the evaluation of nabilone (14) [43], with the remainder including dronabinol (3), nabiximol (1), levonantradol (4), and THC (6). Interestingly, only one clinical trial to date has compared antiemetic and anti-nausea effects of cannabinoids with 5-HT3 antagonists. All the studies included comparators that included a placebo or an alternative antiemetic agent (i.e., prochloperazine, metoclopramide, chlorpromazine, domperidone). Added, there have not been any comparative trials involving cannabinoids and aprepitant, an NK1 antagonist. Meiri et al. [61] compared dronabinol, ondansetron, or the combination for delayed chemotherapy-induced nausea and vomiting (in a double-blind placebo-controlled study) among cancer patients receiving moderate-severe emetogenic chemotherapy. The study demonstrated that dronabinol alone was comparable to ondansetron in the treatment of delayed nausea and vomiting, while the combined treatment was no more effective than either agent. This study was not designed to evaluate acute nausea and vomiting; however, the combination group did report less nausea and vomiting on the chemotherapy treatment day than placebo.

It has been noted that there is a strong preference of smoked marijuana over alternative forms of oral cannabinoids or sublingual forms. Suggested reasons for these have included ability to self-titrate smoked marijuana, ease of administration, short latency of onset for inhaled over alternatives, and the combination of action of other elements (including THC) in smoked forms. Many marijuana users have claimed that smoked marijuana is more efficacious than oral cannabinoid; however, all clinical trials thus far for the purposes of antiemesis in chemotherapy-induced nausea and vomiting have only investigated the effectiveness of oral cannabinoids (versus their counterparts of the sublingual or smoked form) largely in part due to the ability to titrate doses [36].

In the use of cannabis in the cancer population of children, it has been suggested that they may be effective in treating more difficult to control symptoms of nausea and delayed nausea and vomiting. Abrahamov et al. [2] evaluated Delta8-THC, a less psychoactive relative to Delta9-THC in children receiving chemotherapy. In their study, Abrahamov demonstrated mild irritability as a side effect and had effective acute and delayed nausea and vomiting.

In summary of the trials performed thus far, there was a suggested benefit in the use of cannabinoids but without any statistical significance. In all major national guidelines, there is no current recommendation for the use of cannabis or cannabinoid derivatives for the prevention of nausea and vomiting in this population, however, can be used as an alternative for breakthrough treatment in one guideline [7]. Added, in the pediatric guidelines due to limited evidence, there is no active recommendation for cannabinoid use [30, 99].

Chemotherapy agents have been demonstrated to stimulate the chemoreceptor trigger zone with subsequent sensory information being conveyed to the nucleus tractus solitarius and initiation of vomiting via the dorsal monitor nucleus of the vagus and the nucleus ambiguous. The dopamine (D2) receptors, histamine (H1) receptors, and muscarinic cholinergic receptors have been elucidated to be involved with regulating the process of emesis. The chemoreceptor trigger zone is initially stimulated in the area postrema in the floor of the fourth ventricle with impulses passed onto the vomiting center that includes the nucleus tractus solitarius as well as the nucleus ambiguous. Although these centers involve dopamine (D2), histamine (H1), and muscarinic receptors, antiemetic medications available vary in their ability to bind to these receptors. Anticholinergics and antihistaminergic have minimal effect on CINV. Phenothiazines, butyrophenones/butyrophenone derivatives, as well as substituted benzamides are potent dopamine receptor antagonists with varying abilities to block cytotoxic-induced emesis. Additionally, domperidone and metoclopramide's effect on dopamine gut receptors are believed to have a dual site of action via promotion of gastric motility. Mechanism of benzodiazepines may alleviate anxiety and produce amnesia in chemotherapy-treated patients as there is no demonstration of true antiemetic activity.

Conversely, cannabinoids do not address any of these three receptors previously outlined. Nabilone has been suggested to act on opiate-type receptors in the forebrain resulting in inhibition of vomiting center via descending connections. It was proposed that associated encephalin release played a role in maintaining antiemetic center in the medulla wherein steroids similarly protect this center.

Adverse Events

Contrary to popular opinion that cannabis is a harmless pleasure, there are well-documented observed effects from an immediate to long-term basis [52]. Fatalities due to cannabis use in humans has not been substantiated since cannabinoid receptors (unlike opioid receptors) are not located in areas governing respiration. Since cannabinoid receptors are present in other tissues throughout the body beyond the central nervous system, associated symptoms of tachycardia, bronchodilation, muscle relaxation, decreased gastrointestinal motility, hypotension, and tachycardia are regularly experienced.

Cannabis is listed as a schedule 1 class drug with high potential for abuse by the drug enforcement agency. Although their addictive potential was previously lower than that of other prescription agents or substances of abuse [13, 32, 36], the rate has increased to as high as 30% [39], largely due in part from the increased availability of higher-potency cannabis [106].

Cannabinoids are stored in adipose tissue and are excreted with a half-life of 1–3 days. Abrupt discontinuation of cannabis or cannabinoid has not been seen with life-threatening withdrawal that would otherwise be seen in opiates or benzodiazepines [9].

Cannabidiol (CBD) has been demonstrated to be an inhibitor of cytochrome P450, thus concurrent therapy of antineoplastic therapy (which are often metabolized by the same enzymes) has an associated concern for potential increase in toxicity or decreased effectiveness of these therapies [42, 100].

As cannabis is commonly inhaled, questions of associated lung disease and respiratory compromise are inherent as a potential nidus for disease or exacerbation of a chronic issue. The long-term effect of low levels of marijuana exposure in a non-cancer population of 5115 patients did not make any significant impact on pulmonary function testing [75]. Smoked cannabis has also been demonstrated to contain Aspergillus, described previously in cannabis smokers undergoing renal transplant, treated for leukemia or solid tumors with AIDS, and in patients undergoing chronic steroid therapy [81]. Thus in the cancer population, a well-educated discussion of alternative routes of administration beyond smoking cannabis is important.

Cannabis use has been seen to impair driving capability in both the immediate and long-term use. Cannabis has been the most frequently associated with impaired driving-related fatalities among illicit drugs. In a meta-analysis, the risk of accident involvement increased by a factor of two following immediate use of cannabis [38]. In a culpability analysis, those who had tested positive for THC were 2.7–6.6 times as likely to be responsible for a motor vehicle accident versus those who had not been using drugs or alcohol before driving [79]. In an annual report published by a drug trafficking program in the state of Colorado (where recreational marijuana was legalized in 2012), cannabis-related traffic deaths have slowly increased from 15% to 23% between 2013 and 2018 [80].

Cannabis has well-known antiemetic properties. The emergence of cannabinoid hyperemesis syndrome (CHS) has added to the list of centrally mediated adverse effects that cannabinoids can incur that includes cyclical vomiting. Although the mechanism is unclear, several theories have included that the CB1 receptors in the enteric nervous system superseded those of the central nervous system, chronic regular use desensitizes or downregulates the antiemetic properties of cannabinoids and a disrupted Hypothalamic-pituitary-adrenal axis from upregulated ACTH secretion. Reported cases that have included CHS as potential cause of death or as a contributing factor to death have been documented [67] from complications of nonspecific electrolyte disturbances.

Interestingly, CHS is associated with a chronic excessive daily use of cannabis for at least 2 years that is often relieved by sustained cessation of cannabis use, although temporarily symptomatic relief is found with acute cannabis use. Therein creating cycle of failed attempts to maintain abstinence and unrelenting CHS with bouts of emesis. Indeed there could be some concern for ambiguity between emesis secondary to chemotherapy and CHS in patients using cannabis; however, all reported cases thus far have only included smoked cannabis [64, 90]. In addition to suggesting alternative routes of administration, ensuring that a patient has not exhausted other avenues to address their symptom care with the assistance of their treating physician is paramount (in efforts to prevent chronic habitual use).

The increasing attention of cannabis and marijuana derivatives has stimulated the rise of recreational designer drugs particularly spice/K2, which has been responsible for serious adverse effects [102], toxicity, and cases of fatalities in combination with other substances.

Future Directions

The role of cannabis and cannabinoids has potential to take on a greater role in cancer medicine as a therapeutic option for cancer-related disease and sequela of treatment. In a national survey conducted by the American Society of Clinical Oncology, 62% of cancer patients wished they had more information on the benefits and risks of medical cannabis [5]. Current government restrictions on the use of cannabis in the United States include classification as a schedule 1 drug (high potential of abuse and no accepted medical use), thereby limiting the progress of the development of drugs with cannabis components. Most major cancer societies (including the American Society of Clinical Oncology and the National Cancer Institute) [21] have declined to take position on the use of medical marijuana; however, the American Cancer Society has stated that they support the need for more scientific research on the potential risks and benefits.

By current convention, food and drugs are regulated at both the state and federal level. Without federal or state support, dispensaries are often the last line of defense for monitoring and enforcing safety of cannabis production for consumers. This should be further emphasized in a cancer population that is particularly vulnerable to infection and intoxication that seeks this avenue of treatment; this is in reference to a case of a fatal ending for a young cancer patient that had a treatable cancer and passed away from a fungal infection that stemmed from their use of contaminated medical cannabis.

Lastly, increasing changes in the social and political climate toward legalization of cannabis would allow randomized studies to address risks and benefits of cannabis while addressing measures of quality control, administration methods, and addressing optimal dosing. Added, improved regulations would allow future studies to better assess patient outcomes (i.e., disease-specific endpoints, quality of life and adverse events) using standardized measures at similar time points to insure inclusion in future meta-analysis.

Summary and Conclusion

The use of cannabis has historically been used for recreational purposes in the inhaled or vaporized format and until recently has gained traction for their potential medicinal properties. In cancer patients, there have been a total of 10 clinical trials in the use of inhaled cannabis, all of which were for chemotherapy-induced nausea and emesis. Unfortunately, the data was insufficient to provide any evidence for use of this mode of delivery. Added, there are no published controlled clinical trials for any other cancer treatment-related symptoms or cancer-related symptoms for that matter.

On the basis of cannabis derivatives, several controlled trials and meta-analyses have demonstrated support for the use of cannabinoids (dronabinol and nabilone), specifically for chemotherapy-induced nausea and vomiting. Currently, dronabinol and nabilone are approved in the United States by the FDA for only use as treatment or prevention of chemotherapy-induced nausea and vomiting. An increasing number of trials are actively evaluating the use of oral mucosal administration (in the form of a nabiximol spray) in parts of Canada, New Zealand, and other European countries.

Despite the exponential rise in cannabis use, research for a cure to cancer with cannabis has been limited to animal studies with favorable and meaningful conclusions for potential translation into human cancer research. Unfortunately research is further limited and scarce in the clinical setting as only a handful of trials have been conducted, with only one of these with published results [35].

Although many uses of cannabis and their derivatives seem potentially favorable beyond antiemesis in areas (including pain, treatment of cancer, and beyond), limitations to their analysis (specifically in the United Sates) in this context resides in barriers associated with regulation as a schedule 1 substance, finances for funding and access to research-grade product for use on a research scale [65].

References

1. Aapro MS, Kirchner V, Terrey JP. The incidence of anticipatory nausea and vomiting after repeat cycle chemotherapy: the effect of granisetron. Br J Cancer. 1994;69:957–60.
2. Abrahamov A, Abrahamov A, Mechoulam R. An efficient new cannabinoid antiemetic in pediatric oncology. Life Sci. 1995;56:2097–102.
3. Abrams DI, Hilton JF, Leiser RJ, Shade SB, Elbeik TA, Aweeka FT, Benowitz NL, Bredt BM, Korel B, Aberg JA, Deeks SG, Mitchell TF, Mulligan K, Baccheti P, McCune JM, Schambelan M. Short-term effects of cannabinoids in patients with HIV-1 infection. A randomized, placebo-controlled clinical trial. Ann Intern Med. 2003;139:258–66. Ahmedzai S, Carlyle DL, Calder IT, Moran F. Anti-emetic efficacy and toxicity of nabilone, a synthetic cannabinoid, in lung cancer chemotherapy. Br J Cancer 1983;48:657–663.
4. Abrams DI, Couey P, Shade SB, Kelly ME, Benowitz NL. Cannabinoid-opioid interaction in chronic pain. Clin Pharmacl Ther. 2011;90(6):844–51.
5. ASCO's National Cancer Opinion Survey. Harris poll on behalf of ASCO. Alexandria: American Society of Clinical Oncology; 2019.
6. Beal JE, Olson R, Laubenstein L, Morales JO, et al. Dronabinol as a treatment for anorexia associated with weight loss in patients with AIDS. J Pain Symptom Manag. 1995;10:89–7.
7. Berger MJ, Ettinger DS, Aston J, et al. NCCN Guidelines Insights: Antiemesis, Version 2.2017. J Natl Compr Canc Netw. 2017;15(7):883–93. https://doi.org/10.6004/jnccn.2017.0117.
8. Blazquez C, et al. Inhibition of tumor angiogenesis by cannabinoids. FASEB J. 2003;17:529–31.
9. Bonnet U, Preuss UW. The cannabis withdrawal syndrome: current insights. Subst Abus Rehabil. 2017;8:9–37.
10. Bottorff JL, et al. Perceptions of cannabis as a stigamatized medicine: a qualitative descriptive study. Harm Reduct J. 2013;10:2.
11. Brisbois T, de Kock IH, Watanabe SM, et al. Delta-9-tetrahydrocannabinol may palliate altered chemosensory perception in cancer patients: results of a randomized, double-blind, placebo-controlled pilot trial. Ann Oncol. 2011;22(9):2086–93.

12. Brown MRD, Farquhar-Smith P. Cannabinoids and cancer pain: a new hope or a false dawn? Eur J Intern Med. 2018;49:30.
13. Calhoun SR, Galloway GP, Smith DE. Abuse potential of dronabinol. J Psychoactive Drugs. 1998;30(2):187.
14. Casanova ML, et al. Inhibition of skin tumor growth and angiogenesis *in vivo* by activation of cannabinoid receptors. J Clin Invest. 2003;111:43–50.
15. Cichewicz DL, Welch SP. Modulation of Oral morphine Antinociceptive tolerance and naloxone-precipitated withdrawal signs by Oral delta9-tetrahydrocannabinol. J Pharmacol Exp Ther. 2003;305(3):812–7.
16. Cortellini A, et al. What cancer patients actually know regarding medical cannabis? A cross-sectional survey with a critical analysis of the current attitudes. J Oncol Pharm Pract. 2019;25(6):1439–44.
17. Costall B, Domeney AM, Naylor RJ, Tattersall FD. 5-Hydroxytryptamine receptor antagonism to prevent cisplatin-induced emesis. Neuropharmacology. 1986;25:959–61.
18. Crawford SM, Buckman R. Nabilone and metoclopramide in the treatment of nausea and vomiting due to cisplatin: a double blind study. Med Oncol Tumor Pharmacother. 1986;3:39–42.
19. Darmani NA, Johnson CJ. Central and peripheral mechanisms contribute to the antiemetic actions of delta-9-tetrahydrocannabinol against 5-hydroxytryptophan-induced emesis. Eur J Pharmacol. 2004;488:201–12.
20. De Petrocellis L, et al. The endogenous cannabinoid anandamide inhibits human breast cancer cell proliferation. Proc Natl Acad Sci U S A. 1998;95:8375–80.
21. DiGrande S. Medical marijuana in cancer treatment: no standards of care, and so far, no coverage. https://www.ajmc.com/journals/evidence-based-oncology/2018/october-2018/medical-marijuana-in-cancer-treatment-no-standards-of-care-and-so-far-no-coverage?p=2. Visited 6 Nov 2019.
22. Dranitsaris G, Molassiotis A, Clemson M, Roeland E, Schwartzberg L, Dielenseger P, Jordan K, Young A, Aapro M. The development of a prediction tool to identify cancer patients at high risk for chemotherapy-induced nausea and vomiting. Ann Oncol. 2017;28(6):1260–7.
23. Elikottil J, Gupta P, Gupta K. The analgesic potential of cannabinoids. J Opioid Manag. 2009;5:341–57.
24. Fallon MT, Lux EA, McQuade R, Rossetti S, Sanchez R, Sun W, Wright S, Lichtman AH, Kornyeyeva E. Sativex oromucosal spray as adjunctive therapy in advanced cancer patients with chronic pain unalleviated by optimized opioid therapy: two double-blind, randomized, placebo-controlled phase 3 studies. Br J Pain. 2017;11(3):119–33.
25. Fan P. Cannabinoid agonists inhibit the activation of 5-HT3 receptors in rat nodose ganglion neurons. J Neurophysiol. 1995;73:907–10.
26. Felder CC, Glass M. Cannabinoid receptors and their endogenous agoinsts. Annu Rev Pharmacol Toxicol. 1998;38:179–200.
27. Foroughi M, Hendson G, Sargent MA, et al. Spontaneous regression of septum pellucidum/forniceal pilocytic astrocytomas—possible role of cannabis inhalation. Childs Nerv Syst. 2011;27(4):671–9.
28. Frytak S, Moertel CG, O'Fallon JR, et al. Delta-9-tetrahydrocannabinol as an antiemetic for patients receiving cancer chemotherapy. A comparison with prochlorperazine and a placebo. Ann Intern Med. 1979;91:825–30.
29. Galve-Roperh I, et al. Anti-tumoral action of cannabinoids: involvement of sustained ceramide accumulation and extracellular signal-regulated kinase activation. Nat Med. 2000;6:313–9.
30. Garcia JM, Shamliyan TA. Cannabinoids in patients with nausea and vomiting associated with malignancy and its treatments. Am J Med. 2018;131:755.
31. Gomez del Pulgar T, Velasco G, Sanchez C, Haro A, Guzman M. *De novo*-synthesized ceramide is involved in cannabinoid-induced apoptosis. Biochem J. 2002;363:183–8.
32. Grotenhermen F, Russo E. Cannabis and cannabindoids: pharmacology, toxicology, and therapeutic potential. Binghamton: The Haworth Press; 2002.

33. Guerrero AV, Quang P, Dekker N, Jordan RC, Schmidt BL. Peripheral cannabinoids attenuate carcinoma-induced nociception in mice. Neurosci Lett. 2007;433:77–81.
34. Guzman M. Cannabinoids: potential anticancer agents. Nat Rev Cancer. 2003;3(10):745–55.
35. Guzman M, Duarte MJ, Blazquez C. A pilot clinical study of Delta9-tetrahydrocannabinol in patients with recurrent glioblastoma multiforme. Br J Cancer. 2006;95(2):197–203.
36. Hall W, Christie M, Currow D. Cannabinoids and cancer: causation, remediation, and palliation. Lancet Oncol. 2005;6:35–42.
37. Hamamoto DT, Giridharagopalan S, Simone DA. Acute and chronic administration of the cannabinoid receptor agonist CP 55,940 attenuates tumor-evoked hyperalgesia. Eur J Pharmacol. 2007;558:73–87.
38. Hartman RL, Huestis MA. Cannabis effects on driving skills. Clin Chem. 2013;59:478–92.
39. Hasin DS, Saha TD, Kerridge BT, et al. Prevalence of marijuana use disorders in the United States between 2001-2002 and 2012-2013. JAMA Psychiatry. 2015;72(12):1235–42. https://doi.org/10.1001/jamapsychiatry.2015.1858.
40. Howlett AC. Pharmacology of cannabinoid receptors. Annu Rev Pharmacol Toxicol. 1995;35:607–34.
41. Jatoi A, Windschitl HE, Loprinzi CL, Sloan JA, Dakhil SR, Mail-liard JA, Pundaleeka S, Kardinal CG, Fitch TR, Krook JE, Novotny PJ, Christensen B. Dronabinol versus megestrol acetateversus combination therapy for cancer-associated anorexia: a north centralcancer treatment group study. J Clin Oncol. 2002;20:567–73.
42. Jiang R, Yamaori S, Okamoto Y, et al. Cannabidiol is a potent inhibitor of the phytocannabinoid, as a potent inhibitor for CYP2D6. Drug Metab Dispos. 2013;39(11):2049–56.
43. Johansson R, Kilkku P, Groenroos M. A double-blind, controlled trial of nabilone vs. prochlorperazine for refractory emesis induced by cancer chemotherapy. Cancer Treat Rev. 1982;9(suppl B):25–33.
44. Johnson JR, Burnell-Nugent M, Lossignol D, et al. Multicenter, double-blind, randomized, placebo-controlled, parallel-group study of the efficacy, safety, and tolerability of THC:CBD extract and THC extract in patients with intractable cancer related pain. J Pain Symptom Manag. 2010;39(2):167–79.
45. Johnson JR, Lossignol D, Burnell-Nugent M, Fallon MT. An open-label extension study to investigate the long-term safety and tolerability of THC/CBD oromucosal spray and oromucosal THC spray in patients with terminal cancer-related pain refractory to strong opioid analgesics. J Pain Symptom Manag. 2013;46(2):207–18.
46. Johnson SB, Park HS, Gross CP, Yu JB. Use of alternative medicine for Cancer and its impact on survival. JNCI. 2018;110(1):121–4.
47. Kehl L, Hamamoto DT, Wacnik PW, Croft DL, Norsted BD, Wilcox GL, Simone DA. A cannabinoid agonist differentially attenuates deep tissue hyperalgesia in animal models of cancer and inflammatory muscle pain. Pain. 2003;103:175–86.
48. Khasabova IA, Khasabov SG, Harding-Rose C, Coicou LG, Seybold BA, Lindberg AE, et al. A decrease in anandamide signaling contributes to the maintenance of cutaneous mechanical hyperalgesia in a model of bone cancer pain. J Neurosci. 2008;28:11141–52. https://doi.org/10.1523/JNEUROSCI.2847-08.
49. Khasabova IA, Gielissen J, Chandiramani A, Harding-Rose C, Odeh DA, Simone DA, et al. CB1 and CB2 receptor agonists promote analgesia through synergy in a murine model of tumor pain. Behav Pharmacol. 2011;22:607–16. https://doi.org/10.1097/FBP.0b013e3283474a6d.
50. Khasabova IA, Khasabov S, Paz J, Harding-Rose C, Simone DA, Seybold VS. Cannabinoid type-1 receptor reduces pain and neurotoxicity produced by chemotherapy. J Neurosci. 2012;32:7091–101. https://doi.org/10.1523/JNEUROSCI.0403-12.2012.
51. Kimura T, Ohta T, Watanabe K, Yoshimura H, Yamamoto I. Anandamide, an endogenous cannabinoid receptor ligand, also interacts with 5-hydroxytryptamine (5HT) receptor. Biol Pharm Bull. 1998;21:224–6.
52. Kingswood JC. Cannabis based drugs: finding the balance between benefit and harm. BMJ. 2018;363:k5213.

53. Kwaitkowska M, Parker LA, Burton P, Mechoulam R. A comparative analysis of the potential of cannabinoids and ondansetron to suppress cisplatin-induced emesis in the Suncus murinus (house musk shrew). Psychopharmacology. 2004;174:254–9.
54. Layeeque R, Siegel E, Kass R, Henry-Tillman RS, Colvert M, Mancino A, et al. Prevention of nausea and vomiting following breast surgery. Am J Surg. 2006;191:767–72.
55. Lichtman AH, Lux EA, McQuade R, Rossetti S, Sanchez R, Sun W, Wright S, Kornyeyeva E, Fallon MT. Results of a double-blind, randomized, placebo-controlled study of THC:CBD spray oromucosal spray as an adjunctive therapy in advanced cancer patients with chronic uncontrolled pain. J Pain Symptom Manage. 2018;55(2):179–188.e1.
56. Limebeer CL, Parker LA. Delta-9-tetrahydrocannabinol interferes with the establishment and the expression of conditioned disgust reactions produced by cyclophosphamide: a rat model of nausea. Neuroreport. 1999;26:371–84.
57. Lynch ME, Cesar-Rittenberg P, Hohmann AG. A double-blind, placebo-controlled, crossover pilot trial with extension using an oral mucosal cannabinoid extract for treatment of chemotherapy-induced neuropathic pain. J Pain Symptom Manag. 2014;47(1):166–73.
58. Maida V, Ennis M, Irani S, Corbo M, Dolzhykov M. Adjunctive nabilone in cancer pain and symptom management: a prospective observational study using propensity scoring. J Support Oncol. 2008;6(3):119–24.
59. Matsuki N, Ueno S, Kaji T, Ishihara A, Wang CH, Saito H. Emesis induced by cancer chemotherapeutic agents in the Suncus murinus: a new experimental model. Jpn J Pharmacol. 1988;48:303–6.
60. Mechoulam R, Parker LA, Gallily R. Cannabidiol: an overview of some pharmacological aspects. J Clin Pharmacol. 2002;42:11S–9S.
61. Meiri E, Jhangiani H, Vredenburgh JJ, Barbato LM, Carter FJ, Yang HM, et al. Efficacy of dronabinol alone and in combination with ondansetron versus ondansetron alone for delayed chemotherapy-induced nausea and vomiting. Curr Med Res Opin. 2007;23:533–43.
62. Melck D, et al. Involvement of the cAMP/protein kinase a pathway and of mitogen-activated protein kinase in the antiproliferative effects of anandamide in human breast cancer cells. FEBS Lett. 1999;463:235–40.
63. Melck D, et al. Suppression of nerve growth factor trk receptors and prolactin receptors by endocannabinoids leads to inhibition of human breast and prostate cancer cell proliferation. Endocrinology. 2000;141:118–26.
64. Monte AA, Shelton SK, Saben J, et al. Acute illness associated with cannabis use, by route of exposure an observational study. Ann Intern Med. 2019;170(8):531–7.
65. National Academies of Sciences, Engineering, and Medicine, Health and Medicine Division, Board on Population Health and Public Health Practice. Committee on the Health Effects of Marijuana: an evidence review and research agenda. Washington, D.C.: National Academies Press (US); 2017.
66. Niiranen A, Mattson K. A cross-over comparison of nabilone and prochlorperazine for emesis induced by cancer chemotherapy. Am J Clin Oncol. 1985;8(4):336–40.
67. Nourbakhsh M, Miller A, Gofton J. Cannabinoid hyperemesis syndrome: reports of fatal cases. J Forensic Sci. 2019;64(1):270–4. https://doi.org/10.1111/1556-4029.13819.
68. Noyes RJ, Brunk SF, Baram DA, Canter A. Analgesic effect of delta-9-tetrahydrocannabinol. J Clin Pharmacol. 1975a;15(2–3):139–43.
69. Parker LA, Mechoulam R. Cannabinoid agonists and an antagonist modulate conditioned gaping in rats. Integr Physiol Behav Sci. 2003;38:134–46.
70. Parker LA, Mechoulam R, Schlievert C. Cannabidiol, a non-psychoactive component of cannabis, and its dimethylheptyl homolog suppress nausea in an experimental model with rats. Neuroreport. 2002;13:567–70.
71. Pergam SA, Woodfield MC, Lee CM, et al. Cannabis use among patients at a comprehensive cancer center in a state with legalized medicinal and recreational use. Cancer. 2017;123(22):4488–97.
72. Pertwee RG. Cannabinoid receptors and pain. Prog Neurobiol. 2001a;63(5):569.

73. Pertwee RG. Cannabinoids and the gastrointestinal tract. Gut. 2001b;48:859–67.
74. Pertwee RG. Emerging strategies for exploiting cannabinoid receptor agonists as medicines. Br J Pharmacol. 2009;156:397–411.
75. Pletcher MJ, Vittinghoff E, Kalhan R. Association between marijuana exposure and pulmonary function over 20 years. JAMA. 2012;307:173–81.
76. Portella G, et al. Inhibitory effects of cannabinoid CB1receptor stimulation on tumor growth and metastatic spreading: actions on signals involved in angiogenesis and metastasis. FASEB J. 2003;17:1771. https://doi.org/10.1096/fj.02-1129fje.
77. Portenoy RK, Ganae-Motan ED, Allende S, Yanagihara R, Shaiova L, Weinstein S, McQuade R, Wright S, Fallon MT. THC:CBD spray for opioid-treated cancer patients with poorly-controlled chronic pain: a randomized, placebo-controlled, graded-dose trial. J Pain. 2012;13(5):438–49.
78. Rahn EJ, Makriyannis A, Hohmann AG. Activation of cannabinoid CB1 and CB2 receptors suppresses neuropathic nociception evoked by the chemotherapeutic agent vincristine in rats. Br J Pharmacol. 2007;152:765.
79. Ramaekers JG, Berghaus G, van Laar M, Drummer OH. Dose related risk of motor vehicle crashes after cannabis use. Drug Alcohol Depend. 2004;73:109–19.
80. Rocky Mountain high Intensity Drug Trafficking Area (RMHIDTA). The legalization of marijuana in Colorado: the impact. 2019. Volume 6. https://rmhidta.org/files/D2DF/FINAL-Volume6.pdf. Accessed 11 Nov 2019.
81. Ruchlemer R, Amit-Kohn M, Raveh D, Havnus L. Inhaled medicinal cannabis and the immunoscomprimsed patient. Support Care Cancer. 2015;23:819–22.
82. Russo EB. History of Cannabis and its preparations in saga, science and sobriquet. Chem Biodivers. 2007;4:1614–48.
83. Sanchez C, et al. Inhibition of glioma growth *in vivo* by selective activation of the CB2 cannabinoid receptor. Cancer Res. 2001;61:5784–9.
84. Schmidt BL, Hamamoto DT, Simone DA, Wilcox GL. Mechanisms of cancer pain. Mol Interv. 2010;10:3.
85. Schultz S, Beyer M. GW pharmaceuticals achieves positive results in phase 2 proof of concept study in glioma. 2017. Available online at: http://ir.gwpharm.com/static-files/cde942fe-555c-4b2f-9cc9-f34df24c7ad27.
86. Schwartzberg LS. Chemotherapy-induced nausea and vomiting: clinician and patient persepectives. J Support Oncol. 2007;5(2):5–12.
87. Shi S, Brant AR, Sabolch A, Pollom E. False news of a cannabis cancer cure. Cureus. 2019;11(1):e3918.
88. Singh Y, Bali C. Cannabis extract treatment for terminal acute lymphoblastic leukemia with a Philadelphia chromosome mutation. Case Rep Oncol. 2013;6(3):585–92.
89. Smith LA, Azariah F, Lavender VT, Stoner NS, Bettiol S. Cannabinoids for nausea and vomiting in adults with cancer receiving chemotherapy. Cochrane Database Syst Rev. 2015;(11):CD009464.
90. Sorensen CJ, DeSanto K, Borgelt L, et al. Cannabinoid hyperemesis syndrome: diagnosis, pathophysiology, and treatment- a systematic review. J Med Toxicol. 2017;13(1):71–87.
91. St-Amant H, Ware MA, Julien N, Lacasse A. Prevalence and determinants of cannabinoid prescription for the management of chronic noncancer pain: a postal survey of physicians in the Abitibi-Temiscamingue region of Quebec. CMAJ Open. 2015;3:E251–7.
92. Struwe M, Kaempfer SH, Geiger CJ, Pavia AT, Plasse TF, Shepard KV, Ries K, Evans TG. Effect of dronabinol on nutritional status in HIV infection. Ann Pharmacother. 1993;27:827–31.
93. Van Sickle MD, Oland LD, Ho W, Hillard CJ, Mackie K, Davison JS, Sharkey KA. Cannabinoids inhibit emesis through CB1 receptors in the brainstem of the ferret. Gastroenterology. 2001;121:767–74.

94. Van Sickle MD, Oland LD, Mackie K, Davison JS, Sharkey KA. Δ9-tetrahydrocannabinol selectively acts on CB1 receptors in specific regions of dorsal vagal complex to inhibit emesis in ferrets. Am J Physiol Gastrointest Liver Physiol. 2003;285:G566–76.
95. Velasco G, Sanchez C, Guzman M. Towards the use of cannabinoids as antitumor agents. Nat Rev Cancer. 2012;12(6):436–44.
96. Vuckovic S, Srebro D, et al. Cannabinoids and pain: new insights from old molecules. Front Pharmacol. 2018;9:1259.
97. Waissengrin B, Urban D, Leshem Y, et al. Patterns of use of medical cannabis among Israeli cancer patients: a single institution experience. J Pain Symptom Manag. 2015;49:223–30.
98. Ward SJ, McAllister SD, Kawamura R, Murase R, Neelakantan H, Walker EA. Cannabidiol inhibits paclitaxel-induced neuropathic pain through 5-HT(1A) receptors without diminishing nervous system function or chemotherapy efficacy. Br J Pharmacol. 2014;171:636–45. https://doi.org/10.1111/bph.12439.
99. Whiting PF, et al. Cannabinoids for medical use – a systematic review and meta-analysis. JAMA. 2015;313:2456.
100. Yamaori S, Okamoto Y, Yamamoto I. Cannabidiol, a major phytocannabinoid, as a potent atypical inhibitor for CYP2D6. Drug Metab Dispos. 2011;39(11):2049–56.
101. Yeshurun M, Shpilberg O, Herscovici C. Cannabidiol for the prevention of graft-versus-host-disease after allogenic hematopoietic cell transplantation: results of a phase II study. Biol Blood Marrow Transplant. 2015;21(10):1770–5.
102. Freeman M, Rose D, Myers M, et al. Ischemic stroke after use of the synthetic marijuana "spice." Neurology. 2013;81:2090–3.
103. Solheim TS, Blum D, Fayers PM, et al. Weight loss, appetite loss and food intake in cancer patients with cancer cachexia: three peas in a pod? - analysis from a multicenter cross sectional study. Acta Oncole. 2014;53:539–46.
104. Janelsins MC, Tejani MA, Kamen C. Current pharmacotherapy for chemotherapy-induced nausea and vomiting in cancer patients. Expert Opin Pharmacother. 2013;14:757–66.
105. Bakowski MT. Advances in anti-emetic therapy. Cancer Treat Rev. 1984;11(3):237–56.
106. Mehmedic Z, Chandra S, Slade D, et al. Potency trends of Δ9-THC and other cannabinoids in confiscated cannabis preparations from 1993 to 2008. J Forensic Sci. 2010; 55:1209–17.

Chapter 13
Cannabis in Palliative Medicine

Fabienne Saint-Preux, Arpit Arora, Derek Moriyama, Esther Kim, and Arum Kim

Abbreviations

2-AG	2-arachidonoylglycerol
$5HT_{1A}$	Serotonin 1A receptor
AAN	American Academy of Neurology
AEA	Anandamide
ALT	Alanine aminotransferase
AST	Aspartate aminotransferase
CACS	Cancer-related anorexia-cachexia syndrome
CAPC	Center to Advance Palliative Care
CB_1	Cannabinoid receptor 1
CB_2	Cannabinoid receptor 2
CBD	Cannabidiol

F. Saint-Preux
Department of Rehabilitation Medicine, New York University School of Medicine,
New York, NY, USA
e-mail: Fabienne.Saint-Preux@nyulangone.org

A. Arora · A. Kim (✉)
Department of Medicine, Division of Hematology-Oncology, Division of Geriatric-Palliative
Medicine, Department of Rehabilitation Medicine, New York University School of Medicine,
New York, NY, USA
e-mail: Arpit.Arora@nyulangone.org; Arum.Kim@nyulangone.org

D. Moriyama
Department of Medicine, Division of Geriatric-Palliative Medicine, New York University
School of Medicine, New York, NY, USA
e-mail: Derek.Moriyama@nyulangone.org

E. Kim
Department of Radiation Oncology, New York University Langone Health,
New York, NY, USA

© Springer Nature Switzerland AG 2020
K. Finn (ed.), *Cannabis in Medicine*,
https://doi.org/10.1007/978-3-030-45968-0_13

CDC   Center for Disease Control
CINV   Chemotherapy-induced nausea and vomiting
CNS   Central nervous system
CYP   Cytochrome P450
ECS   Endocannabinoid system
FEV1   Forced expiratory volume
GAD   Generalized anxiety disorder
HPA   Hypothalamic-pituitary-adrenal
INR   International normalized ratio
MDD   Major depressive disorder
NNT   Number needed to treat
NREM   Non-rapid eye movement
NRS   Numerical rating scale
PD   Panic disorder
PTSD   Post-traumatic stress disorder
QOL   Quality of life
RCT   Randomized control trial
REM   Rapid eye movement
SAD   Social anxiety disorder
SPST   Simulated public speaking test
TCA   Tricyclic antidepressant
THC   Delta-9-tetrahydrocannabinol
VAS   Visual analogue scale

What Is Palliative Care?

The Center to Advance Palliative Care (CAPC) defines palliative care as "specialized care for people living with a serious illness" [1]. Palliative care aims to relieve symptoms and stress in multiple domains – physical, psychological, social, and spiritual – with the goal to improve overall quality of life (QOL). Typical symptoms in patients living with serious illness include pain, fatigue, nausea, vomiting, dyspnea, anorexia, and cachexia, among others. A multidisciplinary palliative care team may consist of physicians (who practice Palliative Medicine, an American Board of Medical Specialties), nurses, social workers, aides, therapists, pharmacists, chaplains, and volunteers and serves as an extra layer of support for patients and their families. Palliative care can be provided alongside curative or non-curative treatment and at any stage of disease. While it was traditionally provided in the inpatient setting, palliative care is moving upstream to include the ambulatory, facility, and home settings as well. Palliative care providers help patients and their families navigate complex medical decisions by learning about their patients and focusing on aligning treatment options with patients' life philosophies and value systems.

The recent resurgence of interest in medical cannabis and support for its use started predominantly with palliative care applications. Compassionate use programs across most states are reflective of this, and of programs that have qualifying criteria, serious illness, and refractory symptoms are common indications for medical marijuana use. As such, palliative medicine specialists may play an important role for those patients who seek medical cannabis treatments.

Role for Cannabis in Symptom Management

Pain

Palliative medicine specialists are experts in managing pain in the setting of active cancers and nonmalignant pain in the setting of a life-limiting serious illness. Chronic nonmalignant pain does not fall within the scope of palliative medicine and is preferably managed by pain medicine specialists.

The role of cannabinoids in pain management is based on the current understanding of the endocannabinoid system (ECS) and its putative role in pain modulation. Cannabinoid 1 (CB_1) and cannabinoid 2 (CB_2) receptors are well-studied components of the ECS. CB_1 receptors are found on peripheral nerve terminals, and elevated levels are found in areas of the brain that regulate nociceptive processing [2, 3]. CB_1 agonists alone produce analgesic effects in the central nervous system (CNS), while both CB_1 and CB_2 agonists exert analgesic effects peripherally. CB_2 is largely located on anti-inflammatory tissues; through modulation of CB_2, cannabinoids may exert their anti-inflammatory effects by acting on mast cell receptors to attenuate the release of histamine and serotonin and also antinociceptive effects by stimulating keratinocytes to release endogenous opioids [4, 5]. Endocannabinoids, anandamide (AEA), and 2-arachidonoylglycerol (2-AG) modulate nociceptive signaling through local activation of CB_1 receptors. Exogenous phytocannabinoids may regulate neurotransmission and pain signaling within the CNS and immune system.

Cancer Pain

Cancer pain may result from nerve injury, mechanical invasion of pain-sensitive structures, and inflammation. As early as 1975, Noyes et al. explored the effects of synthetic oral delta-9-tetrahydrocannabinol (THC) capsules on cancer pain. The first of two double-blind, placebo-controlled trials measured the pain intensity and pain relief of 10 advanced cancer patients who took 5 mg, 10 mg, 15 mg, and 20 mg of THC or placebo over a 6-hour observation period. It was found that 15 mg and 20 mg doses produced analgesia, though with significant fatigue [6]. Their follow-up study on 34 patients showed that 10 mg of THC produced analgesic effects comparable to 60 mg of codeine [7]. These early studies were limited by small sample sizes, but they led to continued research on cannabinoids for pain management as characterized further. Additionally, these results may inform clinicians about the limited efficacy of cannabinoids in the setting of cancer pain syndromes that often require significant morphine equivalent daily dosing regimens.

Although these early studies used synthetic THC, a more recent study of phytocannabinoids was performed in 2010. This 2-week, multicenter, double-blind trial in Europe investigated the effects of whole-plant extract preparations, nabiximols, in a 1:1 ratio of THC:CBD (cannabidiol) in patients with intractable cancer pain despite optimized opioid therapy. The study showed that the 1:1 extract was superior to THC extract alone or placebo in reducing pain by at least 30% [8]. The follow-up phase III trials of nabiximols for cancer pain demonstrated no improvement in the primary outcome of numerical rating scale (NRS) for pain. However, the experimental group did show improvement in several QOL questionnaires and improvement in sleep with fewer disruptions. This effect was particularly observed in patients from the United States under the age of 65 who were on lower doses of opioids [9]. While evidence for efficacy in cancer-related pain is limited, there may be a possible role of cannabis therapy to address QOL issues.

Further review of the literature reveals distinctions between the patterns of cannabis use between cancer and noncancer patients. In a large cross-sectional study, cancer patients were more likely to use sublingual preparation of cannabis as compared to noncancer patients who were more likely to use an inhaled form [10]. Potential advantages of sublingual preparation of cannabis over inhaled forms include longer duration of action, avoidance of potentially negative pulmonary side effects, and ease of use [10, 11]. This large-scale study showed that medical cannabis users that did not have cancer were more likely to favor inhalation forms through vaporizers, which may raise concerns for potential vaping-related lung injury [10, 12, 13].

Chronic Pain

The data on cannabis use for the treatment of chronic pain conditions is inconclusive. A systematic review of cannabinoids (nabiximols, nabilone, and a fatty acid amide hydrolase inhibitor) found that no studies had a beneficial effect for pain in patients with rheumatoid arthritis, fibromyalgia, or osteoarthritis. Treatment groups also experienced frequent side effects and withdrawals due to those side effects [14]. A randomized, double-blind, placebo-controlled, parallel-design clinical study on the use of oral THC in a dose-escalation fashion in patients with chronic abdominal pain secondary to chronic pancreatitis or surgery showed that, despite adequate absorption of THC, pain intensity did not reduce [15]. A 2017 systematic review on the effects of cannabis among adults for chronic pain concluded that there was insufficient evidence to support its use for non-neuropathic chronic pain conditions, as well as limited evidence showing increased risk for adverse mental health effects [16]. Based on this data, cannabis does not appear to be effective for chronic, nonmalignant, nociceptive pain conditions.

Neuropathic Pain

The most compelling data to support cannabis use for pain management is for neuropathic pain, with several high-quality studies demonstrating its efficacy. A 2015 systematic review and meta-analysis of mostly cannabinoids for neuropathic pain showed greater reduction in pain as compared to the placebo condition [17]. It must be noted, however, that more than half of these studies used synthetic compounds or nabiximols, which may be vastly different from dispensary cannabis products that are available with differing potency and variable oversight. Furthermore, the pain reduction seen in cancer pain syndromes was later debunked with phase III trials of nabiximols.

In 2016, a placebo-controlled, crossover, randomized control trial (RCT) using vaporized cannabis in patients with central neuropathic pain from spinal cord injury showed reduction in neuropathic pain scale ratings without a dose-dependent effect [18]. A similar phase I study on vaporized cannabis for central pain demonstrated similar analgesic effects for both low (2.9%) and high (6.7%) THC concentrations of cannabis with dose-dependent psychoactive side effects (feelings of drunkenness, confusion, difficulty paying attention). Based on this, the investigators concluded that lower potency of THC strains may be preferable due to the similar efficacy with fewer adverse side effects [19]. Another study comparing low (3.5%) versus high (7%) THC levels in smoked cannabis on central and peripheral neuropathic pain demonstrated similar antinociceptive effects, but both groups had increased feelings of impairment, desire for more drug, sedation, and confusion when compared to placebo. Feelings of being "high" and "stoned" and neurocognitive impairments in attention, learning, memory, and psychomotor speed were significantly greater in the higher concentration group as compared to the lower concentration group that exhibited only a decline in learning and memory [20]. These studies suggest a narrow therapeutic window for THC between 2.9% and 3.5% to achieve neuropathic pain relief and minimize potential psychoactive and neurocognitive side effects. The national average of THC potency, however, ranges from 14% to 17% and rising from 4% in 1995 to 12% in 2014 and 17.1% in 2017 [21, 22]. Marijuana concentrates are even more potent, the 2017 Colorado Marijuana Market Size and Demand Study reveals, and THC potency in concentrates jumped from 56.6% in 2014 to 68.6% in 2017 [23]. Shatter and wax, which are forms of concentrates, boast a THC potency as high as 80% [23]. These figures are way above the therapeutic window for pain relief.

In addition to these studies that focus on central pain, there are others that examine peripheral neuropathic conditions. A recent meta-analysis of inhaled cannabis in chronic painful neuropathy showed that inhaled cannabis reduces pain by at least 30% with a number needed to treat (NNT) of one out every five to six patients [24]. While this is promising evidence, the analysis was limited by the small number of studies, potential detection, and performance biases, and the investigators were unable to draw firm conclusions regarding sustained long-term benefits and risk in the community setting [24]. A small, randomized, double-blinded, placebo-controlled, crossover clinical study of patients with diabetic neuropathy showed that vaporized cannabis reduced pain in a dose-dependent manner, with the most consistent effect observed in patients receiving 28 mg THC (CBD content <1%). Medium- and low-dose (16 mg and 4 mg, respectively) THC also resulted in significant reduction in pain intensity scores. Pain reduction was observed as early as 15 minutes and effects were sustained for at least 4 hours [25]. A prospective, placebo-controlled RCT demonstrated efficacy of smoked cannabis cigarettes (THC concentration of 3.56%) in reducing chronic neuropathic pain in HIV-associated peripheral neuropathy [26]. These results were replicated in later studies; however, these studies were small, had short durations, and were not placebo-controlled.

At the time of this writing, the American Academy of Neurology (AAN) position statement on medical marijuana "recognizes that medical marijuana may be useful in treating neurological disorders" and associated symptoms such as pain but also calls for rigorous research to evaluate long-term safety and efficacy of medical marijuana and its compounds. Its favorable position is based on a systematic review of cannabis extract showing efficacy in pain and spasticity management in multiple sclerosis [27, 28]. However, because the safety and efficacy profiles are still uncertain, the AAN further states that it "does not support or advocate for the legalization of medical marijuana for use in neurological disorders at this time." Further research is needed to determine the long-term safety and potential benefits [29].

Nausea

Nausea, the unpleasant sensation of needing to vomit, can occur with or without accompanying vomiting. It is present in up to 80% of cancer patients and even higher in the last days of life [30]. Nausea in the palliative care setting, can result from many causes: drug-induced, conditioned responses (i.e., anticipatory nausea), gastrointestinal origin (e.g., hepatic stretch, gastroparesis, peritoneal inflammation), or central origin (e.g., vestibular dysfunction and brain metastases), among others. The ECS is widely distributed along the gut-brain axis and is purported to play a role in regulating the nausea-vomiting pathway [31].

Chemotherapy-induced nausea and vomiting (CINV) in particular can develop in up to 80% of those receiving chemotherapy and has been well studied [32]. CINV is divided into anticipatory, acute (within 24 hours of medication administration), delayed (greater than 24 hours after medication administration), breakthrough, and refractory. Chemotherapy is thought to induce nausea and vomiting by way of many neurophysiological pathways such as direct stimulation of the chemoreceptor trigger zone, activation of the area postrema, activation of cortical pathways, and activation of peripheral pathways.

There are studies from as early as the 1970s showing the benefits of cannabis-based medications, with the synthetic cannabinoid THC being most commonly studied. Chang et al. performed a placebo-controlled, clinical RCT with 15 patients that showed an incidence of nausea and vomiting of 6–44% depending on the plasma concentration of THC, as compared to 72% for the control group [33]. Since the availability of nabilone, a synthetic THC analogue, and dronabinol, synthetic THC, for treatment of CINV in 1985 and 2006, respectively, several studies and reviews have confirmed the efficacy of cannabinoids for CINV.

A systematic review by Tramer et al. analyzed 30 clinical trials which studied oral dronabinol, oral nabilone, and intramuscular levonantradol [34]. Cannabinoids were found to be more effective than prochlorperazine, metoclopramide, chlorpromazine, thiethylperazine, haloperidol, domperidone, or alizapride for complete control of nausea, though not for very low or very high emetogenic chemotherapy. A later review by Amar in 2006 evaluated 15 studies with nabilone and 14 with dronabinol. Nabilone was superior to prochlorperazine, domperidone, and alizapride for treating CINV, leading to its FDA approval [35].

A more recent Cochrane Review in 2015 looked at 23 RCTs performed between 1975 and 1991 with moderate to highly emetogenic chemotherapy regimens. It found that, compared with placebo, patients were more likely to report absence of nausea and vomiting when cannabinoids were administered, though also more likely to withdraw from the experiments for adverse effects. Furthermore, patients reported a preference of cannabinoids over placebo. There was no evidence of difference between cannabinoids and prochlorperazine or other antiemetics. To note, however, the quality of evidence was rated as low. Another review showed that cannabinoids were more effective than the more typical antiemetics prochlorperazine, metoclopramide, chlorpromazine, and haloperidol [36]. Despite the efficacy of these medications, it should be noted that side effects can also limit widespread use.

While there are sufficient data for the efficacy of synthetic cannabinoids, the evidence for phytocannabinoids is more limited. A 2015 review by Kramer et al. reviewed two studies that looked at smoked marijuana: one study of 15 patients showed benefit in reducing nausea and vomiting, while the other study of 8 patients did not [37]. Medical cannabis may play a role in palliation of nausea and vomiting despite optimized trials of standard antiemetics including synthetic cannabinoids. Further studies are needed to demonstrate comparative efficacy and safety to standard antiemetics.

Anorexia and Cachexia (Dysgeusia)

The ECS may play a role in modulating appetite via CB_1 receptors [38, 39] by reinforcing the motivation to find and consume food with high-incentive value and regulating levels and actions of orexigenic and anorectic mediators [40, 41]. Cannabinoids or, more specifically, pharmaceutical THC drugs have been shown to stimulate appetite in patients with AIDS [42]. However, studies of patients with cancer-related anorexia-cachexia syndrome (CACS) do not demonstrate efficacy [43]. One phase III trial did show that patients with CACS had increased appetite with cannabis extract and THC; however, there was no significant difference compared to placebo in appetite, QOL, mood, or nausea [43]. In patients with CACS, megestrol was found to be superior to dronabinol (2.5 mg twice daily) alone or as adjunctive treatment of megestrol for palliation of anorexia [44].

Dysgeusia is a major complaint of patients on chemotherapy that contributes to anorexia and negatively impacts QOL. In 2011, a double-blind, placebo-controlled, pilot RCT showed that administration of dronabinol to advanced cancer patients with poor appetite and chemosensory alterations resulted in improved and enhanced chemosensory perception and food taste, but no significant differences were seen in appetite, caloric consumption, or QOL scores between the control and treatment groups [45].

Shortness of Breath

Dyspnea is a very commonly reported symptom in palliative care patients. A study done by Pickering et al. found no statistical difference in visual analogue scale (VAS) dyspnea scores in a small RCT in 2011 [45]. While there is no evidence to link smoking marijuana and lung cancer as there is with cigarette smoking, several studies have shown an association between smoking marijuana and the development of chronic bronchitis symptoms [46]. At the time of this writing, there is also a growing concern for the association between vaping devices and lung illness; there have been 380 reported cases and 6 deaths and all cases have a history of using vape devices [47]. Current evidence does not support the use of cannabinoids for dyspnea.

Fatigue

There is evidence that suggests that cannabis may also help alleviate symptoms associated with fatigue. Frequent users report that marijuana gives them mental clarity and focus, but larger-scale controlled studies are lacking. A small 2017 study looking at performance and mood disruptions during simulated night shift work showed that smoking THC reduced disruptions in inhibitory control, recall, sustained attention, and reaction time in a dose- and time-dependent manner and that its participants reported feeling markedly more stimulated and less tired [48]. A caveat to this study is that it was very small with only 10 subjects, and the simulated conditions of shift work may not be reflective of the fatigue that often accompanies serious illness. Another survey study of 538 people with Parkinson's disease and multiple sclerosis found that, compared to non-cannabis users, cannabis users reported less fatigue [49].

However, there is conflicting data that excessive daytime sleepiness is also associated with cannabis use [50]. This seemingly contradictory effect may be explained by recent work demonstrating CBD as a wake-promoting agent and its ability to counteract the sedative effect of THC [51, 52]. The various effects of cannabis on fatigue may be attributed to the different composition of cannabinoids between cannabis products. Further research is needed to better understand the optimal cannabinoid profiles to help with fatigue management.

Insomnia

Studies of medicinal cannabis users have identified insomnia as a common indication for its use. Cannabinoid concentration, dose, and route of administration may have different effects on sleep quality and insomnia symptoms as evidenced by the conflicting and mixed results found in the literature. According to some studies, the role of CBD in the sleep-wake cycle is dose-dependent, with higher doses resulting in increased sleep duration and decreased arousal [53], while lower doses of CBD increases wakefulness, producing a stimulating effect [52, 54]. For THC, a dose of 15 mg resulted in increased sleepiness and delayed sleep onset on the following day after administration [52], and chronic administration of THC was associated with tolerance to its soporific effects [55]. A cross-sectional study of medical cannabis users with insomnia and sleep latency was more likely to use higher CBD concentrations, and there was an association between higher THC doses and decreased hypnotic medication use [56]. Another study found that medicinal cannabis users, both with and without reported sleep problems, experienced decreased sleep latency after cannabis use [57].

Studies of individual cannabinoids (THC and CBD) on sleep quality and insomnia show conflicting results. Both phytocannabinoids and synthetic THC were associated with decreased sleep latency [52, 58], but one study with synthetic THC administration found that the overall amount of nighttime sleep decreased over time, suggestive of a tolerance effect [58]. One of these studies found that, when combined with CBD, THC decreased stage 3 non-rapid eye movement (NREM) sleep, which is the most restorative stage of sleep [54]. Another study on CBD found that it blocked anxiety-induced rapid eye movement (REM) sleep suppression with no effect on NREM sleep [59]. Similarly, anecdotal evidence showed that administration of CBD oil reduced insomnia symptoms and sleep disturbances related to post-traumatic stress disorder (PTSD) [60], suggesting that CBD may impact sleep quality through its anxiolytic effects.

Conclusive data on cannabis for sleep is lacking and further evidence is needed to determine efficacy and duration of treatment for different sleep disorders before this can be a recommended treatment for insomnia.

Anxiety

As with the management of other symptoms, the effects of cannabis on mood are dependent on the composition of its various cannabinoids. Previous studies garnered evidence supporting the anxiolytic and antipsychotic effects of CBD that seem to counteract THC-induced anxiety [61, 62] with lower doses of THC producing anxiolytic effects and higher doses produce anxiogenic effects [63].

THC doses between 1.25 and 30 mg were shown to decrease anxiety in a biphasic, dose-dependent manner in healthy adults [64]. Studies of dronabinol showed that administration of 7.5 mg resulted in reduced limbic reactivity in the lateral amygdala, which is the brain's emotion processing center, to angry or fearful faces [65]. CBD has been shown to produce anxiolytic effects and counteracts the anxiogenic effects of THC, with doses of 300–400 mg producing the same effects as ipsapirone, a serotonin 1A ($5HT_{1A}$) receptor partial agonist in healthy participants [66, 67]. While it may be known that cannabis may induce feelings of dysphoria, anxiety, and panic, studies demonstrate that cannabis generally reduces anxiety when administered at lower doses with CBD activating CB_1 receptors on glutamatergic cortical neurons, offsetting anxiogenic effects of THC regulated by CB_1 receptors on GABAergic forebrain activity [68].

A 2019 systematic review evaluating cannabidiol use in psychiatric disorders identified two completed RCTs exploring the efficacy of acute administration of CBD on anxiety symptoms in patients with social anxiety disorder (SAD). The first, a double-blind RCT with 24 never-treated SAD patients who received 600 mg CBD versus placebo and compared to healthy controls after a simulated public speaking test (SPST) showed significant inhibition in fear of public speaking in the CBD group when compared to placebo [69]. A second within-subject, crossover design RCT with 10 participants compared 400 mg of CBD versus placebo with CBD being associated with significantly decreased levels of anxiety compared to placebo [70]. Currently, a double-blind, placebo-controlled RCT of 50 adults with primary SAD, generalized anxiety disorder (GAD), and panic disorder (PD) is comparing the efficacy and safety of flexibly dosed CBD oil capsules versus placebo [71]. As mentioned earlier, a double-blind placebo RCT of 40 healthy individuals showed that compared to ipsapirone (5 mg) and diazepam (10 mg), 300 mg CBD successfully decreased anxiety after SPST [66]. More recently, in another double-blind study in healthy volunteers, 300 mg of CBD in powder form was identified as the optimal therapeutic dose when compared to placebo to treat SPST-induced anxiety [72]. Taken together, it is likely that any anxiolytic effects of cannabis are primarily CBD-mediated.

Depression

One of the most common known effects of cannabis is a sense of euphoria. Although there is much interest in using these possible euphoric effects to treat depression, there are only case reports [65, 73–75], and large clinical studies do not support cannabis-based medicines for this indication. Furthermore, use of rimonabant, a CB_1 receptor antagonist, increased indices of depression and suicidal ideation in healthy individuals, and rimonabant was subsequently taken off the market due to its severe side effects [64].

The ECS is involved in the clinical effect of various antidepressants. Studies have shown that chronic treatment with tricyclic antidepressants (TCAs) is associated with increased CB_1 receptor density in the hippocampus and hypothalamus and reduced hypothalamic-pituitary-adrenal (HPA) axis activation by stressing stimuli [75, 76]. 2-AG is one of the main endocannabinoids and has its own mimetic phytocannabinoid, CBD; AEA is another endocannabinoid with THC as its mimetic phytocannabinoid. Reduced circulating levels of both endocannabinoids 2-AG and AEA were found in patients with major depressive disorder (MDD) [77, 78]. There are studies that also implicate that genetic variability in ECS regulation can influence susceptibility to mood disorders [79]. Genetic polymorphisms of the ECS have been associated with depressive symptoms and may influence response to antidepressant treatment [80–83]. Despite this preclinical data, there is no high-quality evidence to support the use of phytocannabinoids for depression.

Delirium and Agitation

Prevalence of delirium in the inpatient palliative care setting is reported to be as high as 42% and can be burdensome for patients as well as their caregivers [84]. Treatment of delirium includes both nonpharmacologic and pharmacologic approaches to address modifiable risk factors. There have been a few studies that show that dronabinol can be a good adjunct to standard regimens to decrease the neuropsychiatric symptoms of dementia, including decrease in negative affect, agitation, motor behavior, nighttime disturbances, irritability, and sundowning [85, 86]. A retrospective cohort study published in 2014 showed an association between addition of dronabinol to standard treatment regimens and decreased aberrant vocalizations, motor agitation, aggressiveness, and resistance to care in geriatric patients with dementia [87].

An important note to consider is that synthetic cannabinoids, particularly THC, can worsen psychosis in those with underlying disease or cause new-onset delirium or psychosis in those without underlying mental health disorders [88]. Interestingly, cannabinoid use may be helpful in the treatment of delirium secondary to cannabis intoxication. Levin et al. showed decreased withdrawal symptoms when 10–20 mg of dronabinol was administered daily [89]. Allsop et al. in 2014 found similar results with administration of THC (maximum daily dose of 86.4 mg) and 80 mg of CBD [90]. While there is some literature to support use for cannabis intoxication, evidence to support its use in other settings is more limited. Concern for potential neurotoxic excitation and agitated delirium caused by excessive doses of cannabinoids need to be considered in palliative care patients with potentially limited CNS reserve, especially with unregulated doses of THC that are becoming more widely available [91].

Quality of Life and Existential Distress

Patients living with serious illnesses and accompanying functional loss often experience spiritual and/or existential distress which can be manifested as meaninglessness, hopelessness, being a burden on others, or questioning life itself. Survey-based studies that elicit motivations for cannabis use in the cancer population, such as that done by Pergam et al., reveal that people admit to using cannabis for stress reduction, improvement of QOL, and dealing with this type of distress [92]. Current approaches to relieving existential distress include cognitive behavioral interventions, hypnotically facilitated therapy, meaning-centered psychotherapy, and dignity therapy. These interventions often aim to discuss concerns regarding death and dying openly and clarify new life goals to help create new meaning for patients [93, 94]. Anecdotally and based on clinical experience, there is a subset of patients that appreciates that the euphoric effects of cannabis can create similar results. SK Aggarwal also suggests that "a mild euphoria," "reduction of psychological trauma," and the "increased introspection and meditation" that can result from cannabis use may be helpful in alleviating existential distress [95]. This is an important domain of palliative care for which medical cannabis may provide benefit and more research is needed.

Precautions for Cannabis Use in Palliative Care

For as long as cannabis has been used, adverse effects have been reported. For example, in 1883, Dr. James Oliver described the "cerebral symptoms" from cannabis use in the British Medical Journal as "peculiar indescribable sensations in the head, by no means pleasant in nature," with some of his patients having "an irresistible desire to be always on the move" while others lost "control over the muscles" [96]. Over 100 years later, we now understand a great deal more about how cannabis interacts with different organ systems within the body, including the cardiovascular, pulmonary, and gastrointestinal systems (Table 13.1).

Naturally occurring cannabis plant species produce a group of molecules called phytocannabinoids (plant-based cannabinoids), of which there are over 100 types, and they have varying degrees of effects on the human body [97]. Two of the most active and abundant phytocannabinoids are THC and CBD [96, 98]. THC is known to exert most of the known psychoactive and physiological effects by acting on two endogenous receptors, CB_1 and CB_2. Unlike THC, CBD lacks detectable psychoactive properties and is believed to have lower affinity for CB_1 and CB_2. CBD is thought to counteract some of the effects of THC [99]. While the actions exerted on

Table 13.1 Possible side effects of cannabis by organ system

Psychiatric	Alteration of perception, time distortion, paranoia, anxiety, hallucinations [99]
Neurological	Somnolence, fatigue, memory impairment, dizziness. Cardiovascular events including cerebral vasoconstriction can lead to cerebral ischemia and sleep disturbance [61–63, 155, 156]
Eyes, ears, nose, throat	Reddened eyes, reduced tear flow, photophobia, xerostomia, dental caries [124, 129, 157, 158]
Cardiovascular	Hyperadrenergic state, hypertension, tachycardia, orthostasis, arrhythmia, selective vasodilation/vasoconstriction [100–103]
Pulmonary	Bronchodilation – all forms Cough, wheezes, shortness of breath, increased sputum – when smoked [129, 139, 157, 159]
Gastrointestinal	Nausea, vomiting, increased appetite [145]
Genitourinary	Sperm impairment, possibly erectile dysfunction [8, 118, 148, 160]
Immunologic	Infections [152, 154]

CB_1 and CB_2 by THC and CBD account for their therapeutic effects, they are also the cause of many side effects that we will discuss in this section.

Side Effects

The side effects of cannabis described in the literature generally occur within 30 minutes to 1 hour of consumption and last 2–4 hours after. Eye redness, caused by dilation of blood vessels in the eye, is one of the most notorious side effects associated with cannabis use [100]. THC also has other effects on the eyes, such as reducing intraocular pressure, decreasing tear flow, and causing photophobia. The mechanism by which photophobia occurs is not entirely clear, but it may be due to palpebral fissure narrowing and eyelid ptosis.

Dry mouth (xerostomia) is another very common side effect experienced by cannabis users. This is thought to be caused by the parasympatholytic properties seen in cannabis [101]. Xerostomia has been found to be beneficial in some palliative care patients, namely, head and neck cancer patients who benefit from decreased secretions [102]. This can, however, increase the incidence rate of dental caries and may also be a negative side effect in patients who already suffer from dry mouth [101].

Less commonly known side effects of cannabis include its effects on the reproductive system. Early research supported the idea that marijuana use increased sexual desire, quality of orgasms, and emotional intimacy [103]. Over time, some of the negative effects have come to light as more recent data suggests that chronic cannabis use can reduce sperm count, concentration, and motility, in addition to causing abnormalities in sperm morphology [104]. Animal studies on rats have shown that CB_1 activation by THC can cause erectile dysfunction, but there has not yet been sufficient data to show either beneficial or detrimental effects on erectile function in humans [105].

Psychological

In 2006, 12 students from the University of California at Berkeley were taken to a local hospital after eating marijuana cookies, brownies, and cookie dough. They were described as having severe anxiety and "feelings of doom" due to the ingestion [106]. In 2016, two young men became paranoid after ingesting large amounts of marijuana and called 911 on themselves; they were convinced that they were surrounded by undercover police officers [107]. A study from 2015 showed definitively that intravenous THC increases paranoia when compared to the placebo treatment [108]. Interestingly, informing subjects that THC can cause paranoia increased the likelihood of the event. Subjects that had THC-induced anxiety were more likely to have paranoid ideations.

There is a dose-dependent effect of THC on anxiety, with low doses potentially having an anxiolytic effect and higher doses leading to increased rates of anxiety [109]. It is hypothesized that the complex interaction of the ECS with the amygdala, dopaminergic-dependent brain regions, and HPA axis are responsible for inducing and relieving anxiety. Among studies looking at medical cannabis use for pain, anxiety remains a common side effect, while frank paranoia and psychosis are reported to a lesser degree [110].

Special care should be taken to inform patients about these potentially distressing side effects when starting medical cannabinoids. Recommending medical cannabis to patients with schizophrenia, schizoaffective disorder, or other psychotic disorders should be avoided. Despite associations between schizophrenia and recreational marijuana use, a causal link has not been established. However, there is a concerning association between cannabis use and earlier onset of psychosis, adverse course of psychotic symptoms with exacerbation of symptoms, and negative course of illness [111, 112]. Acute cannabinoid use can induce psychotic symptoms including suspicious and persecutory paranoia, grandiose delusions, conceptual disorganization, fragmented thinking, and perceptual alterations, which can be indistinguishable from those seen in schizophrenia [113]. Additionally, individuals who use large amounts of cannabis at younger ages are more likely to develop mental health disorders in the future [114]. While these psychiatric side effects are often short-lived, prolonged symptoms may occur depending on the method of delivery. Given the dose-dependent nature of psychiatric side effects, it is generally recommended that patients start at a low dose and increase as tolerated.

Neurological

The distribution of the CB_1 receptors throughout the brain is generally considered to be the culprit of the neurological side effects seen mainly with THC. Early RCTs of nabilone for CINV revealed dizziness as one of the most common side effects of the medication [50, 115]. Over time, trials assessing the therapeutic benefits of synthetic cannabinoids for a variety of uses in palliative care populations support the findings from these early trials [116–118]. The dizziness induced by cannabinoids is thought to be caused by the CB_1 receptors located within cells of the cerebellum [119]. Dizziness should always be considered and discussed when recommending cannabinoids, and it is especially important in palliative care patients who often have underlying mobility impairment and increased frailty.

Among palliative care patients, the other extremely important side effect to consider is sleep disturbance. In general, studies have shown that cannabinoids increase sleep quality and can decrease sleep disturbances [120]. Drowsiness is one of the most common side effects described in multiple clinical trials [110]. While this may be helpful in patients that cannot sleep because of severe pain, it may be detrimental to patients with fatigue from end-stage diseases. Furthermore, chronic cannabis users may experience worse sleep when coming off the substance, so patients should be counseled on this aspect if they plan to stop or decrease use of cannabis.

Memory is another area that is highly affected by THC. Among the many aspects of memory, both delayed and immediate word list recall seem to be affected the most [121]. In adults, working memory worsens with marijuana use, with higher use correlating with worse working memory (multiple tasks on the Wechsler Adult Intelligence Scale) [122]. These issues seem to resolve with periods of abstinence. Other domains of executive functioning also seem to be affected by both acute and chronic cannabis use. Planning, attention, reasoning, and problem-solving each seem to be affected to varying degrees. These effects seem to be more pronounced in older adults and, only rarely, within particular domains, may persist after discontinuation of use [122, 123]. Further studies are needed to better understand the impact of these side effects, particularly in geriatric populations of cannabis users who may be more susceptible due to underlying baseline cognitive and mobility dysfunction.

Cerebrovascular

Another major neurological side effect to consider is strokes, with which marijuana use has been loosely associated. There have been case reports and case series of patients presenting with strokes after ingestion of marijuana [124–127]. In an epidemiologic study looking at young patients presenting with cerebral infarction, 6% of 422 patients reported cannabis as the only drug that was taken prior to the event [128]. Furthermore, animal studies have shown that THC exerts a concentration-dependent vasoconstriction effect on blood vessels in the brain [129]. This could be a potential mechanism for marijuana to cause ischemic stroke. Relative hypotension from systemic vasodilation or sympathetic surge after ingestion could also be contributing factors. The data supporting an association between cannabis use and cerebrovascular events at this time remains scant, and more studies are required to clearly delineate a causative effect.

Cardiovascular

One of the first physiologic studies pertaining to cannabis use was from 1969, where it was noted that there was a moderate increase in heart rate after using marijuana [130]. Since that time, it has become clear that this increase in heart rate is likely due to THC's effects on the autonomic nervous system, namely, simultaneous stimulation of the sympathetic system and inhibition of the parasympathetic system [131]. The effects cause an increase in cardiac output with catecholamine release that can last up to 2 hours [132]. Cannabis generally causes a slight increase in systolic blood pressure and a slight decrease in diastolic blood pressure because it also has vasodilatory effects on the peripheral vasculature [133]. This drop in diastolic pressure can lead to orthostatic hypotension, dizziness, and syncope [134]. It should be noted that these physiologic changes seem to diminish with chronic cannabis use [134, 135].

The increase in sympathetic tone during THC ingestion inevitably increases the heart's oxygen requirements and can therefore worsen underlying angina [136, 137]. Many studies looking at cardiac ischemia from marijuana use had subjects smoke marijuana which can increase carboxyhemoglobin and worsen blood oxygen levels. There have also been numerous case reports and case series on marijuana-inducing cardiac arrhythmias from atrial fibrillation to ventricular tachycardia, and this is thought to be from increased sinoatrial and atrioventricular nodal conduction in addition to enhanced sinus automaticity [138–142]. It is unknown whether or not these cardiovascular effects can occur in non-smoking forms of cannabis.

Given that patients seen in palliative care usually have multiple chronic comorbidities, it is very important to assess a patient's underlying cardiac function. Patients should be counseled on the possible cardiac side effects and make sure to contact providers if they experience any symptoms that could indicate an arrhythmia or cardiac ischemia. It may be reasonable to forgo treatment with medical cannabis if a patient has underlying arrhythmias, heart failure, or hypotension, depending on their goals of care. For example, if one's goal is solely QOL for which cannabis may be beneficial, they may opt to use cannabis despite its potential impact on shortening quantity of life.

Pulmonary

While cannabis can be ingested in multiple ways, smoking has historically been the most common mode of ingestion. Countless publications from throughout the 1900s looked at how smoking cannabis affects the lungs. Studies have shown that smoking marijuana chronically correlates with higher rates of asthma, bronchitis, cough, shortness of breath, and wheezing [143]. While smoking marijuana does have implications on the respiratory tract, this does not necessarily apply to FDA-approved cannabinoid formulations.

There have not been any studies looking specifically at orally ingested cannabinoids and effects on the pulmonary system. We can extrapolate from past studies on aerosolized THC inhalation to infer that orally ingested cannabis likely causes a similar effect on bronchodilation, with increases in forced expiratory volume (FEV1) [144, 145]. In multiple clinical trials looking at orally ingested cannabis medications, there does not seem to be any common pulmonary side effects [8, 17, 117, 118, 146].

Electronic cigarettes (e-cigarettes) are a new form of inhaling nicotine and marijuana oils and are commonly referred to as "vaping." The electronic devices aerosolize oils containing THC or nicotine, flavoring, and other chemicals that are then inhaled [147]. As of September 2019, an ongoing multistate investigation by the Center of Disease Control (CDC) on cases of severe pulmonary disease related to "vaping" was underway with the first cases sprouting in Wisconsin and Illinois [12]. More than 25 states have reported at least 215 possible cases, and rising, of severe pulmonary disease associated with vaping THC, nicotine, or both; at least two reported deaths have also been reported to the CDC [13]. As such, while the safety, or lack thereof, of vaping is being investigated, users should consider discontinuing this form of THC administration. At the very least, if vaping is continued, users should monitor themselves for symptoms and seek prompt medical attention if needed.

Gastrointestinal

Cannabinoids may help with appetite and alleviate nausea and vomiting. While there seems to be an improvement in nausea and vomiting in multiple studies, there is also a paradoxical increase in nausea and vomiting in some chronic cannabis users [148]. Long-term cannabis use may cause increased secretion and activation of corticotropin-release leading to this paradoxical increase in nausea and vomiting [149]. These effects are exaggerated in cannabinoid hyperemesis syndrome.

There are many studies of cannabis for different pain indications. In a number of these studies, nausea, dizziness, and vomiting are some of the most common adverse events. For example, in a 2010 placebo-controlled RCT investigating the efficacy of THC:CBD in patients with advanced cancer, there was a significant worsening of nausea and vomiting scores in the treatment group when compared to placebo. A trial from the Journal of Pain looking at the effects of various doses of nabiximols on cancer-related symptoms showed a dose-related incidence of adverse outcomes [118]. Subjects who received higher doses of nabiximols had higher rates of both nausea and vomiting. For subjects who received any dose of nabiximols, 22% had nausea and 16% had vomiting. This was higher than the placebo group where 13% of subjects reported nausea and 8% reported vomiting [118]. In a meta-analysis looking at cannabinoids as compared to placebo, a total of 3,529 subjects (from 30 different studies) reported nausea, giving it a summary odds ratio of 2.08 [17].

Orexigenic effects of cannabis may help cancer patients. Animal models and clinical studies demonstrate a role for the ECS in eating motivation [17, 150]. While these effects are often desired in palliative care patients, for others this may worsen obesity and metabolic syndrome.

Recent data on Epidiolex, a CBD oral solution derived from plant extract that is FDA-approved for seizures in Lennox-Gastaut syndrome and Dravet syndrome, is concerning for effects on the liver [151–153]. Up to 10% of patients showed alanine aminotransferase (ALT) and aspartate aminotransferase (AST) levels greater than three times the upper limit of normal. Of these patients, 78% were also on valproic acid while 22% were not [151]. Liver enzyme levels returned to normal after stopping or decreasing the dose of Epidiolex or other anti-seizure medications like valproic acid. There was no significant increase in bilirubin to indicate severe drug-induced liver injury [99]. As new indications for using CBD arise, its effects on the liver, especially for those who may have underlying dysfunction, will be important to monitor.

Immunologic

The ECS plays a role in the immune system. Concern that cannabinoids may affect the immune system derives from studies of nabiximols. In clinical studies of this marijuana-derived CBD extract, patients had up to a 41% chance of infections, greater than that of the placebo group [152]. Potential immune system dysregulation should be considered when offering cannabis-based medicines to frail palliative care patients.

Additionally, there have been reports of contaminated cannabis at dispensaries [43–45]. In 2017, CBS News reported on a California man undergoing intensive chemotherapy treatment with concurrent medical marijuana use to stave off treatment effects. The patient died from a rare lethal fungal infection as a result of medicinal marijuana use. Physician researchers at UC Davis performed a study on 20 marijuana samples and found them to contain multiple contaminants of bacterial and fungal pathogens including *Cryptococcus*, *Mucor*, *Aspergillus*, *Escherichia coli*, *Klebsiella pneumoniae*, and *Acinetobacter baumannii* [154]. In an already immunocompromised individual, such as a cancer patient undergoing chemotherapy, exposure to such pathogens may be fatal. These potential risks should be discussed with patients before initiating cannabis-based treatments.

Drug-Drug Interactions

Drug metabolism is an extremely complex system by which active components of medications are broken down by enzymes. Both THC and CBD are metabolized in the liver. THC, for example, is oxidized by the enzyme cytochrome P450 (CYP) 2C9 to the primary psychoactive metabolite 11-hydroxy-THC [161], and then further broken down by CYP3A4. THC is known to inhibit the hepatic CYP2C9 enzyme, and this could potentially lead to an increased level of the medications that this enzyme would otherwise metabolize (including but not limited to NSAIDs, sulfonylureas, warfarin, antidepressants, and antiepileptics) [161]. There have been case reports of patients with high international normalized ratio (INR) values due to CYP inhibition by THC [162]. CBD exerts an inhibitory effect on both CYP2C19 and CYP3A4. Data on CBD's interaction with typical medications is scant, but there is an emerging body of evidence that Epidiolex can increase levels of valproic acid, phenytoin, and clobazam [161].

At this time, formal pharmacokinetic studies on how cannabinoids interact with commonly prescribed medications are lacking. Additionally, the inconsistent formulation of various products makes predicting drug interactions difficult. With the availability of more concentrated formulations of CBD, caution should be used with patients on medications that are metabolized by CYP2C19 and CYP3A4. Similarly, with the rise of THC concentrations in some preparations of cannabis, patients may need careful monitoring for potential drug interactions.

Best Practices for the Palliative Care Provider

While discussing the role of cannabis in addressing patient symptoms, it is important to keep the prognosis and intent of treatment (e.g., curative or palliative) in mind. Some cancer- or treatment-related side effects may subside after treatments are completed or treatment dosages are reduced. For instance, a patient receiving radiation therapy can have acute pain that should improve by several weeks after radiation. This patient may be an appropriate candidate for medical cannabis but for a time-limited period. Discussions about treatment duration and expectations are important to set appropriate boundaries and indications for cannabis use. Due to the limited data on the safety profile of medical cannabis, goals of care conversations are necessary to weigh the potential benefits based on limited data versus theoretical and known risks before continuation of cannabis-based treatments.

Although patient counseling guidelines regarding medical cannabis have not been standardized, treatment discussions should include type (such as strain, formulation, etc.), expected benefits and adverse effects, onset of action, dose (doses of cannabinoids if known), route of administration, precautions, and interactions [163]. One way to augment counseling efforts regarding medical cannabis would be to extrapolate from the concepts derived from opioid pain management and use a written agreement. Although the liability and legal ramifications of cannabis agreement forms are yet unknown, examples of such can be found and should be considered by cannabis practitioners [164].

References

1. CAPC. What is palliative care? [Internet]. Available from: https://getpalliativecare.org/whatis/.
2. Pertwee RG, editor. Handbook of cannabis. Oxford: Oxford University Press; 2014.

3. Fine PG, Rosenfeld MJ. The endocannabinoid system, cannabinoids, and pain. Rambam Maimonides Med J. 2013;4(4):e0022.
4. Facci L, Toso RD, Romanello S, Buriani A, Skaper SD, Leon A. Mast cells express a peripheral cannabinoid receptor with differential sensitivity to anandamide and palmitoylethanolamide. Proc Natl Acad Sci U S A. 1995;92(8):3376–80.
5. Ibrahim MM, Porreca F, Lai J, Albrecht PJ, Rice FL, Khodorova A, et al. CB2 cannabinoid receptor activation produces antinociception by stimulating peripheral release of endogenous opioids. Proc Natl Acad Sci U S A. 2005;102(8):3093–8.
6. Noyes R, Brunk SF, Baram DA, Canter A. Analgesic effect of delta-9-tetrahydrocannabinol. J Clin Pharmacol. 1975;15(2–3):139–43.
7. Noyes R, Brunk SF, Avery DH, Canter A. The analgesic properties of delta-9-tertrahydrocannabinol and codeine. Clin Pharmacol Ther. 1975;18(1):84–9.
8. Johnson JR, Burnell-Nugent M, Lossignol D, Ganae-Motan ED, Potts R, Fallon MT. Multicenter, double-blind, randomized, placebo-controlled, parallel-group study of the efficacy, safety and tolerability of THC:CBD extract and THC extract in patients with intractable cancer-related pain. J Pain Symptom Manag. 2010;39(2):167–79.
9. Fallon MT, Lux EA, McQuade R, Rossetti S, Sanchez R, Sun W, et al. Sativex oromucosal spray as adjunctive therapy in advanced cancer patients with chronic pain unalleviated by optimized opioid therapy: two double-blind, randomized, placebo-controlled phase 3 studies. Br J Pain. 2017;11(3):119–33.
10. Kim A, Kaufmann CN, Ko R, Li Z, Han BH. Patterns of medical cannabis use among cancer patients from a medical cannabis dispensary in New York state. J Palliat Med. 2019;22(10):1196–201.
11. Huestis MA. Human cannabinoid pharmacokinetics. Chem Biodivers. 2007;4(8):1770–804.
12. Layden JE, Ghinai I, Pray I, Kimball A, Layer M, Tenforde M, et al. Pulmonary Illness Related to E-Cigarette Use in Illinois and Wisconsin — Final Report. N Engl J Med. 2020; 382:903–16.
13. Schier JG, Meiman JG, Layden J, Mikosz CA, Vanfrank B, King BA, et al. Severe pulmonary disease associated with electronic-cigarette–product–use — interim guidance. MMWR Morb Mortal Wkly Rep. 2019;68(36):787–90.
14. Fitzcharles MA, Ste-Marie PA, Hauser W, Clauw DJ, Jamal S, Karsh J, et al. Efficacy, tolerability, and safety of cannabinoid treatments in the rheumatic diseases: a systematic review of randomized controlled trials. Arthritis Care Res. 2016;68(5):681–8.
15. de Vries M, van Rijckevorsel DC, Vissers KC, Wilder-Smith OH, van Goor H. Tetrahydrocannabinol does not reduce pain in patients with chronic abdominal pain in a phase 2 placebo-controlled study. Clin Gastroenterol Hepatol. 2017;15(7):1079–86.
16. Nugent SM, Morasco BJ, O'Neil ME, Freeman M, Low A, Kondo K, et al. The effects of cannabis among adults with chronic pain and an overview of general harms: a systematic review. Ann Intern Med. 2017;167(5):319–31.
17. Whiting PF, Wolff RF, Deshpande S, Di Nisio M, Duffy S, Hernandez AV, et al. Cannabinoids for medical use: a systematic review and meta-analysis. JAMA. 2015;313(24):2456–73.
18. Wallace M, Schulteis G, Atkinson JH, Wolfson T, Lazzaretto D, Bentley H, et al. Dose-dependent effects of smoked cannabis on capsaicin-induced pain and hyperalgesia in healthy volunteers. Anesthesiology. 2007;107(5):785–96.
19. Wilsey B, Marcotte TD, Deutsch R, Zhao H, Prasad H, Phan A. An exploratory human laboratory experiment evaluating vaporized cannabis in the treatment of neuropathic pain from spinal cord injury and disease. J Pain. 2016;17(9):982–1000.
20. Wilsey B, Marcotte T, Tsodikov A, Millman J, Bentley H, Gouaux B, et al. Randomized, placebo-controlled, crossover trial of cannabis cigarettes in neuropathic pain. J Pain. 2008;9(6):506–21.
21. ElSohly MA, Mehmedic Z, Foster S, Gon C, Chandra S, Church JC. Changes in cannabis potency over the last 2 decades (1995-2014): analysis of current data in the United States. Biol Psychiatry. 2016;79(7):613–9.

22. Chandra S, Radwan MM, Majumdar CG, Church JC, Freeman TP, ElSohly MA. New trends in cannabis potency in USA and Europe during the last decade (2008–2017). Eur Arch Psychiatry Clin Neurosci. 2019;269(1):5–15.

23. Orens A, Light M, Lewandowski B, Rowberry J, Saloga C. Market size and demand for marijuana in Colorado 2017 market update. Boulder: Marijuana Policy Group; 2018. p. 1–51.

24. Andreae MH, Carter GM, Shaparin N, Suslov K, Ellis RJ, Ware MA, et al. Inhaled cannabis for chronic neuropathic pain: a meta-analysis of individual patient data. J Pain. 2015;16(12):1221–32.

25. Wallace MS, Marcotte TD, Umlauf A, Gouaux B, Atkinson JH. Efficacy of inhaled cannabis on painful diabetic neuropathy. J Pain. 2015;16(7):616–27.

26. Abrams DI, Jay CA, Shade SB, Vizoso H, Reda H, Press S, et al. Cannabis in painful HIV-associated sensory neuropathy: a randomized placebo-controlled trial. Neurology. 2007;68(7):515–21.

27. Yadav V, Bever C, Bowen J, Bowling A, Weinstock-Guttman B, Cameron M, et al. Summary of evidence-based guideline: complementary and alternative medicine in multiple sclerosis: report of the guideline development subcommittee of the American Academy of Neurology. Neurology. 2014;82(12):1083–92.

28. Koppel BS, Brust JC, Fife T, Bronstein J, Youssof S, Gronseth G, et al. Systematic review: efficacy and safety of medical marijuana in selected neurologic disorders: report of the guideline development subcommittee of the American Academy of Neurology. Neurology. 2014;82(17):1556–63.

29. Patel FD, Brust J, Song S, Miller T, Narayanaswami P. Position statement: use of medical marijuana for neurologic disorders [Internet]. The American Academy of Neurology; 2014 [cited 2019 Sep 10]. Available from: https://www.aan.com/uploadedFiles/Website_Library_Assets/Documents/6.Public_Policy/1.Stay_Informed/2.Position_Statements/3.PDFs_of_all_Position_Statements/Final%20Medical%20Marijuana%20Position%20Statement.pdf.

30. Morran C, Smith DC, Anderson DA, McArdle CS. Incidence of nausea and vomiting with cytotoxic chemotherapy: a prospective randomized trial of antiemetics. Br Med J. 1979;1(6174):1323–4.

31. Sharkey KA, Wiley JW. The role of the endocannabinoid system in the brain-gut axis. Gastroenterology. 2016;151(2):252–66.

32. Sommariva S, Pongiglione B, Tarricone R. Impact of chemotherapy-induced nausea and vomiting on health-related quality of life and resource utilization: a systematic review. Crit Rev Oncol Hematol. 2016;99:13–36.

33. Chang AE, Shiling DJ, Stillman RC, Goldberg NH, Seipp CA, Barofsky I, Simon RM, Rosenberg SA. Delata-9-tetrahydrocannabinol as an antiemetic in cancer patients receiving high-dose methotrexate. A prospective, randomized evaluation. Ann Intern Med. 1979;91(6):819–24.

34. Tramer MR, Carroll D, Campbell FA, Reynolds DJM, Moore RA, McQuay HJ. Cannabinoids for control of chemotherapy induced nausea and vomiting: quantitative systematic review. BMJ. 2001;323(7303):16–21.

35. Ben M. Cannabinoids in medicine: a review of their therapeutic potential. J Ethnopharmacol. 2006;105(1–2):1–25.

36. Kramer JL. Medical marijuana for cancer. CA Cancer J Clin. 2015;65(2):109–22.

37. Williams CM, Kirkham TC. Anandamide induces overeating: mediation by central cannabinoid (CB1) receptors. Psychopharmacology. 1999;143(3):315–7.

38. Kirkham TC, Williams CM, Fezza F, Di Marzo V. Endocannabinoid levels in rat limbic forebrain and hypothalamus in relation to fasting, feeding and satiation: stimulation of eating by 2-arachidonoyl glycerol. Br J Pharmacol. 2002;136(4):550–7.

39. Di Marzo V, Matias I. Endocannabinoid control of food intake and energy balance. Nat Neurosci. 2005;8(5):585–9.

40. Monteleone P, Matias I, Martiadis V, De Petrocellis L, Maj M, Di Marzo V. Blood levels of the endocannabinoid anandamide are increased in anorexia nervosa and in binge-eating disorder, but not in bulimia nervosa. Neuropsychopharmacology. 2005;30(6):1216–21.

41. Beal JE, Olson R, Laubenstein L, Morales JO, Bellman P, Yangco B, et al. Dronabinol as a treatment for anorexia associated with weight loss in patients with AIDS. J Pain Symptom Manag. 1995;10(2):89–97.

42. Strasser F, Luftner D, Possinger K, Ernst G, Ruhstaller T, Meissner W, et al. Comparison of orally administered cannabis extract and delta-9-tetrahydrocannabinol in treating patients with cancer-related anorexia-cachexia syndrome: a multicenter, phase III, randomized, double-blind, placebo-controlled clinical trial from the Cannabis-In-Cachexia-Study-Group. J Clin Oncol. 2006;24(21):3394–400.

43. Jatoi A, Windschitl HE, Loprinzi CL, Sloan JA, Dakhil SR, Mailliard JA, et al. Dronabinol versus megestrol acetate versus combination therapy for cancer-associated anorexia: a North Central Cancer Treatment Group study. J Clin Oncol. 2002;20(2):567–73.

44. Brisbois TD, de Kock IH, Watanabe SM, Mirhosseini M, Lamoureux DC, Chasen M, et al. Delta-9-tetrahydrocannabinol may palliate altered chemosensory perception in cancer patients: results of a randomized, double-blind, placebo-controlled pilot trial. Ann Oncol. 2011;22(9):2086–93.

45. Pickering EE, Semple SJ, Nazir MS, Murphy K, Snow T, Cummin A, et al. Cannabinoid effects on ventilation and breathlessness: a pilot study of efficacy and safety. Chron Respir Dis. 2011;8(2):109–18.

46. Tashkin DP. Marijuana and lung disease. Chest. 2018;154(3):653–63.

47. CDC. Outbreak of lung disease associated with e-cigarette use, or vaping [Internet]. Center for Disease Control and Prevention; 2019 [cited 2019 Oct 1]. Available from: https://www.cdc.gov/tobacco/basic_information/e-cigarettes/severe-lung-disease.html.

48. Keith DR, Gunderson EW, Haney M, Foltin RW, Hart CL. Smoked marijuana attenuates performance and mood disruptions during simulated night shift work. Drug Alcohol Depend. 2017;178:534–43.

49. Kindred JH, Li K, Ketelhut NB, Proessl F, Fling BW, Honce JM, et al. Cannabis use in people with Parkinson's disease and multiple sclerosis: A web-based investigation. Complement Ther Med. 2017;33:99–104.

50. Niiranen A, Mattson K. A cross-over comparison of nabilone and prochlorperazine for emesis induced by cancer chemotherapy. Am J Clin Oncol [Internet]. 1985 [cited 2019 Jun 13];8(4):336–40. Available from: http://www.ncbi.nlm.nih.gov/pubmed/3002167.

51. Dzodzomenyo S, Stolfi A, Splaingard D, Earley E, Onadeko O, Splaingard M. Urine toxicology screen in multiple sleep latency test: the correlation of positive tetrahydrocannabinol, drug negative patients, and narcolepsy. J Clin Sleep Med. 2015;11(2):93–9.

52. Murillo-Rodriguez E, Sarro-Ramirez A, Sanchez D, Mijangos-Moreno S, Tejeda-Padron A, Poot-Ake A, et al. Potential effects of cannabidiol as a wake-promoting agent. Curr Neuropharmacol. 2014;12(3):269–72.

53. Nicholson AN, Turner C, Stone BM, Robson PJ. Effect of delta-9-tetrahydrocannabinol and cannabidiol on nocturnal sleep and early-morning behavior in young adults. J Clin Psychopharmacol. 2004;24(3):305–13.

54. Carlini EA, Cunha JM. Hypnotic and antiepileptic effects of cannabidiol. J Clin Pharmacol. 1981;21(S1):417S–27S.

55. Zuardi AW. Cannabidiol: from an inactive cannabinoid to a drug with wide spectrum of action. Braz J Psychiatry. 2008;30(3):271–80.

56. Vaughn LK, Denning G, Stuhr KL, de Wit H, Hill MN, Hillard CJ. Endocannabinoid signalling: has it got rhythm? Br J Pharmacol. 2010;160(3):530–43.

57. Belendiuk KA, Babson KA, Vandrey R, Bonn-Miller MO. Cannabis species and cannabinoid concentration preference among sleep-disturbed medicinal cannabis users. Addict Behav. 2015;50:178–81.

58. Tringale R, Jensen C. Cannabis and insomnia. Depression. 2011;4(12):0–68.
59. Gorelick DA, Goodwin RS, Schwilke E, Schwope DM, Darwin WD, Kelly DL, et al. Tolerance to effects of high-dose oral delta9-tetrahydrocannabinol and plasma cannabinoid concentrations in male daily cannabis smokers. J Anal Toxicol. 2013;37(1):11–6.
60. Hsiao YT, Yi PL, Li CL, Chang FC. Effect of cannabidiol on sleep disruption induced by the repeated combination tests consisting of open field and elevated plus-maze in rats. Neuropharmacology. 2012;62(1):373–84.
61. Englund A, Freeman TP, Murray RM, McGuire P. Can we make cannabis safer? Lancet Psychiatry. 2017;4(8):643–8.
62. Boggs DL, Nguyen JD, Morgenson D, Taffe MA, Ranganathan M. Clinical and preclinical evidence for functional interactions of cannabidiol and delta9-tetrahydrocannabinol. Neuropsychopharmacology. 2018;43(1):142–54.
63. Rey AA, Purrio M, Viveros MP, Lutz B. Biphasic effects of cannabinoids in anxiety responses: CB1 and GABA(B) receptors in the balance of GABAergic and glutamatergic neurotransmission. Neuropsychopharmacology. 2012;37(12):2624–34.
64. Christensen R, Kristensen PK, Bartels EM, Bliddal H, Astrup A. Efficacy and safety of the weight-loss drug rimonabant: a meta-analysis of randomised trials. Lancet. 2007;370(9600):1706–13.
65. Gruber AJ, Pope HG, Brown ME. Do patients use marijuana as an antidepressant? Depression. 1996;4(2):77–80.
66. Zuardi AW, Cosme RA, Graeff FG, Guimaraes FS. Effects of ipsapirone and cannabidiol on human experimental anxiety. J Psychopharmacol. 1993;7(1 Suppl):82–8.
67. Phan KL, Angstadt M, Golden J, Onyewuenyi I, Popovska A, de Wit H. Cannabinoid modulation of amygdala reactivity to social signals of threat in humans. J Neurosci. 2008;28(10):2313–9.
68. Lutz B, Marsicano G, Maldonado R, Hillard CJ. The endocannabinoid system in guarding against fear, anxiety and stress. Nat Rev Neurosci. 2015;16(12):705–18.
69. Bergamaschi MM, Queiroz R, Chagas M, Oliveira D, Martinis B, Kapczinski F, et al. Cannabidiol reduces the anxiety induced by simulated public speaking in treatment-naïve social phobia patients. Neuropsychopharmacology. 2011;36(6):1219–26.
70. Crippa J, Derenusson G, Ferrari T, Wichert-Ana L, Duran F, Martin-Santos R, et al. Neural basis of anxiolytic effects of cannabidiol (CBD) in generalized social anxiety disorder: a preliminary report. J Psychopharmacol. 2011;25(1):121–30.
71. ClinicalTrials.gov. Cannabidiol for the treatment of anxiety disorders: an 8-Week pilot study [Internet]. ClinicalTrials.gov. 2019 [cited 2019 Oct 1]. Available from: https://clinicaltrials.gov/show/nct03549819.
72. Linares IM, Zuardi AW, Pereira LC, Queiroz RH, Mechoulam R, Guimarães F, et al. Cannabidiol presents an inverted U-shaped dose-response curve in a simulated public speaking test. Eur Neuropsychopharmacol. 2019;41(1):9–14.
73. Blass K. Treating depression with cannabinoids (Cannabinoids 3). Can Underwrit. 2008;3:8–10.
74. Stockings GT. A new euphoriant for depressive mental states. Br Med J. 1947;1(4512):918–22.
75. Hill MN, Hillard CJ, Bambico FR, Patel S, Gorzalka BB, Gobbi G. The therapeutic potential of the endocannabinoid system for the development of a novel class of antidepressants. Trends Pharmacol Sci. 2009;30(9):484–93.
76. Hill MN, Ho WS, Sinopoli KJ, Viau V, Hillard CJ, Gorzalka BB. Involvement of the endocannabinoid system in the ability of long-term tricyclic antidepressant treatment to suppress stress-induced activation of the hypothalamic-pituitary-adrenal axis. Neuropsychopharmacology. 2006;31(12):2591–9.
77. Hill MN, Miller GE, Ho WS, Gorzalka BB, Hillard CJ. Serum endocannabinoid content is altered in females with depressive disorders: a preliminary report. Pharmacopsychiatry. 2008;41(2):48–53.

78. Hill MN, Miller GE, Carrier EJ, Gorzalka BB, Hillard CJ. Circulating endocannabinoids and N-acyl ethanolamines are differentially regulated in major depression and following exposure to social stress. Psychoneuroendocrinology. 2009;34(8):1257–62.
79. Monteleone P, Bifulco M, Maina G, Tortorella A, Gazzerro P, Proto MC, et al. Investigation of CNR1 and FAAH endocannabinoid gene polymorphisms in bipolar disorder and major depression. Pharmacol Res. 2010;61(5):400–4.
80. Barrero FJ, Ampuero I, Morales B, Vives F, de Dios Luna Del Castillo J, Hoenicka J, et al. Depression in Parkinson's disease is related to a genetic polymorphism of the cannabinoid receptor gene (CNR1). Pharmacogenomics J. 2005;5(2):135–41.
81. Domschke K, Dannlowski U, Ohrmann P, Lawford B, Bauer J, Kugel H, et al. Cannabinoid receptor 1 (CNR1) gene: impact on antidepressant treatment response and emotion processing in major depression. Eur Neuropsychopharmacol. 2008;18(10):751–9.
82. Mitjans M, Serretti A, Fabbri C, Gastó C, Catalán R, Fañanás L, et al. Screening genetic variability at the CNR1 gene in both major depression etiology and clinical response to citalopram treatment. Psychopharmacology. 2013;227(3):509–19.
83. Juhasz G, Chase D, Pegg E, Downey D, Toth ZG, Stones K, et al. CNR1 gene is associated with high neuroticism and low agreeableness and interacts with recent negative life events to predict current depressive symptoms. Neuropsychopharmacology. 2009;34(8):2019–27.
84. Hosie A, Davidson PM, Agar M, Sanderson CR, Phillips J. Delirium prevalence, incidence, and implications for screening in specialist palliative care inpatient settings: a systematic review. Palliat Med. 2013;27(6):486–98.
85. Volicer L, Stelly M, Morris J, McLaughlin J, Volicer BJ. Effects of dronabinol on anorexia and disturbed behavior in patients with Alzheimer's disease. Int J Geriatr Psychiatry. 1997;12(9):913–9.
86. Walther S, Mahlberg R, Eichmann U, Kunz D. Delta-9-tetrahydrocannabinol for nighttime agitation in severe dementia. Psychopharmacology. 2006;185(4):524–8.
87. Woodward MR, Harper DG, Stolyar A, Forester BP, Ellison JM. Dronabinol for the treatment of agitation and aggressive behavior in acutely hospitalized severely demented patients with noncognitive behavioral symptoms. Am J Geriatr Psychiatry. 2014;22(4):415–9.
88. Fattore L. Synthetic cannabinoids-further evidence supporting the relationship between cannabinoids and psychosis. Biol Psychiatry. 2016;79(7):539–48.
89. Levin FR, Mariani JJ, Brooks DJ, Pavlicova M, Cheng W, Nunes EV. Dronabinol for the treatment of cannabis dependence: a randomized, double-blind, placebo-controlled trial. Drug Alcohol Depend. 2011;116(1–3):142–50.
90. Allsop DJ, Copeland J, Lintzeris N, Dunlop AJ, Montebello M, Sadler C, et al. Nabiximols as an agonist replacement therapy during cannabis withdrawal: a randomized clinical trial. JAMA Psychiat. 2014;71(3):281–91.
91. Noble MJ, Hedberg K, Hendrickson RG. Acute cannabis toxicity. Clin Toxicol (Phila). 2019;57(8):735–42.
92. Pergam SA, Woodfield MC, Lee CM, Cheng GS, Baker KK, Marquis SR, et al. Cannabis use among patients at a comprehensive cancer center in a state with legalized medicinal and recreational use. Cancer. 2017;123(22):4488–97.
93. Boston P, Bruce A, Schreiber R. Existential suffering in the palliative care setting: an integrated literature review. J Pain Symptom Manag. 2011;41(3):604–18.
94. Vehling S, Phillip R. Existential distress and meaning-focused interventions in cancer survivorship. Curr Opin Support Palliat Care. 2018;12(1):46–51.
95. Aggarwal SK. Use of cannabinoids in cancer care: palliative care. Curr Oncol. 2016;23(2):S33–6.
96. Oliver J. On the action of Cannabis indica. Br Med J. 1883;1(1167):905–6.
97. Hanus LO, Meyer SM, Munoz E, Taglialatela-Scafati O, Appendino G. Phytocannabinoids: a unified critical inventory. Nat Prod Rep. 2016;33(12):1357–92.

98. Bouquie R, Deslandes G, Mazare H, Cogne M, Mahe J, Gregoire M, et al. Cannabis and anti-cancer drugs: societal usage and expected pharmacological interactions – a review. Fundam Clin Pharmacol. 2018;32(5):462–84.

99. Sekar K, Pack A. Epidiolex as adjunct therapy for treatment of refractory epilepsy: a comprehensive review with a focus on adverse effects. F1000Res. 2019;8:F1000.

100. Korczyn AD. The ocular effects of cannabinoids. Gen Pharmacol. 1980;11(5):419–23.

101. Versteeg PA, Slot DE, van der Velden U, van der Weijden GA. Effect of cannabis usage on the oral environment: a review. Int J Dent Hyg. 2008;6(4):315–20.

102. Elliott DA, Nabavizadeh N, Romer JL, Chen Y, Holland JM. Medical marijuana use in head and neck squamous cell carcinoma patients treated with radiotherapy. Support Care Cancer. 2016;24(8):3517–24.

103. Halikas J, Weller R, Morse C. Effects of regular marijuana use on sexual performance. J Psychoactive Drugs. 1982;14(1–2):59–70.

104. Payne KS, Mazur DJ, Hotaling JM, Pastuszak AW. Cannabis and male fertility: a systematic review. J Urol. 2019;202(4):674–81. https://doi.org/10.1097/JU.0000000000000248.

105. Shamloul R, Bella AJ. Impact of cannabis use on male sexual health. J Sex Med. 2011;8(4):971–5.

106. Lee H. 3 arrested after 16 sickened on pot cookies [Internet]. SF Gate; 2006 [cited 2019 Jun 13]. Available from: https://www.sfgate.com/bayarea/article/BERKELEY-3-arrested-after-16-sickened-on-pot-2552816.php.

107. Levin S. Paranoid men driving high with 20lb of marijuana call police on themselves [Internet]. The Guardian; 2016 [cited 2019 Jun 13]. Available from: https://www.theguardian.com/us-news/2016/jan/21/idaho-men-driving-high-marijuana-call-police.

108. Freeman D, Dunn G, Murray RM, Evans N, Lister R, Antley A, et al. How cannabis causes paranoia: using the intravenous administration of Δ 9 -tetrahydrocannabinol (THC) to identify key cognitive mechanisms leading to paranoia. Schizophr Bull. 2015;41(2):391–9.

109. Turna J, Patterson B, Van Ameringen M. Is cannabis treatment for anxiety, mood, and related disorders ready for prime time? Depress Anxiety. 2017;34(11):1006–17.

110. MacCallum CA, Russo EB. Practical considerations in medical cannabis administration and dosing. Eur J Intern Med. 2018;49:12–9.

111. Foti DJ, Kotov R, Guey LT, Bromet EJ. Cannabis use and the course of schizophrenia: 10-year follow-up after first hospitalization. Am J Psychiatry. 2010;167(8):987–93.

112. D'Souza DC, Sewell RA, Ranganathan M. Cannabis and psychosis/schizophrenia: human studies. Eur Arch Psychiatry Clin Neurosci. 2009;259(7):413–31.

113. Sherif M, Radhakrishnan R, D'Souza DC, Ranganathan M. Human laboratory studies on cannabinoids and psychosis. Biol Psychiatry. 2016;79(7):526–38.

114. Ksir C, Hart CL. Cannabis and psychosis: a critical overview of the relationship. Curr Psychiatry Rep. 2016;18(2):12.

115. Einhorn LH, Nagy C, Furnas B, Williams SD. Nabilone: an effective antiemetic in patients receiving cancer chemotherapy. J Clin Pharmacol [Internet]. 1982 [cited 2019 Jun 13];21(S1):64S–9S. Available from: http://www.ncbi.nlm.nih.gov/pubmed/6271844.

116. Serpell M, Ratcliffe S, Hovorka J, Schofield M, Taylor L, Lauder H, et al. A double-blind, randomized, placebo-controlled, parallel group study of THC/CBD spray in peripheral neuropathic pain treatment. Eur J Pain (United Kingdom). 2014;18(7):999–1012.

117. Collin C, Davies P, Mutiboko IK, Ratcliffe S. Randomized controlled trial of cannabis-based medicine in spasticity caused by multiple sclerosis. Eur J Neurol. 2007;14(3):290–6.

118. Portenoy RK, Ganae-Motan ED, Allende S, Yanagihara R, Shaiova L, Weinstein S, et al. Nabiximols for opioid-treated cancer patients with poorly-controlled chronic pain: a randomized, placebo-controlled, graded-dose trial. J Pain. 2012;13(5):438–49.

119. Svíženská I, Dubový P, Šulcová A. Cannabinoid receptors 1 and 2 (CB1 and CB2), their distribution, ligands and functional involvement in nervous system structures – a short review. Pharmacol Biochem Behav. 2008;90(4):501–11.

120. Kuhathasan N, Dufort A, MacKillop J, Gottschalk R, Minuzzi L, Frey BN. The use of cannabinoids for sleep: a critical review on clinical trials. Exp Clin Psychopharmacol [Internet]. 2019 [cited 2019 Jun 8]; Available from: http://www.ncbi.nlm.nih.gov/pubmed/31120284.

121. Broyd SJ, Van Hell HH, Beale C, Yücel M, Solowij N. Acute and chronic effects of cannabinoids on human cognition — a systematic review. Biol Psychiatry. 2016;79(7):557–67.

122. Thames AD, Arbid N, Sayegh P. Cannabis use and neurocognitive functioning in a non-clinical sample of users. Addict Behav. 2014;39(5):994–9.

123. Lyons MJ, Bar JL, Panizzon MS, Toomey R, Eisen S, Xian H, et al. Neuropsychological consequences of regular marijuana use: a twin study. Psychol Med. 2004;34(7):1239–50.

124. Zachariah SB. Stroke after heavy marijuana smoking. Stroke. 1991;22(3):406–9.

125. Singh NN, Pan Y, Muengtaweeponsa S, Geller TJ, Cruz-Flores S. Cannabis-related stroke: case series and review of literature. J Stroke Cerebrovasc Dis [Internet]. 2012 [cited 2019 Jun 8];21(7):555–60. Available from: https://linkinghub.elsevier.com/retrieve/pii/S1052305710002892.

126. Atchaneeyasakul K, Torres LF, Malik AM. Large amount of cannabis ingestion resulting in spontaneous intracerebral hemorrhage: a case report. J Stroke Cerebrovasc Dis [Internet]. 2017 [cited 2019 Jun 8];26(7):e138–9. Available from: https://linkinghub.elsevier.com/retrieve/pii/S1052305717301751.

127. Mesec A, Rot U, Grad A. Cerebrovascular disease associated with marijuana abuse: a case report. Cerebrovasc Dis [Internet]. 2001 [cited 2019 Jun 8];11(3):284–5. Available from: http://www.ncbi.nlm.nih.gov/pubmed/11306781.

128. Sloan MA, Kittner SJ, Feeser BR, Gardner J, Epstein A, Wozniak MA, et al. Illicit drug-associated ischemic stroke in the Baltimore-Washington young stroke study. Neurology. 1998;50(6):1688–93.

129. Moussouttas M. Cannabis use and cerebrovascular disease. Neurologist. 2004;10(1):47–53.

130. Weil AT, Zinberg NE, Nelsen JM. Clinical and psychological effects of marihuana in man. Science. 1968;162(3859):1234–42.

131. Benowitz NL, Rosenberg J, Rogers W, Bachman J, Jones RT. Cardiovascular effects of intravenous delta-9-tetrahydrocannabinol: autonomic nervous mechanisms. Clin Pharmacol Ther. 1979;25(4):440–6.

132. Gash A, Karliner JS, Janowsky D, Lake CR. Effects of smoking marihuana on left ventricular performance and plasma norepinephrine: studies in normal men. Ann Intern Med. 1978;89(4):448–52.

133. Karschner EL, Darwin WD, McMahon RP, Liu F, Wright S, Goodwin RS, et al. Subjective and physiological effects after controlled sativex and oral THC administration. Clin Pharmacol Ther. 2011;89(3):400–7.

134. Goyal H, Awad HH, Ghali JK. Role of cannabis in cardiovascular disorders. J Thorac Dis. 2017;9(7):2079–92.

135. Jones RT. Cardiovascular system effects of marijuana. J Clin Pharmacol. 2002;42(S1):58S–63S.

136. Prakash R, Aronow WS, Warren M, Laverty W, Gottschalk LA. Effects of marihuana and placebo marihuana smoking on hemodynamics in coronary disease. Clin Pharmacol Ther. 1975;18(1):90–5.

137. Aronow WS, Cassidy J. Effect of smoking marihuana and of a high-nicotine cigarette on angina pectoris. Clin Pharmacol Ther. 1975;17(5):549–54.

138. Miller RH, Dhingra RC, Kanakis C, Amat-y-Leon F, Rosen KM. The electrophysiological effects of delta-9-tetrahydrocannabinol (cannabis) on cardiac conduction in man. Am Heart J. 1977;94(6):740–7.

139. Kosior DA, Filipiak KJ, Stolarz P, Opolski G. Paroxysmal atrial fibrillation following marijuana intoxication: a two-case report of possible association. Int J Cardiol. 2001;78(2):183–4.

140. Fernández-Fernández FJ, Caínzos-Romero T, Mesías PA. Ectopic atrial rhythm associated with cannabis use. Minerva Cardioangiol. 2011;59(1):119–20.

141. Kosior DA, Filipiak KJ, Stolarz P, Opolski G. Paroxysmal atrial fibrillation in a young female patient following marijuana intoxication--a case report of possible association. Med Sci Monit. 2000;6(2):386–9.

142. Charbonney E, Sztajzel JM, Poletti PA, Rutschmann O. Paroxysmal atrial fibrillation after recreational marijuana smoking: another "holiday heart"? Swiss Med Wkly. 2005;135(27–28):412–4.

143. Moore BA, Augustson EM, Moser RP, Budney AJ. Respiratory effects of marijuana and tobacco use in a U.S. sample. J Gen Intern Med. 2005;20(1):33–7.

144. Tashkin DP, Reiss S, Shapiro BJ, Calvarese B, Olsen JL, Lodge JW. Bronchial effects of aerosolized delta 9-tetrahydrocannabinol in healthy and asthmatic subjects. Am Rev Respir Dis. 1977;115(1):57–65.

145. Owen KP, Sutter ME, Albertson TE. Marijuana: respiratory tract effects. Clin Rev Allergy Immunol. 2014;46(1):65–81.

146. Berman JS, Symonds C, Birch R. Efficacy of two cannabis based medicinal extracts for relief of central neuropathic pain from brachial plexus avulsion: results of a randomised controlled trial. Pain. 2004;112(3):299–306.

147. Davidson K, Brancato A, Heetderks P, Mansour W, Matheis E, Nario M, et al. Outbreak of electronic-cigarette–associated acute lipoid pneumonia — North Carolina, July–August 2019. MMWR Morb Mortal Wkly Rep [Internet]. 2019 [cited 2019 Sep 18];68(36):784–6. Available from: http://www.ncbi.nlm.nih.gov/pubmed/31513559.

148. Todaro B. Cannabinoids in the treatment of chemotherapy-induced nausea and vomiting. J Natl Compr Cancer Netw. 2012;10(4):487–92.

149. Simonetto DA, Oxentenko AS, Herman ML, Szostek JH. Cannabinoid hyperemesis: a case series of 98 patients. Mayo Clin Proc. 2012;87(2):114–9.

150. Kirkham TC. Cannabinoids and appetite: food craving and food pleasure. Int Rev Psychiatry. 2009;21(2):163–71.

151. Thiele EA, Marsh ED, French JA, Mazurkiewicz MB, Benbadis SR, Joshi C, et al. Cannabidiol in patients with seizures associated with Lennox-Gastaut syndrome (GWPCARE4): a randomised, double-blind, placebo-controlled phase 3 trial. Lancet. 2018;391(10125):1085–96.

152. FDA. Full Prescribing Information: Epidolex [Internet]. 2018. Available from: https://www.accessdata.fda.gov/drugsatfda_docs/label/2018/210365lbl.pdf.

153. Taylor L, Crockett J, Tayo B, Morrison G. A phase 1, open-label, parallel-group, single-dose trial of the pharmacokinetics and safety of cannabidiol (CBD) in subjects with mild to severe hepatic impairment. J Clin Pharmacol. 2019;59(8):1110–9.

154. Thompson G, Tuscano J, Dennis M, Singapuri A, Libertini S, Gaudino R, et al. A microbiome assessment of medical marijuana. Clin Microbiol Infect. 2017;23(4):269–70.

155. Chadwick B, Miller ML, Hurd YL. Cannabis use during adolescent development: susceptibility to psychiatric illness. Front Psych. 2013;4:129.

156. Levine A, Clemenza K, Rynn M, Lieberman J. Evidence for the risks and consequences of adolescent cannabis exposure. J Am Acad Child Adolesc Psychopharmacol. 2017;56(3):214–25.

157. Caldicott DG, Holmes J, Roberts-Thomson KC, Mahar L. Keep off the grass: marijuana use and acute cardiovascular events. Eur J Emerg Med. 2005;12(5):236–44.

158. Singh A, Saluja S, Kumar A, Agrawal S, Thind M, Nanda S, et al. Cardiovascular complications of marijuana and related substances: a review. Cardiol Ther. 2018;7(1):45–59.

159. Ware MA, Wang T, Shapiro S, Collet JP. COMPASS study team. Cannabis for the management of pain: assessment of safety study (COMPASS). J Pain. 2015;16(12):1233–42.

160. Lu ML, Agito MD. Cannabinoid hyperemesis syndrome: marijuana is both antiemetic and proemetic. Cleve Clin J Med. 2015;82(7):429–34.

161. Cox EJ, Maharao N, Patilea-Vrana G, Unadkat JD, Rettie AE, McCune JS, et al. A marijuana-drug interaction primer: precipitants, pharmacology, and pharmacokinetics. Pharmacol Ther. 2019;201:25–38;S0163-7258(19)30075-0.

162. Damkier P, Lassen D, Christensen MMH, Madsen KG, Hellfritzsch M, Pottegard A. Interaction between warfarin and cannabis. Basic Clin Pharmacol Toxicol. 2019;124(1):28–31.

163. Makary P, Parmar JR, Mims N, Khanfar NM, Freeman RA. Patient counseling guidelines for the use of cannabis for the treatment of chemotherapy-induced nausea/vomiting and chronic pain. J Pain Palliat Care Pharmacother. 2018;32(4):216–25.

164. Wilsey B, Atkinson JH, Marcotte TD, Grant I. The medicinal cannabis treatment agreement: providing information to chronic pain patients through a written document. Clin J Pain. 2015;31(12):1087–96.

Chapter 14
Charting the Pathways Taken by Older Adults Who Use Cannabis: Where Are the Baby Boomers Going Now?

Brian P. Kaskie and Amanjot Mona Sidhu

For the past two decades, American state governments have operated policy-making laboratories that have created a variety of approaches to legalizing cannabis [1, 2]. Meanwhile, the population continues to grow older, and the total number of Americans who are over 65 years old will soon outnumber children under the age of 18 for the first time in history [3]. Within this dynamic national context, several researchers have observed how cannabis use among older adults has outpaced all other age groups [4, 5]. Initially, the remarkable growth was attributed to the entry of the more "cannabis-tolerant" baby boom cohort into old age, but more recent work has suggested the reasons behind increasing cannabis use are more complex [6–8]. Older persons have responded to changing legal environments, and some are now more comfortable with taking cannabis recreationally. Persons over 65 also are experiencing age-related health-care needs and may use cannabis for symptom management and other "medical" or "therapeutic" purposes. We know little else about the expanding intersection between cannabis and older persons.

In this chapter, we account recent trends in cannabis use among persons over 50 and, when possible, consider trends specific to those over 65. We then review research studies illuminating how older adults have taken different pathways to using cannabis – with some being lifelong users and others who only recently started using cannabis for the first time ever [9, 10]. We also observe outcomes experienced by older persons who use cannabis, making a special effort to present a range of health-related outcomes rather than other outcomes such as school performance. At last, we turn to the critical role physicians and other health-care providers

B. P. Kaskie (✉)
University of Iowa, Department of Health Management & Policy, Iowa City, IA, USA
e-mail: brian-kaskie@uiowa.edu

A. M. Sidhu
McMaster University, Hamilton, ON, Canada
e-mail: Sidhua4@mcmaster.ca

© Springer Nature Switzerland AG 2020
K. Finn (ed.), *Cannabis in Medicine*,
https://doi.org/10.1007/978-3-030-45968-0_14

assume in evaluating and advising older persons about cannabis, particularly relative to the use of opioids and other pain management medications.

At this point, it is worth declaring how there is a lack of empirically based knowledge about cannabis and older persons. The research presented in this chapter including the studies reviewed as part of the National Academies of Sciences, Engineering, and Medicine report [11] or based on national surveys such as the National Survey on Drug Use and Health [4, 5, 12–15] falls short in several key ways. For example, most of the research we present does not account for the varieties of cannabis exposure and reveals little about dose, potencies, or routes of administration (e.g., smoking, vaping, edibles), nor do these studies capture substantial differences between marijuana used in clinical trials and commercially available products which are more likely to have increased Δ9-THC (tetrahydrocannabinol) concentrations [16, 17]. We also recognize that most basic and clinical cannabis research rarely includes older adults and those studies which do mostly rely on small samples recruited from limited geographic areas (i.e., states where cannabis is legal). However, rather than concluding this chapter with a standard discussion about the need for more basic and clinical research focusing on cannabis use among older adults, we consider the role of state government policy in further illuminating the intersection between cannabis and older persons.

Cannabis Use Among Older Persons

Cannabis use among older persons has been increasing at a faster rate compared to all other age groups. Data from the National Survey of Drug Use and Health (NSDUH) showed the rate of past-year cannabis use among persons 50 years and older increased by 71.4% between 2006 and 2017. In 2000, the percentage of older persons who had tried cannabis at least once in their lifetime reached 23% among 50–64-year-olds and 3% among those aged 65 and older. By 2011, lifetime usage rates increased to 44% among those between 50 and 64 years old and 17% for persons older than 65 years. The proportion of all persons between 50 and 64 who used in the past year climbed from 2.9% in 2002 to 10.2% in 2016, and among persons over 65, there was more than a tenfold increase as past-year rates grew from 0.2% to 3.7% [4, 5].

While the overwhelming majority of the estimated four million Americans older than 50 years who currently use cannabis are healthy, well-educated, and white, researchers have observed several significant individual differences among these users [13–15]. The NSDUH data indicated that older persons who used cannabis in the past year (i.e., current users) were statistically more likely to have started taking cannabis before the age of 30, with many starting before the age of 18 although researchers also have observed a growing number of older users re-engaging after stopping in midlife or who are naïve, first-time users [18]. Others [19] reported past-year marijuana users identified smoking/inhaling as their preferred method, but a large and growing number of older adults also use edibles and topical formulations (i.e., creams and ointments).

Nearly half of older persons who used consistently in the past year are lifetime users, and nearly a quarter of these consistent users took cannabis at least three times per week. The majority of all persons older than 50 years who took cannabis in the past year used less than once every 10 days, and 25% of these persons used less than five times during the past year [10, 15]. Past-year cannabis use also has been associated with gender (men are more likely to use than women), marital status (those who are not married are more likely to use), and race (nonwhites are more likely to use than whites). Persons older than 50 years who take cannabis are more likely to smoke cigarettes, drink alcohol, and use cocaine and other illicit drugs including opioids [13, 14, 20].

Cannabis use also is more likely to occur among older persons who experience chronic health conditions and look for cannabis for "medical" or "therapeutic" purposes [18, 19, 21]. Since the NSDUH did not collect data on such an exhaustive range of medical conditions, we looked to clinical observations of smaller patient samples to learn more about the conditions associated with cannabis use. For example, these clinical studies have reported cannabis use by older adults to treat glaucoma-related ocular pressure as well as chronic pain, spasticity associated with multiple sclerosis as well as anxiety and depression [19, 21].

Cannabis use among older adults will continue to increase as more of America's baby boomers, whose attitudes toward cannabis and other psychoactive drugs historically have been more favorable than their predecessors, reach and surpass their 65th birthdays [8]. Another perspective suggests the decision to take cannabis is based on subjective calculations concerning reward and risk [6], and older individuals living in states with legal marijuana may perceive less risk and may be more likely to use cannabis. As of June 2019, 34 states and the District of Columbia (DC) had approved comprehensive medical marijuana laws (MMLs), and 13 states and DC had laws legalizing recreational cannabis for adult use [2]. In Canada, older persons were the only age-based group to increase use after cannabis was legalized nationally in 2018 [22].

Outcomes of Cannabis Use

Older adults who use cannabis experience a range of outcomes, some beneficial and others harmful. In an effort to organize the variety of outcomes experienced by older cannabis users, we found the *Proximal/Distal Model of Health Outcomes* to be helpful [23]. This model places health outcomes into four categories: (1) clinical measures, (2) general well-being reports, (3) general functioning reports, and (4) functioning reports specific to disease state or treatment intervention. Regardless of the category they belong to, outcomes fall along a continuum from positive to negative in directionality and in terms of proximity to the individual. For example, a positive proximal outcome for medical cannabis use includes reduction of pain symptoms or sleep issues, and a negative proximal outcome includes increased cognitive impairments. *Distal outcomes* include the broader areas of mobility, role performance, and life satisfaction, and positive distal outcomes include self-reported improvements in wellness, social engagement, and quality of life, and negative distal outcomes include reduced productivity and adverse event such as emergency room use.

In January 2017, the National Academies of Sciences, Engineering, and Medicine reviewed the health effects of cannabis and its potential for therapeutic use in humans [11]. Most notable, the Academies report found *conclusive* evidence that cannabis or cannabinoids are effective as an antiemetic in the treatment of nausea and vomiting resulting from chemotherapy. There is *substantial* evidence that cannabis is effective for the treatment of chronic pain in adult patients and effective for improving patient-reported MS spasticity symptoms. *Moderate* evidence was found that cannabis is effective for improving short-term outcomes for condition-related sleep disturbances, in addition to improving symptoms of anxiety and PTSD. Other clinical studies completed since then have found cannabis to be effective for relieving pain related to chronic conditions. While few of these studies directly observed persons over 65, one recent survey [24] of 2736 patients above age 65 who were taking cannabis primarily for cancer and chronic pain found participants reported reduced pain and increased quality of life.

Alternatively, the Academies report [11] identified *substantial* evidence of worsened respiratory symptoms and more frequent chronic bronchitis episodes from long-term marijuana smoking and *limited* evidence that cannabis use increases the risk of COPD, acute myocardial infarction, ischemic stroke, and prediabetes, particularly for those who intake cannabis through smoking or some other form of combustion. The Academies report also provided *substantial* and *moderate* amounts of evidence concerning marijuana's adverse effects on mental and cognitive health, via the development of schizophrenia or other psychoses, especially due to frequent use during adolescence; impairments in the cognitive domains of learning, memory, and attention from acute use; increased symptoms of mania/hypomania among regular marijuana users with bipolar disorder; increased incidences of social anxiety disorder among regular users; and a slightly elevated risk of depressive disorders and suicide ideation, attempts, and completion among heavier users. Though much of this research rarely included older adults, these adverse effects may be applicable to long-term cannabis users as they grow older.

Other researchers who have deliberately observed older cannabis users have found several problematic outcomes. For example, compared to non-cannabis users, older users have increased psychiatric conditions including anxiety, post-traumatic stress disorder, and bipolar disorder with manic or hypomanic episodes. Cannabis use also has been associated with having more life stressors (interpersonal, financial, legal problems, and being a crime victim), though it remains unclear if cannabis is a cause or correlate to these conditions and episodes [13, 14]. Older adults also were significantly more likely than their non-using age peers to experience an injury, having problems related to driving, and increased use of the emergency department [25, 26]. While the exact mechanisms of injury related to marijuana use are not known, researchers have suggested that cannabis-induced mental status alterations, acute intoxication, and other psychophysiological effects, especially when combined with alcohol and other illicit drugs, may increase users' vulnerability to injury [27]. According to the Substance Abuse and Mental Health Services Administration, Center for Behavioral Health Statistics and Quality's Treatment Episode Data [28] on admissions to treatment centers, the proportion of admissions for any substance use problem/disorder among those 50 and over increased from 11.0% in 2006 to 17.9% in 2017. While marijuana was identified as the primary substance in just 3.0% of all older-adult admissions, researchers determined that cannabis use was common among the majority of older adults who are seeking treatment for alcohol, tobacco, and other drug problems.

There certainly is reason to be concerned that increasing cannabis use among older persons may contribute to increasing rates of substance misuse or other undesirable outcomes. However, it is important to note how the overwhelming majority of older cannabis users do not experience any negative outcomes. More than 9 out of 10 of all older persons who took cannabis in the past year reported having no emotional or functional problems, and the majority indicated they placed no self-limit on their use [7].

The Doctor Patient Relationship

As cannabis legalization continues to spread across the United States and the aging population continues to grow, health-care and other service providers increasingly will come into contact with older patients who are (a) continuing their lifetime use of cannabis; (b) restarting cannabis use after not using since early adulthood; or (c) initiating cannabis use for the first time (so-called naive users). As products become more appealing (e.g., edibles and oils), older patients increasingly will seek guidance from a trusted source to learn about using cannabis. Based on focus groups conducted with 137 older adults in Colorado, researchers identified a strong preference among older persons to discuss cannabis with their health-care providers with whom they have ongoing relationships and share their medical histories. The older adults added they would consider personal physicians to be the most appropriate to provide a referral to the state medical cannabis program [21].

As such, medical doctors and other health professionals should become familiar with the varied pathways of cannabis use among older adults and the corresponding range of outcomes to which these pathways lead. Routine patient evaluations should incorporate questions about cannabis use, like other medications (prescribed and over the counter) and other substances (herbs, supplements, and legal and illegal recreational drugs). Alternatively, if providers do not collect such essential decision-making information, patients using cannabis may experience negative outcomes such as drug interactions and medical complications that could otherwise have been prevented.

In addition, providers should be aware that older adults may be misusing or abusing cannabis, as rates of cannabis use disorder (CUD), as defined in the *Diagnostic and Statistical Manual of Mental Disorders, 5th edition* (American Psychiatric Association, 2017), among users over 50 years old are slightly less than 5.0%, and several reports have shown cannabis use often co-occurs with other substance use disorders (https://www.drugabuse.gov/publications/).

In fact, older adults who used pain relievers nonmedically were more than three times as likely to be cannabis users, in comparison with those who did not use pain relievers [28].

Opioids, Cannabis, and Pain

Pain is one of the most common health-related conditions experienced by Americans over the age of 65, and the most common approach to addressing pain in older adults is to prescribe medications approved by the US Food and Drug Administration [29–31]. Acetaminophen and nonsteroidal anti-inflammatory drugs are often used to treat mild to moderate levels of pain, whereas older adults with more moderate to severe levels of pain are more likely to be prescribed stronger pain relief in the form of opioids [31]. One study reported that between 1999 and 2010, opioid prescriptions for older-adult outpatients increased from 4% to 9% [32]. In a nationwide study of over 250,000 individuals, the use of prescription opioids was highest among white, educated females between the ages of 70 and 75 [33], and women over age 65 also have higher rates of long-term use of prescription opioids than all other groups over 18 [34]. However, the use of anti-inflammatories and opioids can be problematic. Anti-inflammatory medications have been associated with cardiovascular, gastrointestinal, and renal problems [31, 34]. Opioid use by older adults can result in problematic side effects such as nausea, constipation, sedation, and confusion [34].

Alternatively, the primary use of medical cannabis among older adults has been to alleviate pain, and more than 30 states now include pain as a qualifying condition for medical cannabis program participation [8]. Four states (e.g., Illinois, New Jersey, New York, Colorado) have gone as far to integrate opioid replacement as a qualifying condition for their medical cannabis programs – allowing for participants to choose medical cannabis as a complement to, or substitute for, taking opioids. Within these contexts, provider attitudes toward the use of cannabis and opioids certainly can be critical in shaping patient choices, and researchers have found a lack of provider knowledge or an unwillingness to discuss cannabis kept older patients from accessing cannabis as a method of pain control [21].

The Public Interest

By 2000, as the leading edge of the baby boom cohort reached and surpassed their 50th birthdays, 34% were in favor of legalizing cannabis, and such favorable attitudes reached 52% by 2014 as more boomers entered older age [7]. Other researchers have found that as general public opinion about cannabis has become less negative, older individuals have become more likely to adopt favorable attitudes [35]. These changing attitudes among older adults also have been tied to perceptions about the medical benefits of cannabis as nearly 60% of persons over the age of 45 years believed cannabis provided a medical benefit and 72% believed doctors should be allowed to recommend medical cannabis [36]. Although such attitudes were higher among those who previously had taken cannabis, nearly two out of every three who never took cannabis at any point during their life also held such favorable attitudes about medical benefits. Similarly, in conducting focus groups across Colorado, other researchers found that a large portion of non-using older adults believed cannabis contributed to positive outcomes based on the reported experiences of loved ones and friends who used cannabis [21]. Health-care providers also seem to hold positive attitudes about cannabis use for medical purposes. In a survey of 1446 readers of the *New England Journal of Medicine*, researchers [37] found that 76% supported the use of medical cannabis in a case study in which an older woman was diagnosed with metastatic cancer and suffering with nausea and pain.

Both older adults and physicians have indicated the need for information and education about the use of medical cannabis for age-related medical conditions and symptoms, as well as education about methods for consumption, and both groups lament the lack of research on cannabis use [21]. While several provider organizations (e.g., the American Medical Association, American Nurses Association, American Pharmacists Association) have stopped short of endorsing medical cannabis use [8], they all have called for more public education for patients and training for their provider constituencies, with a particular emphasis placed on differentiating the legal risks associated with a doctor prescribing cannabis (i.e., a Food and Drug Administration [FDA] violation) relative to the risks of a doctor discussing or recommending it (i.e., as protected by free speech).

Ultimately, the lack of research and education is problematic, creating a situation in which older adults access potentially unreliable information primarily from non-professionals such as dispensary staff, friends, or acquaintances. Given the current context in which medical providers and the health-care systems in which they work may not offer such patient education and provider training, public health officials should consider providing evidence-based, standardized information, education, and training through the national network of Area Agencies on Aging, the National Library of Medicine, and university-based outreach programs.

Concluding Remarks

In this chapter, we explored the rapidly growing intersection between cannabis and older persons. While initial research has been illuminating, we still have a lot more to learn and need more rigorous studies that examine cannabis across the life course and conduct large experimental (basic and clinical) studies that focus exclusively on age-related disorders. Meanwhile, states continue to expand cannabis legalization, and several critical issues remain unclear. Why are some doctors underinformed or discouraged from talking to older patients about medical cannabis? Should insurance coverage be offered to older adults who take a proven cannabinoid as a substitute for opioids? At this time, these sorts of critical public health policy issues cannot be addressed largely because there is a pervasive lack of reliable and representative information being collected about cannabis and older persons.

In looking forward, we see the critical role state governments assume in shaping the intersection between cannabis and older persons. State authorities can support public education; define provider training requirements; monitor the development, distribution, and dispensation of cannabis; and support research that examines these issues. Indeed, American state governments already have extended cannabis program eligibility for several age-specific neurologic and muscular conditions including amyotrophic lateral sclerosis (covered in 16 states), multiple sclerosis (19 states), and Parkinson's disease (12 states), with little scientific evidence; other states have extended eligibility for persons with terminal illness and support applications submitted by caregivers. As we look to better understand cannabis and older persons, perhaps we should look to state governments for leadership in supporting research, designing evidence-based programs, and protecting older adults.

Acknowledgments This effort was supported by the University of Iowa, College of Public Health, and by the Division of Geriatric Medicine, McMaster University.

References

1. Cerdá M, Wall M, Keyes KM, Galea S, Hasin D. Medical marijuana laws in 50 states: investigating the relationship between state legalization of medical marijuana and marijuana use, abuse and dependence. Drug Alcohol Depend. 2012;120:22–7. https://doi.org/10.1016/j.drugalcdep.2011.06.011.
2. Karmen Hanson AG. State medical marijuana laws. 2019, June 17. Retrieved from http://www.ncsl.org/research/health/state-medical-marijuana-laws.aspx.
3. U.S Census Bureau. The graying of America: more older adults than kids by 2035. 2019, June 17. Retrieved from https://www.census.gov/library/stories/2018/03/graying-america.html.
4. Han BH, Sherman S, Mauro PM, Martins SS, Rotenberg J, Palamar JJ. Demographic trends among older cannabis users in the United States, 2006–13. Addiction. 2017;112:516–25. https://doi.org/10.1111/add.13670.
5. Salas-Wright CP, Vaughn MG, Cummings-Vaughn LA, Holzer KJ, Nelson EJ, AbiNader M, Oh S. Trends and correlates of marijuana use among late middle-aged and older adults in the United States, 2002–2014. Drug Alcohol Depend. 2017;171:97–106. https://doi.org/10.1016/j.drugalcdep.2016.11.031.
6. Ahmed AIA, van den Elsen GA, van der Marck MA, Olde Rikkert MG. Medicinal use of cannabis and cannabinoids in older adults: where is the evidence? J Am Geriatr Soc. 2014;62:410–1. https://doi.org/10.1111/jgs.12661.
7. Black P, Joseph LJ. Still dazed and confused: midlife marijuana use by the baby boom generation. Deviant Behav. 2014;35(10):822–41. https://doi.org/10.1080/01639625.2014.889994.

8. Kaskie B, Ayyagari P, Milavetz G, Shane D, Arora K. The increasing use of cannabis among older Americans: a public health crisis or viable policy alternative? Gerontologist. 2017;57:1166–72. https://doi.org/10.1093/geront/gnw166.
9. Briscoe J, Casarett D. Medical marijuana use in older adults. J Am Geriatr Soc. 2018;66:59–863. https://doi.org/10.1111/jgs.15346.
10. Haug NA, Padula CB, Sottile JE, Vandrey R, Heinz AJ, Bonn-Miller MO. Cannabis use patterns and motives: a comparison of younger, middle-aged, and older medical cannabis dispensary patients. Addict Behav. 2017;72:14–20. https://doi.org/10.1016/j.addbeh.2017.03.006.
11. National Academies of Sciences, Engineering, and Medicine. The health effects of cannabis and cannabinoids: the current state of evidence and recommendations for research. Washington, DC: The National Academies Press; 2017. https://doi.org/10.17226/24625.
12. Agrawal A, Lynskey MT. Correlates of later-onset cannabis use in the National Epidemiological Survey on Alcohol and Related Conditions (NESARC). Drug Alcohol Depend. 2009;105:71–5. https://doi.org/10.1016/j.drugalcdep.2009.06.017.
13. Choi NG, DiNitto DM, Marti CN. Older-adult marijuana users and ex-users: comparisons of sociodemographic characteristics and mental and substance use disorders. Drug Alcohol Depend. 2016;165:94–102. https://doi.org/10.1016/j.drugalcdep.2016.05.023.
14. Choi NG, DiNitto DM, Marti CN. Nonmedical versus medical marijuana use among three age groups of adults: associations with mental and physical health status. Am J Addict. 2017;26(7):697–706. https://doi.org/10.1111/ajad.12598.
15. Han BH, Palamar JJ. Marijuana use by middle-aged and older adults in the United States, 2015–2016. Drug Alcohol Depend. 2018;191:374–81. https://doi.org/10.1016/j.drugalcdep.2018.07.006.
16. Chandra S, Radwan MM, Majumdar CG, Church JC, Freeman TP, ElSohly MA. New trends in cannabis potency in USA and Europe during the last decade (2008–2017). Eur Arch Psychiatry Clin Neurosci. 2019;269(1):5–15. https://doi.org/10.1007/s00406-019-00983-5.
17. ElSohly MA, Mehmedic Z, Foster S, Gon C, Chandra S, Church JC. Changes in cannabis potency over the last two decades (1995–2014) – analysis of current data in the United States. Biol Psychiatry. 2016;79:613–9. https://doi.org/10.1016/j.biopsych.2016.01.004.
18. Arora K, Qualls SH, Bobitt J, Lum HD, Milavetz G, Croker J, Kaskie B. Measuring attitudes toward medical and recreational cannabis among older adults in Colorado. Gerontologist. 2019. https://doi.org/10.1093/geront/gnz054.
19. Lum HD, Arora K, Croker JA, Qualls SH, Schuchman M, Bobitt J, et al. Patterns of marijuana use and health impact: a survey among older Coloradans. Gerontol Geriatr Med. 2019;5. https://doi.org/10.1177/2333721419843707.
20. Wu L, Blazer DG. Illicit and nonmedical drug use among older adults: a review. J Aging Health. 2011;23(3):481–504. https://doi.org/10.1177/0898264310386224.
21. Bobitt J, Qualls SH, Schuchman M, Wickersham R, Lum HD, Arora K, et al. Qualitative analysis of cannabis use among older adults in Colorado. Drugs Aging. 2019. https://doi.org/10.1007/s40266-019-00665-w.
22. Retrieved: https://www.theglobeandmail.com/cannabis/article-seniors-were-the-only-group-to-report-slightly-higher-rates-of/.
23. The Proximal-Distal Continuum of Multiple Health Outcome Measures: The Case of Cataract Surgery Author(s): M. Harvey Brenner, Barbara Curbow and Marcia West Legro Source: Medical Care, 33(4), The Proceedings of the Conference on Measuring the Effects of Medical Treatment (Apr., 1995), pp. AS236–AS244 Published by: Lippincott Williams & Wilkins Stable URL: https://www.jstor.org/stable/3766632 Accessed: 27-04-2020 21:58 UTC
24. Abuhasira R, Schleider LB-L, Mechoulam R, Novack V. Epidemiological characteristics, safety and efficacy of medical cannabis in the elderly. Eur J Intern Med. 2018;49:44–50. https://doi.org/10.1016/j.ejim.2018.01.019.
25. Choi NG, DiNitto DM, Marti CN, Choi BY. Association of traffic injuries, substance use disorders, and ED visit outcomes among individuals aged 50+ years. J Psychoactive Drugs. 2016;48:369–76.

26. Choi NG, Marti CN, DiNitto DM, Choi BY. Older adults' marijuana use, injuries, and emergency department visits. Am J Drug Alcohol Abuse. 2018;44(2):215–23. https://doi.org/1 0.1080/00952990.2017.1318891.
27. World Health Organization. The health and social effects of nonmedical cannabis use. Geneva: World Health Organization; 2016. Retrieved from http://www.who.int/sub stance_abuse/publications/msbcannabis.pdf.
28. Choi NG, DiNitto DM, Marti CN. Older adults who use or have used marijuana: help-seeking for marijuana and other substance use problems. J Subst Abus Treat. 2017c;77:185–92. https://doi.org/10.1016/j.jsat.2017.02.005.
29. Guerriero F. Guidance on opioids prescribing for the management of persistent non-cancer pain in older adults. World J Clin Cases. 2017;5(3):73–81. https://doi.org/10.12998/wjcc. v5.i3.73. PMID: 28352631; PMCID: PMC5352962.
30. Patel KV, Guralnik JM, Dansie EJ, Turk DC. Prevalence and impact of pain among older adults in the United States: findings from the 2011 National Health and Aging Trends Study. Pain. 2013;154(12):2649–57. https://doi.org/10.1016/j.pain.2013.07.029. PMID: 24287107; PMCID: PMC3843850.
31. American Geriatrics Society Panel on the Pharmacological Management of Persistent Pain in Older Persons. Pharmacological management of persistent pain in older persons. Pain Med. 2009;10(6):1062–83. https://doi.org/10.1111/j.1526-4637.2009.00699.x.
32. Steinman MA, Komaiko KD, Fung KZ, Ritchie CS. Use of opioids and other analgesics by older adults in the United States, 1999–2010. Pain Med. 2015;16(2):319–27. https://doi.org/10.1111/pme.12613. Epub 2014 Oct 28. PMID: 25352175; PMCID: PMC4733650.
33. Musich S, Wang SS, Slindee L, Kraemer S, Yeh CS. Prevalence and characteristics associated with high dose opioid users among older adults. Geriatr Nurs. 2019;40(1):31–6. https://doi.org/10.1016/j.gerinurse.2018.06.001.
34. Bruckenthal P, Reid MC, Reisner L. Special issues in the management of chronic pain in older adults. Pain Med. 2009;10:S67–78. https://doi.org/10.1111/j.1526-4637.2009.00667.x.
35. Schuermeyer J, Salomonsen-Sautel S, Price RK, Balan S, Thurstone C, Min SJ, Sakai JT. Temporal trends in marijuana attitudes, availability and use in Colorado compared to non-medical marijuana states: 2003–11. Drug Alcohol Depend. 2014;140:145–55. https://doi.org/10.1016/j.drugalcdep.2014.04.016.
36. Kalata J. Medical uses of marijuana: opinions of US residents 45+. Washington, DC: AARP; 2004.
37. Adler J, Colbert J. Medicinal use of marijuana. N Engl J Med. 2013;368:866–8. https://doi.org/10.1007/s11136-009-9496-9.

Chapter 15
Cannabis in Dermatology

Catherine Murer Antley, Reagan Anderson, and Judith Margulies

Introduction

Use of cannabinoids (cannabidiol [CBD], delta-9-tetrahydrocannabinol [THC], and others) has increased since recent changes in state and federal cannabis laws. Dermatologic consequences of increased environmental, occupational, and personal use exposure to cannabis and its derivatives, both intentional and secondhand, have also been reported. This chapter focuses on dermatologic conditions associated with cannabis and cannabinoid use. Some of the proposed mechanisms of action are considered. A sampling of potential disease states that may or may not be influenced by these products is reviewed, and issues of safety and efficacy are discussed.

The use of cannabis for skin conditions is in its infancy. The clinical relevance of in vitro or animal models is unsure in the absence of clinical human studies of sufficient quality, size, and duration to accurately inform the physician.

Cannabis industries are not routinely forced to follow Food and Drug Administration (FDA) quality and safety standards; problems of purity and effectiveness exist. Although early in 2019 the FDA announced a desire to address the problems related to loosely controlled, state-sanctioned cannabis products, few federal enforcement actions have been taken to date.

Although dermatologic uses may be found for certain cannabis compounds and from a better understanding of the endocannabinoid system, adequate

C. M. Antley (✉)
Vermont Dermatopathology, South Burlington, VT, USA
e-mail: cantley@CHSI.org

R. Anderson
Dermatology, Rocky Vista University, Colorado Springs, CO, USA

J. Margulies
Pharmacology, Timbre Health, Cambridge, MA, USA
e-mail: Judith@judymargulies.com

© Springer Nature Switzerland AG 2020
K. Finn (ed.), *Cannabis in Medicine*,
https://doi.org/10.1007/978-3-030-45968-0_15

evidence-based, medical indication is currently lacking. Conflicts due to funding or sponsorship may exist. Currently, there is not sufficient evidence to warrant or support responsible clinical recommendation of cannabis products for dermatologic uses.

Cannabis as an Allergen

Cannabis allergy may result when there is sensitization to plant-derived allergens through a variety of ways including personal consumption, secondhand smoke, and vape exposure or while handling plant material or product. Symptoms manifest as urticaria, periorbital angioedema, rhinoconjunctivitis, pruritus, and/or severe anaphylaxis.

After decriminalization, legalization, and commercialization of cannabis in several states in the United States and in Canada, allergic hypersensitivity to cannabis allergens has greater recognition as a public health concern [1, 2]. Exposure through increased individual and industrial production, occupational sensitization, consumption of both ingested and smoked products, and passive exposure via airborne cannabis smoke and indirect cutaneous transmission have all been described. Decuyper et al. reported on a 5-year-old boy and two other patients, who suffered from cannabis-related allergies in which sensitization was believed to have occurred through mere passive, secondhand exposure to airborne cannabis allergen and/or skin contact [3].

Environmental exposure is also reported. Cannabis pollen grains are able to float for long distances and thus are widely distributed. In northern Pakistan, where the plant is native and grows easily, 22% of patients in Islamabad showed sensitization by a positive skin test reaction of greater than 2 mm to *Cannabis sativa* pollen; however, the relationship between the skin prick tests and the individual's clinical presentation was not investigated by the clinicians. In and around Omaha, Nebraska, where feral cannabis, usually with low THC content, grows widely around former hemp fields, individuals with allergic rhinoconjunctivitis and/or asthma symptoms had a positive scratch test to hemp 61% of the time [4]. Silvers and Bernard [2] surveyed an allergy practice's exposure to cannabis in Colorado and found that 12% of people who never smoked cannabis had symptoms from secondhand smoke. Of those who had ever smoked, 26% experienced symptoms, while 50% of those who actively smoked reported symptoms that were described as "respiratory, ocular, and skin." Rabinovitch et al. stated that, with legalization and commercialization, these trends are concerning and suggest cannabis use and exposure could become an increasing public health hazard [5].

Cannabis allergy was first described by Liskow et al., who reported an "anaphylactoid" response to cannabis in a young woman after she inhaled cannabis for the first time. Skin prick testing and passive transfer studies at the time suggested but did not prove a response to THC [6].

Consumption of hemp seed was described by Stadtmauer as leading to an episode of anaphylaxis in a patient who previously smoked cannabis regularly [7]. Smoking cannabis after the event did not elicit an allergic response in the patient. The authors speculate hemp seed may be allergenic when ingested. A series of five pediatric and adult patients suffering anaphylaxis after consuming hemp seed has been described by Bortolin et al. [8]. A Canadian study by Alkhammash et al. described a series of 15 patients who presented with an allergic reaction to hemp seed, cannabis, or both. Eleven individuals experienced an allergic reaction when they first encountered hemp seed; seven of the patients were anaphylactic at presentation. The authors surmise past experience with cannabis allergen may have sensitized these individuals. The results point to a possible clinical cross-reactivity in sensitivity to hemp seed allergy and cannabis. They also suggest anaphylaxis may be a presenting sign or symptom of hemp allergy [9].

In December 2018, the FDA approved as generally recognized as safe (GRAS) the use of hulled hemp seed, hemp seed, and hemp seed protein powder for human consumption, products reportedly with no intrinsic THC (https://www.fda.gov/food/cfsan-constituent-updates/fda-responds-three-gras-notices-hemp-seed-derived-ingredients-use-human-food).

Occupational exposure is increasingly recognized worldwide. Contact urticaria, a hypersensitivity reaction, has resulted from cannabis allergen exposure in a forensic laboratory workplace, as described by Majmudar et al. in their 2006 case report [10]. Another report, published in 2008, involved a technician sensitized by exposure to cannabis while working in a law enforcement laboratory. It was noted three other individuals in the laboratory also showed symptoms resembling this patient's contact urticaria [11].

Exposed workers in a hemp factory in Croatia had a 64.2% prevalence of positive skin reactions to extracts of hemp organic dust. Fifty-six percent of these workers were noted to have had nasal symptoms, and 22% had asthma associated with their workplace, both values greater than the nonexposed controls. Impaired respiratory function was documented in exposed individuals but not linked to their increased antibody marker levels (IgE) or positive skin testing [12].

The mechanism of the cannabis allergic response in humans and the characterization of the allergens are not yet completely understood. Much research is still needed for the development of meaningful diagnostic testing and recommendations for treatment [4]. Gamboa et al. suggested sensitization to cannabis might be caused by an allergenic lipid transfer protein (LTP) labeled Can s 3 [13]. LTP is an important allergen in plant and food allergies. Ebo noted LTP allergens can induce symptoms by ingestion, inhalation, or even contact and that they are highly stable and cross-react with a number of pollens and foods, especially fruits [14].

Armentia et al. [15] noted that, among their study group of 340 individuals addicted to drugs and with histories of atopy/asthma, tomato and tobacco sensitization appeared to be significant risk factors for cannabis sensitization. The authors noted cannabis consumption may be associated with measurable allergic response. Using cannabis-specific IgE determination, they describe a sensitivity of 88.1% and a specificity of 96% for cannabis sensitization. The authors claim prick tests using cannabis extracts and specific IgE determination using biotinylated cannabis extracts were efficient in detecting sensitization to cannabis and positivity was related to clinical profiles (anaphylaxis, asthma, angioedema) severe enough to require emergency medical attention.

Ebo [14] and others described that, in 21 northern European patients with plant food allergies, those who also tested positive for cannabis allergy using skin testing and basophil activation testing also had more severe reactions than patients without cannabis allergy. Unusual food allergies for this northern European cohort were also seen, such as allergies to banana, tomato, citrus, and others. The authors speculate this is possibly because nonspecific ns-LTPs are stable, ubiquitous allergenic proteins and cross-react with these foods. Sensitization toward ns-LTP from cannabis may explain these unusual allergies, as well as the more severe plant food allergies encountered. One patient with cannabis allergy was not sensitized toward ns-LTP; therefore, more work is required to fully describe all the pathogenic allergens at play in cannabis allergy.

Min and Min's study [1] of 2671 individuals including 316 current cannabis users describes how cannabis-using patients were found to be more likely than nonusers to be sensitized to allergens unrelated to cannabis, such as molds *(Alternaria alternata)*, dust mites *(Dermatophagoides farinae* and *Dermatophagoides pteronyssinus)*, plants (ragweed, rye grass, Bermuda grass, oak, birch, and peanut), and cat dander. Higher blood lead and cadmium levels were also found in cannabis-using individuals. Some of these findings may be spurious or possibly due to the known problem of contamination of cannabis with molds, bacteria, and heavy metals [16]. Cross-sectional and observational design also limits the study. Regardless, the authors conclude that cannabis exposure through use or cultivation may be associated with an increased risk of allergen-specific sensitization to cannabis and/or other allergens.

Avoidance of cannabis is the recommended treatment of choice for this allergy.

To date, there is no universally approved and standardized test for cannabis sensitivity, but cannabis as a possible allergen should be kept in the clinician's differential diagnosis. More clinical studies will be needed to accurately evaluate the presence and severity of the risk cannabis allergy poses to users and/or the public.

Cannabinoids in the Treatment of Allergic Contact Dermatitis

The possible immunosuppressive effects of cannabinoids have been explored as a way to improve the symptoms of allergic contact dermatitis in animal models [17]. Evidence from several studies suggests that the endocannabinoid system may regulate allergic dermatitis by altering the animal's chemokine system.

Topical and subcutaneous THC has been shown to decrease inflammation in animal models of allergic contact dermatitis [18, 19]. Further investigations revealed the action of THC was independent of cannabinoid receptor 1 (CB1) and/or cannabinoid receptor 2 (CB2) [17]. (The cannabinoid receptors are also referred to as CR1 and CR2) [20]. Subsequent in vitro studies by this group suggested the anti-inflammatory mechanism involves decreased *interferon-γ* dependent chemokines of the T lymphocytes. Similarly, THC-treated keratinocytes from an allergic contact dermatitis mouse model showed, in the setting of THC treatment, those chemokines associated with increased inflammation were less prominent regardless of the presence of CB1 or CB2. The mechanism of action of THC in these models is unclear, but Katchan et al. [21] suggest it may involve either direct action or action through CB1 and/or CB2 or through receptors other than CB1 and CB2, such as peroxisome proliferator-activated receptors (PPARs) or the G-protein-coupled receptor (GPR55) or another messaging pathway.

In addition to THC and analogues, del Rio et al. have assessed the role CBD may play in decreasing inflammation [22]. An in vitro model of allergic contact dermatitis using human cells appeared to show the addition of CBD decreased chemokines (monocyte chemotactic protein 2, interleukin-6 and interleukin-8, and tumor necrosis factor alpha) made by human keratinocytes. Another in vitro study also appeared to show that, in this model, arachidonylethanolamide/anandamide (AEA, the endocannabinoid analogue to THC) and related [14] compounds increased in CBD-treated human keratinocytes [23]. Although, currently, the roles of CB1, CB2, and related receptors do not appear clear, the authors believe this is the first demonstration of the anti-inflammatory properties of CBD in an experimental human model of allergic contact dermatitis.

Cannabis and Acne

Acne vulgaris is the most prevalent human skin disorder, afflicting around 50 million Americans. The condition is multifactorial, and pathogenesis is related to hormonal influences (both systemic and locally produced and mediated by the pilosebaceous gland), sebum production, infectious agents, inflammation, altered hyperkeratinization, and associated cytokine production [24]. IL-6, tumor necrosis factor-α, IL-12, IL-8, and IL-1β have been shown to underlie this multifactorial and seemingly ubiquitous disease [25].

Cannabinoid receptors have been found to be present in human sebaceous glands, pilosebaceous units, and adnexal structures and on sensory nerve fibers in the human skin [26]. These receptors may be involved in lipid production and apoptosis, reportedly mediated by CB2-coupled signaling involving the MAPK (mitogen-activated protein kinase) pathway [27]. In vitro studies have demonstrated, in addition to other mechanisms, CBD modulates a complex signaling network involving tetrahydrocannabivarin-4 (TRPV4) ion channels, adenosine A2a receptors, and multiple downstream elements, thereby exerting sebostatic and anti-inflammatory effects in a human cellular/organ culture model of acne vulgaris [28, 29]. Olah et al. concluded from another in vitro study [30] that THCV4 and CBD had lipostatic actions and suppressed proliferative fibrocytes; however, the cannabinoids cannabigerol (CBG), cannabichromene (CBC), and cannabidivarin (CBDV) increased sebaceous lipid synthesis. All cannabinoids studied exhibited what the authors described as remarkable anti-inflammatory changes, including decreased inflammatory cytokines.

In another in vitro study, authors Solee Jin and Mi-Young Lee described hemp seed hexane extracts displaying antimicrobial, anti-inflammatory, and anti-lipogenic-promoting properties on *P. acnes*-induced inflammation in HaCaT cells and IGF-1-stimulated lipogenesis in sebocyte tissue culture [31].

By late 2019, there were no published trials with large numbers of human subjects on CBD for the clinical management of acne [32]. One human trial, a single-blind study of 3% cannabis seed extract cream versus vehicle, was evaluated in 11 normal men followed for safety and efficacy. The authors reported significant reduction in sebum and erythema after 12 weeks of follow-up to the well-tolerated cream [33]. Notwithstanding this clinical study on topical hemp seed cream, it is known that hemp seed extract has a 3:1 omega-6 to omega-3 ratio [34]. Given that omega-6 is a known pro-inflammatory agent [35], it is unknown if or under which circumstances ingesting hemp seed extract may exacerbate outbreaks of acne.

With more than 400 components within the cannabis plant, the real-world use of the product differs from that of a purified drug in the laboratory or clinical setting. Similarly, real-world results differ significantly from in vitro models and human studies. In the clinical setting, dermatologists have noticed that some of their most difficult to control acne cases have involved patients who use cannabis. This is supported by a French survey [36] that found regular use of cannabis was highly associated with acne, with an odds ratio of 2.88 (95% CI: 1.55–5.37) in more than 10,000 subjects. In addition, Dréno et al. [37] stated they could not find more published studies on the topic, but their experience supports the impression there is a relationship between cannabis use and acne outbreaks.

The current lack of clarity as to whether cannabis prevents or exacerbates acne in patients is likely influenced by several factors. Financial incentives in the cannabis industry conceivably play a role in study selection, methods, and outcomes. There is no standard cannabis isolate; therefore, differences in active ingredients make it difficult to gather consistent data. Well-documented effects from the use of cannabis products, like increased appetite or mood change, could make a patient more acne prone or otherwise create an environment conducive to a flare.

Regardless of the above considerations, there are currently enough conflicting data from both studies and clinical experience to preclude formation of solid conclusions about the effects of cannabinoids on acne.

Cannabinoids and Autoimmune Disorders

Lupus Erythematosus, Dermatomyositis, and Systemic Sclerosis

The endocannabinoid system may be an important actor within the human immune response. Because of this possible role, the immune-moderating effects of endocannabinoids and cannabinoids more generally have increasingly been objects of investigation, with resources appropriated to possible use of cannabinoids to treat autoimmune diseases and/or to shed light on the mechanisms of disease.

Autoimmune-mediated dermatological diseases afflict a minority of patients but are of considerable importance to the dermatologist's practice due to their significant morbidity and mortality. Cannabinoids generally display immunosuppressive properties as they impact the human immune response. Specifically, cannabinoids cause apoptosis in inflammatory cells such as T cells, macrophages, and others; they orchestrate and moderate the production of numerous cytokines; and they reduce an array of pro-inflammatory leukocytes [21]. One of the receptors through which the cannabinoids act is CB2, which is widely represented on inflammatory cells, especially lymphocytes, macrophages, mast cells, natural killer cells, peripheral mononuclear cells, and microglia, and it may be through this receptor that the immune response is modified or decreased [38]. On the other hand, in addition to the apparent anti-inflammatory actions, there are also some indications that point to cannabinoids increasing the propensity for development or exacerbation of an inflammatory response. These include evidence of cannabinoids associated with amplifying B-cell proliferation [39]. Notwithstanding these findings, in vitro and animal studies have begun to evaluate the possible use of cannabinoids as an immunosuppressive for the treatment of autoimmune disease.

Lupus Erythematosus

Systemic lupus erythematosus (SLE) is a multi-organ autoimmune disease that involves the skin, with classic features such as "butterfly" malar rash. SLE is characterized by autoantibodies and a dysregulated immune response. Increased endocannabinoids have recently been demonstrated in the serum of lupus patients. Navarini et al. [40] found increased plasma levels of the endocannabinoid 2-arachidonoylglycerol (2-AG) in patients with SLE when compared to controls. Their laboratory analysis of patient sera also suggests the presence of an altered 2-AG metabolism. Other endocannabinoids such as N-arachidonoylethanolamine (AEA) and N-palmitoylethanolamine (PEA) were unaltered in the SLE patients. The authors believe the findings suggest a deranged endocannabinoid system in SLE patients, which may prove pathogenetically significant. They note these studies are preliminary, and more studies are needed to confirm or refute the conclusions and to explore possible clinical implications.

Dermatomyositis

Dermatomyositis (DM) is an autoimmune disease with prominent cutaneous features, including Gottron's papules and facial violaceous poikiloderma. In patients with DM, it has been shown that inflammatory cytokines are elevated in their skin lesions but not their sera; these cytokines include increased interferons alpha and beta (INF-a, INF-b) and tumor necrosis factor-a (TNF-a) [41]. Peripheral blood mononuclear cells (PWBC) from patients with DM have been studied with an in vitro assay using synthetic cannabinoid ajulemic acid, which has very low affinity for CB1 (generally found in the central nervous system) but high affinity for CB2 (found on immune cells) [42]. CB2 agonists have been shown to play a role in suppressing inflammation. Compared to healthy controls, the ajulemic acid-treated DM cells showed a decrease in IFN-a and IFN-b and TNF-a, consistent with possibly serving an anti-inflammatory role in ameliorating this disease process [43]. More investigation and phase II clinical trials are required to ascertain the clinical significance of this finding.

Systemic Sclerosis

Systemic sclerosis is an autoimmune connective tissue disease of unclear etiology characterized by increased fibroblast activity/dysfunction, increased extracellular matrix deposition, microvascular endothelial cell damage, and autoimmunity associated with immune dysregulation. Women are affected almost 15 times more frequently than men. The condition nearly always impacts the skin but is also seen in multiple internal organs such as the gastrointestinal tract or lungs. Fibroblasts undergo myofibroblast differentiation, show decreased apoptosis, and release increased extracellular matrix [44].

The endocannabinoid system acts through receptors and receptor pathways to impact a wide range of biologic effects, including inflammation, cell turnover, and apoptosis. Some of these involve binding the two protein G-coupled specific receptors: CB1 and CB2 [45]. The transient receptor potential of vanilloid type 1 (TRPV1) channels, the peroxisome proliferator-activating receptors (PPARs) [46], and the adenosine A2A receptors have also been shown to be involved in (endo)cannabinoid action [47]. Because the inflammatory cell infiltrate, macrophages, mast cells, lymphocytes, and associated cytokines are believed to be involved in the development of systemic sclerosis and are linked to the fibroblasts' growth and increased production of extracellular material, a number of studies have begun to try to elucidate the modulating role that the endocannabinoid system may play in this disease progression.

Inactivation of CB1 has been associated with decreased fibrosis in murine models and in vitro [48]. The same study indicated A2A receptor activation in a tissue culture model stimulated an increased deposition of collagen, apparently mediated through the cannabinoid system, a coupling already described in the central nervous system. On the other hand, CB2 stimulation by agonist led to decreased fibrosis and leukocyte infiltration in an animal model [49].

Further studies showed the activated fibroblasts in systemic sclerosis had decreased apoptotic cells, and this was reversed with cannabinoid exposure. A non-CB1, non-CB2 messaging path (the PPARs) was demonstrated to work alone to decrease inflammation and fibrosis when activated by a THC-like analogue [50].

The immunosuppressive, anti-inflammatory, and pro-apoptotic properties of cannabinoids, coupled with the presence of cannabinoid responsiveness in fibroblasts, make cannabinoids logical candidates for further study. Human trials have been initiated to further explore the role cannabinoids may be able to play in ameliorating the clinical course of the disease. At the time of publication, however, these promising and provocative findings remain preliminary.

Cannabis and Infection

There is some evidence smoking or ingesting cannabis may result in increased susceptibility to cutaneous viral infection. Cannabis use has been associated with a report of increased herpes simplex virus outbreak [51]. An in vitro study by Zhang et al. [52] also demonstrated increased viral load in Kaposi's sarcoma-associated herpesvirus (KSHV) in the presence of THC, as well as increased Kaposi's sarcoma cell proliferation. The authors suggest THC may enhance KSHV infection and replication and foster KSHV-mediated endothelial transformation. They also postulate cannabis use may put patients at increased risk for development and progression of Kaposi's sarcoma. Lastly, there are studies indicating use of cannabis is associated with a decreased immune response to live virus immunization, such as being used in smallpox vaccination [53]. In animal studies, cannabis resin and THC each worsened and prolonged symptoms of viral infection in mice in conjunction with an observed decrease in specific antibody production [54]. At this time, these findings are preliminary, and further study is needed to confirm or refute their clinical significance.

Cannabis and Arteritis

Within the differential diagnosis of arterial ulcers, particularly involving lower extremities, cannabis arteritis may be a consideration, a fact that may conceivably be overlooked in the United States. A recent French study found cannabis use was associated with thromboangiitis obliterans in patients under 50, accounting for 40% of afflicted patients in one study [55]. Timlin et al. [56] stated they believe that over 50 cases they reviewed were an underestimation of the actual prevalence of this condition. With the potential for increased use of cannabis, it is possible this entity could become more common.

Cannabis use has been linked to cardiovascular disease, including myocardial infarction and stroke [57, 58]. The etiology of this phenomenon may be multifactorial but involves, in addition to a dose-dependent increase in heart rate of 20–100% [59, 60], arrhythmias, vasoconstriction (vasospasm), and vasculopathy such as arteritis. While the etiology of the vasculopathy is unclear, the following elements appear to participate: direct vasoconstrictor/vasospasm effect of THC and the effect of possible arsenic, which has been associated with thromboangiitis obliterans and has been found in cannabis and homemade cigarettes [61]. It is also possible THC may act directly on platelets and activate the clotting cascade [62].

The clinical hallmark of cannabis arteritis is a painful necrotic lesion on a distal extremity accompanied by reduced to absent palpable pedal pulses, particularly in young males using cannabis. Symptoms characteristically improve upon cessation of cannabis use but recur with resumption. A negative workup is found for hypercoagulable factors such as proteins C and S, antithrombin III, factor II mutation, resistance to activated C protein, anticardiolipid, and/or cryoglobulins, with no stigmata of emboli or pseudoxanthoma elasticum (PXE) [63]. Studies show narrowing of the involved vessels, but the calcific atherosclerosis typically seen in tobacco smokers is not present in these young patients. The disease generally resolves completely with aspirin and cessation of cannabis use. However, a painful and unrelenting course is observed in reported cases if cannabis use is continued, even involving amputation in 40% of patients in at least one series [63]. More clinical studies will be required to understand the practical clinical significance and actual prevalence or rarity of cannabis arteritis.

Cannabis and Neoplasia

Cannabis and Melanoma and Nonmelanoma Skin Cancer

In the laboratory, endocannabinoids, cannabinoids, and their receptors (CB1/CB2, TRPV1, and others) are linked to the development, growth, spread, regulation, and control of skin cancer, but the exact roles remain unclear. CB1/CB2 ligands are present on normal skin and to a greater degree on malignant tumors that develop in the skin. The development of skin tumors is also associated with an altered endocannabinoid system. Therefore, numerous studies have been aimed at untangling the role of cannabinoids and the various receptors as regulators of cutaneous malignancy, yielding compelling but conflicting results.

While animal and in vitro studies have disclosed information that appears to point toward the possible future use of cannabis derivatives or laboratory-created cannabinoids in the treatment of dermatologic neoplasia, a review of currently available treatments by Li and Kamp [64] found, at this time, for both melanoma and nonmelanoma skin cancers, adequate clinical studies proving efficacy are either insufficient or nonexistent or show negative evidence. The authors found a dearth of clinical trials that would support medical claims when evaluated using the Oxford Centre for Evidence-Based Medicine grading system, making it impossible for them to recommend cannabis as a treatment for skin cancer. Studies adequately exploring toxicity or contraindications that the skin cancer patient may encounter when using cannabis are not generally available. Furthermore, some clinicians have reported harm to patients self-treating their skin cancer with cannabis-derived products purchased over the counter or sourced on the Internet. In fact, use of cannabis during immunotherapy with nivolumab appeared to decrease tumor response rates in a recent preliminary study [65] in patients with advanced malignancies. Response rate decreased from 37% to 15% for nonmelanoma skin cancer and from 40% to 10% for melanoma skin cancer; while overall survival was not affected, the findings prompt caution and further study. In other cases, patients have delayed treatment or surgery in favor of cannabis products that were advertised as remedies for cancer.

Melanoma

Blazquez et al. [66] described how, in human melanoma and melanoma cell lines expressing CB1 and CB2, in vitro THC reduces melanoma cell growth in proportion to the number of CB receptors. Armstrong et al. [67] suggested THC-related melanoma cell death in tissue culture is mediated through apoptosis, and they report this effect is increased when the cells are also exposed to CBD in addition to THC.

Conversely, other studies have found evidence suggesting activation of the endocannabinoid system via CB1 may promote melanoma growth. These studies by Carpi et al. [68] found silencing/reduction of CB1 receptors on human melanoma cells arrested the cells in G1/S phase and decreased expression of P-Akt and p-ERK, both of which work to decrease the number of viable melanoma cells. These findings suggest a possible role of intact CB1 in promoting human melanoma cell growth in vitro. While Glodde et al. [69] found that THC treatment of transplanted melanoma cell tumors in an in vivo mouse model significantly decreased the size of the tumors, the treatment did not impact melanoma cell growth in vitro, nor did the authors find any relationship to the presence of CB1/CB2 receptors. They suggest the effect is mediated through changes to the pro-inflammatory microenvironment.

Sailler et al. [70] studied the altered local endocannabinoid microenvironment in an in vivo mouse melanoma model and were able to translate their observations to humans by assessing cancer-associated changes in circulating endocannabinoids in 298 patients with several types and stages of cancer. In the mouse model, they found plasma 2-arachidonoylglycerol (2-AG) levels were increased in mice with tumors. In the human cancer patients, oleoylethanolamide (OEA) and palmitoylethanolamide (PEA) levels rose as the number of metastases increased. While the findings are not yet clear enough to qualify as a measurable marker for cancer prognosis, the statistically significant changes to the endocannabinoid system in the setting of cancer suggest the system may play a role in the regulation of cancer progression.

Arachidonylethanolamide/anandamide (AEA, the endocannabinoid analogue to THC) may act differently at different concentrations: In vitro studies at high doses showed AEA is associated with apoptosis of melanoma cells via TRPV1-dependent pathway. At low levels however, AEA stimulates melanogenesis in a CB1-dependent fashion [71].

Nonmelanoma Skin Cancer

In vitro studies demonstrated that activation of cannabinoid receptors results in cell death through apoptosis of malignant epidermal cells but not benign cells. Casanova et al. [72] also described significant tumor growth inhibition of malignant tumors when treated with a mixed CB1/CB2 agonist. In addition to increased apoptosis, the treated tumors demonstrated reduced tumor vascularization in the setting of decreased expression of pro-angiogenic factors such as vascular endothelial growth factor (VEGF), placental growth factor, and angiopoietin 2. However, Zheng et al. [73] have shown how CB1 and CB2 appear to be required for the development of UV-induced inflammation and resulting skin cancer in a mouse model of UV solar irradiation and cutaneous tumors. Mice without CB1/CB2 receptors were resistant to the development of inflammation and tumors.

Synthetic cannabinoid ligands (both street drugs and selected cannabinoids JWH-018, JWH-122 and JWH-210) appear to have significant anti-inflammatory and antitumor characteristics in one reported mouse cancer model [74].

Nonmelanoma skin cancer overexpresses cyclooxygenase 2 (COX-2). AEA-programmed cell death occurs after AEA is metabolized by COX-2 to a prostaglandin (15d-PGJ2-EA) required for AEA-programmed cell death. Impeding AEA metabolism with FAAH inhibitor renders AEA more cytotoxic to the tumor cells. Since noncancerous cells have low COX-2, this AEA-mediated cell death is elegantly selective for malignant cells. The apoptotic pathway also appears to be independent of cannabinoid receptors (CB1/CB2 or TRPV1) [75].

Clearly the relationship between neoplasia and cannabinoids is complex. In laboratory studies and murine models, cannabinoids and manipulation of the endocannabinoid system have shown mixed results as candidates for fighting neoplasia. Currently, none of the mechanisms involved are completely understood, and conflicting results are noted. More studies, including controlled clinical human trials, are needed before cannabinoids should be considered for skin cancer treatment.

Cannabis: Product Reliability and Safety

Drug Delivery and Unreliable Product

The clinical response to cannabis-derived dermatological products relies on good manufacturing practices that assure the quality, purity, identity, and strength of drug products. Products applied as creams, ointments, sprays, gels, transdermal patches, lip balms, oils, moisturizers, and others offer a variety of options for drug delivery. The transdermal, nasal, and oral mucosal products including sprays, chewing gum, patches, and sublingual tablets have been shown to increase patient tolerance of cannabinoids while also avoiding first-pass hepatic metabolism [76].

As with any drug product, adverse events associated with cannabinoid formulations may result from the active ingredients, the inactive ingredients, and the vehicle or delivery system. Yet at the crux of the topic of cannabinoid use in dermatology is the question of safety, reliability, and reproducibility of the final manufactured product achieved by obtaining quality raw materials, ensuring dependable manufacturing operating systems, investigating deviations from quality standards, maintaining reliable testing laboratories and records, and incorporating safe practices for packaging, labeling, and storage of the consumer product [77]. Moreover, if the cannabis plant material from which the drug product is derived contains other compounds, the resulting adulterated product may lead to additional untoward events. The raw plant materials are well known for a propensity for fungal and heavy metal contamination [16]. Since in some areas in the United States the cannabis industry is currently less responsive to regulation, concerns over microbial, mycotoxin, heavy metal, and pesticide contamination persist [78].

The discussion is further complicated by differing individual state standards for purity testing. In California, 18% of cannabis product was found to not meet accuracy standards for product labeling, meaning the product sold had greater than 10% more or less THC or CBD than the label indicated [77, 78]. In another example, Oregon was able to test only 3% of products on sale and 33% of growers for safety and reliability for the state's cannabis program [79]. Cannabis testing laboratory fraud has been shown to contribute to unreliable consumer product in several states [80]. Therefore, healthcare practitioners need to be aware not only of concentration and content concerns about active ingredients, they also need to be concerned about potential contamination from a wide variety of pathogens and about false or deceptive labeling practices.

Between 2014 and mid-2019, the FDA issued 21 warning letters for cannabis misbranded and adulterated product due to inaccurate label claims for THC, CBD, or hemp. Several examples of similar CBD product issues were presented in oral testimony during the FDA's May 31, 2019, Public Hearing for Scientific Data and Information on Cannabis and Cannabis-Derived Compounds [81].

To assess how reliable the labels are for CBD products, specifically those claiming to contain pure CBD, Bonn-Miller et al. [82] purchased 84 products sold online from 31 companies. This independent and blinded analysis for cannabinoid content and concentration for CBD found 42.85% of the products were under-labeled by more than 10%, 26.19% were over-labeled by more than 10%, and 30.95% were labeled within 10%, which they considered could be called accurate. In addition, assessment for adulteration with THC found 21.43% of the tested product had up to 6.43 mg/ml of THC, a concentration sufficient to induce intoxication or impairment especially in children with lower body mass indexes. Last, many of the products contained other cannabinoids: 15.48% contained cannabidiolic acid and 2.38% contained cannabigerol.

With a heightened public interest in CBD, some cosmetic manufacturers are exploring marketing strategies to navigate the less stringent cosmetic regulations of the FDA as they introduce new CBD or cannabinoid-containing cosmetic products [83]. Because transdermal absorption of these cannabinoids can occur, a consumer may unwittingly experience psychoactive effects, decreased intellectual and motor performance, and/or a positive drug screen. At this time, it is unclear if limits or outright restrictions will be imposed by the FDA on the cannabinoid content of topical cosmetics.

Unintended Consequences of Increased Cannabis Use in Dermatology

This review of the dermatologic literature suggests a possible emphasis on investigation of cannabinoids as future medications for dermatologic conditions. In comparison, the public's cannabis exposure as a possible etiology of dermatologic disease has generally been given less investigational attention and resources. Yet, as the likelihood of cannabis-related allergens becomes greater and more individuals are passively, occupationally, environmentally, or intentionally exposed and sensitized, the dermatologist can reasonably expect to see increased cannabis allergy or urticarial cases in clinical practice. It is possible this may also be true for other cannabis-related dermatologic disorders including acne and cannabis arteritis, as previously discussed [36, 55, 56, 63]. More studies will be needed to ascertain the practical clinical prevalence of these and other entities.

Absorption of cannabinoids from dermatological use may also be a cause of impaired or dysregulated immune responses. Infection has resulted from moldy or contaminated cannabis plant material [84, 85]. Studies will need to determine not only how cannabinoids may be used to suppress an overactive immune system but also what ramifications possible immunosuppression by cannabinoids will have on the innate and acquired immune system's ability to fight infections and mount appropriate host response, particularly in previously immunocompromised individuals such as transplant patients. Assessment of actual clinical relevance and prevalence will also be needed.

Cannabinoids are absorbed through the skin making them potentially available for systemic effects. Anecdotal reports from Colorado and elsewhere include cases where THC skin patches are used to wean users from the smoking and vaping of cannabis and to control withdrawal symptoms such as rebound anxiety attacks (personal communication). Reports of transdermal systemic absorption underline the need for human studies to document possible toxicities and side effects of topical cannabis products in order to protect public health and accurately inform patients and providers alike.

Of concern in the context of potential treatment for acne, dermatitis, and other skin conditions are reports of adults and children experiencing psychoactive effects such as somnolence and disorientation during or after application of CBD oils and creams (personal communication). This could be due to the action of CBD itself or from adulteration of the product with higher than the 0.3% THC levels allowed for legalized products. In addition to somnolence and sedation, the known adverse effects of orally administered CBD include hepatotoxicity, increased suicidal behavior and ideation, increased incidence of infection, vomiting, and diarrhea [86]. It is not well studied if systemic absorption of topical cannabis products could also lead to addiction.

Lastly, it appears largely unmeasured if, or to what extent, patients are forgoing lifesaving treatment because of false medical promises. For example, a patient may arrive at the clinic after having delayed treatment of a skin cancer because it has been "treated" with cannabis oil, which Internet sources claimed would "cure cancer." Clinical studies have not yet assessed the morbidity or mortality resulting from this delay of treatment due to false medical promises of topical dermatologic cannabis products.

In summary, adverse dermatological effects have been reported from cannabis exposure. More research is needed to accurately measure and describe the characteristics and clinical significance of these untoward events. While the potential for the discovery and development of effective dermatological treatments using cannabis-derived products is clear, thoughtful and comprehensive research is required before medical recommendations should be advanced.

References

1. Min J, Min K. Marijuana use is associated with hypersensitivity to multiple allergens in US adults. Drug Alcohol Depend. 2018;182:74–7.
2. Silvers WS, Bernard T. Spectrum and prevalence of reactions to marijuana in a Colorado allergy practice. Ann Allergy Asthma Immunol. 2017;119(6):570–1.
3. Decuyper I, et al. Where there's smoke, there's fire: cannabis allergy through passive exposure. J Allergy Clin Immunol Pract. 2016;5(3):864–5.
4. Ocampo T, Rans T. Cannabis sativa: the unconventional "weed" allergen. Ann Allergy Asthma Immunol. 2015;114:187–92.
5. Rabinovitch N, et al. The highs and lows of marijuana use in allergy. Ann Allergy Asthma Immunol. 2018;121(1):14–7.
6. Liskow B, et al. Allergy to marihuana. Ann Intern Med. 1971;75(4):571–3.
7. Stadtmauer G, et al. Anaphylaxis to ingestion of hempseed (Cannabis sativa). J Allergy Clin Immunol. 2003;112(1):216–7.
8. Bortolin K, et al. Case series of 5 patients with anaphylaxis to hemp seed ingestion. J Allergy Clin Immunol. 2016;137(2):AB239.
9. Alkhammash S, et al. Cannabis and hemp seed allergy. J Allergy Clin Immunol Pract. 2019;7(7):2429–2430.e1.
10. Majmudar V, et al. Contact urticaria to Cannabis sativa. Contact Dermatitis. 2006; 54(2):127.
11. Williams C, et al. Work-related contact urticaria to Cannabis sativa. Contact Dermatitis. 2008;58(1):62–3.
12. Kanceljak-Macan B, et al. Organic aerosols and the development of allergic disorders. Arh Hig Rada Toksikol. 2004;55:213–20.
13. Gamboa P, et al. Sensitization to cannabis sativa by a novel allergenic lipid transfer protein, Can s 3. J Allergy Clin Immunol. 2007;120(6):1459–60.
14. Ebo DG. New food allergies in a European non-Mediterranean region: is Cannabis sativa to blame? Int Arch Allergy Immunol. 2013;161:220–8.
15. Armentia A, et al. Allergic hypersensitivity to cannabis in patients with allergy and illicit drug users. Allergol Immunopathol (Madr). 2011;39(5):271–9.
16. Nie B, et al. The role of mass spectrometry in the cannabis industry. J Am Soc Mass Spectrom. 2019;30(5):719–30.
17. Gaffal E, et al. Anti-inflammatory activity of topical THC in DNFB-mediated mouse allergic contact dermatitis independent of CB1 and CB2 receptors. Allergy. 2013;68:994–1000.
18. Karsak M, et al. Attenuation of allergic contact dermatitis through the endocannabinoid system. Science. 2007;316:1494–7.

19. Diaz P, et al. 6-Methoxy-N-alkyl isatin acylhydrazone derivatives as a novel series of potent selective cannabinoid receptor 2 inverse agonists: design, synthesis and binding mode prediction. J Med Chem. 2009;52(2):433–44.
20. Bobrov M, et al. Expression of Type I Cannabinoid Receptors at Different Stages of Neuronal Differentiation of Human Fibroblasts. Bull Exp Biol Med. 2017;163:272–5.
21. Katchan V, et al. Cannabinoids and autoimmune diseases: a systematic review. Autoimmun Rev. 2016;15:513–28.
22. del Rio C, et al. The endocannabinoid system of the skin. A potential approach for the treatment of skin disorders. Biochem Pharmacol. 2018;157:122–33.
23. Petrosino S, et al. Anti-inflammatory properties of cannabidiol, a non-psychotropic cannabinoid, in experimental allergic contact dermatitis. J Pharmacol Exp Ther. 2018;365:652–63.
24. Makrantonaki E, et al. An update on the role of the sebaceous gland in the pathogenesis of acne. Dermatoendocrinol. 2011;3(1):41–9. https://doi.org/10.4161/derm.3.1.13900.
25. Kistowska M, et al. Propionibacterium acnes promotes Th17 and Th17/Th1 responses in acne patients. J Investig Dermatol. 2015;135(1):110–8.
26. Stander S, et al. Distribution of cannabinoid receptor 1 (CB1) and 2 (CB2). J Dermatol Sci. 2005;38:177–88.
27. Dobrosi N, et al. Endocannabinoids enhance lipid synthesis and apoptosis of human sebocytes via cannabinoid receptor-2-mediated signaling. FASEB J. 2008;22:3685–95.
28. Maccarrone M, et al. Endocannabinoid signaling at the periphery: 50 years after THC. Trends Pharmacol Sci. 2015;36(5):277–96.
29. Olah A, et al. Cannabidiol exerts sebostatic and anti-inflammatory effects of human sebocytes. J Clin Invest. 2014;124:3713–24.
30. Olah A, et al. Differential effectiveness of selected non-psychotropic phytocannabinoids on human sebocyte functions implicates their introduction in dry seborrheic skin and acne treatment. Exp Dermatol. 2016;25:701–7.
31. Jin S, Lee M. The ameliorative effect of hemp seed hexane extracts on Propionibacterium acnes-induced inflammation and lipogenesis in sebocytes. PLoS One. 2018;13(8):e0202933. Published online 2018 Aug 27. https://doi.org/10.1371/journal.pone.0202933.
32. Jhawar N, et al. The growing trend of cannabidiol in skincare products. Clin Dermatol. 2019;37:279–81.
33. Ali A, Akhtar N. The safety and efficacy of 3% cannabis seeds extract cream for reduction of human cheek skin sebum and erythema content. Pak J Pharm Sci. 2015;28(4):1389–95.
34. Siano F, et al. Comparative study of chemical, biochemical characteristic and ATR-FTIR analysis of seeds, oil and flour of the edible fedora cultivar hemp (Cannabis sativa L.). Molecules. 2018;24(1):83.
35. Ghosh S, et al. Fish oil attenuates omega-6 polyunsaturated fatty acid-induced dysbiosis and infectious colitis but impairs LPS dephosphorylation activity causing sepsis. PLoS One. 2013;8(2):e55464.
36. Wolkenstein P, et al. Smoking and dietary factors associated with moderate-to-severe acne in French adolescents and young adults: results of a survey using a representative sample. Dermatology. 2015;230:34–9.
37. Dréno B, et al. The influence of exposome on acne. J Eur Acad Dermatol Venereol. 2018;32(5):812–9.
38. Iversen L. Cannabis and the brain. Brain. 2003;126:1252–70.
39. Rieder S, et al. Cannabinoid-induced apoptosis in immune cells as a pathway to immunosuppression. Immunobiology. 2010;215:598–605.
40. Navarini L, et al. Endocannabinoid system in systemic lupus erythematosus: first evidence for a deranged 2-arachidonoylglycerol metabolism. Int J Biochem Cell Biol. 2018;99:161–8.
41. Nabatian A, et al. Tumor necrosis factor alpha release in peripheral blood mononuclear cells of cutaneous lupus and dermatomyositis patients. Arthritis Res Ther. 2012;14(1):1–11.
42. Tepper M, et al. Ultrapure ajulemic acid has improved CD2 selectivity with reduced CD1 activity. Bioorg Med Chem. 2014;22:3245–51.

43. Robinson E, et al. Cannabinoid reduces inflammatory cytokines, tumor necrosis factor alpha, and type I interferons in dermatomyositis in vitro. J Investig Dermatol. 2017;137:2445–7.
44. Marquart S, et al. Inactivation of the cannabinoid receptor CB1 prevents leukocyte infiltration and experimental fibrosis. Arthritis Rheum. 2010;62(11):3467–76.
45. Servettaz A, et al. Targeting the cannabinoid pathway limits the development of fibrosis and autoimmunity in a mouse model of systemic sclerosis. Am J Pathol. 2010;177(1):187–96.
46. Juknat A, et al. Differential transcriptional profiles mediated by exposure to the cannabinoids cannabidiol and delta nine tetrahydrocannabinol in BV-2 microglial cells. Br J Pharmacol. 2012;165(8):2512–28.
47. Klein TW. Cannabinoid-based drugs as anti-inflammatory therapeutics. Nat Rev Immunol. 2005;5:400–11.
48. Lazzerini P, et al. Adenosine A2A receptor activation stimulates collagen production in sclerodermic dermal fibroblast either directly and through a cross-talk with the cannabinoid system. J Mol Med. 2012;90:331–42.
49. Akhmetshina A, et al. The cannabinoid receptor CB2 exerts antifibrotic effects in experimental dermal fibrosis. Arthritis Rheum. 2009;60(4):1129–36.
50. Garcia-Gonzalez E, et al. Can cannabinoids modulate fibrotic progression in systemic sclerosis? Isr Med Assoc J. 2016;18:156–8.
51. Juel-Jensen B. Cannabis and recurrent herpes simplex. BMJ. 1972;4(5835):296.
52. Zhang X, et al. Cannabinoid modulation of Kaposi's sarcoma-associated herpes virus infection and transformation. Cancer Res. 2007;67(15):7230–7.
53. Huemer H, et al. "Recreational" drug abuse associated with failure to mount a proper antibody response after a generalised orthopoxvirus infection. Infection. 2007;35(6):469–71.
54. Huemer H, et al. Cannabinoids lead to enhanced virulence of smallpox vaccine (vaccinia) virus. Immunobiology. 2011;216:670–7.
55. Sauvanier M, et al. Lower limb occlusive arteriopathy: retrospective analysis of 73 patients with onset before the age of 50 years. J Mal Vasc. 2002;27:69–76.
56. Timlin H, et al. Vascular effects of cannabis: case report and review of literature. J Rheumatol Arthritis Dis. 2017;2:1–3.
57. Jouanjus E, et al. Cannabis use: signal of increasing risk of serious cardiovascular disorders. J Am Heart Assoc. 2014;3:e000638. https://doi.org/10.1161/JAHA.113.000638.
58. Kalla A, et al. Cannabis use predicts risks of heart failure and cerebrovascular accidents: results from the National Inpatient Sample. J Cardiovasc Med. 2018;19:480–4. https://doi.org/10.2459/JCM.0000000000000681.
59. Cappelli F, et al. Cannabis: a trigger for acute myocardial infarction? A case report. J Cardiovasc Med. 2008;9(7):725–8.
60. Middleman MA, et al. Triggering myocardial infarction by marijuana. Circulation. 2001;103:2805–9.
61. Noel B. Thromboangiitis obliterans a new look for an old disease. Int J Cardiol. 2001;78:199.
62. Dahdouh Z, et al. Cannabis and coronary thrombosis: what is the role of platelets? Platelets. 2012;23:243–5.
63. Combemale P, et al. Cannabis arteritis. Br J Dermatol. 2005;152:166–9.
64. Li J, Kampp J. Review of common alternative herbal "remedies" for skin cancer. Dermatol Surg. 2019;45(1):58–67.
65. Taha T, et al. Cannabis impacts tumor response rate to nivolumab in patients with advanced malignancies. Oncologist. 2019;24(4):549–54.
66. Blazquez C, et al. Cannabinoid receptors as novel targets for the treatment of melanoma. FASEB J. 2006;20:2633–5.
67. Armstrong J, et al. Exploiting cannabinoid induced cytotoxic autophagy to drive melanoma cell death. J Invest Dermatol. 2015;135:1629–37.
68. Carpi S, et al. Tumor promoting effects of cannabinoid receptor type 1 in human melanoma cells. Toxicol In Vitro. 2017;40:272–9.

69. Glodde N, et al. Differential role of cannabinoids in the pathogenesis of skin cancer. Life Sci. 2015;138:35–40.
70. Sailler S, et al. Regulation of circulating endocannabinoids associated with cancer and metastases in mice and humans. Onco Targets Ther. 2014;1:272–82.
71. Pucci M, et al. Endocannabinoids stimulate human melanogenesis via type-1 cannabinoid receptor. J Biol Chem. 2012;287:15466–78.
72. Casanova M, et al. Inhibition of skin tumor growth and angiogenesis in vivo by activation of cannabinoid receptors. J Clin Invest. 2003;111:43–50.
73. Zheng D, et al. The cannabinoid receptors are required for ultraviolet-induced inflammation and skin cancer development. Cancer Res. 2008;68(10):3992–8.
74. Nakajima J, et al. Structure-dependent inhibitory effects of synthetic cannabinoids against 12-0-tetradecanoylphorbol-13-acetate-induced inflammation and skin tumor promotion in mice. J Pharm Pharmacol. 2013;65(8):1223–30.
75. Soliman E, Van Dross R. Anandamide-induced endoplasmic reticulum stress and apoptosis are mediated by oxidative stress in non-melanoma skin cancer: receptor-independent endocannabinoid signaling. Mol Carcinog. 2016;55:1807–21.
76. Bruni N, et al. Cannabinoid delivery systems for pain and inflammation treatment. Molecules. 2018;10:2478.
77. USFDA. Facts about the current good manufacturing practices (CGMPs). https://www.fda.gov/drugs/pharmaceutical-quality-resources/facts-about-current-good-manufacturing-practices-cgmps. Accessed 30 Aug 2019.
78. https://apnews.com/2cb04323f9074c1ca28001693f6e2a8a. Accessed 25 Aug 2019.
79. Oregon Secretary of State. 2019. https://sos.oregon.gov/audits/Documents/2019-04.pdf. Accessed 25 Aug 2019.
80. https://www.nbcbayarea.com/news/local/Industry-Insiders-Warn-of-Fraud-at-Marijuana-Testing-Labs-458125743.html. Accessed 25 Aug 2019.
81. USFDA. Scientific data and information about products containing cannabis or cannabis-derived compounds; Public Hearing. https://www.fda.gov/news-events/fda-meetings-conferences-and-workshops/scientific-data-and-information-about-products-containing-cannabis-or-cannabis-derived-compounds. Accessed 30 Aug 2019.
82. Bonn-Miller MO, et al. Labeling accuracy of cannabidiol extracts sold online. JAMA. 2017;318(17):1708–9.
83. Fulton A, Blitz S. Into the weeds: walking the regulatory line of CBD in cosmetics. Cosmetics and Toiletries https://www.cosmeticsandtoiletries.com/regulatory/claims/Into-the-Weeds-Walking-the-Regulatory-Line-of-CBD-in-Cosmetics-511854642.html. Accessed 20 Aug 2019.
84. Shapiro BB, et al. Cryptococcal meningitis in a daily cannabis smoker without evidence of immunodeficiency. BMJ Case Rep. 2018;2018:bcr-2017-221435.
85. Thompson GR, et al. A microbiome assessment of medical marijuana. Clin Microbiol Infect. 2017;23(4):269–70.
86. Szaflarski JP, et al. CBD EAP study group. Long-term safety and treatment effects of cannabidiol in children and adults with treatment-resistant epilepsies: expanded access program results. Epilepsia. 2018;59(8):1540–8.

Chapter 16
Fetal and Neonatal Marijuana Exposure

Leeann M. Blaskowsky

Conceptualizing Neonatal Development

Concept analysis is essential in the creation of theory [1]. By defining terms or concepts, within the context of the theory presented, clarity and understanding can be assured. For providers caring for neonates (infants up to 28 days of life) in neonatal intensive care (NICU), development serves as the core of the care decisions made every day [2]. Developmental psychology recognized the ability for the brain to adapt to varying circumstances many years ago, but its application to practice continues to evolve, examining development, scientifically, over the lifespan with a large number of theories focusing on childhood; the time when the largest amount of change occurs. For the neonatal population, Newman et al. report that early, specifically fetal and neonatal, development markedly affects mental health in later life [3].

Although the study of brain development has only recently, in the past 30–50 years according to the experts, begun to expand, the information being examined and shared is increasing exponentially. Kolb and Gibb describe the multilayered processes involved beginning with neurogenesis as a sequence of events including mitosis, neuronal formation and migration, synaptogenesis, pruning, and myelin formation [4]. While the exact numbers vary according to author and study, suffice it to say these cells number in the hundreds of billions by term, defined as ≥37 completed weeks of gestation (Fig. 16.1). Using structural and physiological imaging methods, Vasung et al. have been able to demonstrate the vast changes in the fetal and neonatal brain [5]. Admittedly, not all of these cells survive, undergoing a process referred to as pruning through programmed cell death to eliminate those parts no longer deemed essential. Similar, in function at least, to the programmed cell death, known as apoptosis, that changes a fetal mitt to a hand with fingers by

L. M. Blaskowsky (✉)
University of Colorado School of Medicine, Department of Pediatrics, Aurora, CO, USA

© Springer Nature Switzerland AG 2020
K. Finn (ed.), *Cannabis in Medicine*,
https://doi.org/10.1007/978-3-030-45968-0_16

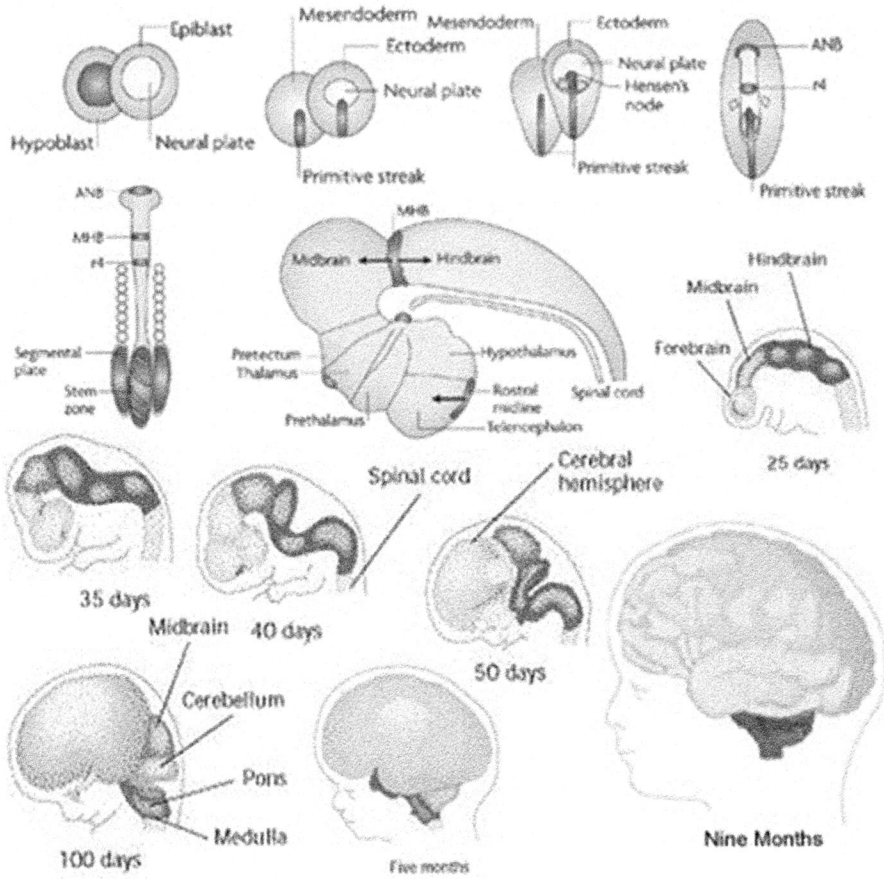

Fig. 16.1 Fetal brain structure development with approximate gestational landmarks. (Reproduced with permission. Source: researchgate.net/publication/327222314)

destroying a predetermined number of the epithelial cells surrounding the bony structures. While examining hippocampal changes with the presence or absence of certain chemical elements in postnatal development, Chwiej and colleagues concluded that brain development involves numerous complex processes that, when disrupted, may lead to serious brain pathology [6].

Through the study of those born too soon, we can explain and compare this vulnerable period for any infant. Als, through her work designated as synactive theory, developed a program for assessment and care known as the Newborn Individualized Developmental Care and Assessment Program (NIDCAP®) after demonstrating a reduction of neurodevelopmental disabilities [7, 8, 9]. Bingham conveys the benefits of this specialized care decreased length-of-stay, improved nipple feeding transitions, and improved family interactions. Als furthered her research with an additional study of her program's ability to improve brain function and structure in preterm infants. Correcting the effects of intrauterine growth restriction, a known comorbidity of neonatal neurodevelopmental issues, by hypothesizing the reduction of noxious stimuli resets the physiologic responses to pain and stress, thereby reducing the release of damaging free radicals which cause toxic damage resulting in inappropriate cell death along with changes in sensory thresholds, activity, and sensitivity.

Haumont examined the effects of developmentally supportive care by measuring cerebral hemodynamics with near-infrared spectroscopy (NIRS) and noted significant variations during a routine diaper change. Even a procedure not typically viewed as painful, like a routine diaper change, had an impact [9]. Ackerman's work studying the developing brain examined the influences of norepinephrine and serotonin and the roles; these endogenous chemicals play in the perception of pain and the physiological responses to it [10]. If even changing a diaper can be viewed by a newborn, in this case a premature one, as affecting cerebral hemodynamics similar to a procedure known to cause pain [9], does it not stand to reason that a noxious exposure could contribute to at least an equal disturbance? A developing fetus, within the womb, is very much like the preterm infant except that we are afforded the ability to study the reactions of an infant whose physiology is expected to function before it would be if carried to term. Noting that habituation, through exposure and chemically mediated responses, can play a large part in the modeling of the brain during development; Ackerman's preliminary conclusions are now being studied in much greater detail.

Perinatal Exposure to Cannabinoids Through Pregnancy and Breastfeeding

Science has clearly demonstrated that Δ-9 tetrahydrocannabinol (THC), the psychoactive compound found in the *Cannabis sativa* (marijuana) plant, is absorbed into the lungs when smoked and the gastrointestinal tract when ingested and readily distributed to brain and fat cells [11]. Distribution within the brain and activation of endocannabinoid receptors produces the psychoactive effect reported with marijuana use (Fig. 16.2). The preferential distribution within the fat confirms the molecular attraction to fat, also known as lipophilic. As a fetus develops, the placenta serves as the critical interface for exchanging gas and nutrients (e.g., oxygen and glucose) as well as the transmission of noxious substances like marijuana, nicotine, alcohol, or other drugs of abuse [4, 11].

The American College of Obstetrics and Gynecology (ACOG) committee opinion on marijuana use during pregnancy and lactation details the studies with animal models that demonstrated placental transmission of THC with fetal levels reaching 10% of maternal levels after an acute exposure and even higher for repeated exposures [11]. In their 2017 committee opinion, ACOG made the following recommendations:

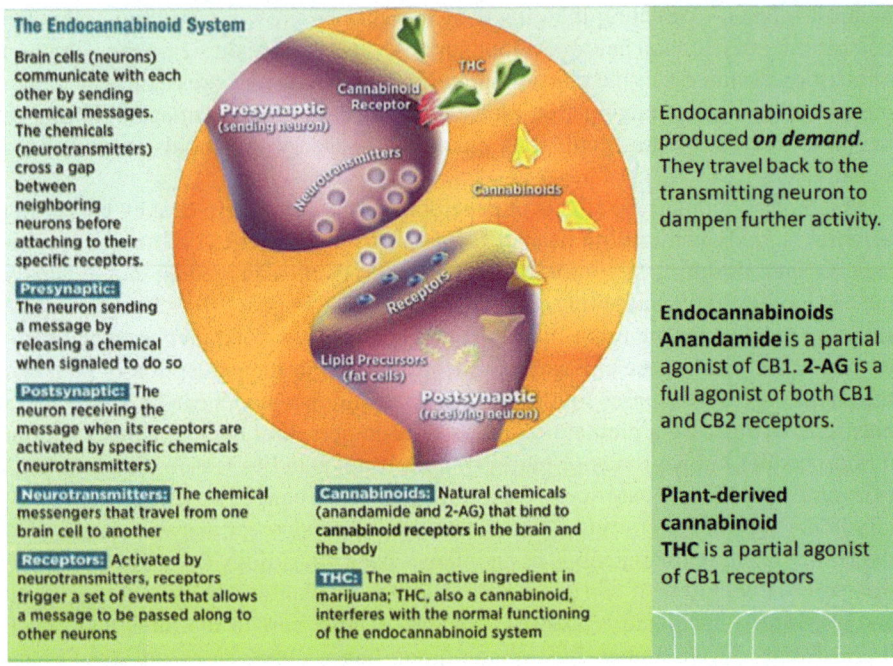

The Endocannabinoid System

Brain cells (neurons) communicate with each other by sending chemical messages. The chemicals (neurotransmitters) cross a gap between neighboring neurons before attaching to their specific receptors.

Presynaptic: The neuron sending a message by releasing a chemical when signaled to do so

Postsynaptic: The neuron receiving the message when its receptors are activated by specific chemicals (neurotransmitters)

Neurotransmitters: The chemical messengers that travel from one brain cell to another

Receptors: Activated by neurotransmitters, receptors trigger a set of events that allows a message to be passed along to other neurons

Cannabinoids: Natural chemicals (anandamide and 2-AG) that bind to cannabinoid receptors in the brain and the body

THC: The main active ingredient in marijuana; THC, also a cannabinoid, interferes with the normal functioning of the endocannabinoid system

Endocannabinoids are produced **on demand**. They travel back to the transmitting neuron to dampen further activity.

Endocannabinoids Anandamide is a partial agonist of CB1. **2-AG** is a full agonist of both CB1 and CB2 receptors.

Plant-derived cannabinoid THC is a partial agonist of CB1 receptors

Fig. 16.2 Endocannabinoid system. (Reproduced with permission. Source: March of Dimes)

- All women should be asked about alcohol, tobacco, and other drug use, including marijuana and other medications used for nonmedical reasons, before and in early pregnancy.
- Women reporting marijuana use should be educated about the potential adverse consequences of use during pregnancy.
- Women who are pregnant or considering pregnancy should be encouraged to discontinue marijuana use.
- Pregnant women should be encouraged to discontinue marijuana use for medicinal purposes in favor of alternative therapies with pregnancy-specific safety data.
- There are insufficient data to evaluate infant safety during lactation and breastfeeding, and, in the absence of this data, marijuana use is discouraged.

Since THC is lipophilic, understanding that breastmilk contains increasing concentrations of fat during each feeding/pumping session, then its presence in breastmilk is certain. What is not certain are the absolute transmission concentrations as they appear both dose (amount of maternal use) and proximity (to sampling) dependent. Historically, the evidence for documenting has been old and limited, but the presumption for proximity to maternal use and dosing should be relatively self-evident and is now emerging in the literature.

Because marijuana is still federally regulated as a schedule I controlled substance, effective trials to study THC concentrations in breastmilk have historically been severely limited. More recent trials are measuring the transmission of THC in mother's milk, and some have even detected the cannabidiol found in CBD oils purportedly not containing anything transmissible. Even if the transmission levels are studied and documented, how will safety be assured? Marijuana, whether medical or recreational, has not been subjected to Food and Drug Administration (FDA) efficacy testing and approval with safety monitoring. It is also not subject to stringent prescribing guidelines, with some states only permitting usage recommendations, and supply chain safety of other currently scheduled drugs [12]. And let us not forget the cannabidiol (CBD) being marketed as safe for all because it contains no THC, or does it? Without regulation, consumers may be exposing themselves and their children to levels that may be "acceptable" to the industry but far from zero.

Developmental Impact for the Newborn Period and beyond

Understanding the delicacies associated with fetal neuronal development, although the evidence is lacking, does not rely solely upon hard data. There are known psychoactive effects on the adult, fully formed neurons through THC exposure (Fig. 16.3). With data demonstrating that THC does cross the placenta, even more damage is likely being done to the neurons still forming, whether inside or outside the womb. The fetal brain, which begins as the tip of the 3 mm neuronal tube, forms approximately 15 million cells per hour during the first 12–14 weeks of gestation and continues throughout the pregnancy arriving at the more than 100 billion nerve cells present in the term newborn (Fig. 16.1). Neurons continue to proliferate until about 18 months of age [10].

Outside the womb, babies are further exposed through breastmilk if mothers continue to use marijuana following delivery. Historically data was limited and antiquated with relatively little information on THC concentrations available. But, more is emerging that demonstrates THC is passed into the milk of mothers who use marijuana [13, 14]. Δ^9 tetrahydrocannabinol, not metabolites, are found in varying concentrations in maternal milk. Levels found vary based on the amount and route of consumption as well as timing of sample collection. Keeping in mind the lipophilic nature of THC, it can be found in maternal milk for several weeks after last use if the mother is a chronic user. To a lesser extent, cannabidiol (CBD) has also been found in detectable levels in maternal milk [15].

The emergence of epigenetics has presented us with an even more detailed examination of the physiologic properties associated with development,

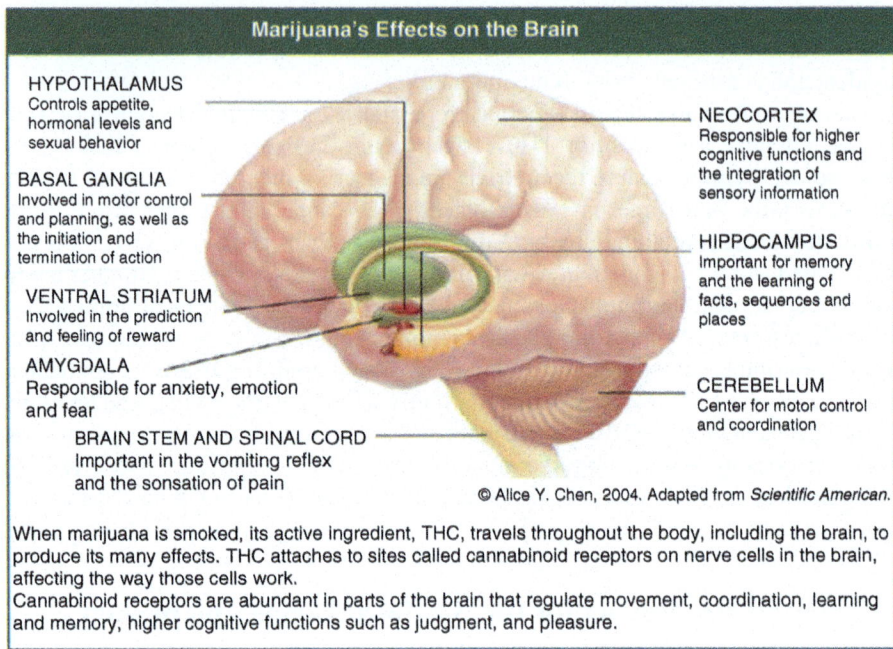

Marijuana's Effects on the Brain

HYPOTHALAMUS
Controls appetite,
hormonal levels and
sexual behavior

BASAL GANGLIA
Involved in motor control
and planning, as well as
the initiation and
termination of action

VENTRAL STRIATUM
Involved in the prediction
and feeling of reward

AMYGDALA
Responsible for anxiety, emotion
and fear

BRAIN STEM AND SPINAL CORD
Important in the vomiting reflex
and the sonsation of pain

NEOCORTEX
Responsible for higher
cognitive functions and
the integration of
sensory information

HIPPOCAMPUS
Important for memory
and the learning of
facts, sequences and
places

CEREBELLUM
Center for motor control
and coordination

© Alice Y. Chen, 2004. Adapted from *Scientific American.*

When marijuana is smoked, its active ingredient, THC, travels throughout the body, including the brain, to produce its many effects. THC attaches to sites called cannabinoid receptors on nerve cells in the brain, affecting the way those cells work.
Cannabinoid receptors are abundant in parts of the brain that regulate movement, coordination, learning and memory, higher cognitive functions such as judgment, and pleasure.

Fig. 16.3 Marijuana's effects on the brain. (Reproduced with permission. Source: National Institute on Drug Abuse www.drugabuse.gov)

specifically the hypothalamic-pituitary-adrenal (HPA) axis. Many studies have been published and reviewed to present the data alluding to the connections between various exposures during the perinatal and neonatal periods and the impact they have on later life. Montenegro et al. discussed the importance of understanding this relationship in their 2019 systematic review of the literature. They discussed Roseboom's 2001 landmark work that detailed the observations of mortality in adults who had been exposed to the Amsterdam famine in the mid-1940s during their fetal period [16]. Whether DNA methylation, noncoding RNAs, or histone modifications, the associations with disease many years after exposure are continuing to emerge [3].

The exact mechanisms for this development are very complicated, involving both genetic and environmental factors, and its study continues to evolve [17]. Improving upon the epidemiological theories from the 1950s with the fetus being characterized the fetus as a "perfect parasite," Dr. David Barker theorized that in utero programming was the major contributor leading to future disease issues in his fetal origins hypothesis. Although birthweight was found to be the most commonly available and easily compared measure of fetal well-being, it was found not to be as entirely sensitive as initially proposed [18]. Developmental experts have further added environmental exposures to the list of factors impacting later life [7, 8, 9]. Interestingly, it has been concluded, the most vulnerable period for this remodeling is in the first 3 months of development. A period correlating directly with either the time before pregnancy awareness or the time when women are most vulnerable to seeking marijuana as an alternative to combat the effects of nausea and vomiting associated with the first trimester of pregnancy [12].

Numerous studies coinciding with the medical and recreational legalization of marijuana have examined the still-developing adolescent brain. The National Institutes of Health is currently following approximately 10,000 children ages 9–10 into adulthood to facilitate understanding the many factors that can disrupt development with the ABCD study [19]. In October 2019, Frau et al. published data linking prenatal cannabis exposure in rat dams to long-term synaptic plasticity changes in dopaminergic neurons in male, but not female, offspring. These changes were displayed as altered balance in excitatory and inhibitory neuronal stimulation which led to amplified preadolescent THC exposure sensitivity [20]. Duke University scientists also found a sex-based difference in DNA methylation in human brain tissues with males having more alteration and exhibiting more neurobehavioral symptoms through the gene's known link to autism [21]. Their study examined hypomethylation in the sperm of THC exposed male rats which was also detected in the forebrains of the offspring. By studying various aspects of pharmacokinetics, structural and psychological impacts, and global function, they all reach similar conclusions—marijuana affects brain cells. Even the adult studies examining cortical thinning, owing to continued pruning, are demonstrating the impact the drug has on existing, fully-developed neurons [4].

Impact of Legalization on Use in Pregnancy

As the legalization of both medical and recreational marijuana use has moved across the country, the medical community is dealing with the far-reaching implications. In the state of Colorado, for example, where marijuana was legalized for medical use in 2001 and recreational use in 2014, marijuana usage among pregnant women has risen dramatically [22]. Additionally, the potency of available products has also risen in recent years, further raising the concerns for exposure to the developing fetus and neonate. In the 1970s, the THC potency available in most marijuana was around 2%. With advanced cloning techniques, the concentration is currently consistently found at 20–25% [23]. The rise of edibles and vaping has introduced entirely new compounds and concentrates, known by a variety of names based upon the extraction techniques used. Processing concentrates, known as budder, kief, or shatter/scatter, can have concentrations of 40–80% THC, with some even approaching 100%. Users are "accenting" their typical smoking method with the addition of one of these concentrates, known as "topping your flower," and is only one of several ways to markedly increase the THC concentrations they are consuming. If the user is a pregnant or breastfeeding woman, their child is also exposed to much more THC. As states begin to legalize both medical and recreational marijuana, more data will become available. Sadly, it will only be available *after* the damage has been done.

Drs. Reece and Hulse have reviewed the implications for prenatal cannabis exposure from three major cohort studies. These studies, with a notable agreement, detailed impaired brain growth, intellectual deficits, as demonstrated on school tests, as well as cardiovascular anomalies, in addition to others. The effects of cannabis exposure were suggestive of a dysfunction spectrum ranging from mild or moderate to very severe [24]. In another study, they directly linked rising autism rates to both the increasing use and concentrations of cannabinoids in the United States and Australia, citing several very large studies and data compiled by the Centers for Disease Control and Prevention [25]. By comparing data regarding cannabinoid concentrations from federal seizures and CDC data on autism rates, they were able to demonstrate a potential causality, using Hill criteria, across the United States linked directly with what they termed high-use states and legalization in those states. In high-use states like Colorado, Alaska, and Washington, rates of autism spectrum disorder (ASD) were rising faster than low-use states at rates reaching statistical significance. Although not experimental studies, which would be ethically unfeasible, these are the first to detail true teratogenic implications with marijuana exposure. Historically reports were limited to in utero growth restriction and lower birthweights as these were the only data available for comparison and noted previously. Newer information, however, is also demonstrating lower postnatal growth rates and increased morbidity [25, 26]. Even the US Food and Drug Administration (FDA) issued a statement in October 2019 strongly advising against using cannabis in any form, including CBD, while pregnant or breastfeeding [27].

Despite all the emerging, and largely very concerning information for safety and developmental impacts, Colorado lawmakers advanced and signed into law, on World Autism Day 2019, House Bill 1028, which adds autism to the list of approved conditions for the use of medical marijuana. Although the legislation had been proposed and passed by the assembly in two previous sessions, it had been vetoed by the previous administration, citing a lack of evidence to support its use, especially for children. To date, the FDA has only approved one form (Epidiolex—cannabidiol) to treat a rare, severe seizure disorder variant in children [27]. Providers will now be dealing with the requests from parents to use something to treat autism that may, in fact, according to the latest data, have had a hand in the creation of the condition in the first place [28, 29]. Unless the parents choose to accept the risks and give their child what they have been able to purchase for recreational use without any awareness of safe prescribing and dosing.

Discussion Points for Education and Management

As legalization continues, so does the rise of pregnant women choosing to continue their prepregnancy use or seek ways to alleviate pregnancy symptoms. In 2016, Volkow and associates reported a more than 60% rise among pregnant women from 2002 to 2014 [30]. Citing "some sources on the internet" as recommending cannabis products to combat nausea and vomiting associated with early pregnancy; the discussion about exposure and risks needs to start before women ever conceive

(Fig. 16.4). In clinical practice, if a pregnant woman reports persistent or recurrent nausea and vomiting beyond the typical first-trimester expectations, are they reporting unusual pregnancy-related symptoms, or have they crossed the threshold for cannabinoid hyperemesis syndrome and worsening their symptoms with continued use [31]? A simple Internet search produces many links to information supporting the use and how to get marijuana products, but credible sources that discourage use take a little more digging. The less-than-credible sources cite the lack of data and growing legalization as a support for their cause. The points they appear to be missing are the experiences of the past.

An illustration of this point is found in thalidomide. When first introduced as an anticonvulsant, most taking the drug noted that it made the users sleepy. This agent was marketed as a mild sleeping agent safe for pregnant women and readily prescribed as such, although none of the safety testing involved pregnant animals. In 1962, limb anomalies were linked to the use of the drug, and its use in pregnancy was deemed unsafe, too late for the thousands affected. This shift from presuming safety to proving it began a lengthy process involving clinical trials and testing that are now commonplace in medical practice [32]. The difficulty for marijuana is the schedule I classification that may impact drug study as well as the ethical feasibility of designing a trial. However, it is not only the study of cannabis itself. A Utah legislative subcommittee recently declined fund appropriation to study the prevalence of cannabis and opioid use among pregnant women, a study anticipated to assist in designing educational programs [33]. As the legalization wave continues, so, too, does the normalization of its use without understanding the dangers it may be imposing.

In their 2015 review, Drs. Metz and Stickrath sought to provide clinicians with a practical review of existing literature and recommendations for practice [34]. They discussed the variable opinions surrounding marijuana as producing little or no harm among pregnant women as a barrier to education and likely contributing to its use in pregnancy. They further detail many of the aforementioned concerns for developmental and neurobiologic alterations found in fetal brains as further support for the teratogenic effects imposed by prenatal cannabis exposure. There is also evidence that marijuana use can inhibit prolactin, essential for maternal milk production, in addition to continued exposure if the mother does not discontinue use while breastfeeding [13].

We are, then, left to determine the effects *after* children have already been affected. Fine et al. examined the complexity of early neurological development by examining the effects of maternal mental illness as an example of child risk [3]. These effects were evident not only in infancy but through to adolescence as structural brain changes, emotional and behavioral problems, as well as infant temperament, development, and cognitive functioning in later years. Because fetal/neonatal/infant development can be impacted by a host of environmental, teratogenic, and neurobiologic factors, it is difficult to isolate a sole causative source, but the data surrounding the effects of cannabis is emerging. From overall birthweight to heart defects and links to rising rates of autism, study after study is demonstrating more convincing evidence that cannabis is harming our children. Although more study is warranted to facilitate evidence-based education for families, we should be sharing what we do know.

Conclusion

Despite the difficulties with effectively studying the effects of marijuana exposure during the perinatal and neonatal periods, the available data is troubling at best. Concerns for learning, attention, focus, and even placement on the autism spectrum mentioned earlier in this chapter *must* be the focus as the medical community seeks to educate prospective and new parents. The information from outside medicine most certainly exists and can make marijuana and THC appear harmless, and even helpful, as an alternative to the standards of obstetrical and newborn care, as evidenced by the 70% of Colorado marijuana shop owners recommending its use in the first trimester of pregnancy [35], although some states are now requiring signs warning of the dangers posed by THC use during pregnancy and breastfeeding be posted. From combating first-trimester nausea to relieving the aches and pains of changing physiology and help with sleeping, marijuana is being advertised and, in some cases, being recommended as a panacea 'fix-it-all'. Data is also emerging about the occurrence of intractable vomiting and psychosis associated with marijuana presenting to emergency departments across the country, which begs the question of safety for anyone.

The challenge will continue to be battling the information available to all on the Internet. Providers will be tasked with asking specific questions, distributing information, and tracking for future study. Hospitals must begin and continue data collection to provide information to be used for further study and reporting. The US Surgeon General issued an advisory in October of 2019 which confirms the potential harm to the developing fetal and neonatal brain [36]. The CDC,

Fig. 16.4 Maternal educational exemplar from state of Washington. (https://www. knowthisaboutcannabis. org/your-health/)

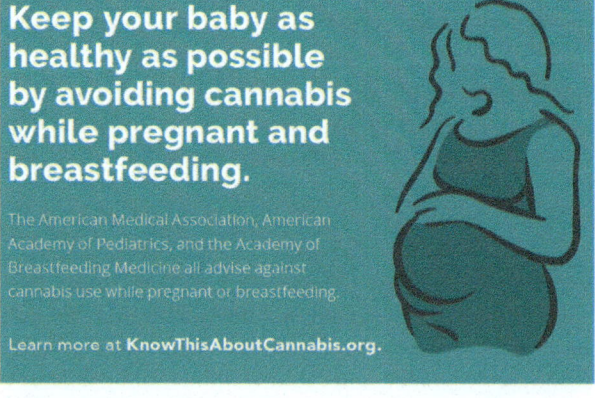

Keep your baby as healthy as possible by avoiding cannabis while pregnant and breastfeeding.

The American Medical Association, American Academy of Pediatrics, and the Academy of Breastfeeding Medicine all advise against cannabis use while pregnant or breastfeeding.

Learn more at **KnowThisAboutCannabis.org.**

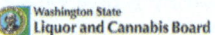

Washington State
Liquor and Cannabis Board

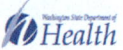

For people with disabilities, this document is available on request in other formats. To submit a request, please call 1-800-525-0127 (TDD/TTY call 711).   340-340 May 2019

AAP, and ACOG are also recognizing this as an issue (Fig. 16.4), but will it be too late for an entire generation? It is incumbent upon the medical community to educate patients by asking questions, addressing concerns, clarifying misconceptions, and continuing to seek answers through continued research and reporting and following the ACOG recommendations, using well-studied alternatives, and discouraging use not only while pregnant and breastfeeding but also before pregnancy begins.

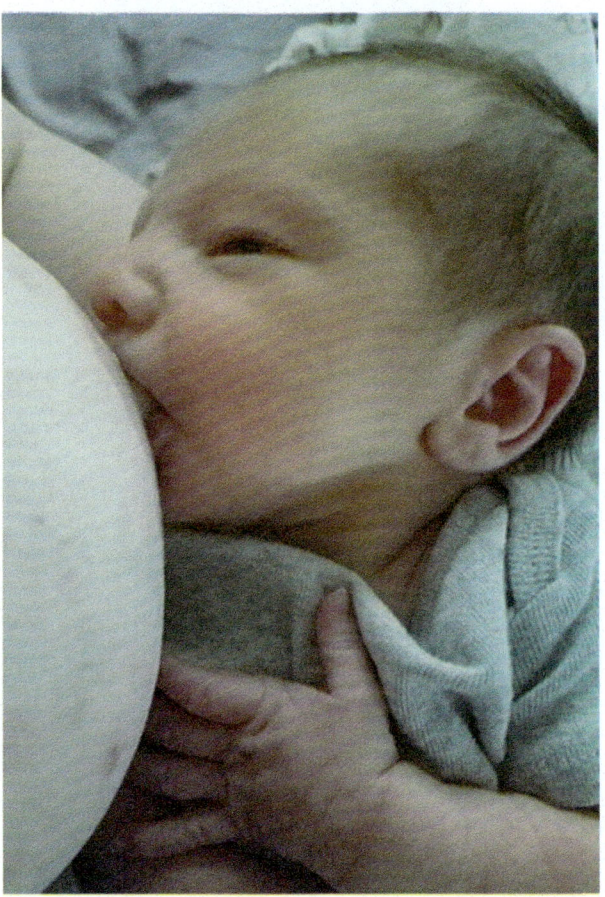

At chapter header, at **breast**

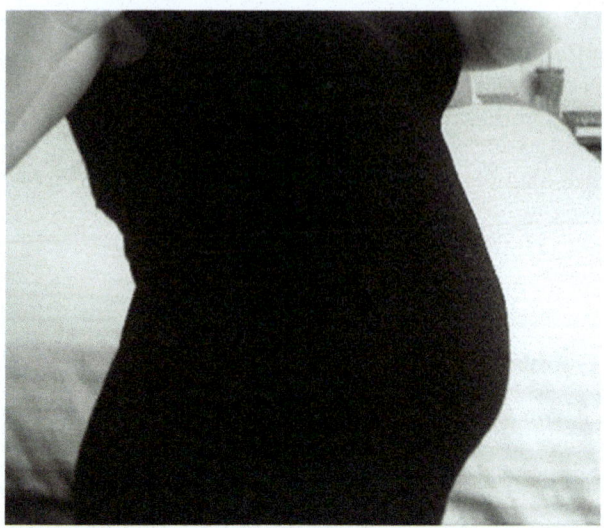

At chapter header, **30 weeks**

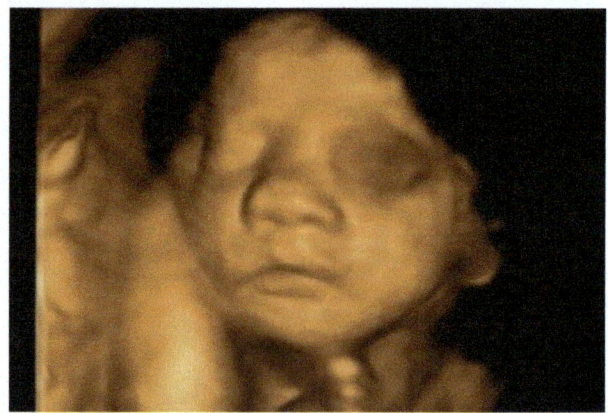

At chapter header, **4**D ultrasound **36 weeks**

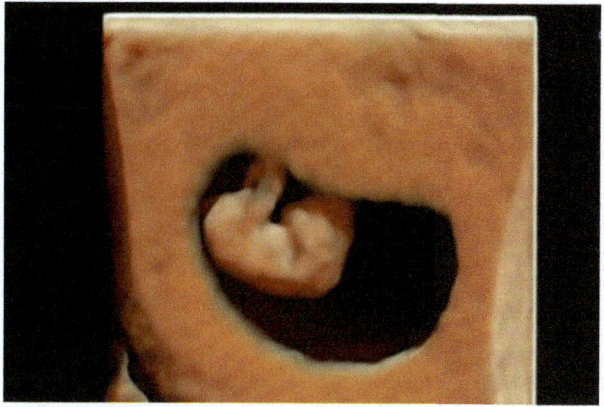

At chapter header, **4D** ultrasound **6 weeks**

References

1. Alligood M. Nursing theorists and their work. 8th ed. St. Louis: Mosby; 2014.
2. McGrath JM, Cone S, Samra HA. Neuroprotection in the preterm infant: further understanding of the short and long-term implications for brain development. Newborn Infant Nurs Rev. 2011;11(3):109–12.
3. Newman L, Judd F, Olsson CA, Castle D, Bousman C, Sheehan P, et al. Early origins of mental disorder – risk factors in the perinatal and infant period. BMC Psychiatry. 2016;16:270. https://doi.org/10.1186/s12888-016-0982-7.
4. Kolb B, Gibb R. Brain plasticity and behaviour in the developing brain. J Can Acad Child Adolesc Psychiatry. 2011;20(4):265–76.
5. Vasung L, Abaci Turk E, Ferradal SL, Sutin J, Stout JN, Ahtam B, et al. Exploring early human brain development with structural and physiological neuroimaging. NeuroImage. 2019;187:226–54.
6. Chwiej J, Palczynska M, Skoczen A, Janeczko K, Cieslak J, Simon R, et al. Elemental changes of hippocampal formation occurring during postnatal brain development. J Trace Elem Med Biol. 2018;49:1.
7. Als H, Duffy FH, McAnulty G, Butler SC, Lightbody L, Kosta S, et al. NIDCAP improves brain function and structure in preterm infants with severe intrauterine growth restriction. J Perinatol. 2012;32(10):797–803.
8. Bingham RJ. Evidence matters: research on developmental dare. Nurs Womens Health. 2012;16:45–50.
9. Haumont D. NIDCAP and developmental care. J Pediatr Neonat Individual Med. 2014;3(2):e030240. https://doi.org/10.7363/030240. Retrieved from: http://www.jpnim.com/index.php/jpnim/article/view/030240/199.
10. Ackerman S. Chapter 6: The development and shaping of the brain. In: Discovering the brain. Washington, DC: National Academies Press (US); 2006.
11. American College of Obstetricians and Gynecologists. Marijuana use during pregnancy and lactation. Committee Opinion No. 722. Obstet Gynecol. 2017;130:e205–9.
12. Klieger SB, Gutman A, Allen L, Pacula RL, Ibrahim JK, Burris S. Mapping medical marijuana: state laws regulating patients, product safety, supply chains and dispensaries. Addiction. 2016;112(12):2206–16.

13. Paramore B, Paramore BS. Marijuana and breastfeeding. Internat J Childbirth Edu. 2017;32(3):37–40.
14. Baker T, Datta P, Rewers-Felkins K, Thompson H, Kallem RR, et al. Transfer of inhaled cannabis into human breast milk. Am J Obstet Gynecol. 2018;131(5):783–8.
15. Bertrand KA, Hanan NJ, Honerkamp-Smith G, Best BM, Chambers CD. Marijuana use by breastfeeding mothers and cannabinoid concentrations in breast milk. Pediatrics. 2018;142(3):1–8.
16. Montenegro YHA, Nascimento DQ, Assis TO, Santos-Lopes SSD. The epigenetics of the hypothalamic-pituitary-adrenal axis in fetal development. Ann Hum Genet. 2019;83:195–213.
17. Kunes J, Vaneckova I, Mikulaskova B, Behuliak M, Maletinska L, Zicha J. Epigenetics and a new look on metabolic syndrome. Physiol Res. 2015;64:611–20.
18. Almond D, Currie J. Killing me softly: the fetal origins hypothesis. J Econ Perspect. 2011;25(3):153–72.
19. National Institutes of Health. Adolescent brain cognitive development study. Collab Res Addict NIH. 2019. From: https://www.addictionresearch.nih.gov/abcd-study.
20. Frau R, Miczan V, Traccis F, Aroni S, Pongor C, Saba P, et al. Prenatal THC exposure produces a hyperdopaminergic phenotype rescued by pregnenolone. Nat Neurosci. 2019. Retrieved from: https://doi.org/10.1038/s41593-019-0512-2.
21. Duke University Medical Center. Gene linked to autism undergoes changes I n men's sperm after pot use. 2019. Retrieved from: https://www.sciencedaily.com/releases/2019/08/190827123515.htm?fbclid=IwAR2-pSW5vhfg1ZTjDpt_f5hW6hdeGNoUislOR8uRkvJIKVxmmw-zJ44cPycQ.
22. Monte AA, Zane RD, Heard KJ. The implications of marijuana legalization in Colorado. JAMA. 2015;313(3):241–2.
23. Doctors for Disaster Preparedness Newsletter. Health effects of marijuana. 2019. Retrieved from: https://www.ddponline.org/2019/05/28/health-effect-of-marijuana/#more-639.
24. Reece A, Hulse G. Explaining contemporary patterns of teratology. Clin Pediatr. 2019;4(1):46.
25. Arevalo-Marcano S, Buyukgoz C, Zia M, Rajegowda B. Prevalence of maternal marijuana use and its effects on neonatal growth and breastfeeding in an urban "Babyfriendly" hospital. Neonatal Intensive Care. 2019;32(4):16–9.
26. Metz TD, Allshouse AA, Hogue CJ, Goldenberg RL, Dudley DJ, et al. Maternal marijuana use, adverse pregnancy outcomes, and neonatal morbidity. Am J Obstet Gynecol. 2017;217(4):478.
27. US Food & Drug Administration.
28. Reece A, Hulse G. Epidemiological associations of various substances and multiple cannabinoids with autism in USA. Clin Pediatr OA. 2019;4(2):155.
29. Hadland SE, Knight JR, Harris SK. Medical marijuana: review of the science and implications for developmental behavioral pediatric practice. J Dev Behav Pediatr. 2015;36(2):115–23.
30. Volkow N, Compton W, Wargo E. The risks of marijuana use during pregnancy. JAMA, published online December 19, 2016. Retrieved from: http://jamanetwork.com.
31. Chocron Y, Zuber JP, Vaucher J. Cannabinoid hyperemesis syndrome. BMJ. 2019:366:l4366 from: https://www.bmj.com/content/366/bmj.l4336.
32. Science Museum. Brought to life: exploring the history of medicine. 2019. https://broughttol-life.sciencemuseum.org.uk/broughttolife/themes/controversies/thalidomide.
33. Cortez M. Utah panel recommends no money for study to determine prevalence of maternal cannabis. 2019. https://www.deseret.com/2019/2/18/20666166/utah-panel-recommends-no-money-for-study-to-determine-prevalence-of-maternal-cannabis-use.
34. Metz T, Stickrath E. Marijuana use in pregnancy and lactation: a review of the evidence. Am J Obstet Gynecol. 2015;213(6):761–78.
35. Daley J. Study: dispensaries recommend marijuana to pregnant women against medical advice. CPR News, 9 May 2018. 2019. https://www.cpr.org/2018/05/09/study-dispensaries-recommend-marijuana-to-pregnant-women-against-medical-advice/.
36. Adams J. US Surgeon General's advisory: marijuana use and the developing brain. Office of the Surgeon General. 2019. https://www.hhs.gov/surgeongeneral/reports-and-publications/addiction-and-substance-misuse/advisory-on-marijuana-use-and-developing-brain/index.html.

Chapter 17
Cannabinoids in Gastrointestinal Disorders

Michelle Kem Su Hor, Monica Dzwonkowski, Tesia Kolodziejczyk, Lorne Muir, Nazar Dubchak, Sabina Hochroth, Bhaktasharan Patel, Aaron Wu, Sean Knight, Garrett Smith, Uday Patel, Quentin Remley, and Cicily Hummer

Investigation of Cannabinoid Hyperemesis Syndrome: Pathophysiology, Treatment, and Burden

Monica Dzwonkowski, Michelle Kem Su Hor, Tesia Kolodziejczyk, and Lorne Muir

First reported in 2004, cannabis hyperemesis syndrome (CHS) is a condition that is characterized by repeated bouts of severe vomiting in the setting of chronic, daily cannabis use. It is frequently associated with compulsive hot baths or showers in an attempt to control symptoms. Patients with CHS visit various healthcare settings with complaints of intractable nausea and vomiting, though these patients often go misdiagnosed or have delayed diagnosis in many instances. CHS is under-recognized and unsuspected due to the paradox that cannabis is utilized to control or prevent nausea and vomiting in some patients, and also the fact that cannabis remains federally illegal in the United States, which leads to underreporting or dishonesty about use. Patients

M. K. S. Hor
Springs Gastroenterology, PLLC Colorado Springs, CO, USA

Rocky Vista University, Parker, CO, USA

M. Dzwonkowski (✉) · T. Kolodziejczyk · L. Muir · N. Dubchak · S. Hochroth · A. Wu
S. Knight · G. Smith · U. Patel · Q. Remley · C. Hummer
Rocky Vista University, Parker, CO, USA
e-mail: monica.dzwonkowski@rvu.edu; Tesia.kolodziejczyk@rvu.edu; Lorne.muir@rvu.edu;
Nazar.dubchak@rvu.edu; Sabina.hochroth@rvu.edu; aaron.wu@rvu.edu;
sean.knight@rvu.edu; garrett.smith@rvu.edu; uday.patel@rvu.edu;
quentin.remley@rvu.edu; cicily.hummer@rvu.edu

B. Patel
Peak Gastroenterology Associates, Colorado Springs, CO, USA
bpatel@peakgastro.com

© Springer Nature Switzerland AG 2020
K. Finn (ed.), *Cannabis in Medicine*,
https://doi.org/10.1007/978-3-030-45968-0_17

often undergo various expensive medical tests and workups. In an observational study of CHS patients followed over two years, the median charge for emergency visits and hospital admissions for CHS was $95,023 [1]. Another study analyzed the costs for 17 patients diagnosed with CHS. The total cost for combined emergency department visits and radiological studies averaged out to over $76,000 per patient. On average, these patients had almost 18 emergency room visits before the diagnosis was made. Patients were exposed to an average of 5.94 X-rays, 4.94 CT scans, and 2.41 ultrasounds. Among the 17 patients, there were 48 total hospital admissions, an appendectomy and two cholecystectomies, 8 colonoscopies, and 17 esophagoduodenoscopies (EGDs) [2]. A retrospective observational study of patients seen in a Colorado hospital emergency department conducted from 2009 to 2014 looked at patients with cannabis-related diagnoses and positive urine drug analyses (matched with hospital billing records). During the study period, the authors found that the hospital incurred a loss of twenty million dollars in uncollected charges [3]. Thus, cannabis use and CHS present a significant financial burden in addition to a physical one.

Dr. Andrew Monte, an associate professor of Emergency Medicine, and his research team at the University of Colorado School of Medicine led a large study published in the *Annals of Internal Medicine* in March 2019 which analyzed emergency visits related to cannabis use between January 2012 and December 2016. Their findings showed that according to billing codes, 9973 emergency department visits were tied to patients who were smoking or ingesting marijuana. Emergency physicians determined that over 25% of these patients were dealing with symptoms related, at least partially, to their marijuana use. In addition, researchers found a threefold increase in marijuana-related emergency department visits between 2012 and 2016. Patients often suffered from nausea and vomiting, but also reported psychiatric symptoms such as psychosis and hallucinations. Other common symptoms reported included acute anxiety, panic attacks, and tachycardia, with heart rates increased from 20 to 50 beats/min. Marijuana users that sought help were generally young males. Women who sought treatment, however, compromised more of the users who used edibles and many came from outside of Colorado, suggesting that they were not regular users. Visits attributable to inhaled cannabis were more likely to be for CHS or CHS-like symptoms (18.0% versus 8.4%), while visits attributable to edible cannabis were more likely to be due to acute psychiatric symptoms (18.0% versus 10.9%), intoxication (48% versus 28%), and cardiovascular symptoms (8.0% versus 3.1%). When controlled for product sales statewide, visits due to the use of edibles were 33 times higher than expected, though overall, more users sought help after smoking marijuana, and only about 10% of emergency visits were linked to edibles. Sales of edibles represent a much smaller share of Colorado's marijuana sales; therefore, a disproportionate number of patients using edibles seemed to suffer toxic side effects and reported more long-lasting effects than smokers and vapers [4].

Deaths tied to cannabis consumption are difficult to quantify and may go unrecognized, but have been reported, particularly with vaping and edibles. One man killed his wife while intoxicated on cannabis edibles. Another man jumped to his death from a balcony after consuming cannabis cookies. A third person who ate marijuana edibles committed suicide [3]. Deaths related to vaping have been discussed in the GERD portion of this chapter. Deaths related to CHS have also been reported. The first was a 27-year-old female who had an 8-year history of nausea and vomiting in the setting of chronic marijuana use, with negative laboratory, radiographic, and endoscopic results. Two days before her death, she was seen in the ED for an episode of severe nausea and vomiting. This supports the notion that emergency rooms and healthcare providers need to be aware of the signs and symptoms of CHS to prevent devastating consequences. Her cause of death was reported as a complication of cannabinoid hyperemesis syndrome and the manner as natural. The second death, a 27-year-old male, was found deceased at a drug rehabilitation and recovery home. He had been vomiting ten times per day for five days prior to his death, initially attributed to food poisoning. He had a history of long-term cannabis use and cyclical episodes of vomiting in the past. Interestingly, he had a period of apparent cessation of vomiting when he was initially admitted to the drug rehabilitation program. His death was determined to be related to chronic cannabis use and reported as natural. A third case reports a 31-year-old male with a history of seizure disorders and multiple sclerosis diagnosed 6 years before his death (but neurologically stable prior to his death), with a history of chronic vomiting and nausea of unknown etiology. He had a long-standing history of cannabis consumption since age 18. CHS was appreciated in this case but was not listed as the cause of death [5].

Other deaths related to cannabis use include metabolic disturbances, motor vehicle accidents related to marijuana use, and increased risk of myocardial dysfunction and worse outcomes with myocardial infarction related to marijuana use. One study in 2001 conducted by Mittleman et al. interviewed 3882 patients with acute MI about the use of marijuana. The authors found that the risk for developing acute MI was 4.8 times higher than average in the hour immediately after marijuana use [6]. A study by Mukamal et al. found a 4.2-fold increased risk of mortality in hospitalized MI patients who reported marijuana use more than once per week before the onset of MI compared with nonusers [7]. More data on the cardiac effects of marijuana are discussed in the cardiac portion of this book.

The fraction of fatal accidents in which at least one driver tested positive for marijuana (THC) has increased nationwide from 2013 to 2016 by an average of 10% [8]. Identifying a causal effect for these accidents is difficult due to the presence of various confounding variables. Studies report increasing fatalities related to the legalization of marijuana; however, one study by Hansen et al. used a synthetic control group approach which showed that control groups had similar increases in marijuana-related fatalities despite not having legalized recreational marijuana. This study was generated using data from the Fatal Analysis and Reporting System from 2000 to 2016. This does not suggest that marijuana-related motor vehicle fatalities have not increased, but rather there may not be a correlation between the legalization of marijuana and the increase in drivers who are abusing marijuana, and that causal effect is hard to determine [8]. Nevertheless, the increase in marijuana-related motor vehicle fatalities is significant in a world where cannabis use is becoming more commonplace, and enhances the point that cannabis-related deaths are difficult to quantify and likely underreported.

The epidemiology of CHS has also been examined. A study conducted by Bollom et al. collected data from the National Emergency Department Sample (NEDS) records that included primary diagnosis codes for vomiting in combination with cannabis use or dependence observed in emergency departments between 2006 and 2013. This data was collected from over 25 million visits in almost 1000 emergency departments and was weighted to provide national estimates. Men between the ages of 20 and 29 were the most common group to present to the ED for vomiting with cannabis use disorder (CUD); yet, all age groups showed an increase in patients with these symptoms, presenting to EDs over the years. Compared to Northeast and Southern regions of the United States, the Midwest and West had higher rates of ED visits for vomiting with CUD. The greatest increase between 2006 and 2013 was in the West, with 22.8 out of 100,000 ED visits comprising of patients with vomiting and cannabis use disorder [9].

Though CHS is becoming more common as cannabis is legalized around the United States and other countries, the pathophysiological mechanism behind CHS is still unknown. Various hypotheses have been proposed to explain the pathophysiology, though data is lacking and none show high quality of evidence to support their theories.

It is unknown why cannabis appears to suppress nausea and vomiting in some patient populations, while inducing it in others. One theory is that CHS is caused by dysregulation of the endocannabinoid system, composed of CB1 and CB2 receptors, their substrates, and the enzymes responsible for their degradation. There is limited evidence that emetogenic and antiemetic properties of THC and its analogs are mediated through CB1 receptors in humans; however, this theory is supported by various animal and in vitro studies. Depending on future studies and their design, this theory may prove to be more feasible down the line. Another hypothesis was that genetic variation in metabolic enzymes accounts for the appearance of CHS. This theory may explain why not all chronic cannabis users develop CHS, though evidence was again lacking. Animal studies showed some evidence that cannabinoids interact with CB1 receptors throughout the GI tract and alter GI motility, including slowing of gastric emptying which could lead to nausea and vomiting; however, the results were not consistently reproducible in human studies [1]. In summary, the pathophysiology of CHS remains unknown, and further research studying the exact mechanism of the condition is needed to better understand why some chronic users suffer from it while other users are spared.

Due to CHS not being recognized until 2004, the diagnosis and treatment practices vary widely among practitioners. Seven authors have proposed various diagnostic criteria, though it remains unclear whether or not these diagnostic criteria consistently identify patients with the diagnosis. In addition, the criteria vary slightly, making it difficult for practitioners to accurately identify and diagnose the condition. One study, conducted by Sorensen et al., looked at the various diagnostic criteria proposed by the seven authors and the overlap of the criteria among them. The major diagnostic characteristics that had overlapped at least 75% of the time among the seven proposed criteria included history of regular cannabis use for >1 year, severe nausea and vomiting, vomiting that recurs in a cyclical pattern over months, resolution of symptoms after stopping cannabis, compulsive hot bath/showers with symptom relief, male predominance, abdominal pain, at least weekly cannabis use, history of daily cannabis use, and age <50 at time of evaluation. The symptoms that were inconsistent among the proposed diagnostic criteria were normal bowel habits, negative medical workup, weight loss >5 kg, and reliable return of symptoms within weeks of resuming use. After analyzing various case reports and case series utilizing the diagnostic criteria, the results of the study suggest that the characteristics with the highest sensitivity for identifying patients with CHS include the following: at least weekly cannabis use for greater than 1 year, severe nausea and vomiting that recurs in a cyclic pattern over months and is usually accompanied by abdominal pain, resolution of symptoms after stopping cannabis use, and compulsive hot baths/showers with symptom relief [1]. It is unknown whether higher potency cannabis has a higher risk of causing CHS, as most sources only report "chronic" and "regular" cannabis use. As mentioned in the IBS chapter, potency of marijuana has increased over the years, with the average potency in the United States rising from 4% to 12% between 1995 and 2014. This value is likely even higher now [10]. One study done in Europe between May 2010 and April 2015 showed that use of high-potency cannabis (>10% THC) was a strong predictor of psychotic disorder in Amsterdam, London, and Paris, where high-potency cannabis is widely available. This study compared 901 patients with first-episode psychosis with 1237 population controls from 11 different sites across Europe. The study found that daily cannabis use was associated with an increased risk of psychotic disorder compared with never users and that daily use of high-potency strains of cannabis was associated with a nearly fivefold increase odds of psychotic disorder [11]. This suggests higher potency cannabis can have more detrimental effects, but more research is warranted to determine whether high potency is a factor in developing CHS or not.

It is not completely known why hot showers seem to help patients with CHS. A case report from Bernard and Trappey in 2017 reported a 24-year-old male presenting with CHS, who noticed that running helped relieve his CHS symptoms. The mechanism behind this unique treatment is not clear, but the increased and redistributed blood flow via exercise may be an explanation. THC causes an elevated core body temperature, and the hot shower treatment employed by many afflicted is thought to increase blood flow to the skin thus allowing body heat to dissipate through the skin. Exercise also increases blood flow to the skin, and so may be another means of body temperature regulation and control of symptoms. Other studies have shown that CB1 and CB2 receptors are present on presynaptic parasympathetic ganglia resulting in increased vasodilation to the visceral organs. It is proposed that exercise helps redistribute blood flow away from the GI system toward the exercising muscle, which may also help relieve the GI-predominant symptoms of CHS [12].

Treatment for CHS is limited to symptomatic control and abstinence from cannabis use, though many studies displaying evidence toward the latter have very small sample sizes. Wallace et al. reported that among the 25 patients with CHS who abstained, 24 had complete symptom resolution. Three other studies, conducted by Allen et al. ($n = 7$), Simonetto et al. ($n = 6$), Patterson et al. ($n = 4$), reported symptom resolution in 100% of patients; however, sample sizes were dismal. Sorenson et al. reported that out of a cumulative synthesis of 85 patients, 64 of which had abstained, and 21 who did not, 62 patients had complete resolution of symptoms. The 21 patients who did not abstain all had ongoing symptoms. Though this sample size is still small, it could motivate further research to provide insight on whether or not abstaining from cannabis will completely resolve symptoms of CHS [1].

An expert consensus panel made up of The San Diego Emergency Medicine Oversight Commission, County of San Diego Health and Human Services Agency, and the San Diego Kaiser Permanente Division of Medical Toxicology published guidelines in 2017 to help ED physicians in the treatment of CHS. The primary treatment of CHS is cannabis cessation and patients should be educated on the importance of abstinence from cannabis. Supportive care can be offered in the ED and consists of fluid and electrolyte replacement PRN, as well as traditional anti-emetics such as diphenhydramine 25–50 mg IV, ondansetron 4–8 mg IV, and meto-clopramide 10 mg IV. Some case reports indicate that haloperidol 5 mg or olanzapine 5 mg may also be beneficial in symptom management. Use of benzodiazepines have mixed results, and opioids should be avoided as they are not effective and can lead to opioid dependence as well as nausea. Patients can also be educated on the use of hot showers for symptom relief, or in lieu of showering, topical capsaicin can be applied three times daily to the abdomen or posterior surface of arms [13].

Research evaluating the role of supportive care and symptomatic control in CHS patients is small, but beneficial. Patients may present with acute renal injury and severe dehydration secondary to ongoing cyclical vomiting and high-temperature baths or showers, and as such may require aggressive fluid resuscitation. The use of dopamine antagonists, such as haloperidol, and antiemetics, such as aprepitant, has been shown to be useful in managing CHS symptoms; however, the evidence is based out of case studies only. One study, conducted by Hickey et al., reported complete resolution of CHS-related vomiting one hour after administration of 5 mg haloperidol. According to Sorenson et al., THC has been shown to increase dopamine synthesis, turnover, reflux, and dopamine cell firing, which could explain clinical improvement with dopamine antagonist administration [1]. A recent case report from Swetha et al. in June 2019 reported a 30-year-old female presenting with CHS symptoms refractory to traditional antiemetic medications who had significant improvement after starting aprepitant (Emend). Aprepitant is an FDA-approved NK1 antagonist for the treatment of chemotherapy-induced nausea and vomiting. NK1 receptors play a role in vagal feedback promoting vomiting. The antagonism of NK1 receptors thus results in cessation of vomiting. This case report suggests that aprepitant should be further explored as a potential treatment option for CHS [14].

A case report from Phillip et al. in 2016 reported a 27-year-old male with a history of Bipolar I who presented to the emergency department for a manic episode, which was preceded by a 3-week history of daily nausea and vomiting. The patient was a chronic cannabis user, and his GI symptoms were attributed to CHS. The manic episode was thought to be caused by decreased absorption of his oral mood stabilizers related to the daily vomiting. This case report demonstrates that it is important for physicians to consider the decreased absorption of critical medications in those presenting with CHS, and further strengthens the demand for ongoing research on this condition [15].

Conclusion

Further research into the greater understanding of the endocannabinoid system in human subjects is needed to better understand the pathophysiology of CHS and thus provide appropriate therapies, in addition to protecting patients from other undesirable outcomes such as decreased medication absorption or dehydration. For over a decade, physicians have had minimal knowledge about the potential side effects of long-term cannabis use manifesting as CHS. Research expansion and education producers will facilitate greater awareness of CHS and expedite its diagnosis, therefore avoiding unnecessary cost burden, avoiding delaying of treatment, and improve physician-patient relationships. Studies are needed that include close follow-up of patients diagnosed with CHS, the method of cannabis use, the length of time of cannabis use, among other factors including genetic variables. Early referral to substance abuse services may help to reduce relapses among this difficult-to-treat group of patients, as abstinence is speculated to be the only sustaining treatment option at this time.

Investigation of the Endocannabinoid System in the Pathophysiology of Irritable Bowel Syndrome and the Potential Use of Cannabis as a Complementary and Alternative Medicine Therapy

Michelle Kem Su Hor, Monica Dzwonkowski, Lorne Muir, Tesia Kolodziejczyk, Nazar Dubchak, and Sabina Hochroth

Irritable bowel syndrome (IBS) is the most common functional gastrointestinal (GI) disorders with a global prevalence of about 11%, depending on the population investigated and the diagnostic criteria used. It affects about 15% of the US population [16]. IBS is a disorder characterized by abdominal discomfort, pain, and altered bowel habits. It is more commonly diagnosed in women than men and in people younger than 50 years. There is no gold standard for diagnosing IBS, and standard clinical investigations such as endoscopy and biochemical studies produce unremarkable results for IBS patients. The most recent Rome IV criteria for the diagnosis of IBS requires that patients have had recurrent abdominal pain on average of at least one day per week in the past three months that is associated with two or more of the following: pain related to defecation (increased or unchanged by defecation), change in stool frequency, or change in stool form or appearance [17]. Another diagnostic model is the Manning Criteria, which focuses on pain relief after the passage of stool, incomplete bowel movements, mucus in the stool, and changes in stool consistency. According to the Manning Criteria, the more symptoms you have, the greater the likelihood of IBS. Symptom patterns of IBS can be divided into four main subtypes: diarrhea predominant (IBS-D), constipation predominant (IBS-C), mixed pattern (IBS-M), or unclassified (IBS-U) [18].

The pathophysiology of IBS is complex and not completely understood but it appears to involve the gut microbiome; altered intestinal permeability; immune activation; autonomic, hormonal, psychological, environmental, and genetic factors; and brain-gut interactions [19]. Storr et al. showed that endocannabinoids are crucially involved in the control of motility, secretion, inflammation, visceral hypersensitivity, pain control, and microbiome, and as such may provide a potential therapeutic benefit for IBS [20].

Briefly, the endogenous endocannabinoid system is made up of "classical" cannabinoid receptors (CB1, CB2), "non-classical" receptors (TRPV1, GRP55), endocannabinoids (anandamide, AEA; 2-arachidonyloglycerol, 2-AG) that bind to cannabinoid receptors, and a group of enzymes which are responsible for cannabinoid synthesis and degradation [21]. CB1 and CB2 receptors are expressed in the human colon and colonic epithelium is biochemically and functionally responsive to cannabis [22]. CB1 and CB2 are also activated by tetrahydrocannabinol (THC), the psychoactive component of marijuana. THC and other direct CB1 agonists have been recognized to possess medicinally beneficial properties; however, these agents also produce undesirable side effects such as impaired cognition and motor control, which limits their utility as therapeutic agents. One potential approach to retaining beneficial effects of cannabinoid activation, while limiting undesirable effects of global cannabinoid activation, is to elevate endogenous endocannabinoid tone by inhibiting hydrolytic degradation [23].

Two important enzymes that are responsible for the metabolism of AEA and 2-AG are fatty acid amide hydrolase (FAAH) and monoacylglycerol lipase (MAGL). MAGL is a serine hydrolase that hydrolyzes 2-arachidonoylglycerol (2-AG), an endocannabinoid-like anandamide. FAAH is an intracellular enzyme, located in the brain, liver, and GI tract. FAAH is involved in the degradation of endocannabinoids and cannabinoid-like fatty acid amides, including palmitoylethanolamide (PEA) and oleoylethanolamide (OEA), which may bind to both, "classical" and "non-classical" cannabinoid receptors, and can also exert biological activity via non-cannabinoid pathways. FAAH inhibitors and FAAH knockout mice have displayed analgesic properties without disruptions in motility, cognition, or body temperature. These findings suggest that FAAH may represent a potential therapeutic target for treating IBS through reduction of pain and inflammation [23].

Fichna et al. conducted a pilot study in 2013 and the aim of his research team was to investigate whether IBS-defining symptoms correlate with changes in endocannabinoids or cannabinoid-like fatty acid levels in IBS patients. The researchers measured the AEA, 2-AG, OEA, and PEA plasma levels of diarrhea-predominant (IBS-D) and constipation-predominant (IBS-C) patients and compared them with healthy subjects following the establishment of correlations between biolipid contents and disease symptoms. FAAH mRNA levels were evaluated in colonic biopsies from IBS-D and IBS-C patients and matched controls. Their results showed that patients with IBS-D had higher levels of 2-AG and lower levels of OEA and PEA. In contrast, patients with IBS-C have higher levels of OEA. Multivariate analysis found that lower PEA levels are associated with cramping abdominal pain. FAAH mRNA levels were lower in patients with IBS-C. The researchers concluded that IBS subtypes and their symptoms show distinct alterations of endocannabinoid and endocannabinoid-like fatty acid levels. These changes may partially result from reduced FAAH expression. The above reported changes support the notion that the endogenous cannabinoid system (ECS) is involved in the pathophysiology of IBS and the development of IBS symptoms [21].

Another study, conducted by Cremon et al., hypothesized that an imbalance of the endocannabinoid system is partly responsible for IBS, and that endocannabinoid-like dietary compounds may improve IBS symptoms such as abdominal pain. In particular, PEA is a dietary component commonly found in egg yolks and peanuts, two foods consistently reported to exert anti-inflammatory and analgesic properties in both in vitro and in vivo. Another compound, polydatin, is derived from grapes and may act synergistically with PEA to reduce mast cell activation and local oxidative stress. Cremon et al. conducted a pilot study evaluating the efficacy and safety of dietary PEA and polydatin in patients with IBS. The primary discovery of the study was that the PEA/polydatin treatment was markedly effective in reducing the severity of abdominal pain and discomfort in IBS patients. Unselected patients with IBS had an increased infiltration and activation of mast cells in the colonic mucosa, compared with control group. The study also showed that OEA was significantly reduced in people with IBS, while the CB2 receptor was significantly increased in patients with IBS as compared with controls. This suggests an altered endocannabinoid system and endocannabinoid-like mediators in IBS [24].

Based on the above studies, IBS subtypes and their symptoms show distinct alterations of the endocannabinoid system. These changes may result from reduced FAAH expression. These studies support the notion that the endocannabinoid system is involved in the pathophysiology of IBS and the symptoms involved with the condition.

The current pharmacological treatments available for IBS focus on reducing symptom severity; unfortunately, some of these drugs also produce side effects which affect quality of life. The limited benefit from current drug therapy has led many IBS patients to seek further relief thus increase their quality of life through complementary and alternative medicines (CAM). This includes herbal and probiotic therapies, mind-body therapies such as hypnotherapy, cognitive-behavioral therapy (CBT), biofeedback therapy, muscle relaxation, stress management, acupuncture, and osteopathic manipulation treatments [25].

The cannabis plant has a long history of utilization as a fiber and seed crop in China. Use of cannabis seeds as well as other plants parts have been recorded in Chinese medical text books for nearly 2000 years, but the use of the plant could have been present for much longer [26]. From a pollen study conducted in May of 2019, cannabis pollen appeared in northwestern China 19.6 million years ago. From there, cannabis pollen dispersed to Europe (6 million years ago), then to eastern China (1.2 million years ago), and India (32.6 thousand years ago). Thus, it is likely that cannabis use, whether medically or recreationally, has been ongoing for many years [27]. Chinese surgeon, Hua Tuo, used mafeisin, an herbal anesthetic made with a mixture of hemp and wine, to help make his patients insensitive to pain [28]. In the United States, cannabis was utilized during the nineteenth and twentieth centuries, and was described in the *United States Pharmacopoeia* for the first time in 1850. In 1996, California became the first state to legalize the use of medical cannabis under physician supervision [29]. Cannabis treatment continues to be investigated as a potential CAM in the twenty-first century, and as the substance is legalized across the United States and around the world, more practitioners need to be aware of potential implications of its use.

According to the World Health Organization (WHO), marijuana/cannabis use has an annual prevalence rate of approximately 147 million people (nearly 2.5% of global population). In 2014, approximately 22.2 million Americans aged 12 years or older reported current cannabis use, and 8.4% of this population reported use within the previous month. Of note, strains used today are much more potent than those used in ancient times. One study sampled marijuana confiscated by the Drug Enforcement Administration from 1995 to 2014. Over 38,600 samples were tested. Analysis of the samples found that average THC potency has risen from 4% to 12%, and the CBD content has decreased from 0.28% to <0.15%. This shifts the ratio of THC:CBD in many strains from 14× to 80× in just 20 years [10]. Marijuana concentrates contain THC levels that could range from 40% to 80%, according to the Drug Enforcement Agency. This form of marijuana can be up to four times more potent than high-grade marijuana plants, which normally contain around 20% of THC. These products do not resemble the same products of ancient medicine 2000 years ago, yet have gained popularity among marijuana users. Concentrates are vaporized, leading to an odorless and easier to conceal method of using cannabis [30].

There are few studies that conclude cannabis therapy is effective for treating certain medical conditions. More prospective studies are needed to achieve this sort of evidence, if it exists. The National Academies of Science, Engineering, and Medicine appointed an ad hoc committee in 2017 to investigate and create a comprehensive, in-depth review of existing evidence regarding the health effects of marijuana or its constituents. The study reviewed 22 conditions. Out of these 22, only 4 had positive outcomes. These included substantial evidence for neuropathic and cancer-related pain (but not other forms of chronic pain), chemotherapy-induced nausea and vomiting, spasticity associated with multiple sclerosis, and moderate evidence that cannabinoids, particularly nabiximols, are an effective treatment to improve short-term sleep outcomes in patients with obstructive sleep apnea, fibromyalgia, neuropathic and cancer-related pain, and multiple sclerosis suffering from condition-related sleep disturbances [31]. It is important to note that nabiximols (natural, purified cannabis extracts) are not available in the United States, and that this data was also based on synthetic THC, not dispensary cannabis. More research is needed to examine the role of dispensary grade cannabis before any sort of recommendations can be made as this research is based on synthetic products or nabiximols. Cannabis products with high doses of CBD have been recommended by some neurologists to children with epilepsy to reduce seizure frequency or severity. The National Academies study concluded that there is insufficient evidence to support or refute the conclusion that cannabis is an effective treatment for epilepsy [31]. According to a July 2019 statement from the American Epilepsy Society (AES), pharmaceutical grade CBD demonstrates moderate efficacy in specific types of seizures. The AES warns against potential adverse effects of CBD, as well as the unregulated and difficult-to-control artisanal CBD which is made readily available and is highly advertised to consumers. Multiple published reports have discussed the mislabeling of cannabis-derived compounds, and many of the products tested were artisanal. These products were shown to contain different levels of THC, CBD, or other cannabis compounds than stated on the labels, and were contaminated with various microbes, herbicides, pesticides, heavy metals, and other harmful products. There is need for rescheduling of CBD and cannabis-derived compounds so that further research can be done not only in epilepsy, but for other diseases. Rescheduling these products could allow for more control over the contents of these products and give providers the reassurance that what they are recommending to their patients is controlled and accurately labeled [32].

Though cannabis is speculated to provide benefits to some patients, it also can cause undesirable side effects. Short-term side effects include diminished motor skills, decreased reaction time, fatigue, anxiety, increased heart rate, decreased blood pressure, dry mouth, among others. Long-term side effects include depression, anxiety, and dependence. Abrupt cessation may cause withdrawal. Symptoms of withdrawal can include insomnia, anxiety, depression, appetite changes, abdominal pain, headache, tremor, and restlessness. Patients and providers should be aware of any potential side effects when using or prescribing cannabis, whether it be for medical or recreational purposes [33]. Cannabis use disorder is now a recognized ICD-10 code, with available billable codes including cannabis dependence with psychotic disorder, cannabis dependence with withdrawal, and cannabis dependence with other cannabis-induced disorder, among quite a few others [34]. The route of intake is also an important component to consider in terms of long-term health complications. Smoking or vaping can cause damage to lungs, chronic cough, bronchitis, or other lung infections. In certain patient populations, long-term cannabis use can cause a disorder called cannabinoid hyperemesis syndrome, which will be discussed in another portion of this chapter. This syndrome leads to uncontrollable nausea and vomiting. Certain populations of patients, such as pregnant women, should avoid cannabis use altogether as there is a lack of research on how cannabis affects a developing fetus [33].

Adejumo A. et al.'s poster presentation at the World Congress of Gastroenterology at ACG 2017 discussed the association between long-term cannabis use and the endogenous cannabinoid system (ECS). The researchers analyzed 4,709,043 patients from a 2014 National Inpatient Survey. They found 0.03% had a primary admission for IBS and 1.32% for cannabis use disorder (CUD). CUD was correlated with an increased risk for IBS. The risk increased for men was higher compared with women and among Caucasians compared with African-Americans. Following propensity matched analysis, the researchers found that CUD was correlated with an 80% increased risk for IBS [35].

A randomized pharmacodynamic and pharmacogenetic trial, conducted in November of 2011 by Wong BS et al., analyzed the effects of dronabinol (DRO), a nonselective cannabinoid receptor agonist, on colon transit in IBS-D patients. The researchers randomly assigned 36 adult patients (34 females, 2 males) to receive two different doses of DRO or placebo for two days' duration. Results of the study showed that DRO did not significantly affect colonic transit; however, a second study conducted in 2012 by the same researchers, Wong et al., found that DRO may inhibit colonic transit in a subset of IBS-D patients who have a genetic variation in CB1 receptors. The researchers proposed that a selective CB1 agonist may have potential as a therapy in IBS-D-predominant patients [36]. More research is warranted on whether medications such as dronabinol would be more favorable over dispensary cannabis.

Another study, by Klooker et al., tested the effects of DRO (up to 10 mg) on visceral perception of rectal distension in ten IBS patients versus twelve healthy controls. This study showed that DRO did not affect baseline rectal perception to distension compared to placebo in either group [37].

The above small trials found no effect on the two low doses of dronabinol on gastrointestinal transit. The quality of evidence for the finding of no effect for IBS is insufficient based on the short treatment duration, small sample size ($n = 36$), disproportionate gender representation, short-term follow-up, and lack of patient-reported outcomes. In addition, there is the conclusion from the National Academy of Sciences which reported insufficient evidence to support or refute the conclusion that cannabis is an effective treatment for the symptoms of IBS.

Conclusion

IBS is the most common GI disorders encountered worldwide. There is no test to definitively diagnose IBS, it is thought to be a diagnosis of exclusion. The pathophysiology of IBS is not completely understood, but it appears to involve, in part, the endocannabinoid system, in addition to psychosocial, environmental, and genetic factors, and brain-gut interactions. Current treatment strategies for IBS focus on symptom reduction using various medications and dietary modifications, though the therapies often are accompanied by undesirable side effects. As a result, many IBS patients remain undertreated or dissatisfied with their quality of life and seek alternative and complementary therapies, such as cannabis. The endocannabinoid system has been shown to be involved in altering gut motility, and is speculated to be involved in the pathophysiology of IBS. Unfortunately, a few studies have been conducted on exploring cannabis use as a potential treatment for IBS, and those that have been conducted have small sample sizes and investigated dronabinol, an oral cannabis agent. More research is required to appropriately analyze whether or not cannabis is useful in treating symptoms of IBS. These studies should focus on various routes of administration, doses, type of cannabinoid (CBD, THC, etc.), and have larger sample sizes. A regulated, purified product would be more favorable over an artisanal one to limit contamination, mislabeling, and potential dangerous adverse effects from taking an unregulated substance.

Inflammatory Bowel Disease and Cannabis

Michelle Kem Su Hor, Bhaktasharan Patel, Monica Dzwonkowski, Aaron Wu, Sean Knight, Garrett Smith, and Uday Patel

Epidemiology Ulcerative colitis (UC) and Crohn's disease (CD) are diseases characterized by chronic inflammation of the gastrointestinal tract and are collectively known as inflammatory bowel disease (IBD). According to the CDC, in 2015, the estimated prevalence of adults reporting a diagnosis of IBD in the United States was about 3 million (1.3%). Those more likely to report a diagnosis of IBD were adults aged 45 years or older, Hispanic or non-Hispanic whites, unemployed, less than high school level of education, born in the United States, living in poverty, and those living in suburban areas. This data is based on the National Health Interview Survey (NHIS). The NHIS is a household survey that provides estimates which are nationally representative on a broad range of health measures for civilian, noninstitutionalized populations. These data are limited by various factors, including recall bias, exclusion of active-duty military and incarcerated persons, exclusion of residents of long-term care facilities, and about a 50% response rate for the 2015 NHIS. All of these factors can lead to an underestimation of the true prevalence of IBD in the United States [38].

A study published in *Gastroenterology* in April 2019 reported estimates of the prevalence of IBD in Canada. Using population-based data from 7 provinces, which make up around 95% of Canada's total population, the estimated prevalence of IBD in 2008 was 0.5%. By 2018, the authors estimated the prevalence increased to 0.7% and by 2030, the authors estimate it will increase to 1.0%. The authors state they estimate approximately 270,000 Canadians are currently living with IBD [39].

Another study, published in 2011 in *Gastroenterology* reports that the highest incidences of IBD have been reported in northern Europe, the United Kingdom and North America. IBD has been emerging in countries that had previously had rare cases reported, including South Korea, China, India, Iran, Lebanon, Thailand, the French West Indies, Japan, and North Africa. More research is needed to estimate the prevalence worldwide, though the consensus is that the prevalence has been increasing globally over the years [40].

There Are Three Important Pathophysiological Factors Involved in Inflammatory Bowel Disease: Microbes, Genetics, and Immune Dysregulation

Microbes

Host-microbial interactions are critical for pathogenesis of inflammatory bowel disease. Every individual has unique microbial flora. Microbial alteration from a variety of mechanisms (diet, parasites, antibiotics exposure) modulates inflammatory outcomes and increase the prevalence of IBD. Dysregulated T-cell responses have been noted due to alteration in density and diversity of bacteria. Certain probiotics have been associated with improvement of inflammation by inducing Treg cells and modulating growth factors. Many of the genes associated with IBD overlap with genes involved in responses to mycobacterium, i.e., tuberculosis and Leprae. This overlaps with the histopathology [41].

Genetics

The risk of IBD is increased with affected family members. For Crohn's disease, the concordance rate for monozygotic twins is 50%, and for ulcerative colitis, the concordance rate is 15%. There are 160 IBD-associated genes shared between Crohn's disease and ulcerative colitis. NOD2 (Nucleotide Oligomerization bing Domain 2) encodes intracellular protein that binds bacterial peptidoglycan which activates NF-Kb (inflammatory pathway). Less than 10% of patients who have a NOD 2 variant (mutation) develop Crohn's at an earlier age and have worse outcomes after ileoanal anastomosis in ulcerative colitis. Presence of NOD 2 variant confers susceptibility. Other genes of interest are ATG16L1 (Autophagy related 16 like) and IRGM (immunity-related GTPase M) [41].

Inflammatory Bowel Disease

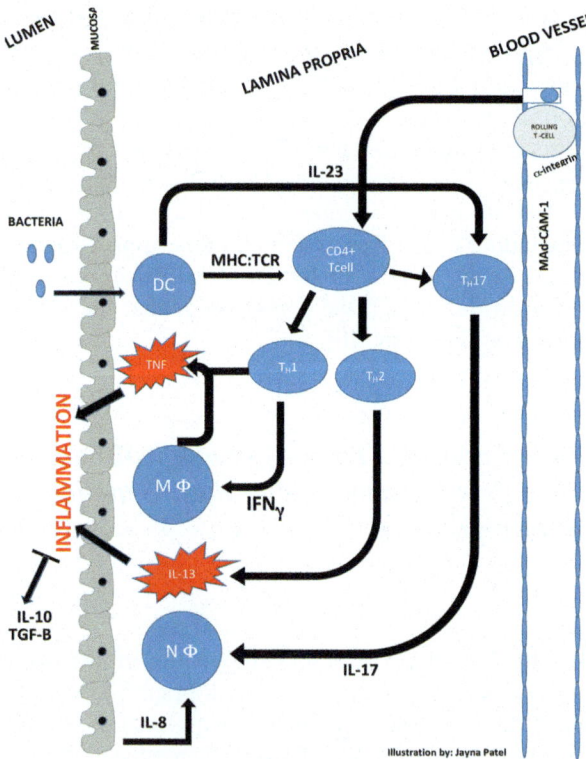

DC dendritic cell (antigen-presenting cell); *Mφ* activated macrophage; *Nφ* neutrophil; *MHC* major histocompatibility complex; *TCR* T-cell receptor; *TNF* tumor necrosis factor; *IFNγ* interferon gamma; *TGFβ* transforming growth factor beta

Inflammation in the gut mucosa begins with the recognition of foreign antigen by antigen-presenting cell (APC), the dendritic cells. Dendritic cells propagate the cycle of inflammation via activating CD4 T helper cell differentiation. Dendritic cells directly bind CD4 T cell through MHC-TCR. Dendritic cells also release IL23 to influence TH17 differentiation. Mutations in IL 23 receptors have been linked to susceptibility for IBD. TH17 recruits neutrophils to the area of inflammation via release of IL17. Clinical trials show IL17 blockage do not help in preventing inflammation [41, 42, 57].

CD4 cells can also differentiate into TH1, which also mediates inflammation via IFN-gamma 1, activating macrohages which release TNF, a direct mediator of inflammation. TH1 can also directly release TNF. TH1 is additionally influenced by IL12, released by APC (i.e., dendritic cells). TH2 is differentiated from CD4 T-cells by IL4. Differentiated CD4 releases IL13, which is another direct mediator of inflammation. Modulation of inflammation is mediated by IL10 released by TR1 cell and TGF B released by TH3 cells. Mutation of IL10 receptors is linked to severe and early onset of IBD.

Inflammation of the gut mucosa is mainly mediated by TNF and IL13 produced by TH1 and TH2 cells, respectively. TMF can also be influenced by activated macrophages which are mediators of INF (gamma) which is released by TH1 helper T cell.

CD4 T cell is dependent upon integrin and adhesion molecules such as alpha 4-beta 7 and MAdCAM 1. These adhesion molecules mediate leukocyte migration through blood vessel endothelium into lamina propria.

Th17 cells are derivatives of T helper cells and have a critical role in regulating the process of inflammation and interaction at mucosal surfaces and play an important role in autoimmunity [41].

The current conventional therapies for the management of IBD are aimed at induction of remission of the disease mainly through suppression of the immune system. This treatment strategy involves the use of corticosteroids, aminosalicylates, antibiotics, immunomodulators, and biologics. Unfortunately, chronic pharmacologic treatments produce unwanted adverse side effects, which in turn, affect the quality of life of IBD patients. Adverse effects from long-term steroid use include Cushing's syndrome, diabetes, osteoporosis, bruising, acne, and adrenal suppression, among others. A slightly increased risk of lymphoma has been reported with the use of 6-mercaptopurine, an immunomodulator. An immunosuppressive agent, methotrexate, has been shown to induce liver fibrosis and cirrhosis. Biologics pose the risk of activating latent tuberculosis or hepatitis, and screening for these diseases prior to initiation of therapy is imperative [43]. Sulfasalazine, an aminosalicylate agent, commonly causes adverse reactions in up to 30% of patients, including gastrointestinal, central nervous system, cutaneous, and hematologic reactions. These adverse reactions are either immune/hypersensitivity related or dose related [44].

In addition to medications, IBD patients who are refractory to medical therapies often resort to more aggressive therapies, such as surgery with resection of the diseased bowel [45]. IBD patients may be dissatisfied with the conventional therapies due to their limited options and unwanted adverse side effects. Patients are focusing on complementary and alternative medicine (CAM) for the management of their IBD symptoms, including abdominal pain, cramps, bloating, diarrhea, decreased appetite, weight loss, and extraintestinal symptoms such as joint pain, depression, and anxiety. The media – as well as more relaxed marijuana laws – in the United States have paved the way for IBD patients to seek cannabis for symptomatic control of their symptoms. Many IBD patients are now leaning toward cannabis for reduction of their symptoms, in hopes of improving their quality of life. Lin et al. reported a study by Storr et al. that up to 17.6% of patients with IBD report prior or current use of cannabis for their symptoms, with 84% of these users reporting improvement in abdominal pain. Between 10 and 15% of patients with IBD reported active use for relief of nausea, abdominal pain, and diarrhea. Those patients with active use had a more active disease process and a history of prior abdominal surgeries, and also use chronic pain medications in addition to other CAM therapies [46]. The reported study was based on a Canadian study by Storr et al. which demonstrated improvements in the quality of life as well as a reduction in Harvey-Bradshaw Indices [47]. The Harvey-Bradshaw Index has five parameters that include previous day well-being, previous day abdominal pain, previous day number of liquid, abdominal mass, and complications (e.g., arthralgia, uveitis, erythema nodosum, aphthous ulcer, pyoderma gangrenosum, anal fissures, appearance of a new fistula, and/or abscess) [48]. Cigarette smoking has been shown to be a strong predictor for surgery in patients with Crohn's disease. The same study conducted by Storr et al. from 2008 to 2009 observed a similar effect with cannabis use. The authors administered an anonymous questionnaire to 313 consecutive IBD patients seen at the University of Calgary. The questionnaire asked about the motives, pattern of use, and subjective beneficial and adverse effects of cannabis. Cannabis users versus nonusers were compared to identify variables predictive of poor IBD outcomes, specifically hospitalization or surgery. The authors found that the use of cannabis for more than 6 months at any time for IBD symptoms was a strong predictor of surgical need in Crohn's disease patients, after correcting for other variables such as tobacco smoking, time since diagnosis, and biologic use. Cannabis was not shown to predict hospitalization rates in IBD patients [46, 47]. The healthcare industry, especially physicians, can no longer ignore cannabis as an alternative treatment for IBD patients, though careful consideration is needed in terms of implementing cannabis as a potential therapy.

Several other population studies have reinforced the use of cannabis for symptom relief by IBD patients, which were mentioned in a large review conducted by Ahmed and Katz, published in 2016. Garcia-Planella et al. conducted a survey in 2007 of 214 IBD patients in Spain and found that nearly 10% of patients actively used cannabis or its derivatives [49]. Lal et al. (2011) surveyed 291 IBD patients in Ontario, Canada, and found that patients with UC reported 50.5% lifetime and 11.6% active use of cannabis, while patients with CD reported 48.1% lifetime and 15.9% active cannabis use [49]. Ravikoff Allergretti et al. surveyed the patterns of cannabis use in the US population. Their study was a prospective cohort study involving 292 participants at a specialized IBD center. The authors had a 94%

response rate, with 12.3% of respondents with IBD reporting active cannabis, and 32% reporting lifetime use for IBD symptom control. Symptoms perceived to be effectively controlled by cannabis included abdominal pain, poor appetite, nausea, and, less effectively, relief of diarrhea. The authors also commented that more clinical trials are needed to determine marijuana's therapeutic potential for IBD therapy to guide prescribing decisions as human studies involving objective evidence, including decreased serum biomarkers and endoscopic evidence of disease improvement, are not yet available. Larger, double-blind, randomized controlled trials using serial inflammatory markers, biopsy findings, and disease severity improvement via endoscopic findings are needed before cannabis can be recommended as an option for the treatment of IBD [49].

Weiss and colleagues conducted the first large population-based survey using the National Health and Nutrition Exam Survey (NHNES) in 2015. The authors reviewed over 2 million IBD patients in regard to patterns of cannabis use. The authors' results showed that IBD patients had a higher incidence of having used marijuana or its resin form, hashish (67.3%), versus the matched control subjects (60%). In addition, IBD patients were more likely to use a higher amount of marijuana or hashish per day, but were less likely to use marijuana or hashish every month for 1 year. Males, patients over 40, and IBD were identified to be predictors of marijuana or hashish use, based on multivariable logistic regression analysis. IBD patients tended to score higher on the Median Depression Score and were more likely to have alcohol-use patterns concerning for dependence and abuse. IBD patients also were more likely to have a higher prevalence of smoking and had higher levels of inflammatory markers such as C-reactive protein (CRP) [49].

Ahmed and Katz recognized in their review that many of the smaller studies shared several themes with the large study conducted by Weiss et al. First, cannabis use is common among IBD patients, and these patients report substantial therapeutic effects in the management of symptoms, such as abdominal pain and nausea. Many patients expressed interest in using cannabis for the management of their IBD symptoms, though are afraid to inquire to their physician or admit to using marijuana. This emphasizes the need for the healthcare community to research the potential therapeutic benefits of cannabis in the treatment of IBD. Patients involved in these studies were mainly from tertiary care centers, specialized for IBD, suggesting poor control of their symptoms [49].

Anandamide (AEA), a partial agonist of cannabinoid receptors, CB1 and CB2, is an endogenous bioactive lipid. Experimental colitis has been shown to improve when AEA reuptake is inhibited via the endocannabinoid membrane transport inhibitor VDM111 in animal models [46, 50]. Furthermore, exocannabinoids, with phytocannabinoid cannabidiol (CBD) as the most studied, reduce intestinal inflammation induced by lipopolysaccharides, as measured by TNF alpha. CBD has been shown to reduce inducible nitric oxide synthase (iNOS) expression, which also reduces IL-1beta and increases IL-10 levels [50]. These effects are seen when CBD is administered intraperitoneally or rectally, whereas it was not seen when administered orally. CBD also increases the anti-inflammatory effects of THC in chemical colitis in rat and mice models [50]. CB2 activation has been shown to decrease nitric oxide production by macrophages and reduce reactive oxygen species production by intestinal epithelium in murine models [46]. These murine models are largely what prompted human trials, most of which are coming out of Tel Aviv, though human studies are still lacking. Small observational studies have suggested that cannabis use improves quality of life, general health perceptions, social function, work function, and may reduce corticosteroid use among IBD patients [46].

One small prospective randomized controlled trial (RCT; $n = 21$) analyzed Crohn's patients with Crohn's Disease Activity Index (CDAI) scores >200 who had not responded to conventional medical therapies, including corticosteroids, immunomodulators, or anti-TNF agents. The participants were randomized to receive cannabis cigarettes (115 mg THC) two times per day, or placebo cigarettes with cannabis flower that had THC extracted. The active cannabis cigarettes were made from dried cannabis flowers of genetically identical plants known to contain 23% THC and <0.5% CBD. The placebo cigarettes were made from cannabis flowers with THC extracted using 95% ethanol. The final products showed to contain <0.4% THC and undetectable amounts of other cannabinoids including CBD. The process was repeated and shown to be reproducible and all cigarettes were machine made to ensure quality. Each cigarette contained 0.5 g of dried product. There were no measures to ensure intake was standardized. For example, some patients may not have taken in as deep of breaths as other patients, which may alter the amount of THC they were exposed to. Other participants may have coughed during smoking which could also lower the amount of THC intake, or conversely, some may have been able to hold their breath longer which may have increased the amount of THC intake. Disease activity and laboratory testing were assessed every 2 weeks for 8 weeks of treatment and 2 weeks thereafter [46, 51]. The CDAI score is used in clinical trials to assess disease activity in Crohn's patients, ranging from 0 to 600. Values between 150 and 219 are labeled as mildly active disease, 220–450 are moderately active disease, and <150 indicates clinical remission. The score is based off of various factors including medication use, symptoms, signs, and lab values [52]. CDAI decreased >100 points in 10 of 11 (90%) participants of the cannabis group versus 4 of 10 (40%) in the placebo group, with a significant increase in quality of life in the cannabis group. Clinical remission was not met in a majority of patients; 5 of 11 participants (45%) in the cannabis group versus 1 of 10 (10%) of the placebo participants achieved clinical remission (CDAI <150). Cannabis did not improve CRP levels. Important to note, 19 of the 21 patients were able to distinguish whether they were in the cannabis group or not due to the psychotropic effects of cannabis. This, in addition to the small sample size, can alter the results and usefulness of this study and more research is warranted [46, 52].

Another small RCT ($n = 20$) observed patients with active Crohn's who were randomized to receive 20 mg of cannabidiol per day or placebo. No significant difference in CDAI scores were noted between the two groups after 8 weeks. A third trial, conducted by Irving et al., showed that patients with left-sided or extensive ulcerative colitis who were stable on 5-aminosalicylates (5-ASA) had improved quality of life after cannabidiol-rich botanical extract versus placebo administration. Remission rates at 10 weeks were similar between the two groups [46, 53].

It should be noted that two Cochrane reviews covered the above human clinical trials, looking specifically at cannabis to treat CD and UC separately. Four out of the five studies reviewed were from the one research team led by Dr. Timna Naftali out of Tel Aviv, Israel. Based on Cochrane's GRADE analysis of quality of evidence, the three Naftali, et al. studies on cannabis treatment for CD yielded very low to low quality evidence, with two of the studies at high risk for bias, and one study at low risk. The cannabis used included flower cigarettes, 5% CBD oil and 15% CBD oil with 5% THC. The dependent variables were clinical remission, subjective disease activity index, quality of life, and serum CRP levels (which were unchanged with intervention in all studies that looked) [54]. The two studies on UC yielded moderate to low quality evidence by the Irving et al. team, and low quality evidence from the Naftali team, with both studies at relatively low risk for bias. The cannabis used included capsules with 50–250 mg CBD and up to 4.7% THC, and flower cigarettes with up to 23 mg THC. The dependent variables were measurements of clinical response, quality of life via IBDQ, subjective disease activity index, and biomarkers of serum CRP in both studies, as well as fecal calprotectin levels in one (again no differences in biomarkers seen) [55].

The GRADE criteria include study design, risk of bias, magnitude of effect, inconsistency, imprecision, and indirectness and are applied to each statistical claim in each study [56]. The authors of the Cochrane reviews conclude that no conclusive evidence has yet been concluded as to whether cannabis can treat IBD at the pathophysiologic level, especially since even when the subjective disease activity indices are improved by treatment, scopes and biopsies show no reduction in actual inflammation. This suggests that the benefits seen in three out of the five studies may be caused by a central mechanism, rather than local, or disease-modifying [54, 55]. However, there was some determination that CBD oil, or cannabidiol, is at least safe to use even if its efficacy has yet to be determined without better studies [54, 57].

Current criteria classifying cannabis as a Schedule I drug include the following: not currently having accepted medical use, having a high potential for abuse, and lack of accepted safety for use under medical supervision [58]. This has provided several hurdles to further research including regulatory obstacles, cannabis supply, and research funding. The National Academies of Science (NAS) recognized that most of the research on cannabis is conducted through funding from the National Institute of Drug Abuse (NIDA). Much of this research funding is toward identifying health risks of cannabis and not potential health benefits. Between 2015 and 2016, the National Institutes of Health (NIH) spent over 100 million dollars on cannabis research, of which 60 million dollars was provided by the NIDA. However, there has been a substantial amount of research regarding the use of cannabinoids in murine models that demonstrate reduction in inflammation in colitis [58]. There may be analogous efficacy in humans, although human studies have been limited due to the small sample sizes. These studies have shown improvement in subjective factors, such as quality of life, but no studies have showed objective evidence of true disease modification via improved biomarker profiles or endoscopic evidence of healing. The conflict between federal classification and state laws has led to unstandardized prescription and access to cannabis, limiting the research on benefits of cannabis on the endocannabinoid system, including its effects in IBD patients. It is important to take into consideration these limitations in regard to future studies.

Conclusion

Cannabis is used in almost one-fifth of patients with IBD, especially those with severe disease who use it to relieve symptoms of abdominal pain, nausea, poor appetite, diarrhea, and weight loss. Other motives for using cannabis among IBD patients include ineffectiveness of current conventional therapies, improve quality of life, and a sense of autonomy or gaining control over the disease. Patients may also choose cannabis over conventional therapies to avoid unwanted side effects from medications or complications from surgery, though cannabis use does not come without side effects of its own, as well as issues with legality and standardization. Though cannabis has offered some evidence in murine and other animal models as having potential for being therapeutic for IBD patients, human trials have failed to provide enough objective evidence for healthcare professionals to definitively recommend for or against it. High quality, prospective, randomized trials are needed to assess what portions of the cannabis plant, what dosage, and what preparation is best while minimizing side effects for IBD patients. In addition, studies looking at objective factors, including serial biomarkers, biopsy results, and endoscopic evidence of disease regression, are needed. Furthermore, one study mentioned above by Storr et al. raised the possibility that smoking cannabis can hasten surgical need in Crohn's patients. Thus, patients with Crohn's disease, particularly if fibrostenotic variant, should be cautioned against using cannabis until further research is available to evaluate the safety and efficacy.

Cannabis in Relation to Gastroesophageal Reflux Disease

Monica Dzwonkowski, Michelle Kem Su Hor, and Quentin Remley

Gastroesophageal reflux disease (GERD) is defined as frequent reflux of stomach acid through the lower esophageal sphincter (LES) into the esophagus, which can cause irritation of the lining of the esophagus. It is caused by weakening or improper mechanics of the LES. Common signs and symptoms of GERD include heartburn, usually after eating and may be worse at night, chest pain, regurgitation of food or sour liquid, globus sensation (lump in throat), and bloating [59]. Atypical GERD symptoms include frequent swallowing, chronic cough, laryngitis, difficulty swallowing (dysphagia), dental erosions, new or worsening asthma, discomfort in ears and nose, sleep disturbances, and excessive throat clearing [60]. Risk factors for GERD include obesity, hiatal hernia, pregnancy, connective tissue disorders, and gastroparesis. GERD symptoms can also be exacerbated by smoking, eating large meals, eating late meals, eating certain fatty or fried foods, coffee, alcohol, and medications such as aspirin. Over time, chronic inflammation in the esophagus from GERD can cause esophageal strictures, ulcers, or even Barrett's esophagus (metaplasia of esophageal epithelial tissue from squamous to columnar), which can progress to esophageal cancer [59].

The prevalence of GERD is around 10–20% in the Western world and less than 5% in Asian countries, according to a 2005 systematic review of 15 epidemiological studies. A population-based survey in the United States revealed that 22% of respondents reported heartburn or regurgitation within the last month while 16% reported regurgitation. The incidence in the Western world was approximately 5 per 1000 person years, which suggests GERD is a chronic condition since the prevalence is higher relative to the incidence. The epidemiology of GERD is difficult to estimate since epidemiological studies are based on patient self-reporting of symptoms which pose a potential for bias, and these studies also do not take all of the symptoms of GERD into account when assigning the diagnosis, thus leading to a potential underreporting of cases. For example, patients with objective evidence of GERD seen on EGD do not always have signs and symptoms such as heartburn or regurgitation [61]. Nevertheless, GERD is a fairly common GI condition.

The pathophysiology of GERD is multifactorial and may involve mechanisms such as dysfunctions of the anti-reflux barrier or impaired esophageal clearance, may depend on the type of offensive refluxate, and may also involve defective esophageal tissue resistance [62]. Transient lower esophageal relaxations (TLESRs) are one of the dysfunctions of the anti-reflux barrier and are the predominant mechanism seen in GERD. TLESRs are triggered by postprandial gastric distension to relieve counteracting gastric pressure on the LES. These relaxations are a vago-vagal reflex; signals from the brain stem activate receptors in the proximal stomach [63–65].

Research has shown that the endocannabinoid system may also be involved in some aspects of GERD. Cannabinoids are chemical compounds found endogenously in the human body, known as the endocannabinoid system (ECS), and exogenously in the marijuana plant. The ECS plays an important role in the regulation of synaptic transmission in the central and enteric nervous systems, both excitatory and inhibitory. It is involved in the mediation of a variety of processes including pain sensation and modulation, motor function, inflammation, and immunity of many organ systems, including the gastrointestinal system [63, 66].

Cannabinoid receptors (CBRs) are G-protein coupled receptors (GPCR) that are expressed in two main forms: CB1 and CB2 [67]. CB1 is expressed in central and peripheral neurons, while CB2 is primarily expressed by inflammatory and immune cells including plasma cells and macrophages throughout the GI tract [68–70]. There is a wide distribution of cannabinoid receptors (CBRs) in the enteric nervous system (ENS), highlighting the role of cannabis in GI health and disease [71–73]. CB1 has been shown to play a role in intestinal motility by reducing both large and small intestine muscle tone when activated [74–77]. In the upper GI tract, activation of CB1 has been shown to decrease intra-gastric pressure and concurrently delays gastric emptying via inhibition of excitatory neurons [78, 79]. CB2 receptors located in CNS have been shown to play a role in the emetic pathway, and have also been found in inflammatory and immune cells within the GI tract [80–83]. CB1 is found to be more extensively expressed in the GI tract than CB2 receptors [63, 84].

A study conducted by Calabrese et al. in 2010 demonstrated the presence of CBRs in human esophageal epithelium. The authors compared patients with non-erosive (NERD) and erosive esophageal reflux (ERD) to normal controls. The study included 87 total subjects after screening: 10 controls, 39 NERD, and 38 ERD, all of whom had typical symptoms for at least 1 year and abnormal 24-hour pH parameters. Eight specimens of macroscopically normal mucosa were taken from each patient. None of the patients admitted having used cannabis, and they all had been undergoing cyclical therapy with PPI. They found an increased expression of CB1 mRNA in the esophageal mucosa of both the NERD and ERD patients, but overall less expression compared with normal controls. The study also showed that the NERD patients had a 1.4-fold higher CB1R expression than ERD patients [63, 85].

The presence of CBRs in the esophagus, specifically those affecting TLESRs, offers a potential therapeutic target for treating GERD. One human study by Beumont et al. showed a decreased rate of TLESRs in healthy volunteers who received 10 and 20 mg of a cannabinoid agonist (Δ9-THC) three times a week apart [86]. The agonist significantly reduced the number of TLESRs but caused a non-significant reduction of acid reflux episodes in the first postprandial hour. In addition, the LES pressure and spontaneous swallowing were significantly reduced by the agonist. In high doses, central activity led to increased nausea and vomiting. Centrally acting CB1 receptor agonists produce psychotropic effects, and therefore selective targeting of peripheral CB1 receptors is necessary for effective therapy [87, 88]. An important mechanism in the control of acid exposure or contact time in the esophagus is the swallow reflex. Spontaneous swallow decreases stasis and promotes clearance of reflux, therefore decreasing esophageal mucosal injury [89]. The authors noted that although administration of a CB1 agonist decreased TLESRs, it also decreased spontaneous swallows. This potentially limits the benefit of decreasing TLESRs [63, 90].

In 2011, Scarpellini et al. studied the effects of CB1 receptor antagonist rimonabant on fasting and postprandial LES function in healthy subjects. Twelve healthy volunteers underwent esophageal manometry studies with administration of wet swallows and a meal after 3 days of premedication with placebo or with 20 mg of rimonabant. Results of the study showed that rimonabant enhanced postprandial LES pressure, while preprandial LES pressure, swallow-induced relaxations, and amplitude of peristaltic contractions were not altered. However, rimonabant significantly increased the duration of peristaltic contractions during both periods. In addition, the number of postprandial TLESRs and acid reflux episodes were significantly lower after rimonabant therapy. The authors concluded that rimonabant enhances postprandial LES pressure and decreases TLESRs in healthy subjects, but its therapeutic use is limited by its side effect of major depression and the medication was subsequently taken off the market [63, 91, 92].

As of late 2019, 11 states (Alaska, California, Colorado, Illinois, Maine, Massachusetts, Michigan, Nevada, Oregon, Vermont, Washington) and the District of Columbia have adopted laws legalizing marijuana for recreational use. Americans can buy legal marijuana almost as easily as they could order a pizza or get a cup of coffee.

There are a multitude of ways to consume marijuana, but the most common methods of administering marijuana are inhalation, oral, sublingual, and topical. Each method has its unique characteristics, and the consumer usually picks a method that is most suitable for their use. Smoking has the fastest onset, unfortunately, smoking also irritates the throat and lungs. Vaping, like smoking, provides a quick onset of effects and was thought to not expose users to the harsh effects of smoking [93]. This method of intake could be considered for patients who want a more discreet way of using marijuana; however, recently 49 states, the District of Columbia, and one US territory have reported over 1000 cases of lung injury associated with the use of vaping products. Hundreds of illnesses and dozens of deaths have been reported due to electronic cigarette-related lung damage, particularly with THC vaping. Vaping was previously considered a safer alternative to smoking, but this recent evidence suggests any form of inhalation should be avoided [94]. Tinctures allow patients to measure an exact dose, though as mentioned in the IBS portion of this chapter, artisanal products may contain different contents than what is advertised on the label. Patients can add marijuana tinctures to food or beverages or take them sublingually. Capsules work slower than tinctures taken sublingually, but they may provide effects in more controlled doses, if they are regulated. Capsules may be ideal for patients who do not feel comfortable smoking marijuana. Moreover, it is more socially acceptable to take a pill rather than smoking or vaping [93].

Like most medications/drugs, marijuana may cause side effects, which are discussed in the IBS section of this chapter. More education needs to be provided to the medical community about cannabis products and their potential therapeutic effects, while not ignoring the potential side effects and complications, such as cannabinoid hyperemesis syndrome, so that medical professionals can provide better education for their patients. With this being said, there is a need for more research to be performed not only on the effects of THC on the GI system, but also for dosing. With increased regulation of cannabis products and more research, consumers would be able to reduce the risks of experiencing unpleasant side effects.

Conclusion

Gastroesophageal reflux disease results from the reflux of stomach acid through the lower esophageal sphincter to esophagus, irritating the esophageal tissues and producing symptoms. Lower esophageal sphincter weakening or poor mechanics are usually at the core of this problem. GERD can present with either typical or atypical symptoms. The prevalence of GERD in the western world is estimated to be 10–20%. Cannabinoid receptors are GPCRs that are found within the GI tract, particularly CB1. CB1 agonist administration has been shown to decrease TLESRs significantly, but also significantly reduced LES pressure and spontaneous swallowing. The study by Beumont showed a reduction of acid reflux episodes, although it was at a non-significant level. High doses of CB1 agonists caused an increase in nausea and vomiting. CB1 antagonists (rimonabant) was shown to increase LES pressure, TLESRs, and acid reflux episodes, but its therapeutic use is limited by its side effect of major depression and it has also been taken off the market. Overall, marijuana and THC-based products are becoming more commonplace, with many routes of administration. The presence of cannabinoid receptors within the GI system allows for a potential target for treating various diseases, such as GERD; however, more research is needed to determine whether or not cannabis can be used as a therapy for esophageal disorders. It is important to note that cannabis use can also lead to complications, including cannabinoid hyperemesis syndrome (CHS). The pathophysiology of CHS is not completely understood; it is unknown why some users experience CHS and others are spared. No definitive recommendations can be made at this time on whether or not cannabis use will be a useful therapy for GI disorders until more research is completed.

Nonalcoholic Fatty Liver Disease and Cannabinoids

Michelle Kem Su Hor, Monica Dzwonkowski, and Cicily Hummer

What is NAFLD?

Nonalcoholic fatty liver disease, or NAFLD, is comprised of nonalcoholic fatty liver (NAFL) and nonalcoholic steatohepatitis (NASH). NAFLD is defined by radiologic or histologic evidence of excess fat accumulation (steatosis) in the liver in the absence of alternative etiologies, such as hepatotoxic or steatogenic medication use, hereditary disorders, viral hepatitis, autoimmune liver disease, or significant alcohol consumption [95, 96]. Many patients with NAFLD are asymptomatic and have a normal physical examination [95]. These patients may go undiagnosed for years, having only mildly elevated or normal liver enzymes on routine blood testing. NAFLD is often found incidentally by imaging studies performed for other reasons, for example, abdominal ultrasounds looking for gallbladder pathology, or CT scans for determining the etiology of abdominal pain [95]. Before a diagnosis of NAFLD is made, all other causes of fatty liver must be excluded. NAFL is the most common form of NAFLD and does not cause significant damage to the liver. A fraction of patients with NAFLD may develop chronic cell injury, leading to nonalcoholic steatohepatitis (NASH), which is characterized by inflammation and liver cell death. Patients with NASH are at higher risk of developing end-stage liver diseases, such as cirrhosis, liver failure requiring a liver transplant, and hepatocellular carcinoma, a type of liver cancer. NASH patients are also at a higher risk of death from cardiovascular disease and other types of cancer [97]. Though the exact cause has not been fully established on why extra-hepatic cancer risk increases with NAFLD, it is postulated that there is a link between obesity and metabolic syndrome: common conditions in those with NAFLD and extra-hepatic cancers. Several studies have shown an association between NAFLD and an increased risk for adenomas and colorectal cancer. Two large studies by Hwang et al. with a study population of 2917, and a Korean study by Lee et al. with a study population of 5517, showed a higher prevalence of colorectal lesions compared with patients without NAFLD [97]. A study by Stadlmayr et al. showed that NAFLD is an independent risk factor for colorectal cancer [97]. Other smaller studies have linked NAFLD to other cancers including esophageal, pancreas, kidney, breast, malignant melanoma, lung, and prostate [97]. Even though these are smaller studies, all healthcare providers should be vigilant in screening NAFLD patients for extra-hepatic cancers especially colorectal cancer.

NAFLD is quickly becoming a worldwide epidemic, with global prevalence estimated at 25%. The highest prevalence is in South America and the Middle East, followed by Asia, the United States, and Europe [98]. NAFLD is a part of the metabolic syndrome characterized by diabetes, insulin resistance (pre-diabetes), increased weight/obesity, elevated blood lipids such as cholesterol and triglycerides, and hypertension. Conditions that increase insulin resistance, such as polycystic ovarian syndrome, also contribute to an increased likelihood of developing NAFLD [95]. NAFLD is not only present in obese individuals, there are also people with a BMI <25 kg/m^2 who may present with NAFLD. These people are referred to as having "lean-NAFLD." The prevalence of lean NAFLD varies from 7% in the United States to as high as 19% in Asian countries [99, 100]. Lean NAFLD disproportionately affects older males, with comorbidities including type II diabetes, hypertension, metabolic syndrome, dyslipidemia, chronic kidney disease, and heart disease [99, 100]. People with lean and obese NAFLD share a common altered metabolic and heart disease profile, which in turn, may lead to a collective risk for adverse metabolic and heart disease outcomes, including diabetes and ischemic heart disease [99, 100]. A genetic polymorphism in the patatin-like phospholipase domain-containing 3 (PNPLA3) gene, a gene related to lipid transformation, is now recognized as a major genetic determinant of NAFLD in lean and obese NAFLD patients, and is associated with a greater chance of progression to NASH in both cohorts [99, 100]. Besides genetic predisposition, other risk factors that contribute to the development of NAFLD include environmental factors such as diet, exercise, tobacco consumption, gut microbiome, and lack of access to healthcare [101].

Treatment of NAFLD mainly consists of weight loss regimens, decreasing caloric intake, increasing physical activity, and avoiding alcohol which could potentially cause alcohol-induced fatty liver injury. Recent emerging evidence suggests that cannabinoids also play an important role in the modulation of NAFLD and, pending further studies, may have future therapeutic benefits in management of patients with NAFLD. The endocannabinoid system (ECS) is a biological system postulated to have evolved over 500 million years ago [102]. It is present in all vertebrates and is primarily composed of endocannabinoids (substrates), endocannabinoid receptors, and endocannabinoid-metabolizing enzymes. Initially, researchers suggested endocannabinoid receptors were only present in the central nervous system, but further research has found that these receptors are found throughout the body, including skin, immune cells, bone, adipose tissue, liver, pancreas, skeletal muscles, heart, blood vessels, kidneys, and gastrointestinal tract [102]. Furthermore, research has revealed that the ECS is involved in a wide variety of bodily processes, including nociception, memory, mood, appetite, stress, sleep, metabolism, immune function, and reproductive function.

Endocannabinoids are lipid mediators that interact with endocannabinoid receptors to produce effects similar to those of delta-9-tetrahydrocannabinol, or THC, the main psychoactive component of marijuana. The two main endogenous cannabinoids discovered are 2-arachidonoylglycerol (2-AG) and arachidonoyl ethanolomaide (anandamide, or AEA), which bind to the G-protein coupled cannabinoid receptors, CB1 and CB2. CB1 receptors are highly expressed in the brain and at lower concentrations, in the peripheral tissues. In the liver, CB1 receptors are found in hepatocytes, stellate cells, and sinusoidal epithelial cells [96]. CB2 receptors are also found in brain and peripheral tissues, and in Kupffer and stellate cells in the liver [96].

The role of CB1 receptors in the development of fatty liver is related to high fat consumption and is mediated by liver AEA-induced CB1 receptor activation and upregulation from increased fatty acid synthesis. The role of CB2 in development of NAFLD is still unclear; however, there is higher CB2 receptor expression in people with NAFLD but not in people with normal livers, suggesting a link between CB2 activation in those with risk factors for NAFLD, such as obesity, insulin resistance, type 2 diabetes and hypertriglyceridemia [104].

Various cytochrome P450s (CYPs) are responsible for the metabolism of drugs and other chemicals not naturally found in the body. Different drugs and chemicals undergo different metabolic pathways for breakdown in the liver. The liver detoxifies and facilitates excretion of foreign substances by enzymatically converting fat-soluble compounds to water-soluble compounds, using the CYP system as a catalyst. Some drugs can affect processing times within the CYP system, allowing for faster or slower metabolism of medications. Understanding this system is crucial for healthcare professionals because drug-drug interactions can have devastating consequences [105].

Approximately 79% of prescription and over-the-counter drugs that are metabolized by the liver are metabolized via CYP3A4, CYP3A5, CYP2C9, CYP2D6, and CYP2C19 [105]. Cannabidiol, or CBD, is metabolized primarily by CYP3A4 and CYP2C19 and has also been reported to be an inhibitor of these pathways [106]. Given the effects CBD has on the CYP system, it has the potential to interact with many prescription and over-the-counter drugs that are hepatically metabolized. THC is also metabolized by CYP3A4 as well as CYP2C9, and an inducer of CYP1A2; however, further research is warranted regarding the effects of THC and other components of marijuana on drug metabolism to establish clinical significance and guidance on treatment strategies [107]. Clinical recommendations of reducing other drug dosages, monitoring for adverse reactions, and finding alternative therapies should be considered in those using cannabis and taking prescription or over-the-counter medications [106].

Cannabis components may also have important implications in liver transplant patients. Post-transplant patients are given immunosuppressant drugs, such as tacrolimus, to decrease the risk of rejection. CBD has been reported to cause increased tacrolimus concentrations. In a case report from 2018 about a patient taking 2–2.9 g of CBD daily for refractory epilepsy and tacrolimus for interstitial nephritis, a threefold increase in dose-normalized tacrolimus occurred [108]. Another case report from 2016 discussed tacrolimus toxicity in a patient who was on immunosuppression post-transplant. The patient was taking tacrolimus for a stem cell transplant and developed toxicity, but healthcare professionals could not figure out why. He later admitted to taking edible marijuana gummies brought in by his family member while receiving tacrolimus. Despite decreasing the dose of tacrolimus, the levels continued to rise, and the patient was transferred to the ICU due to the impairment he suffered from combining marijuana with tacrolimus [109]. There is currently no consensus on cannabis use in transplant patients. Though case reports and anecdotal evidence of post-transplant complications attributed to marijuana use exist, studies showing overall survival rates in various transplant patients do not differ among marijuana users and nonusers. More research is needed on cannabis and its effects on immunosuppressant medications, as well as its interactions with other medications and its implications on transplant patient and organ or graft survival [110].

A population-based case-control study conducted by Adejumo et al. looked at the relationship between cannabis use and the prevalence of NAFLD [111]. Using data from the Healthcare Cost and Utilization Project Nationwide Inpatient Sample (HCUP-NIS) database, the study reviewed clinical records for 5,950,391 patients aged 18–90 years old, collected from January 1 to December 31, 2014. The study categorized patients into non-cannabis users (5,833,812), nondependent cannabis users (103,675), and dependent cannabis users (12,904), using data from ICD-9 coding. The study then categorized patients into groups based on age, gender, race, socioeconomic status, insurance type as well as patient-specific conditions such as hypertension, diabetes, high cholesterol, metabolic syndrome, obesity, and tobacco use. Alcohol users were excluded as alcohol could lead to alcoholic steatohepatitis. Chi-square analysis was performed with a p-value of <0.05 considered statistically significant. A crude odds ratio was also performed to determine how cannabis use relates to other risk factors of NAFLD development. The prevalence of NAFLD in dependent cannabis users was 68% less than nonusers, and for non-dependent users the prevalence was 15% less than nonusers, before adjusting for other NAFLD risk factors. Though non-dependent users and dependent users had lower rates of NAFLD when compared to nonusers before adjusting for variables, after adjusting for other NAFLD risk factors (obesity, age, high cholesterol), only dependent user data remained statistically significant. In summary, chronic, dependent cannabis users have lower rates of NAFLD when compared to non-dependent and nonusers, even when adjusting for confounding variables [111].

In 2019, further research was conducted on the association of marijuana use with nonalcoholic fatty liver disease [112]. This study was a population-based epidemiological study. The data was collected in the National Health and Nutrition Examination Survey (NHANES 2005–2014) and NHANES III (1988–1994). This study examined patients who were suspected of having NAFLD, which, using the NHANES data, was determined by serum alanine aminotransferase (ALT) >30 IU/L for men and >19 IU/L for women in the absence of all other liver diseases (significant alcohol consumption, positive HBsAg, positive anti-HCV, etc.). Using the NHANES III data, NAFLD was defined based on ultrasonography. These methods provided 22,366 participants suspected of having NAFLD (NHANES 14,080; NHANES III 8,286). This population was further divided by marijuana use. Never users (NHANES 40.8%; NHANES III 56.1%), past users who used previously but not within the last 30 days (NHANES 47.1%; NHANES III 36.9%), current light users who used at least once in the last 30 days but not on more than four different days (NHANES 4.9%; NHANES III 4.9%), and current heavy users who used at least five different days in the last 30 days (NHANES 7.3%; NHANES III 2.2%). Due to the discrepancy between the current heavy user population in the NHANES and NHANES III, the categories of current light user and current heavy user data from NHANES III were combined for further analysis. This allows for a greater sample size and greater statistical power of the study. Baseline characteristics were compared using the chi-squared test for categorical variables or linear regression for continuous variables. Multivariable logistic models were created to identify predictors of NAFLD after consideration of other potential demographic and clinical confounders. The prevalence of suspected NAFLD and ultrasonographically diagnosed NAFLD were inversely associated with marijuana use ($p < 0.001$). In the younger participants, heavy marijuana use showed a 35% risk reduction in suspected NAFLD compared to nonusers in a fully adjusted model ($P = 0.0001$). This trend was also demonstrated but had marginal significance in persons over 40 years old (risk reduction 26%; $P = 0.067$). Using a multivariate analysis, with an age, gender, ethnicity-adjusted model, researchers found reduced rates of NAFLD in marijuana users when comparing current light or heavy users to nonusers (OR 0.76 (95% CI 0.58–0.98) and 0.70 (95% CI 0.56–0.89)). To further investigate marijuana's predictive value, researchers created an insulin resistance-adjusted model and marijuana use remained an independent predictor of lower risk of suspected NAFLD. These findings suggest that there may be a protective effect of marijuana use with regard to suspected NAFLD independent of metabolic risk factors [112]. However, the researchers did not look at which specific compound in marijuana (THC, CBD, THCV, etc.) was causing the protective effects and instead suggest further investigation into the pathophysiology of marijuana components.

Up until recently, there was no theoretical explanation for why cannabis users have lower BMIs than nonusers, even though they consume on average over 800 calories more than nonusers [103]. Clark et al. published an article discussing a theory about the role that cannabis plays on metabolism in the body. The theory is that since CB1 receptors mediate energy uptake storage and energy conservation, downregulation of CB1 receptors from chronic cannabis exposure leads to a decrease in energy stores and an increase in metabolic rate. This effect lasts up to four weeks after cessation of cannabis use. If this theory is correct, this would help in understanding how cannabis may interact with the human body. Further research needs to be done to investigate how cannabis works on the metabolism, as well as specifically which components of cannabis have this effect. This research would also aid in understanding whether cannabis is protective or not protective against NAFLD, as high BMI is a risk factor for the development of NAFLD [103].

Another research study by Dibba et al. investigated the mechanistic role of the endocannabinoid system in NAFLD [113]. It is well known that insulin resistance is a key contributor to the pathogenesis of NAFLD. Thus, previous treatments revolved around weight reduction, via diet and exercise, to reduce insulin resistance in at-risk populations. Recent studies have suggested that the endocannabinoid system and its associated cannabinoid receptors may have therapeutic effects on the development of NAFLD [113]. Historically, antagonism of the CB1 receptor has demonstrated therapeutic benefits, such as decreasing obesity rates and hepatic steatosis, especially when central nervous system effects were minimalized [113]. A drug designed to antagonize the CB1 receptor, rimonabant, was introduced in 2006. Rimonabant reduced hepatomegaly and hepatic steatosis, reduced markers of liver damage, and reduced levels of hepatic TNFα, suggesting a reduction in hepatic inflammation. Despite these positive effects, the drug was withdrawn from the market in 2008 because of increased risk of central nervous system toxicity, particularly anxiety and depression. Antagonism of CB1 has also demonstrated promising effects with increased resistance to hepatic steatosis, reversal of hepatic steatosis, and improvements in glycemic control, insulin resistance, and dyslipidemia, but further research is needed to determine how to target this receptor without increasing the risk of adverse reactions [113]. The compound tetrahydrocannabivarin (THCV), an analog of THC, can act as a CB1/CB2 agonist in low doses and/or a CB1/CB2 neutral antagonist in high doses; however, further investigation is warranted because alternate studies show that isomers of THCV can induce agonist effects independently [113]. Due to the nature of THCV to potentially act as an antagonist at CB1 receptors, this represents a potential target for pharmacokinetics in the future.

One study by Millar et al. researched articles about CBD administration. Out of 1038 articles found, 35 met the inclusion criteria. The results were inconclusive, as the trials that dealt with assessing diabetes, Crohn's, and fatty liver disease were quite small ($n = 6$–62) and used a very low dose of CBD (2.4 mg/kg/day). More research and clinical trials with higher sample sizes and greater variety of doses of CBD and other cannabis components are needed to assess the link between CBD administration and the protective or risk factors for fatty liver and other medical conditions [114].

Another study published by Ewing et al. in April of 2019 studied the effects of CBD extract on mouse livers. The animals were given 0, 246, 738, or 2460 mg/kg of CBD in 24 hours (noted as acute toxicity) or 0, 61.5, 184.5, or 615 mg/kg CBD for 10 days (noted as subacute toxicity). The doses were based on scaled mouse equivalent doses of the maximum recommended human maintenance dose of

Epidiolex (20 mg/kg), an oral solution of CBD. In the acute phase, ALT, AST, total bilirubin, and liver-to-body weight (LBW) ratios all increased for the 2460 mg/kg dosed mice. In the 615 mg/kg dosed mice in the subacute phase, 75% of the mice developed a moribund condition between days 3 and 4. The 615 mg/kg mice also had increased LBW ratios, ALT, AST, and total bilirubin. Hepatotoxicity gene expression assays revealed CBD regulated more than 50 genes, many linked to lipid metabolism and drug metabolism. This study suggests that CBD may cause hepatotoxicity if administered in high doses and that CBD potentially causes drug-drug interactions [115]. The drug used in this study, Epidiolex, has been shown to increase ALT levels in controlled trials. In human trials, Epidiolex 20 mg/kg/day increased ALT greater than 3 times the upper limit of normal in 30% of patients with already elevated ALT levels, and 12% of subjects with normal baseline ALT levels. Zero patients taking Epidiolex 10 mg/kg/day experienced ALT elevations greater than 3 times the upper limit of normal when ALT was elevated above normal at baseline, compared with 2% of patients in whom ALT was within the normal range at baseline. This elevation is exacerbated in patients taking concomitant antiepileptic medications, such as valproate or clobazam. Reduction in ALT levels occurred in roughly two-thirds of patients when Epidiolex was discontinued or dose adjusted, whereas one-third of patients experienced a reduction in ALT levels despite continuation of Epidiolex at the current dose. Though a link between CBD use and hepatotoxicity has been shown in these trials, more research is still warranted on how exactly CBD is affecting these metabolic pathways in human subjects. Patients taking Epidiolex and other CBD formulations should be monitored closely for hepatotoxic effects [116].

A couple of small studies published in JAMA discussed the inaccuracy of labeling of CBD products purchased online and for edible medical cannabis products, though sample sizes were relatively low. One study ($n = 75$) reported edible cannabis products from 3 major metropolitan areas failed to accurately label over 50% of their products. Many products contained significantly less cannabinoid content than labeled, while others contained significantly more THC than labeled. Of the 75 products from 47 different brands, only 17% were accurately labeled. This can be misleading to purchasers and can pose greater risk of adverse effects if the amounts of active ingredients are inappropriately reported [117]. Another study ($n = 84$), looked at CBD products purchased online. This study resulted in over 42.85% over-labeled products (less actual CBD in product), 26.19% under-labeled products (more actual CBD in product), and 30.95% accurately labeled products. Vaporization liquid was most frequently mislabeled. In addition, THC was detected in 18 of the 84 samples tested [118]. If products contain less CBD than is labeled, potential therapeutic effects may be diminished. On the contrary, if a product contains more CBD than is labeled, potential harmful effects may be amplified. Furthermore, if a CBD product contains psychoactive THC, this could produce intoxication or impairment, a particularly worrisome scenario in children. Caution should be taken with purchasing CBD products from unknown or unregulated sources.

Conclusion

Overall, the studies mentioned above do not offer a definitive argument for or against the use of cannabis as a management strategy for NAFLD. More high quality studies are needed to evaluate the best method of consumption (inhalation, consumption, topical, etc.), the best dosage for therapeutic effect, and the mechanistic details of how various active ingredients in cannabis (e.g., THC, CBD, THCV) modulate the development of NAFLD, hepatotoxicity, and drug-drug interactions. Although cannabinoids have been associated with improved outcomes in NAFLD in epidemiologic studies, there is insufficient data to support their use in this disease at this time until more robustly designed studies of marijuana can be planned/conducted. No recommendations can be made regarding the clinical application or harm of cannabis use in patients with NAFLD until prospective basic and human studies are conducted. Furthermore, if new research points to therapeutic benefits of cannabis use in the management of patient with NAFLD, a pharmaceutical grade, regulated formulation of cannabis should be used in place of over-the-counter or unregulated dispensary formulations to reduce the risk of mislabeled or contaminated products and potential increased adverse outcomes.

References

1. Sorensen CJ, DeSanto K, Borgelt L, Phillips KT, Monte AA. Cannabinoid hyperemesis syndrome: diagnosis, pathophysiology, and treatment—a systematic eeview. J Med Toxicol. 2017;13(1):71–87. Published online 2016 Dec 20. https://doi.org/10.1007/s13181-016-0595-z.
2. Zimmer DI, McCauley R, Konanki V, et al. emergency department and radiological cost of delayed diagnosis of cannabinoid hyperemesis. J Addict. 2019;2019:1307345. Published 2019 Jan 1. https://doi.org/10.1155/2019/1307345.
3. Finn K. The hidden costs of marijuana use in colorado: one emergency department's experience. J Global Drug Pol Pract. http://www.globaldrugpolicy.org/Issues/Vol%2010%20Issue%202/Articles/The%20Hidden%20Costs%20of%20Marijuana%20Use%20in%20Colorado_Final.pdf.
4. Monte AA, Shelton SK, Mills E, et al. Acute illness associated with cannabis use, by route of exposure. Ann Intern Med. 2019;170(8):531. https://doi.org/10.7326/m18-2809.
5. Nourbakhsh M, Miller A, Gofton J, Jones G, Adeagbo B. Cannabinoid hyperemesis syndrome: reports of fatal cases. J Forensic Sci. 2019;64(1) https://doi.org/10.1111/1556-4029.13819.
6. Mittleman MA, Lewis RA, Maclure M, Sherwood JB, Muller JE. Triggering myocardial infarction by marijuana. Circulation. 2001;103:2805e2809.
7. Mukamal KJ, Maclure M, Muller JE, Mittleman MA. An exploratory prospective study of marijuana use and mortality following acute myocardial infarction. Am Heart J. 2008;155:465e470.
8. Hansen B, Miller K, Weber C. Early evidence on recreational marijuana legalization and traffic fatalities. Econ Inq. 2018. https://doi.org/10.1111/ecin.12751.
9. Bollom A, Austrie J, Hirsch W, et al. Emergency department burden of nausea and vomiting associated with cannabis use disorder: us trends from 2006 to 2013. J Clin Gastroenterol. 2018;52(9):778–83. https://doi.org/10.1097/MCG.0000000000000944.

10. Elsohly MA, Mehmedic Z, Foster S, Gon C, Chandra S, Church JC. Changes in cannabis potency over the last 2 decades (1995–2014): analysis of current data in the United States. Biol Psychiatry. 2016;79(7):613–9. https://doi.org/10.1016/j.biopsych.2016.01.004.
11. Di Forti M, Quattrone D, Freeman T, Tripoli G, Gayer-Anderson C, Quiggley H. The contribution of cannabis use to variation in the incidence of psychotic disorder across Europe (EU-GEI): a multicentre case-control study. Lancet Psychiatry. 2019;6(5):427–36. https://doi.org/10.1016/S2215-0366(19)30048-3.
12. Trappey BE, Olson APJ. Running out of options: rhabdomyolysis associated with cannabis hyperemesis syndrome. J Gen Intern Med. 2017;32(12):1407–9. Published online 2017 Jun 29. https://doi.org/10.1007/s11606-017-4111-1.
13. Lapoint J, Meyer S, Yu CK, Koenig KL, Lev R, Thihalolipavan S, Staats K, Kahn CA. Cannabinoid hyperemesis syndrome: public health implications and a novel model treatment guideline. West J Emerg Med. 2018;19(2):380–6. Published online 2017 Nov 8. https://doi.org/10.5811/westjem.2017.11.36368.
14. Parvataneni S, Varela L, Vemuri-Reddy SM, Maneval Cureus ML. Emerging role of aprepitant in cannabis hyperemesis syndrome. 2019;11(6):e4825. Published online 2019 Jun 4. https://doi.org/10.7759/cureus.4825.
15. Gregoire P, Tau M, Robertson D. Cannabinoid hyperemesis syndrome and the onset of a manic episode. BMJ Case Rep. 2016:bcr2016215129. Published online 2016 Apr 27. https://doi.org/10.1136/bcr-2016-215129.
16. Canavan C, West J, Card T. The epidemiology of irritable bowel syndrome. Clin Epidemiol. 2014;6:71–80. Published online 2014 Feb 4. https://doi.org/10.2147/CLEP.S40245.
17. Lehrer J. What is the Rome IV criteria for diagnosis of irritable bowel syndrome (IBS)? https://www.medscape.com/answers/180389-10034/what-is-the-rome-iv-criteria-for-diagnosis-of-irritable-bowel-syndrome-ibs. Published 23 Sep 2019. Accessed 9 Oct 2019.
18. Mayo Clinic Staff. Irritable bowel syndrome. Mayo Clinic. https://www.mayoclinic.org/diseases-conditions/irritable-bowel-syndrome/diagnosis-treatment/drc-20360064. Published March 17, 2018. Accessed 9 Oct 2019.
19. Chong PP, Chin VK, Looi CY, Wong WF, Madhavan P, Yong VC. The microbiome and irritable bowel syndrome – a review on the pathophysiology, current research and future therapy. Front Microbiol. 2019;10. https://doi.org/10.3389/fmicb.2019.01136.
20. Storr MA, Yce B, Andrews CN, Sharkey KA. The role of the endocannabinoid system in the pathophysiology and treatment of irritable bowel syndrome. Neurogastroenterol Mot. 2008;20(8):857–68. https://doi.org/10.1111/j.1365-2982.2008.01175.x.
21. Fichna J, Wood JT, Papanastasiou M, et al. Endocannabinoid and cannabinoid-like fatty acid amide levels correlate with pain-related symptoms in patients with ibs-d and ibs-c: a pilot study. PLoS ONE. 2013;8(12). https://doi.org/10.1371/journal.pone.0085073.
22. Wright K, Rooney N, Feeney M, et al. Differential expression of cannabinoid receptors in the human colon: cannabinoids promote epithelial wound healing. Gastroenterology. 2005;129(2):437–53. https://doi.org/10.1016/j.gastro.2005.05.026.
23. Ahn K, Johnson DS, Cravatt BF. Fatty acid amide hydrolase as a potential therapeutic target for the treatment of pain and CNS disorders. Expert Opin Drug Discovery. 2009;4(7):763–84. https://doi.org/10.1517/17460440903018857.
24. Cremon C, Stanghellini V, Barbaro MR, et al. Randomised clinical trial: the analgesic properties of dietary supplementation with palmitoylethanolamide and polydatin in irritable bowel syndrome. Aliment Pharmacol Ther. 2017;45(7):909–22. https://doi.org/10.1111/apt.13958.
25. Mcpartland JM, Guy GW, Marzo VD. Care and feeding of the endocannabinoid system: a systematic review of potential clinical interventions that upregulate the endocannabinoid system. PLoS ONE. 2014;9(3). https://doi.org/10.1371/journal.pone.0089566.
26. Brand EJ, Zhao Z. Cannabis in Chinese medicine: are some traditional indications referenced in ancient literature related to cannabinoids? Front Pharmacol. 2017;8. https://doi.org/10.3389/fphar.2017.00108.

27. McPartland JM, Hegman W, Long T. Veget Hist Archaeobot. 2019;28:691. https://doi.org/10.1007/s00334-019-00731-8.
28. The Editors of Encyclopaedia Britannica. Hua Tuo. Encyclopædia Britannica. https://www.britannica.com/biography/Hua-Tuo. Published April 29, 2016. Accessed 27 Oct 2019.
29. Bridgeman MB, Abazia DT. Medicinal cannabis: history, pharmacology, and implications for the acute care setting. P T. 2017;42(3):180–8.
30. What You Should Know About Marijuana Concentrates. DEA.gov. https://www.dea.gov/sites/default/files/resource-center/Publications/marijuana-concentrates.pdf. Published December 2014. Accessed 18 Nov 2019.
31. National Academies of Sciences, Engineering, and Medicine. The health effects of cannabis and cannabinoids: The current state of evidence and recommendations for research. Washington: The National Academies Press; 2017. https://doi.org/10.17226/24625.
32. Welty TE, Chapman KE, Faught RE, Kotloski RJ. American Epilepsy Society (AES): written Comments to Norman E. "Ned" Sharpless, MD, Acting Commissioner of Food and Drugs, U.S. Food and Drug Administration (FDA), Department of Health and Human Services (HHS). Epilepsy Curr. 2019;19(6):361–8. https://doi.org/10.1177/1535759719878716.
33. Medical Cannabis. Gastrointestinal Society. https://badgut.org/information-centre/a-z-digestive-topics/cannabis/. Published August 26, 2019. Accessed 27 Oct 2019.
34. ICD-10-CM Codes. 10. https://www.icd10data.com/ICD10CM/Codes/F01-F99/F10-F19/F12-. Published 2018. Accessed 18 Nov 2019.
35. Adejumo A, et al. P1150. Presented at: World Congress of Gastroenterology at American College of Gastroenterology Annual Scientific Meeting; Oct. 13–18, 2017; Orlando.
36. Wong BS, Camilleri M, Eckert D, et al. Randomized pharmacodynamic and pharmacogenetic trial of dronabinol effects on colon transit in irritable bowel syndrome-diarrhea. Neurogastroenterol Mot. 2012;24(4). https://doi.org/10.1111/j.1365-2982.2011.01874.x.
37. Klooker TK, Leliefeld KEM, Wijngaard RMVD, Boeckxstaens GEE. The cannabinoid receptor agonist delta-9-tetrahydrocannabinol does not affect visceral sensitivity to rectal distension in healthy volunteers and IBS patients. Neurogastroenterology & Motility. 2010;23(1). https://doi.org/10.1111/j.1365-2982.2010.01587.x.
38. Dahlhamer JM, Zammitti EP, Ward BW, Wheaton AG, Croft JB. Prevalence of inflammatory bowel disease among adults aged ≥18 years — United States, 2015. MMWR Morb Mortal Wkly Rep. 2016;65:1166–9. https://doi.org/10.15585/mmwr.mm6542a3.
39. Coward S, et al. Past and future burden of inflammatory bowel diseases based on modeling of population-based data. Gastroenterology. 156(5):1345–1353.e4. https://doi.org/10.1053/j.gastro.2019.01.002.
40. Cosnes J, et al. Epidemiology and natural history of inflammatory bowel diseases. Gastroenterology. 140(6):1785–1794.e4. https://doi.org/10.1053/j.gastro.2011.01.055.
41. Hueber W, Sands BE, Lweitzky S, et al. Secukinumab, a human anti-IL 17A monoclonal antibody, for moderate to severe crohn's disease; unexpected results of a randomized , double-blind placebo-controlled trial. Gut. 2012;61:1693.
42. Abbas AK, Aster JC, Kumar V. Robbins and Cotran pathologic basis of disease. 9th ed. Philadelphia: Elsevier/Saunders; 2015. p. 796–8.
43. Feldman PA, Wolfson D, Barkin JS. Medical management of Crohn's disease. Clin Colon Rectal Surg. 2007;20(4):269–81. https://doi.org/10.1055/s-2007-991026.
44. Cheifetz A, Cullen G. Sulfasalazine and 5-aminosalicylates in the treatment of inflammatory bowel disease. UpToDate. https://www.uptodate.com/contents/sulfasalazine-and-5-aminosalicylates-in-the-treatment-of-inflammatory-bowel-disease. Published May 13, 2019. Accessed 5 Dec 2019.
45. Al Hashash J, Regueiro M. Overview of medical management of high-risk, adult patients with moderate to severe Crohn disease. UpToDate. https://www.uptodate.com/contents/overview-of-medical-management-of-high-risk-adult-patients-with-moderate-to-severe-crohn-disease. Published November 25, 2019. Accessed 6 Dec 2019.

46. Lin SC, Cheifetz AS. The use of complementary and alternative medicine in patients with inflammatory bowel disease. Gastroenterol Hepatol. 2018;14(7):415–25.
47. Storr M, Devlin S, Kaplan GG, Panaccione R, Andrews CN. Cannabis use provides symptom relief in patients with inflammatory bowel disease but is associated with worse disease prognosis in patients with Crohn's disease. Inflamm Bowel Dis. 2014;20(3):472–80.
48. Sandborn WJ, Feagan BG, Hanauer SB, et al. A review of activity indices and efficacy endpoints for clinical trials of medical therapy in adults with Crohn's disease. Gastroenterology. 2002;122:512–30.
49. Ahmed W, Katz S. Therapeutic use of cannabis in inflammatory bowel disease. Gastroenterol Hepatol. 2016;12(11):668–79.
50. Ambrose T, Simmons A. Cannabis, cannabinoids, and the endocannabinoid system—is there therapeutic potential for inflammatory bowel disease? J Crohns Colitis. 2018;13(4):525–35. https://doi.org/10.1093/ecco-jcc/jjy185.
51. Naftali T, Bar-Lev Schleider L, Dotan I, Lansky EP, Sklerovsky Benjaminov F, Konikoff FM. Cannabis induces a clinical response in patients with Crohn's disease: a prospective placebo-controlled study. Clin Gastroenterol Hepatol. 2013;11(10):1276–1280.e1. https://doi.org/10.1016/j.cgh.2013.04.034. Epub 2013 May 4
52. Crohn's Disease Activity Index (CDAI). Calculate by QxMD. https://qxmd.com/calculate/calculator_337/crohn-s-disease-activity-index-cdai. Published 2019. Accessed 6 Dec 2019.
53. Irving PM, Iqbal T, Nwokolo C, et al. A randomized, double-blind, placebo-controlled, parallel-group, pilot study of cannabidiol-rich botanical extract in the symptomatic treatment of ulcerative colitis. Inflamm Bowel Dis. 2018;24(4):714–24.
54. Kafil TS, Nguyen TM, MacDonald JK, Chande N. Cannabis for the treatment of Crohn's disease. Cochrane Database Syst Rev. 2018;11. Art. No.: CD012853 https://doi.org/10.1002/14651858.CD012853.pub2.
55. Kafil TS, Nguyen TM, MacDonald JK, Chande N. Cannabis for the treatment of ulcerative colitis. Cochrane Database Syst Rev. 2018;11. Art. No.: CD012954. https://doi.org/10.1002/14651858.CD012954.pub2.
56. Guyatt GH, Oxman AD, Vist GE, Kunz R, Falck-Ytter Y, Alonso-Coello P, et al. GRADE: an emerging consensus on rating quality of evidence and strength of recommendations. BMJ. 2008;336(7650):924–6.
57. Naftali T, Mechulam R, Marii A, Gabay G, Stein A, Bronshtain M, et al. Low-dose cannabidiol is safe but not effective in the treatment for Crohn's Disease, a randomized controlled trial. Dig Dis Sci. 2017;62:1615–20.
58. Swaminath A, Berlin EP, Cheifetz A, Hoffenberg E, Kinnucan J, Wingate L, et al. The role of cannabis in the management of inflammatory bowel disease: a review of clinical, scientific, and regulatory information. Inflamm Bowel Dis. 2018;25(3):427–35. https://doi.org/10.1093/ibd/izy319.
59. Gastroesophageal reflux disease (GERD). Mayo Clinic. https://www.mayoclinic.org/diseases-conditions/gerd/symptoms-causes/syc-20361940. Published October 23, 2019. Accessed 13 Nov 2019.
60. Signs of Gastroesophageal Reflux Disease. Main Line Gastroenterology Associates. https://mainlinegi.com/encounter-health/about-heartburnreflux. Published 2019. Accessed 13 Nov 2019.
61. Kahrilas P. Clinical manifestations and diagnosis of gastroesophageal reflux in adults. UpToDate. https://www.uptodate.com/contents/clinical-manifestations-and-diagnosis-of-gastroesophageal-reflux-in-adults?search=gerd&source=search_result&selectedTitle=3~150&usage_type=default&display_rank=3#H3. Published March 6, 2018. Accessed 13 Nov 2019.
62. Koek GH, Sifrim D, Lerut T, Janssens J, Tack J. Effect of the GABA(B) agonist baclofen in patients with symptoms and duodeno-gastro-oesophageal reflux refractory to proton pump inhibitors. Gut. 2003;52(10):1397–402.

63. Gotfried J, Kataria R, Schey R. Review: the role of cannabinoids on esophageal function—what we know thus far. Cannabis Cannabinoid Res. 2017;2(1):252–8. https://doi.org/10.1089/can.2017.0031.
64. Dent J, Dodds WJ, Friedman RH, et al. Mechanism of gastroesophageal reflux in recumbent asymptomatic human subjects. J Clin Invest. 1980;65:256–67.
65. Mittal RK, Holloway RH, Penagini R, et al. Transient lower esophageal sphincter relaxation. Gastroenterology. 1995;109:601–10.
66. Aizpurua-Olaizola O, Elezgarai I, Rico-Barrio I, et al. Targeting the endocannabinoid system: future therapeutic strategies. Drug Discov Today. 2017;22:105–10.
67. Coutts AA, Irving AJ, Mackie K, et al. Localisation of cannabinoid CB(1) receptor immunoreactivity in the guinea pig and rat myenteric plexus. J Comp Neurol. 2002;448:410–22.
68. Matsuda LA, Bonner TI, Lolait SJ. Localization of cannabinoid receptor mRNA in rat brain. J Comp Neurol. 1993;327:535–50.
69. Duncan M, Mouihate A, Mackie K, et al. Cannabinoid CB2 receptors in the enteric nervous system modulate gastrointestinal contractility in lipopolysaccharide-treated rats. Am J Physiol Gastrointest Liver Physiol. 2008;295:G78–87.
70. Coutts AA, Izzo AA. The gastrointestinal pharmacology of cannabinoids: an update. Curr Opin Pharmacol. 2004;4:572–9.
71. Wright K, Rooney N, Feeney M, et al. Differential expression of cannabinoid receptors in the human colon: cannabinoids promote epithelialwound healing. Gastroenterology. 2005;129:437–53.
72. Pertwee RG. Cannabinoids and the gastrointestinal tract. Gut. 2001;48:859–67.
73. Boesmans W, Ameloot K, van den Abbeel V, et al. Cannabinoid receptor 1 signalling dampens activity and mitochondrial transport in networks of enteric neurones. Neurogastroenterol Motil. 2009;21:958–e77.
74. Hornby PJ, Prouty SM. Involvement of cannabinoid receptors in gut motility and visceral perception. Br J Pharmacol. 2004;141:1335–45.
75. Pinto L, Capasso R, Di Carlo G, et al. Endocannabinoids and the gut. Prostaglandins Leukot Essent Fatty Acids. 2002;66:333–41.
76. Yuece B, Sibaev A, Broedl UC, et al. Cannabinoid type 1 receptor modulates intestinal propulsion by an attenuation of intestinal motor responses within the myenteric part of the peristaltic reflex. Neurogastroenterol Motil. 2007;19:744–53.
77. Izzo AA, Mascolo N, Pinto L, et al. The role of cannabinoid receptors in intestinal motility, defaecation and diarrhoea in rats. Eur J Pharmacol. 1999;384:37–42.
78. Storr MA, Yuce B, Andrews CN, et al. The role of the endocannabinoid system in the pathophysiology and treatment of irritable bowel syndrome. Neurogastroenterol Motil. 2008;20:857–68.
79. Adami M, Zamfirova R, Sotirov E, et al. Gastric antisecretory effects of synthetic cannabinoids after central or peripheral administration in the rat. Brain Res Bull. 2004;64:357–61.
80. Van Sickle MD, Duncan M, Kingsley PJ, et al. Identification and functional characterization of brainstem cannabinoid CB2 receptors. Science. 2005;310:329–32.
81. Onaivi ES. Neuropsychobiological evidence for the functional presence and expression of cannabinoid CB2 receptors in the brain. Neuropsychobiology. 2006;54:231–46.
82. Storr M, Gaffal E, Saur D, et al. Effect of cannabinoids on neural transmission in rat gastric fundus. Can J Physiol Pharmacol. 2002;80:67–76.
83. Berdyshev EV. Cannabinoid receptors and the regulation of immune response. Chem Phys Lipids. 2000;108:169–90.
84. Izzo AA. The cannabinoid CB(2) receptor: a good friend in the gut. NeurogastroenterolMotil. 2007;19:704–8.
85. Calabrese C, Spisni E, Liguori G, et al. Potential role of the cannabinoid receptor CB in the pathogenesis of erosive and non-erosive gastrooesophageal reflux disease. Aliment Pharmacol Ther. 2010;32:603–11.

86. Beaumont H, Jensen J, Carlsson A, et al. Effect of delta9- tetrahydrocannabinol, a cannabinoid receptor agonist, on the triggering of transient lower oesophageal sphincter relaxations in dogs and humans. Br J Pharmacol. 2009;156:153–62.

87. Ameri A. The effects of cannabinoids on the brain. Prog Neurobiol. 1999;58:315–48.

88. Plowright AT, Nilsson K, Antonsson M, et al. Discovery of agonists of cannabinoid receptor 1 with restricted central nervous system penetration aimed for treatment of gastroesophageal reflux disease. J Med Chem. 2013;56:220–40.

89. Dickman R, Shapiro M, Malagon IB, et al. Assessment of 24-h oesophageal pH monitoring should be divided to awake and asleep rather than upright and supine time periods. Neurogastroenterol Motil. 2007;19:709–15.

90. Mostafeezur RM, Zakir HM, Takatsuji H, et al. Cannabinoids facilitate the swallowing reflex elicited by the superior laryngeal nerve stimulation in rats. PLoS One. 2012;7:e50703.

91. Scarpellini E, Blondeau K, Boecxstaens V, et al. Effect of rimonabant on oesophageal motor function in man. Aliment Pharmacol Ther. 2011;33:730–7.

92. Blondeau K, Boecxstaens V, Rommel N, et al. Baclofen improves symptoms and reduces postprandial flow events in patients with rumination and supragastric belching. Clin Gastroenterol Hepatol. 2012;10:379–84.

93. Medical information reviewed by Joseph R. Medical marijuana as an alternative treatment for acid reflux. Marijuanadoctors.com. https://www.marijuanadoctors.com/conditions/acid-reflux/. Published 28 January 2019

94. Update: Interim Guidance for Health Care Providers Evaluating and Caring for Patients with Suspected E-cigarette, or Vaping, Product Use Associated Lung Injury – United States, October 2019. Centers for Disease Control and Prevention. https://www.cdc.gov/mmwr/volumes/68/wr/mm6841e3.htm. Published October 17, 2019. Accessed 18 Nov 2019.

95. Alkhouri N, Kay MH. Non-alcoholic Fatty Liver Disease (NAFLD). American College of Gastroenterology. https://gi.org/topics/fatty-liver-disease-nafld/. Published December 2012. Accessed 20 July 2019.

96. Bazsinsky-Wutschke I, Zipprich A, Dehghani F. Endocannabinoid system in hepatic glucose metabolism, fatty liver disease, and cirrhosis. Int J Mol Sci. 2019;20(10):2516. https://doi.org/10.3390/ijms20102516.

97. Sanna C, Rosso C, Marietti M, Bugianesi E. Non-alcoholic fatty liver disease and extrahepatic cancers. Int J Mol Sci. 2016;17(5):717. Published 2016 May 12. https://doi.org/10.3390/ijms17050717.

98. Araújo AR, Rosso N, Bedogni G, Tiribelli C, Bellentani S. Global epidemiology of non-alcoholic fatty liver disease/non-alcoholic steatohepatitis: What we need in the future. Liver Int. 2018;38:47–51. https://doi.org/10.1111/liv.13643.

99. Younossi ZM, Stepanova M, Negro F, et al. Nonalcoholic fatty liver disease in lean individuals in the United States. Medicine. 2012;91(6):319–27. https://doi.org/10.1097/md.0b013e3182779d49.

100. Golabi P, Paik J, Fukui N, Locklear CT, de Avilla L, Younossi ZM. Patients with lean non-alcoholic fatty liver disease are metabolically abnormal and have a higher risk for mortality. Clin Diab. 2019;37(1):65–72. https://doi.org/10.2337/cd18-0026.

101. Duarte SM, Stefano JT, Oliveira CP. Microbiota and nonalcoholic fatty liver disease/non-alcoholic steatohepatitis (NAFLD/NASH). Ann Hepatol. 2019;18(3):416–21. https://doi.org/10.1016/j.aohep.2019.04.006.

102. Mackie K. Cannabinoid receptors: where they are and what they do. J Neuroendocrinol. 2008;20(s1):10–4. https://doi.org/10.1111/j.1365-2826.2008.01671.x.

103. Clark T, Jones J, Hall A, Tabner S, Kmiec R. Theoretical explanation for reduced body mass index and obesity rates in *cannabis* users. Cannabis Cannabinoid Res. 2018;3(1):259–71. https://doi.org/10.20944/preprints201807.0197.v1.

104. Mallat A, Lotersztajn S. Endocannabinoids and liver disease. I. Endocannabinoids and their receptors in the liver. Am J Physiol-Gastro Liver Physiol. 2008;294(1). https://doi.org/10.1152/ajpgi.00467.2007.

105. McDonnell AM, Dang CH. Basic review of the cytochrome p450 system. J Adv Pract Oncol. 2013;4(4):263–8.
106. Brown JD, Winterstein AG. Potential adverse drug events and drug–drug interactions with Medical and Consumer Cannabidiol (CBD) Use. J Clin Med. 2019;8(7):989. https://doi.org/10.3390/jcm8070989.
107. Alsherbiny MA, Li CG. Medicinal cannabis – potential drug interactions. Med. 2018. https://doi.org/10.20944/preprints201812.0032.v1.
108. Leino AD, Emoto C, Fukuda T, Privitera M, Vinks AA, Alloway RR. Evidence of a clinically significant drug-drug interaction between cannabidiol and tacrolimus. Am J Transplant. 2019. https://doi.org/10.1111/ajt.15398.
109. Hauser N, Sahai T, Richards R, Roberts T. High on cannabis and calcineurin inhibitors: a word of warning in an era of legalized marijuana. Case Reports Transplantat. 2018;2016:1–1. https://doi.org/10.1155/2018/7095846.
110. Rai HS, Winder GS. Curr Psychiatry Rep. 2017;19:91. https://doi.org/10.1007/s11920-017-0843-1.
111. Adejumo AC, Alliu S, Ajayi TO, et al. Cannabis use is associated with reduced prevalence of non-alcoholic fatty liver disease: a cross-sectional study. PLoS One. 2017;12(4):e0176416. Published 2017 Apr 25. https://doi.org/10.1371/journal.pone.0176416.
112. Kim D, Kim W, Kwak M-S, Chung GE, Yim JY, Ahmed A. Inverse association of marijuana use with nonalcoholic fatty liver disease among adults in the United States. Plos One. 2017;12(10). https://doi.org/10.1371/journal.pone.0186702.
113. Dibba P, Li A, Cholankeril G, Iqbal U, Gadiparthi C, Khan MA, Kim D, Ahmed A. Mechanistic potential and therapeutic implications of cannabinoids in nonalcoholic fatty liver disease. Med. 2018;5(2):47.
114. Millar S, Stone N, Bellman Z, Yates A, England T, Osullivan S. A systematic review of cannabidiol dosing in clinical populations. Br J Clin Pharmacol. 2019. https://doi.org/10.1111/bcp.14038.
115. Ewing LE, Skinner CM, Quick CM, et al. Hepatotoxicity of a cannabidiol-rich cannabis extract in the mouse model. Molecules. 2019;24(9):1694. Published 2019 Apr 30. https://doi.org/10.3390/molecules24091694.
116. Epidiolex [package insert]. Carlsbad: Greenwich Biosciences, Inc; 2018.
117. Vandrey R, Raber JC, Raber ME, Douglass B, Miller C, Bonn-Miller MO. Cannabinoid dose and label accuracy in edible medical cannabis products. JAMA. 2015;313(24):2491. https://doi.org/10.1001/jama.2015.6613.
118. Bonn-Miller MO, Loflin MJE, Thomas BF, Marcu JP, Hyke T, Vandrey R. Labeling accuracy of cannabidiol extracts sold online. JAMA. 2017;318(17):1708–9. https://doi.org/10.1001/jama.2017.11909.

Chapter 18
Looking at Marijuana Through the Lens of Public Health

Elizabeth Brooks and Stig Erik Sørheim

Introduction

The rapid pace of marijuana legalization across the United States (US) and Canada presents a significant challenge to public health professionals, who are charged with the responsibility to promote health and community well-being.

The field of public health has historically been driven by science. However, the peer-reviewed evidence base on marijuana-related harms – and benefits – is limited. Numerous studies find association between marijuana use and various adverse outcomes. However, in many cases the evidence for causal effects is inconclusive, and it is difficult to completely discount residual confounding or even reverse causality. Some of the phenomena that we are interested in are relatively recent, and the research simply has not caught up. The legal framework around marijuana is evolving rapidly, new and more potent marijuana products have emerged, marijuana use patterns are changing, and new routes of administration have gained popularity. Thus, some of the evidence we rely on today may already be outdated.

The manufacturing, distribution, and use of cannabis are regulated globally by the International Drug Control Conventions. In the United States, it is regulated by the Controlled Substances Act (CSA), which was passed by Congress in 1970. The CSA outlined a scheduling system which placed marijuana in the most restrictive schedule, thereby limiting the opportunity to carry out marijuana research in the United States.

E. Brooks
University of Colorado, Aurora, CO, USA

Whole Health Innovation, Denver, CO, USA

S. E. Sørheim (✉)
Actis-Norwegian Policy Network on Alcohol and Drugs, Oslo, Norway
e-mail: ses@actis.no

© Springer Nature Switzerland AG 2020
K. Finn (ed.), *Cannabis in Medicine*,
https://doi.org/10.1007/978-3-030-45968-0_18

Under the International Drug Control Conventions, the World Health Organization is charged with conducting medical, scientific, and public health evaluation of substances to reflect new knowledge [1]. In 2018, the WHO Expert Committee on Drug Dependence (ECDD) for the first time reviewed cannabis and cannabis-related substances, including cannabidiol (CBD). They recommended that cannabis be moved from the most restrictive schedule (Schedule IV) of the international drug conventions to the second most restrictive schedule (Schedule I), partly due to the potential medical effects of cannabis and partly because cannabis was regarded as less harmful than other drugs in Schedule IV, such as heroin and fentanyl [2]. Furthermore, they recommended that CBD should not be scheduled under the international drug conventions since it is not psychoactive and there is no evidence of abuse or dependence and since CBD also has medical uses [3].

Despite a growing evidence base, the information that we have about cannabis is still somewhat tentative and preliminary. Research points to a number of possible concerns, and new issues may arise as the situation evolves. The surge of vaping-related lung illness in 2019 is a striking case in point. Careful monitoring is needed to identify public health challenges and strengthen the evidence base. Simultaneously, marijuana legalization efforts are accompanied by disparate, and often outspoken, political and social views about its risks and benefits. Anecdotal reports are commonplace.

We are maneuvering through an era of broad marijuana legalization and decriminalization efforts with limited evidence. However, lessons from other fields of public health can provide some guidance. Experiences with alcohol and tobacco suggest that social norms, price, availability, and exposure influence consumption in a population, and that population-level harm is related to consumption levels.

In 1994, the Centers for Disease Control and Environment (CDC) defined the three core functions of public health: assessing, monitoring, and investigating potential health hazards; developing and enforcing policies to regulate, mobilize, and empower groups or individuals; and assuring the effectiveness of programs while linking and educating communities. Public health professionals must respond to new and evolving conditions and events in order to carry out these core functions. The response must be based on the best available evidence and requires monitoring, policy development, community and individual empowerment, as well as continuous evaluation to improve performance.

In this chapter, we present an overview of the most salient topics in the field today, with consideration for the limitations noted above. Many of these topics will be treated at greater length in other chapters of this book. Using the CDC framework as a backdrop, we discuss how marijuana legalization and decriminalization efforts influence public health monitoring, policy, and assurance. Specifically, we review marijuana use and differential risks; health concerns related to accidents and harm associated with acute intoxication, physical health effects, mental health effects and harm to others; and public health response regarding regulations and campaign messaging.

Marijuana Use and Differential Risks

Consumption Rates

While public health is not primarily occupied with the legal status of marijuana, changes in use and usage patterns are relevant to its mission of ensuring community well-being. Insofar as legal status and regulations impact use, public health and safety can be influenced by the rapid increase in legalization and decriminalization.

Historically, most marijuana research has been done in places with relatively low consumption and low rates of heavy, persistent use. Users primarily smoked low potency marijuana, either alone or with tobacco. A look at marijuana today presents a markedly different picture. Consumption rates today are higher; around one in three young adults uses marijuana regularly in states like Colorado, Oregon, Vermont, and Maine, according to the 2017 NSDUH survey [4], and the share of daily or near-daily users has increased [5].

Differential Use Patterns

Differential use patterns have been noted in specific areas and by specific populations. This preliminary finding stands out as an important area to monitor in public health. Several studies indicate that availability influences marijuana use [6–8]. Experience with alcohol and tobacco shows that there are more outlets in less affluent and minority communities [9–11]; a similar trend has been found with marijuana in recent data from Colorado and Washington [12–14]. There is further concern that consumption of marijuana is skewed toward a small minority of heavy users with low socioeconomic status [5]. Recent data from Monitoring the Future shows that the rate of daily marijuana use is twice as high among young adults who do not attend college, compared to their peers in college [15].

Early evidence suggests that legalization affects social norms, which, in turn, may impact consumption rates. Social norms among young college age adults have changed more rapidly in Colorado than in the country as a whole [16]. One study found that the frequency of marijuana use in Colorado college students was much higher than the national average, particularly daily or near-daily use [17]. A review found media coverage, advertising, and social media overwhelmingly favorable to marijuana and positively correlated with the audience's marijuana-related beliefs and behaviors [18]. Furthermore, a study of adolescents in California found that exposure to marijuana marketing was associated with greater intention to use, higher average use, and more negative consequences over a 7-year period [6].

The NSDUH surveys show that legal states are among the highest consuming states in the United States, with a sharper increase than the rest of the country [19]. Population survey results are supported by other data sources. For example, a recent wastewater analysis from Washington state found a two- to threefold increase in marijuana use since legalization [20].

Potency and Methods of Consumption

Marijuana today is not like marijuana of the past. In the last two decades, tetrahydrocannabinol (THC) potency has risen sharply [21–24], and new products and routes of administration have emerged. Edible products, topical creams, marijuana oils, and various concentrates make up a growing share of the total marijuana market. While the consequences of high THC marijuana are not well documented, studies show that higher potency is associated with a greater severity of dependence [25], an increase in the number of people who seek treatment [26], higher risk of progression to marijuana use disorder [27], and higher rates of psychosis [28–30].

While smoking marijuana remains the most common mode of consumption, vaping and edible use is increasing. Many young people use several modes of administration, which may carry different risks. Most emergency room visits are due to inhaled marijuana; however, edibles seem to carry a greater risk of acute psychiatric visits, intoxication, and cardiovascular symptoms [31]. The shift toward dabbing high concentrate marijuana (such as wax or shatter) carries specific risks, including paranoia, psychosis, burns, and other inhalation injuries [32].

Accidents and Harm Associated with Acute Intoxication

In addition to euphoric effects, marijuana intoxication is associated with impaired thinking and concentration, drowsiness, short-term memory loss, loss of coordination and balance, changes in sensory perception, slower reaction time, and lower ability to perform complex tasks. These acute effects can increase the risk of accidents and harms.

Road Traffic Accidents

Given the temporary physiologic changes that accompany marijuana use, public health is interested in understanding whether the legalization of marijuana increases incidents of impaired driving and accidents. Epidemiological and experimental studies find that marijuana impairs driving performance and increases the risk of crashes. [33] The risk of motor vehicle accidents is 2–3 times higher among marijuana-impaired drivers, with substantially increased risk if the driver also has elevated blood alcohol level [34].

The number of drivers in fatal accidents who tested positive for Delta-9 THC (indicating recent use) in Washington doubled from 2013 to 2017 [35]. Most of these tested above 5 ng/ml and were positive for alcohol or other drugs [36]. Marijuana-related fatalities also increased in Colorado, with a 109% increase in the number of marijuana-related fatalities between 2013 and 2018 [37]. Other studies compared traffic fatalities in neighboring states where marijuana was and was not legalized, finding a temporary increase in Colorado, Washington, and Oregon 1 year after legalization [38].

Survey data suggest that there is an association between people's perception of risk and their willingness to drive after using [35, 39]. Seven in ten marijuana users in Colorado reported driving within 3 hours after using during the past year; 27% of users said they drove under the influence of marijuana almost daily [40].

Marijuana can stay in a person's system anywhere from a few hours to up to several weeks, depending on how much is consumed, frequency of use and individual tolerance. The pharmacology of marijuana makes it difficult to assess impairment levels. While there is a close correspondence between blood alcohol content and alcohol intoxication, the relationship between THC levels and intoxication is less consistent and depends on the route of administration.

Workplace Accidents

Based on road accident research, it is plausible that marijuana impairment increases the risk of workplace accidents, injuries, and fatalities [41]. A study of Egyptian construction workers found increased injury severity and more workdays lost among workers who used marijuana [42]. Empirical data in this area are scarce, and effects would likely be dependent on the job sector.

Marijuana use can be of concern in safety sensitive industries. Some business owners report difficulty finding employees who can pass a drug test [43]. National data from the private drug testing company, Quest, reported an increase in positive urine tests for marijuana among nearly all workforce categories from 2004 to 2018 [44].

Violence

The association between marijuana and violence is controversial. Some studies suggest that marijuana is associated with reduced aggression [45]; others find a higher risk of violence [46, 47]. Aggression, increased hostility, and impulsiveness are linked to withdrawal [48, 49], although the risk is relatively modest compared to alcohol.

There is an association between marijuana and psychosis and an association between psychosis and violence in some patients [50]. Marijuana use disorder has been shown to be a risk factor for violence in the early phase of psychosis and in patients with severe mental illness [51–54]. However, given the limited numbers of patients affected, it is unclear if increased risk estimates are large enough to register on the population level.

Hospital and ER Admissions and Overdose

Despite claims that marijuana is a relatively benign and safe drug, marijuana-related emergency room visits and hospital admissions have increased in the United States in recent years [55]. Providers treat a variety of marijuana-related symptoms, including gastrointestinal problems and cardiorespiratory effects, traumatic injuries, and accidental ingestions [56]. Patients may present with varying degrees of mental health symptomology, such as anxiety, paranoia, and psychosis. Studies show high rates of co-occurring mental health diagnoses in marijuana-related ER and hospital visits [57]. In addition to physical and mental health symptomology, patients present with acute injuries including burns from butane hash oil explosions [58] and inhalational injuries [32].

There is growing concern about increased marijuana-related emergencies in children and teens, particularly in newly legal markets [56]. In recent years, there has been increasing awareness of cannabis hyperemesis syndrome (CHS) – uncontrolled and sustained vomiting that subsides when marijuana use ceases [59]. Studies suggest that CHS is frequently undiagnosed and considerably more common than previously thought, potentially impacting more than two million patients a year [60, 61]. The syndrome can be a costly and potentially serious condition, with documented reports of fatalities [62, 63].

Several studies from Colorado found increases in marijuana-related emergency room visits following legalization, perhaps even tripling in frequency [64, 65]. While the majority of emergency room visits were related to inhaled marijuana, edible products accounted for a disproportionate share. Inhaled marijuana was more likely to result in hospitalization, whereas edibles more often result in acute psychiatric symptoms, intoxication, and cardiovascular symptoms [31]. Finn and Salmore found a steep increase in marijuana-related diagnoses at a Colorado hospital between 2009 and 2014, resulting in significant costs to the facility [66]. Other studies found increases in adolescent marijuana-related visits in recent years [67]. Still, the data is not completely consistent. Research looking at inpatient databases found neutral effects on healthcare utilization in the time immediately following legalization compared to two other states [68]. Many of the hospital studies have a low base rate of visits, and the precise clinical relevance is unclear. Further, the study designs often make it difficult to tease out differences between marijuana-related presentations and recent procedural changes which improved marijuana identification.

According to the CDC, direct overdose deaths due to a lethal dose of marijuana are unlikely. Still, this does not mean that ingestion amount is inconsequential. High dosages of marijuana are typically more severe, and effects may include extreme confusion, anxiety, paranoia, panic, rapid heart rate, delusions or hallucinations, increased blood pressure, and severe nausea or vomiting [69].

Physical Health Effects

From a public health perspective, the legalization and decriminalization of marijuana raises concerns about the potential for adverse health effects

Pulmonary Effects

Even though new ways of ingesting marijuana have increased, smoking remains the most common route of administration. In the legal market in Colorado, researchers found that nearly all young people who use marijuana smoke some or most of the time [70]. Decades of research has demonstrated the harmful effects of cigarette smoking; [71] alarmingly, marijuana smoke contains many of the same substances and carcinogens as tobacco smoke, and inhaling burning plant material may harm the lungs. Currently, however, research on the effects of marijuana smoke on lung cancer, emphysema, and chronic obstructive pulmonary disease (COPD) is unclear and inconsistent [34, 72]. Possible explanations include (1) the effect of smoking marijuana may not be as strong as tobacco, (2) marijuana use traditionally has been less intensive than tobacco smoking, or (3) it is hard to disentangle the harms from marijuana from those of tobacco.

Still, other pulmonary problems appear similar to those found in cigarette smokers; marijuana has been linked to chronic bronchitis, coughing, wheezing, and sputum production [34, 73]. Marijuana was identified as a risk factor for bronchial asthma or use of asthma medication in a Norwegian sample, even when controlling for known confounders [74]. Concurrent use of marijuana and tobacco may increase the risk of respiratory harm [75].

Pulmonary Effects from Vaping

In the summer of 2019, there were almost 200 reports of severe lung illness linked to vaping within a couple of weeks. Patients presented with shortness of breath, breathing problems, vomiting, diarrhea, and fever. Some patients were intubated and required treatment in intensive care units [76]. By the end of September 2019, the CDC were investigating 530 cases, and there were at least 8 confirmed fatalities [77].

The cases involved different types of vaping devices and different vaping liquids. Early reports indicate that a majority of the cases were linked to THC oils [78].

While many of the cases involved black market cannabis oil, at least one of the fatalities was an Oregon man who had used a vaping device containing marijuana bought at a licensed dispensary [79].

Many of the patients were quite young. A study from Wisconsin and Illinois shows that the median age was 19 years [78]. However, harms are not limited to young people. The age range in the study was 16–53 years, and at least one of the fatalities was a person over 50 years.

Little is known about the risks of nicotine vaping, and even less is known about vaping cannabis oil. So far it is unclear whether the cases are linked to specific vaping devices, to vaping in general, or to specific vaping products. While black market THC oils are a strong suspect, other vaping liquids have also been involved [76, 79]. Despite regulation, a study found that 50% of THC vaping products in Washington were over the state's threshold for pesticides [76]. Other possible culprits include harmful substances in commercially available vaping products, such as formaldehyde, tin and lead, as well as certain flavoring and thickening agents.

It is also possible that the phenomenon is not new, but that earlier cases were misclassified or overlooked. Case reports have described similar events before [80, 81].

Further research is needed to understand the mechanisms between vaping and lung illness. However, the recent cases clearly illustrate the need for careful monitoring and evidence-based policy responses.

Cardiovascular Effects

A number of adverse cardiovascular effects are associated with marijuana use, including sudden cardiac death, vascular events, arrhythmias, and stress cardiomyopathy in relatively young users [82–84]. While the most serious cardiovascular events are rare, researchers speculate that they may be underdiagnosed [85]. A population-based study found that marijuana abuse was significantly associated with elevated rates of myocardial infarction in women and young people, even when controlling for known risk factors [86], and that the risk of myocardial infarction increased fourfold for up to an hour after smoking. After controlling for several known confounders, Kalla et al. found that marijuana was an independent predictor of heart failure and cerebrovascular events [87]. Marijuana use has also been shown to produce symptoms of angina in older users [34].

Cancer

Because marijuana contains many of the same carcinogens as tobacco and is often inhaled in the same manner, there may be similar linkages with lung cancer. [88] Research in this area, however, is unclear and often contradictory [34, 89, 90]. A recent meta-analysis [91] finds an association with higher lung cancer rates, although the risk appears to be much lower than with tobacco [92]. Several studies showed an association between marijuana use and testicular cancer [93, 94], particularly among long-term users (>10 years) [91]. There is limited evidence linking marijuana use to other types of cancer [95].

Reproductive Health

Researchers have examined the correlation between marijuana use and infertility in men and women. Smoking marijuana is associated with reduced sperm count, sperm motility, and viability. Evidence from experimental, observational, and animal studies show mixed results concerning fertility among men who use marijuana [96–99]. There is some evidence that cannabinoids can affect the female reproductive system. Studies show that marijuana use can influence ovulation and that exogenous cannabinoids can lower estrogen and progesterone levels [100, 101]. Despite considerable uncertainty, a recent review article concludes that marijuana may reduce the ability to conceive in couples that have difficulties getting pregnant, but not in couples without fertility issues [102].

Mental Health Effects

One of the findings from marijuana research over the past decades is that regular marijuana use is consistently associated with poor psychosocial outcomes and mental health in adulthood [34]. In the absence of randomized trials, it is difficult to tease out causal relationships. However, for some mental health conditions, there is strong evidence for a causal connection and increasing insight into possible biological mechanisms.

Addiction

Despite its reputation as a natural and benign drug, marijuana can be addictive, and those with marijuana dependence may suffer through cycles of use, relapse, and withdrawal, just like any other drug. Earlier studies suggest that around one in nine marijuana users become addicted to marijuana, with risk estimates jumping to one in six among adolescents [34]. Addiction research among recent or current users show even higher rates. NSDUH data indicate that 15% of past month users meet the DSM-IV criteria for a marijuana use disorder [103]; the rate jumps significantly among daily users, with estimates between 30–50% [34, 104].

There is some concern that the rate of marijuana addiction has risen since the most frequently cited studies in the 1990s. THC potency has increased, and new methods of using marijuana have gained popularity. Most sources indicate that marijuana use disorders increased in the United States since 2002 [105], although it is difficult to determine if this is the result of more dependency or better identification of the problem. Analyses show that recent increases were significantly higher in some groups, particularly among men, African Americans, urban residents, and populations who were unmarried or had lower incomes [106]. Somewhat inconsistently, NSDUH data found declining rates of marijuana use disorder among heavy users in the same time period [107, 108]. Changes in addiction rates are not limited to American populations, however. Europe has seen a sharp increase in the number of patients seeking treatment for marijuana use disorders, despite stable use [109]. Marijuana is now the most frequently cited drug among new patients entering treatment in Europe [110]. Marijuana users are significantly more likely to experience addiction than, e.g., psychosis [111].

Marijuana withdrawal is not uncommon. Several studies demonstrate marijuana withdrawal syndrome after cessation of regular use [112]. The symptoms include irritability, anger, aggression, nervousness or anxiety, sleep problems, reduced appetite and weight loss, restlessness, depressed mood, and physical symptoms such as abdominal pain, sweating, fever or chills, and headaches [105, 113]. Symptoms are experienced most during the first week of cessation and can persist up to a month. A study of regular users (>3 times per week) found that 12% reported experiencing withdrawal [114]. Withdrawal increases among heavy users in treatment, with more than half reporting symptoms. Marijuana withdrawal can be debilitating for the user and may present as an obstacle to cessation [105, 114].

Cognitive Effects and the Developing Brain

Acute effects of marijuana use include impaired attention, motor skills, executive functions, and working and episodic memory. Most effects are transitory and cease after less than a month [111, 115–118]. Whereas these short-term effects are well documented, long-term effects are more controversial. It is notoriously difficult to establish causal connections, and even when studies control for known confounders, residual confounding or reverse causality cannot be discounted.

There is strong evidence that marijuana use is associated with poor psychosocial outcomes (e.g., higher risk of dropping out of high school and poorer grades, lower likelihood of enrolling in higher education or attaining a university degree) [119–122]. NSDUH data show that the age of marijuana initiation is associated with unemployment [123]. At least some of these outcomes may be modifiable; research suggests that memory and grades improve upon maintained abstinence [124, 125].

A recent review suggests that long-term cognitive effects have been overstated and that reported deficits can be explained by acute effects or effects of withdrawal [126]. Even if cognitive effects are reversible, persistent marijuana use in formative years can still have long-term effects, because short-term effects could affect educational outcomes or the acquisition of social capital and life skills that are important in adulthood [120].

Growing evidence indicates that the adolescent brain is more vulnerable to marijuana use than the adult brain. The body's own endocannabinoid system plays a key role in neurodevelopment, and the introduction of exogenous cannabinoids could disrupt the balance of the endocannabinoid system. Such a mechanism is further supported by animal studies [115].

IQ and motivation effects are commonly associated with marijuana use. A study from New Zealand found a persistent drop in IQ among adolescent onset heavy marijuana users over a period of several decades [127]. However, a longitudinal study of teenagers failed to find an effect, and two recent twin studies did not find a long-term impact in the late teens [128, 129]. The results in the later three studies may be partly due to shorter observation period than in the New Zealand study. Since the nineteenth century, marijuana has been linked to "amotivation" – a lack of goal-directed behavior, concentration, and perseverance. This effect is supported by Volkow et al. who demonstrated both preclinical and clinical evidence. An acute amotivational effect has also been found in experimental settings [115, 116].

Long-term effects might indicate a change in one's physiology. While brain imaging studies found some alterations in brain structure, the differences are generally limited, and causality is not always established. Many of these studies suffer from small sample sizes, and the clinical relevance is often unclear [115, 118, 130, 131].

Psychosis and Schizophrenia

A number of studies have shown a correlation and a dose-response effect between marijuana use and psychosis or schizophrenia [28, 132]. While rare, marijuana-associated psychosis is a serious outcome for the user. Psychosis, particularly with conversion to schizophrenia, is a significant burden on individuals, families and health services.

Although the absence of randomized controlled trials makes it difficult to establish a causal link between marijuana and psychosis, there is strong evidence supporting such a mechanism. Longitudinal studies show that marijuana use precedes psychotic episodes [115]. Current evidence does not support a self-medication theory [133], and the association between marijuana and psychosis remains after controlling for prodromal symptoms, other drugs, and parental psychosis [134]. Furthermore, a Norwegian study found increased risk of psychotic-like symptoms among marijuana using twins compared to their non-using siblings [135].

The risk of psychosis has been linked to THC in marijuana [136]. THC has been found to cause psychotic symptoms in a laboratory setting [137, 138]. A study by Di Forti et al. found that individuals who used high potency marijuana had elevated rates of psychotic disorders [30]. A European multicenter study demonstrated higher incidence of first episode psychosis in cities with high prevalence of high potency marijuana, and estimated that marijuana is involved in 30% of first episode psychosis in London and 50% in Amsterdam [139]. Population-level estimates indicate that the elimination of marijuana could reduce the incidence of schizophrenia by around 10% [140].

Research has identified some biologically plausible mechanisms between marijuana and psychosis [133, 141, 142]. Marijuana use is linked to earlier onset of psychosis [30], and patients who continue using marijuana after their first psychotic episode have poorer prognosis, increased risk of relapse, and worse outcomes [47, 143–145]. Continued use is also associated with increased conversion to schizophrenia [146–149]. There is likely some interaction between marijuana exposure and individual and genetic vulnerability. Marijuana use is neither a necessary nor a sufficient cause for psychosis and schizophrenia, but current evidence suggests that it is a component cause of psychosis [140].

Other Mental Health Outcomes

Marijuana is associated with a number of other mental health problems, including anxiety and depression. However, the association is less consistent than with psychosis, and the link has not been shown to be causal [95].

A recent review found elevated risk for depression and suicidality, but not for anxiety among young adults [150]. For individuals diagnosed with bipolar disorders, near-daily marijuana use may be linked to greater symptom severity. Regular marijuana use may increase the risk of developing social anxiety disorder [95]. Even though individual risk of mental health problems is moderate in most studies, the association is a public health concern. The relatively large number of marijuana users generates a high potential for elevated risk [150].

Suicide risk is an area of particular alarm. Heavy marijuana users are more likely to report thoughts of suicide than non-users [95, 150, 151]. Teens who use marijuana are more likely to make suicide attempts [150, 152], even in low- and middle-income countries [153]. Data from Colorado shows that marijuana is the most frequently noted substance in toxicological screens of young people who die from suicide [37] and heavy marijuana use is associated with higher suicide risk among army veterans [154].

Use of Other Substances (Alcohol, Opioids, Polydrug Use)

Marijuana use is statistically associated with the use of alcohol, tobacco, and other illicit drugs. People who use tobacco or alcohol are more likely to use marijuana [155]. Although the evidence is still limited, there is early evidence that vaping increases the risk of later marijuana use [156, 157]. Similarly, marijuana users frequently use other substances, particularly alcohol and tobacco [158–160]. The association between marijuana and other substances is sometimes interpreted as a "gateway effect" [161], implying that marijuana use increases the risk of using other substances.

Some evidence from animal studies suggests that marijuana use can alter the brain's susceptibility to other drugs and prime the brain for addiction [92, 162]. This could provide a causal mechanism for a "gateway effect." However, the evidence is still inconclusive. On the other hand, there is strong evidence to suggest that the use of substances is related to underlying personality traits and vulnerabilities. People who are at risk of using drugs use marijuana first because it is most easily available, and some go on to experiment with other drugs later [92, 162].

In recent years, public health experts have expressed concern about a "reverse gateway effect," from marijuana to tobacco use [163]. Recent data show that marijuana is increasingly the first substance used by teens [162]. Marijuana is often used together with tobacco, either mixed in joints, spliffs, or blunts, or, sequentially, as a chaser [164–166]. Survey data show that daily marijuana use occurs predominantly among people who also smoke tobacco [158, 160]. Co-use leads to nicotine exposure, which can result in addiction.

Some studies find a higher risk of later daily tobacco smoking among marijuana users and lower odds of quit attempts [75, 167–169]. If marijuana acts as a gateway to tobacco, an increase in marijuana use could have serious public health consequences by increasing tobacco use [170]. Furthermore, co-use is associated with poorer physical and mental health outcomes in young adults [171]. Some people have hypothesized that increased marijuana use will reduce alcohol consumption and therefore reduce the total burden of substance use problems in society. However, the evidence on substitution is contradictory, suggesting that the effect is unclear and perhaps context dependent [172]. The first states to legalize marijuana have not experienced a decrease in alcohol consumption so far, according to industry data [173]. Simultaneous use of alcohol and marijuana is common [174–176]. Mixing alcohol and marijuana is associated with higher consumption, increased risk of negative outcomes, and greater risk of substance use disorders [176–179]. A longitudinal study found that marijuana use is associated with higher risk of alcohol use disorder, marijuana use disorder, nicotine dependence, and any other drug disorder [180]. Marijuana use is also associated with progression to heavier alcohol involvement [181]. Similarly, marijuana use among young people is associated with higher risk of marijuana use disorder and higher risk of use of other illicit drugs [95, 152]. Polysubstance use patterns are more frequent than single-substance use [182].

Molds and Contaminants

While some tout the use of marijuana as a natural and safe substance, the cultivation of many agricultural products presents possible health risks that are relevant to public health tracking and regulation. The primary concerns associated with marijuana surround molds and contaminants.

Mold appears on marijuana for a variety of reasons. On the production side, mold may develop when the plant is exposed to improper humidity levels, watering, ventilation, or drying techniques. On the consumer side, mold may develop if marijuana is exposed to wet conditions, or there is otherwise improper storage in moist conditions [183]. One recent study found that 90% of 20 marijuana samples purchased from California dispensaries tested positive for bacteria and fungi [184]. Exposure to some molds and bacteria can cause illness, particularly among immunocompromised individuals whose risk of opportunistic lung infections may increase from inhaled molds [185, 186]. In a single study, a case of invasive aspergillosis was associated with marijuana use [187]. Others note a risk to even relatively healthy individuals, as exposure to molds and bacteria is associated with increased symptomology in individuals with asthma [188, 189]. Consistent exposure to some molds may further impair the health of the marijuana industry workers [190].

Like all crops, marijuana plants are vulnerable to pests and disease, sometimes requiring the use of agricultural pesticides [189]. According to researchers, the use of pesticides, particularly when used on unlawful grow operations, is severely underestimated. In one study, researchers found evidence of pesticide residue on 65% of the plants tested [191]. In most countries, pesticides use is regulated by a government agency. In the United States, the federal office of the Environmental Protection Agency (EPA) serves in this capacity. Yet, because the federal government considers marijuana a Schedule I drug, no pesticides have been approved for use on marijuana plants, nor has the EPA provided guidance about levels of "safe" pesticide residues on marijuana products. This has led to concern that growers may apply inappropriate levels of pesticide on marijuana plants [189].

Marijuana is susceptible to contamination by chemicals such as lead, ammonia, and formaldehyde, which have been linked to a handful of adverse health events [192–194]. The process used to create marijuana products such as wax and hash oil is another area of concern. Because of this, many localities with legal marijuana now require contaminant testing, as well as labels that list chemicals used during the growing or production process. However, as regulation policies are established by each separate jurisdiction, safety regulations and subsequent monitoring are not ubiquitous. Exposures represent a potential health hazard not only to the individuals purchasing marijuana but to marijuana industry workers. While more research is needed, some question the safety of workers' exposure to hazards such as dusts, bioaerosols, volatile organic compounds, and ultraviolet radiation during the harvesting and processing phases of marijuana cultivation [195, 196]. While testing requirements and protocols vary between states, evidence suggests that there may be significant shortcomings in this area. An audit by the Oregon Liquor Control Commission determined that the state did not adhere to mandatory inspection schedules, failing to meet even basic standards. In 2018, only 3% of retailers and 32% of growing operations were inspected by regulatory personnel [197].

Harm to Others

Substance use affects not only users, but also the people around them. Secondhand smoke, accidents, fetal effects, and accidental and/or toxic exposure are areas of increased public health concern post-legalization. Further, while we do not expand upon it here, substance use disorders cause considerable stress for children, families, partners, and close friends. Such non-tangible harms are hard to measure, but may have severe emotional, economic, and psychosomatic consequences [198–200].

Secondhand Smoke

Limited evidence on the effects of secondhand smoke from marijuana should not be taken as evidence that it is harmless. Secondhand marijuana smoke shows similar effects to secondhand tobacco smoke in animal studies [82, 201]. Marijuana metabolites can be found in the urine of children who are exposed to marijuana smoke; this risk increases if parents are daily marijuana smokers [202]. Studies found higher likelihood of reporting adverse health outcomes in children who lived in households with marijuana smoking after controlling for cigarette exposure [203] and higher rate of emergency department visits among children who were exposed to a combination of marijuana and tobacco smoke [204].

Social norms surrounding secondhand marijuana smoke have not kept pace with norms surrounding tobacco smoke. The evidence for harmful effects of marijuana smoke is more limited, but inhalation of all kinds of smoke is likely harmful. It may be particularly relevant for cardiovascular effects, which is the main cause of deaths from passive tobacco smoking [205].

Marijuana Use During Pregnancy and Breastfeeding

Several studies have pointed to increasing marijuana use among pregnant women in recent years [206–208]. Volkow et al. documented a twofold increase in marijuana use during pregnancy from 2002/2003 to 2016/2017 [209]. Data from Washington state show a steep increase in marijuana use among pregnant women from 2009 to 2014, accompanied by an increase in the number of maternal inpatients stays related to marijuana use only [210]. Data suggest that marijuana use during pregnancy is more than twice as common among women between 18–25 years than those between 26–44 years [211].

Many women view marijuana as a natural product and therefore believe it is a safer alternative to pharmaceuticals for controlling nausea. However, marijuana use is also increasing among women who do not experience nausea [212–214]. NSDUH data found that 16.2% of pregnant marijuana users report daily or almost daily use, while 18.1% of past year users met the criteria for substance abuse or dependence [212]. National data show an increase in the incidence of marijuana dependence/ abuse among pregnant women from 1999 to 2013 [213].

When marijuana is ingested, cannabinoids cross the placental barrier and may affect the endocannabinoid system of the fetus [214]. Marijuana is associated with a number of adverse outcomes, including increased risk of preterm birth and other complications, such as small size for gestational age, longer hospitalization periods, and transfer to neonatal intensive care unit [213, 215, 216]. Marijuana exposure has been linked to child development and behavior, with evidence of psychosocial, behavioral, and cognitive effects [34]. Animal studies suggest that marijuana affects development and impacts the fetus, with some indication that interaction between alcohol and cannabinoids increases the risk of harm [217–219].

Cannabinoids are easily transferred to breast milk and to the baby. THC can be traced in breast milk several days after last reported marijuana use [220]. Some studies have suggested psychomotor deficits in infants exposed to marijuana in breast milk, although the evidence is yet inconclusive [221]. Breastfeeding guidelines warn against marijuana use during breastfeeding [214].

Perceived risk from regular marijuana use has decreased among both pregnant and nonpregnant women in the United States over the past decade [222]. Ko et al. found that a majority of women believe there is no or little risk of harm from marijuana use once or twice during pregnancy. Bayrampour et al. found that women were uncertain about harmful effects and received little counseling from the health services on the topic [212, 223]. Many women seek medical advice from budtenders regarding the safety of using marijuana during pregnancy. While nonmedical employees are advised to refer clients to healthcare practitioners for these types of conversations, one study documented that an alarming 70% of Colorado dispensaries recommended marijuana for treating nausea in the first trimester [224]. Given the multitude of health risks linked to marijuana use, this indicates the need to improve outreach to both dispensaries and the public about the need to discuss marijuana-related questions with medical professionals.

Accidental Exposure

In recent years there have been numerous reports about children accidentally exposed to cannabinoids, particularly high THC products [225]. One study found that the number of children under the age of 6 who ingested marijuana was stable from 2000 to 2008, but later increased by 27% per year. More than 70% of accidental exposure cases occurred in states with legalized marijuana [226]. An increase in accidental exposure in toddlers was also found in Europe [227].

Many edible products can be hard to distinguish from regular food products and candies, and some products have shapes and colors appealing to young children. Legal access to marijuana could cause more people to store marijuana in their homes, which increases the risk that it could get in the hands of children [228]. Data from Colorado show a doubling in exposure in 2 years after legalization and a higher increase than the rest of the country [229]. A study of accidental exposure among children under 6 years found significantly higher rates in states that legalized medical marijuana [230]. Similarly, a study from Massachusetts found an increase in pediatric marijuana exposure after the introduction of medical marijuana [231].

Health Benefits

The use of marijuana for treating various health conditions is not a new concept, although it has gained attention since the global era of legalization and decriminalization. The use of marijuana for medical purposes stretches thousands of years back in China, Egypt, and India. One example of early use in Western medicine is the treatment of rheumatoid pain and convulsions by Irish physician Sir William O'Shaughnessy in the mid-1800s [232].

The international drug control treaties allow the medical use of marijuana as long as certain requirements are fulfilled. Medical use must be based on scientific evidence, supervised by health personnel and dispensed by prescription, and there must be measures in place to prevent diversion [233].

In Europe, market authorization of medicines requires clinical trials for safety and efficacy. Most European countries allow some medical use of cannabinoids for a limited number of diagnoses or in cases where other treatment options have failed or are causing too many side effects. National medicines authorities have approved different cannabinoid products, mostly medicinal products such as dronabinol or nabiximols (Sativex), but in some cases also standardized marijuana products. No EU country recommends smoking as a mode of consumption [234].

Several countries in Europe also have "early access" or "compassionate" programs that make unauthorized medicines available in certain circumstances. "Early access" medicines must be prescribed by a licensed prescriber, and patients often have to cover the costs of the treatment [234].

The US Food and Drug Administration (FDA) has approved individual components of marijuana or similar synthetic substances for certain conditions. In 2018, the agency authorized the use of the CBD-based drug, Epidiolex, for treating seizures associated with two rare, severe forms of epilepsy. Unlike THC, Epidiolex does not give people the sensation of being "high" when consumed. Furthermore, the FDA has approved the synthetic cannabinoids dronabinol and nabilone for nausea associated with chemotherapy when conventional treatment does not work; dronabinol may also be used for the treatment of weight loss associated with AIDS [235].

The FDA has not approved the marijuana plant as medicine. Nevertheless, a majority of US states allow some form of medical marijuana in addition to the FDA-approved cannabinoids. Many of the state laws have been driven by voter initiatives and passed by referenda. Qualifying conditions vary between the states, and the size of the medical marijuana programs varies widely.

Marijuana has been proposed for a wide range of conditions; however, in most cases the evidence is limited, insufficient, or nonexistent. The strongest evidence for an effect of cannabinoids is for chemotherapy-induced nausea, multiple sclerosis-related spasticity, and neuropathic pain. In all these cases, the effect is described as moderate [95]. More recent reviews have questioned the use of cannabinoids for pain due to limited effect and adverse events [236–238].

There is currently great interest in research on cannabinoids. Researchers in the United States and the rest of the world are conducting medical trials with marijuana and marijuana extracts to examine treatment efficacy for other diseases and symptoms such as multiple sclerosis, pain, and substance use disorders [239]. While there are many anecdotal reports about beneficial effects publicized through popular media outlets [95, 240, 241], some providers are reluctant to recommend a drug whose form, contents, dose, and type cannot be specified, as they would be in a typical prescription [242].

Some studies suggest that access to medical or recreational marijuana can reduce the use of opioids and opioid-related deaths, citing state-level differences in opioid mortality [243, 244]. Still others find self-reported reductions in opioid use among people who use marijuana to manage pain, and fewer opioid prescriptions among Medicaid enrollees who have access to medical marijuana [245–248]. However, Shover et al. [249] analyzed state-level data with a longer time series and found that the differences originally observed reversed over time, suggesting that there is no clear link. This conclusion is supported by a study of national survey data that found no effect on opioid use after legalization of medical marijuana [250].

Furthermore, several studies found that marijuana use is associated with higher opioid use in pain patients and greater risk of medical and nonmedical use of prescription drugs [251–253]. A large prospective study from Australia found no evidence that marijuana improved patient outcomes, no evidence that it reduced opioid use, and no evidence that it reduced pain [254]. A recent US study found greater risk of anxiety, depression, and substance abuse issues among medical marijuana users, but not improved pain experience [255]. Patients who receive more opioid prescriptions are also at higher risk of marijuana use disorder [256].

Public Health Response: Regulations and Messaging

Regulations

In 2014, the American Public Health Association issued a position statement which encouraged the development of comprehensive marijuana regulations as a public health priority [257]. The Association aimed to ensure oversight of the burgeoning legalized marijuana market in order to proactively address the unforeseen effects of legalization. Regulations to prevent marijuana access by minors, to protect and inform consumers, and to guard against unintended consequences to others as a result of marijuana use were encouraged.

Local and state governments play a seminal role in this effort health through mechanisms such as setting age limits; developing and monitoring product packaging, labeling, and warning requirements; invoking retail display and access standards; ensuring product testing and quality standards; setting potency and advertising limits, and revoking motor vehicle operation restrictions while impaired.

Response to marijuana legalization varies considerably around the world [258]. The European Federation of Addiction Societies issued a position statement stressing establishment of regulations at European level. The Federation advised the creation of registration and medical indications information, the development of uniform compounds and strength of products, and rules concerning sales and marketing [259].

In the United States, the regulation of these mechanisms varies by locality and may not be uniformly monitored or enforced. Colorado's regulator, the Marijuana Enforcement Division, updates its policies every year. The public health perspective on regulations is guided by the precautionary principle, which advises that the introduction of a new product whose ultimate effects are disputed or unknown should proceed in such a manner that it serves to protect the community from harm.

Considerations of how regulations will impact the black market are warranted. For example, a legal ban may drive up prices because it introduces inefficiencies in all parts of the supply chain. Taxation of legal products can compensate price drops but may create new incentives for a black market. Furthermore, in legal markets, the marijuana industry is increasingly trying to influence the outcome of policy processes that affect their business interests.

Public Health Messaging

Increasing community knowledge of issues associated with drug use is a key component of public health. Yet, marijuana messaging efforts present a unique challenge, particularly in areas where some form of marijuana legalization or decriminalization has passed. While public health messaging is led by science, it would be ignorant to dismiss the influences of the political and social norms of the time. Public support for marijuana legalization has increased rapidly. According to the Pew Research Center, 62% of Americans believe that marijuana should be legal, compared with about 20% two decades ago [260]. For public health professionals, it can be difficult to provide credible information about known or potential risks to an audience that may be opposed to hearing the message or interpret it as a part of a political debate surrounding legalization.

In the United States, fear tactics have long been used to warn people about the risks associated with tobacco and other drugs [261]. Yet, public health's approach to community-based messaging is changing, and early mistakes in marijuana media campaigns suggest that a different tactic is needed. In Colorado, one of the first community-level campaigns to rollout after legalization was largely deemed to be a failure after the creators erected human-sized rodent cages around the metro area that prominently displayed the tagline "Don't be a Lab Rat." Quickly, the displays became a target of both vandals and skeptics, ultimately backfiring when a school district refused to allow the exhibit on any of their campuses. Simultaneous public outcry focused on the pedantic tone of the campaign, underscoring the evolution of marijuana legalization as a community-backed effort. Within a few short months, the lack of support forced the sponsors to remove the exhibits from public display altogether.

New approaches to public health messaging increasingly focus on teaching the community about personal responsibility and science-based data rather than messages aimed at curtailing use. In alcohol policy, economic operators have tended to favor messaging around "responsible use" – shifting accountability from suppliers to individual consumers – from supply side measures to individual behavior [262]. Critics have described these messages as "strategically ambiguous," since they fail to define "responsible" and may ultimately promote the product [263–265]. In the case of formerly illegal substances, responsible use messages may have the unintended effect of normalizing use.

Harm reduction is a new paradigm in the field of drug education and treatment. Harm reduction works to minimize the hazards associated with drug use rather than the use itself [266]. Increasingly, public health messaging tailors its messaging efforts toward the needs of the intended audience, attempting to answer questions the audience is likely to ask. Campaign messages provide fact-based information, such as educating expecting mothers about research showing there is no safe level of cannabis use during pregnancy, or about how THC remains in breast milk after using marijuana. Outreach to parents, guardians, and adults who work with children (e.g., teachers, coaches, mentors) provides information about how to talk to young people about marijuana. In Colorado's *Protect What's Next Campaign*, adults were given tips about how to start a conversation about marijuana, how to listen to the concerns of youth, and how to share information about the health and legal consequences of underage use. Colorado took a similar approach to messaging adult users with their Good to Know campaign, which prioritized educating the audience about state laws and potential safety issues [267].

In jurisdictions with greater legal access to marijuana and increased social acceptance of marijuana use, it is important to educate the public about the risks of pediatric exposure and provide clear and strong messaging about safe storage of marijuana products. Regulatory measures, including labeling, childproof packaging, and product designs that are less appealing to children (e.g., candy) should be considered.

Conclusion

The marijuana landscape is changing rapidly, and the research is struggling to keep up. Public attitudes toward marijuana have shifted significantly. Decriminalization, medical marijuana laws, and full legalization have transformed the legal landscape.

Changing consumption patterns, new products, and new routes of administration have emerged.

Although the evidence base on marijuana is expanding, there is still limited knowledge about the health and social consequences of marijuana. Based on current knowledge, there are several areas of concern for public health, ranging from physical and mental health to accidents, acute effects, and harm to others. There is also evidence for some medical benefits, although the science is limited. We do not yet know the full impact of these harms and benefits on public health, and careful monitoring is needed.

The changing situation presents public health with new challenges in terms of monitoring, developing adequate regulatory frameworks, responding to new challenges, and communicating effectively about risks and harms. Public health messaging must resonate with shifting public attitudes to marijuana use, and public health policies must be negotiated with consumers as well as economic operators.

While we navigate these unchartered waters, we can draw some lessons from other fields of public health. In the face of uncertainty, public health policy should be based on the best available evidence and guided by the precautionary principle.

References

1. WHO's role under the international drug control conventions [Internet]. 2015 [cited 2019 Sep 12]. Available from: http://www.who.int/medicines/access/controlled-substances/ecdd/en/.
2. WHO Expert Committee on Drug Dependence Forty-first report [Internet]. [cited 2019 Sep 12]. Available from: https://apps.who.int/iris/handle/10665/325073.
3. WHO Expert Committee on Drug Dependence Fortieth report [Internet]. [cited 2019 Sep 12]. Available from: https://apps.who.int/iris/handle/10665/279948.
4. Center for Behavioral Health Statistics S, International R. National survey on drug use and health: comparison of 2008-2009 and 2016-2017 Population Percentages (50 States and the District of Columbia) [Internet]. [cited 2019 Aug 23]. Available from: https://www.samhsa.gov/data/sites/default/files/cbhsq-reports/NSDUHsaeTrendTabs2017/NSDUHsaeLongTermCHG2017.pdf.
5. Davenport SS, Caulkins JP. Evolution of the United States marijuana market in the decade of liberalization before full legalization. J Drug Issues [Internet]. 2016 [cited 2019 Jun 26];46(4):411–27. Available from: http://journals.sagepub.com/doi/10.1177/0022042616659759.
6. D'Amico EJ, Rodriguez A, Tucker JS, Pedersen ER, Shih RA. Planting the seed for marijuana use: changes in exposure to medical marijuana advertising and subsequent adolescent marijuana use, cognitions, and consequences over seven years. Drug Alcohol Depend [Internet]. 2018 [cited 2019 May 10];188:385–91. Available from: https://linkinghub.elsevier.com/retrieve/pii/S037687161830231X.
7. Shih RA, Rodriguez A, Parast L, Pedersen ER, Tucker JS, Troxel WM, et al. Associations between young adult marijuana outcomes and availability of medical marijuana dispensaries and storefront signage. Addiction [Internet]. 2019 [cited 2019 Jul 23];add.14711. Available from: http://www.ncbi.nlm.nih.gov/pubmed/31183908.
8. Mair C, Freisthler B, Ponicki WR, Gaidus A. The impacts of marijuana dispensary density and neighborhood ecology on marijuana abuse and dependence. Drug Alcohol Depend

[Internet]. 2015 [cited 2019 May 7];154:111–6. Available from: http://www.ncbi.nlm.nih.gov/pubmed/26154479.

9. Hyland A, Travers MJ, Cummings KM, Bauer J, Alford T, Wieczorek WF. Tobacco outlet density and demographics in Erie County, New York. Am J Public Health [Internet]. 2003 [cited 2019 Jun 26];93(7):1075–6. Available from: http://ajph.aphapublications.org/doi/10.2105/AJPH.93.7.1075.

10. LaVeist TA, Wallace JM. Health risk and inequitable distribution of liquor stores in African American neighborhood. Soc Sci Med [Internet]. 2000 [cited 2019 Jun 26];51(4):613–7. Available from: https://www.sciencedirect.com/science/article/abs/pii/S0277953600000046.

11. Hackbarth DP, Silvestri B, Cosper W. Tobacco and alcohol billboards in 50 Chicago neighborhoods: market segmentation to sell dangerous products to the poor. J Public Health Policy [Internet]. 1995 [cited 2019 Jun 26];16(2):213. Available from: https://www.jstor.org/stable/3342593?origin=crossref.

12. Shi Y, Meseck K, Jankowska MM. Availability of medical and recreational marijuana stores and neighborhood characteristics in Colorado. J Addict [Internet]. 2016 [cited 2019 May 7];2016:7193740. Available from: http://www.ncbi.nlm.nih.gov/pubmed/27213075.

13. Denver's pot businesses mostly in low-income, minority neighborhoods – The Denver Post [Internet]. [cited 2019 Aug 21]. Available from: https://www.denverpost.com/2016/01/02/denvers-pot-businesses-mostly-in-low-income-minority-neighborhoods/.

14. Tabb LP, Fillmore C, Melly S. Location, location, location: assessing the spatial patterning between marijuana licenses, alcohol outlets and neighborhood characteristics within Washington state. Drug Alcohol Depend [Internet]. 2018 [cited 2019 Jun 26];185:214–8. Available from: https://linkinghub.elsevier.com/retrieve/pii/S037687161830067X.

15. Marijuana use among US college students reaches new 35-year high. University of Michigan News [Internet]. [cited 2019 Sep 10]. Available from: https://news.umich.edu/marijuana-use-among-us-college-students-reaches-new-35-year-high/.

16. Wallace GT, Parnes JE, Prince MA, Conner BT, Riggs NR, George MW, et al. Associations between marijuana use patterns and recreational legislation changes in a large Colorado college student sample. Addict Res Theory [Internet]. 2019 [cited 2019 Jul 22];1–11. Available from: https://www.tandfonline.com/doi/full/10.1080/16066359.2019.1622003.

17. Jones J, Nicole Jones K, Peil J. The impact of the legalization of recreational marijuana on college students. Addict Behav [Internet]. 2018 [cited 2019 Jan 24];77:255–9. Available from: https://www.sciencedirect.com/science/article/abs/pii/S030646031730312X.

18. Park S-Y, Holody KJ. Content, Exposure, and effects of public discourses about marijuana: a systematic review. J Health Commun [Internet]. 2018 [cited 2019 Aug 23];23(12):1036–43. Available from: http://www.ncbi.nlm.nih.gov/pubmed/30395785.

19. Center for Behavioral Health Statistics S, International R. National survey on drug use and health: comparison of 2015-2016 and 2016-2017 population percentages (50 States and the District of Columbia) [Internet]. [cited 2019 Sep 24]. Available from: https://www.samhsa.gov/data/sites/default/files/cbhsq-reports/NSDUHsaeChangeTabs2017/NSDUHsaeShortTermCHG2017.pdf.

20. Burgard DA, Williams J, Westerman D, Rushing R, Carpenter R, LaRock A, et al. Using wastewater-based analysis to monitor the effects of legalized retail sales on cannabis consumption in Washington State, USA. Addiction [Internet]. 2019 [cited 2019 Jun 26]; Available from: http://doi.wiley.com/10.1111/add.14641.

21. Chandra S, Radwan MM, Majumdar CG, Church JC, Freeman TP, ElSohly MA. New trends in cannabis potency in USA and Europe during the last decade (2008–2017). Eur Arch Psychiatry Clin Neurosci [Internet]. 2019 [cited 2019 Apr 30];269(1):5–15. Available from: http://www.ncbi.nlm.nih.gov/pubmed/30671616.

22. Freeman TP, Groshkova T, Cunningham A, Sedefov R, Griffiths P, Lynksey MT. Increasing potency and price of cannabis in Europe, 2006-2016. Addiction [Internet]. 2018 [cited 2019 Jan 4]; Available from: http://doi.wiley.com/10.1111/add.14525.

23. Rømer Thomsen K, Lindholst C, Thylstrup B, Kvamme S, Reitzel LA, Worm-Leonhard M, et al. Changes in the composition of cannabis from 2000–2017 in Denmark: analysis of confiscated samples of cannabis resin. Exp Clin Psychopharmacol [Internet]. 2019 [cited 2019 Jun 25]; Available from: http://www.ncbi.nlm.nih.gov/pubmed/31219274.

24. ElSohly MA, Mehmedic Z, Foster S, Gon C, Chandra S, Church JC. Changes in cannabis potency over the last 2 decades (1995–2014): analysis of current data in the United States. Biol Psychiatry [Internet]. 2016 [cited 2019 May 13];79(7):613–9. Available from: http://www.ncbi.nlm.nih.gov/pubmed/26903403.

25. Freeman TP, Winstock AR. Examining the profile of high-potency cannabis and its association with severity of cannabis dependence. Psychol Med. 2015;45(15):3181–9.

26. Freeman TP, van der Pol P, Kuijpers W, Wisselink J, Das RK, Rigter S, et al. Changes in cannabis potency and first-time admissions to drug treatment: a 16-year study in the Netherlands. Psychol Med [Internet]. 2018 [cited 2018 Feb 6];1–7. Available from: https://www.cambridge.org/core/product/identifier/S0033291717003877/type/journal_article.

27. Arterberry BJ, Treloar Padovano H, Foster KT, Zucker RA, Hicks BM. Higher average potency across the United States is associated with progression to first cannabis use disorder symptom. Drug Alcohol Depend [Internet]. 2018 [cited 2018 Dec 19]; Available from: https://www.sciencedirect.com/science/article/pii/S0376871618308202.

28. Marconi A, Di Forti M, Lewis CM, Murray RM, Vassos E. Meta-analysis of the association between the level of cannabis use and risk of psychosis. Schizophr Bull [Internet]. 2016 [cited 2018 Apr 16];42(5):1262–9. Available from: http://www.ncbi.nlm.nih.gov/pubmed/26884547.

29. Potter DJ, Hammond K, Tuffnell S, Walker C, Di Forti M. Potency of Δ^9-tetrahydrocannabinol and other cannabinoids in cannabis in England in 2016: implications for public health and pharmacology. Drug Test Anal [Internet]. 2018 [cited 2018 Feb 28]; Available from: http://doi.wiley.com/10.1002/dta.2368.

30. Di Forti M, Sallis H, Allegri F, Trotta A, Ferraro L, Stilo SA, et al. Daily Use, Especially of high-potency cannabis, drives the earlier onset of psychosis in cannabis users. Schizophr Bull [Internet]. 2014 [cited 2019 Jul 25];40(6):1509–17. Available from: http://www.ncbi.nlm.nih.gov/pubmed/24345517.

31. Monte AA, Shelton SK, Mills E, Saben J, Hopkinson A, Sonn B, et al. Acute illness associated with cannabis use, by route of exposure. Ann Intern Med [Internet]. 2019 [cited 2019 Apr 25];170(8):531. Available from: http://www.ncbi.nlm.nih.gov/pubmed/30909297.

32. Schneberk T, Sterling GP, Valenzuela R, Mallon WK. 390 "A Little Dab Will Do Ya": an emergency department case series related to a new form of "High-Potency" marijuana known as "Wax." Ann Emerg Med [Internet]. 2014 [cited 2019 Jun 27];64(4):S139. Available from: https://linkinghub.elsevier.com/retrieve/pii/S0196064414010257.

33. Ramaekers JG. Driving Under the Influence of Cannabis. JAMA [Internet]. 2018 [cited 2019 May 14];319(14):1433. Available from: http://jama.jamanetwork.com/article.aspx?doi=10.1001/jama.2018.1334.

34. Hall W. What has research over the past two decades revealed about the adverse health effects of recreational cannabis use? 2014 [cited 2019 Jul 23]; Available from: https://www.drugfree.org.au/images/pdf-files/library/Cannabis/What_has_research_over_the_past_two_decades_revealed_about_the_adverse_health_effects_of_recreational_cannabis_use.pdf.

35. Eichelberger AH. Marijuana use and driving in Washington State: risk perceptions and behaviors before and after implementation of retail sales. Traffic Inj Prev [Internet]. 2019 [cited 2019 Jun 26];20(1):23–9. Available from: https://www.tandfonline.com/doi/full/10.1080/15389588.2018.1530769.

36. Research W, Division D. Cannabis involvement among drivers in fatal crashes [Internet]. Washington Traffic Safety Commission Toxicology Reports. 2019 [cited 2019 Jun 28]. Available from: https://wtsc.wa.gov/research-data/.

37. RMHIDTA. The legalization of marijuana in Colorado: the impact. Mo Med. 116(6):450.

38. Lane TJ, Hall W. Traffic fatalities within US states that have legalized recreational cannabis sales and their neighbours. Addiction [Internet]. 2019 [cited 2019 Jun 28];114(5):847–56. Available from: https://onlinelibrary.wiley.com/doi/abs/10.1111/add.14536.

39. The Daily – National Cannabis Survey, first quarter 2019 [Internet]. [cited 2019 Jun 28]. Available from: https://www150.statcan.gc.ca/n1/daily-quotidien/190502/dq190502a-eng.htm.

40. CDOT survey reveals new insight on marijuana and driving [Internet]. [cited 2019 Aug 7]. Available from: https://www.codot.gov/news/2018/april/cdot-survey-reveals-new-insight-on-marijuana-and-driving.

41. Els C, Jackson TD, Tsuyuki RT, Aidoo H, Wyatt G, Sowah D, et al. Impact of cannabis use on road traffic collisions and safety at work. Can J Addict [Internet]. 2019 Mar [cited 2019 Jun 27];10(1):8–15. Available from: http://insights.ovid.com/crossref?an=02024458-201903000-00003.

42. Khashaba E, El-Helaly M, El-Gilany A, Motawei S, Foda S. Risk factors for non-fatal occupational injuries among construction workers: a case–control study. Toxicol Ind Health [Internet]. 2018 [cited 2019 Jun 27];34(2):83–90. Available from: http://journals.sagepub.com/doi/10.1177/0748233717733853.

43. Employees and execs are failing drug tests at shocking rates [Internet]. [cited 2019 Aug 7]. Available from: https://nypost.com/2018/10/20/employees-and-execs-are-failing-drug-tests-at-shocking-rates/.

44. Quest diagnostics: drug testing index [Internet]. [cited 2019 Aug 8]. Available from: http://www.questdiagnostics.com/home/physicians/health-trends/drug-testing.

45. De Sousa Fernandes Perna EB, Theunissen EL, Kuypers KPC, Toennes SW, Ramaekers JG. Subjective aggression during alcohol and cannabis intoxication before and after aggression exposure. Psychopharmacology (Berl) [Internet]. 2016 [cited 2019 Jul 24];233(18):3331–40. Available from: http://www.ncbi.nlm.nih.gov/pubmed/27422568.

46. Norström T, Rossow I. Cannabis use and violence: is there a link? Scand J Public Health [Internet]. 2014 [cited 2019 Jul 22];42(4):358–63. Available from: http://www.ncbi.nlm.nih.gov/pubmed/24608093.

47. Schoeler T, Monk A, Sami MB, Klamerus E, Foglia E, Brown R, et al. Continued versus discontinued cannabis use in patients with psychosis: a systematic review and meta-analysis. Lancet Psychiatry. 2016;

48. Smith PH, Homish GG, Leonard KE, Collins RL. Marijuana withdrawal and aggression among a representative sample of U.S. marijuana users. Drug Alcohol Depend [Internet]. 2013 [cited 2019 Jul 24];132(1–2):63–8. Available from: https://www.sciencedirect.com/science/article/abs/pii/S0376871613000045?via%3Dihub.

49. Ansell EB, Laws HB, Roche MJ, Sinha R. Effects of marijuana use on impulsivity and hostility in daily life. Drug Alcohol Depend [Internet]. 2015 [cited 2018 May 7];148:136–42. Available from: http://www.ncbi.nlm.nih.gov/pubmed/25595054.

50. Douglas KS, Guy LS, Hart SD. Psychosis as a risk factor for violence to others: a meta-analysis. Psychol Bull [Internet]. 2009 [cited 2019 Jul 24];135(5):679–706. Available from: http://doi.apa.org/getdoi.cfm?doi=10.1037/a0016311

51. Beaudoin M, Potvin S, Dellazizzo L, Luigi M, Giguère C-E, Dumais A. Trajectories of dynamic risk factors as predictors of violence and criminality in patients discharged from mental health services: a longitudinal study using growth mixture modeling. Front Psychiatry [Internet]. 2019 [cited 2019 Jun 4];10:301. Available from: https://www.frontiersin.org/article/10.3389/fpsyt.2019.00301/full.

52. Ware MA, Wang T, Shapiro S, Collet J-P, Boulanger A, Esdaile JM, et al. Cannabis for the management of pain: assessment of safety study (COMPASS). J Pain [Internet]. 2015 [cited 2019 Jan 9];16(12):1233–42. Available from: https://linkinghub.elsevier.com/retrieve/pii/S1526590015008378.

53. Moulin V, Baumann P, Gholamrezaee M, Alameda L, Palix J, Gasser J, et al. Cannabis, a significant risk factor for violent behavior in the early phase psychosis. Two patterns of inter-

action of factors increase the risk of violent behavior: cannabis use disorder and impulsivity; cannabis use disorder, lack of insight and treatment adherence. Front Psychiatry [Internet]. 2018 [cited 2019 Jan 31];9:294. Available from: https://www.frontiersin.org/article/10.3389/fpsyt.2018.00294/full.

54. Lamsma J, Cahn W, Fazel S, investigators G and N. Use of illicit substances and violent behaviour in psychotic disorders: two nationwide case-control studies and meta-analyses. Psychol Med [Internet]. 2019 [cited 2019 Aug 30];1–6. Available from: https://www.cambridge.org/core/product/identifier/S0033291719002125/type/journal_article.

55. Volkow ND, Baler R. Emergency department visits from edible versus inhalable cannabis. Ann Intern Med [Internet]. 2019 [cited 2019 Aug 6];170(8):569–70. Available from: https://annals.org/aim/fullarticle/2729210/emergency-department-visits-from-edible-versus-inhalable-cannabis.

56. Chen Y-C, Klig JE. Cannabis-related emergencies in children and teens. Curr Opin Pediatr [Internet]. 2019 [cited 2019 May 22];31(3):291–6. Available from: http://www.ncbi.nlm.nih.gov/pubmed/31090567.

57. Hall KE, Monte AA, Chang T, Fox J, Brevik C, Vigil DI, et al. Mental health–related emergency department visits associated with cannabis in Colorado. Acad Emerg Med [Internet]. 2018 [cited 2019 Jun 27];25(5):526. Available from: http://www.ncbi.nlm.nih.gov/pubmed/29476688.

58. Bell C, Slim J, Flaten HK, Lindberg G, Arek W, Monte AA. Butane hash oil burns associated with marijuana liberalization in Colorado. J Med Toxicol [Internet]. 2015 [cited 2019 Jan 16];11(4):422–5. Available from: http://link.springer.com/10.1007/s13181-015-0501-0.

59. Sorensen CJ, DeSanto K, Borgelt L, Phillips KT, Monte AA. Cannabinoid hyperemesis syndrome: diagnosis, pathophysiology, and treatment-a systematic review. J Med Toxicol [Internet]. 2017 [cited 2018 Feb 19];13(1):71–87. Available from: http://www.ncbi.nlm.nih.gov/pubmed/28000146.

60. Habboushe J, Rubin A, Liu H, Hoffman RS. The prevalence of cannabinoid hyperemesis syndrome among regular marijuana smokers in an urban public hospital. Basic Clin Pharmacol Toxicol [Internet]. 2018 [cited 2019 Mar 27];122(6):660–2. Available from: http://doi.wiley.com/10.1111/bcpt.12962.

61. Khattar N, Routsolias JC. Emergency department treatment of cannabinoid hyperemesis syndrome. Am J Ther [Internet]. 2018 [cited 2019 Jun 27];25(3):e357–61. Available from: http://insights.ovid.com/crossref?an=00045391-201806000-00009.

62. Nourbakhsh M, Miller A, Gofton J, Jones G, Adeagbo B. Cannabinoid hyperemesis syndrome: reports of fatal cases. J Forensic Sci [Internet]. 2018 [cited 2019 Jan 3]; Available from: http://doi.wiley.com/10.1111/1556-4029.13819.

63. Zimmer DI, McCauley R, Konanki V, Dynako J, Zackariya N, Shariff F, et al. Emergency department and radiological cost of delayed diagnosis of cannabinoid hyperemesis. J Addict [Internet]. 2019 [cited 2019 Apr 30];2019:1–4. Available from: http://www.ncbi.nlm.nih.gov/pubmed/30723570.

64. Kim HS, Monte AA. Colorado cannabis legalization and its effect on emergency care. Ann Emerg Med [Internet]. 2016 [cited 2019 Jun 26];68(1):71–5. Available from: https://linkinghub.elsevier.com/retrieve/pii/S0196064416000056.

65. Wang GS, Hall K, Vigil D, Banerji S, Monte A, VanDyke M. Marijuana and acute health care contacts in Colorado. Prev Med (Baltim) [Internet]. 2017 [cited 2019 Jul 24];104:24–30. Available from: https://www.sciencedirect.com/science/article/pii/S0091743517301202.

66. Finn K. The hidden costs of marijuana use in Colorado: one emergency department's experience. [cited 2018 Feb 6]; Available from: http://www.globaldrugpolicy.org/Issues/Vol 10 Issue 2/Articles/The Hidden Costs of Marijuana Use in Colorado_Final.pdf.

67. Wang GS, Davies SD, Halmo LS, Sass A, Mistry RD. Impact of marijuana legalization in Colorado on adolescent emergency and urgent care visits. J Adolesc Heal [Internet]. 2018 [cited 2019 Mar 28];63(2):239–41. Available from: https://linkinghub.elsevier.com/retrieve/pii/S1054139X18300041.

68. Delling FN, Vittinghoff E, Dewland TA, Pletcher MJ, Olgin JE, Nah G, et al. Does canna-bis legalisation change healthcare utilisation? A population-based study using the healthcare cost and utilisation project in Colorado, USA. BMJ Open [Internet]. 2019 [cited 2019 May 16];9(5):e027432. Available from: https://bmjopen.bmj.com/content/9/5/e027432.
69. Is it possible to "overdose" or have a "bad reaction" to marijuana? FAQs. Marijuana. CDC [Internet]. [cited 2019 Aug 7]. Available from: https://www.cdc.gov/marijuana/faqs/over-dose-bad-reaction.html.
70. Schneider KE, Tormohlen KN, Brooks-Russell A, Johnson RM, Thrul J. Patterns of co-occurring modes of marijuana use among Colorado high school students. J Adolesc Health [Internet]. 2019 [cited 2019 Jun 24];64(6):807–9. Available from: http://www.ncbi.nlm.nih.gov/pubmed/30777637.
71. Department of Health U, Services H. The health consequences of smoking – 50 years of progress: a report of the surgeon general [Internet]. [cited 2019 Aug 27]. Available from: www.cdc.gov/tobacco.
72. Tashkin DP, Roth MD. Pulmonary effects of inhaled cannabis smoke. Am J Drug Alcohol Abuse [Internet]. 2019 [cited 2019 Aug 22];1–14. Available from: https://www.tandfonline.com/doi/full/10.1080/00952990.2019.1627366.
73. Ghasemiesfe M, Ravi D, Vali M, Korenstein D, Arjomandi M, Frank J, et al. Marijuana use, respiratory symptoms, and pulmonary function: a systematic review and meta-analysis. Ann Intern Med [Internet]. 2018 [cited 2019 Feb 11];169(2):106–15. Available from: http://annals.org/article.aspx?doi=10.7326/M18-0522.
74. Bramness JG, von Soest T. A longitudinal study of cannabis use increasing the use of asthma medication in young Norwegian adults. BMC Pulm Med [Internet]. 2019 [cited 2019 Apr 12];19(1):52. Available from: https://bmcpulmmed.biomedcentral.com/articles/10.1186/s12890-019-0814-x.
75. Strong DR, Myers MG, Pulvers K, Noble M, Brikmanis K, Doran N. Marijuana use among US tobacco users: findings from wave 1 of the population assessment of tobacco health (PATH) study. Drug Alcohol Depend [Internet]. 2018 [cited 2019 Jan 17];186:16–22. Available from: https://linkinghub.elsevier.com/retrieve/pii/S0376871618301121.
76. Furlow B. US state governments investigate suspected vaping-associated severe lung disease. Lancet Respir Med [Internet]. 2019 [cited 2019 Sep 5];0(0). Available from: http://www.ncbi.nlm.nih.gov/pubmed/31477520.
77. Eighth death linked to vaping as illnesses surge around the United States - CNN [Internet]. [cited 2019 Sep 24]. Available from: https://edition.cnn.com/2019/09/19/health/vaping-lung-injury-new-cases-530-bn/index.html.
78. Layden JE, Ghinai I, Pray I, Kimball A, Layer M, Tenforde M, et al. Pulmonary illness related to E-cigarette use in Illinois and Wisconsin – preliminary report. N Engl J Med [Internet]. 2019 [cited 2019 Sep 10];NEJMoa1911614. Available from: http://www.nejm.org/doi/10.1056/NEJMoa1911614.
79. Illicit "Pot" oil culprit in vaping disease? Medpage Today [Internet]. [cited 2019 Sep 6]. Available from: https://www.medpagetoday.com/pulmonology/smoking/81924.
80. He T, Oks M, Esposito M, Steinberg H, Makaryus M. "Tree-in-bloom": severe acute lung injury induced by vaping cannabis oil. Ann Am Thorac Soc [Internet]. 2017 [cited 2019 Sep 13];14(3):468–70. Available from: http://www.atsjournals.org/doi/10.1513/AnnalsATS.201612-974LE.
81. Sommerfeld CG, Weiner DJ, Nowalk A, Larkin A. Hypersensitivity pneumonitis and acute respiratory distress syndrome from E-cigarette use. Pediatrics [Internet]. 2018 [cited 2019 Sep 13];141(6):e20163927. Available from: https://pediatrics.aappublications.org/content/141/6/e20163927.
82. Singh A, Saluja S, Kumar A, Agrawal S, Thind M, Nanda S, et al. Cardiovascular complica-tions of marijuana and related substances: a review. Cardiol Ther [Internet]. 2018 [cited 2019 Feb 7];7(1):45–59. Available from: http://www.ncbi.nlm.nih.gov/pubmed/29218644.

83. Pacher P, Steffens S, Haskó G, Schindler TH, Kunos G. Cardiovascular effects of marijuana and synthetic cannabinoids: the good, the bad, and the ugly. Nat Rev Cardiol [Internet]. 2017 [cited 2017 Oct 26]; Available from: http://www.nature.com/doifinder/10.1038/nrcardio.2017.130.
84. Patel RS, Kamil SH, Bachu R, Adikey A, Ravat V, Kaur M, et al. Marijuana use and acute myocardial infarction: a systematic review of published cases in the literature. Trends Cardiovasc Med [Internet]. 2019 [cited 2019 Aug 29]; Available from: http://www.ncbi.nlm.nih.gov/pubmed/31439383.
85. Goyal H, Awad HH, Ghali JK. Role of cannabis in cardiovascular disorders. J Thorac Dis [Internet]. 2017 Jul [cited 2019 Jul 25];9(7):2079–92. Available from: http://www.ncbi.nlm.nih.gov/pubmed/28840009.
86. Chami T, Kim CH. Cannabis abuse and elevated risk of myocardial infarction in the young: a population-based study. Mayo Clin Proc [Internet]. 2019 [cited 2019 Aug 8];94(8):1647–9. Available from: https://www.mayoclinicproceedings.org/article/S0025-6196(19)30464-1/fulltext.
87. Kalla A, Krishnamoorthy PM, Gopalakrishnan A, Figueredo VM. Cannabis use predicts risks of heart failure and cerebrovascular accidents. J Cardiovasc Med [Internet]. 2018 [cited 2019 Apr 24];19(9):480–4. Available from: http://www.ncbi.nlm.nih.gov/pubmed/29879084.
88. Oehha. Evidence on the carcinogenicity of marijuana smoke California Environmental Protection Agency [Internet]. 2009 [cited 2019 Jul 26]. Available from: https://oehha.ca.gov/media/downloads/proposition-65/chemicals/finalmjsmokehid.pdf.
89. Huang Y-HJ, Zhang Z-F, Tashkin DP, Feng B, Straif K, Hashibe M. An epidemiologic review of marijuana and cancer: an update. Cancer Epidemiol Biomarkers Prev [Internet]. 2015 [cited 2019 Aug 5];24(1):15–31. Available from: http://www.ncbi.nlm.nih.gov/pubmed/25587109.
90. Zhang Z, Morgenstern H, Spitz M, Tashkin D, Yu G, Marshall J. Marijuana use and increased risk of squamous cell carcinoma of the head and neck. Cancer Epidemiol Biomarkers Prev [Internet]. 2015 [cited 2019 Aug 5];8(12):1071–8. Available from: http://cebp.aacrjournals.org/content/24/1/15.short#.
91. Park S, Myung S-K. Cannabis smoking and risk of cancer: a meta-analysis of observational studies. J Glob Oncol [Internet]. 2018 [cited 2019 Jul 26];(4_suppl_2):196s. Available from: http://ascopubs.org/doi/10.1200/jgo.18.79302.
92. Volkow ND, Baler RD, Compton WM, Weiss SRB. Adverse health effects of marijuana use. N Engl J Med [Internet]. 2014 [cited 2019 Jul 26];370(23):2219–27. Available from: http://www.nejm.org/doi/10.1056/NEJMra1402309.
93. Lacson JCA, Carroll JD, Tuazon E, Castelao EJ, Bernstein L, Cortessis VK. Population-based case-control study of recreational drug use and testis cancer risk confirms an association between marijuana use and nonseminoma risk. Cancer [Internet]. 2012 [cited 2019 Jul 26];118(21):5374–83. Available from: http://doi.wiley.com/10.1002/cncr.27554
94. Callaghan RC, Allebeck P, Akre O, McGlynn KA, Sidorchuk A. Cannabis use and incidence of testicular cancer: a 42-year follow-up of Swedish men between 1970 and 2011. Cancer Epidemiol Biomarkers Prev [Internet]. 2017 [cited 2019 Jul 26];26(11):1644–52. Available from: http://www.ncbi.nlm.nih.gov/pubmed/29093004.
95. The health effects of cannabis and cannabinoids [Internet]. Washington, D.C.: National Academies Press; 2017 [cited 2019 Jul 26]. Available from: https://www.nap.edu/catalog/24625.
96. Fronczak CM, Kim ED, Barqawi AB. The insults of illicit drug use on male fertility. J Androl [Internet]. 2012 [cited 2019 Aug 13];33(4):515–28. Available from: http://doi.wiley.com/10.2164/jandrol.110.011874
97. Hsiao P, Clavijo RI. Adverse effects of cannabis on male reproduction. Eur Urol Focus [Internet]. 2018 May [cited 2019 Aug 6];4(3):324–8. Available from: https://linkinghub.elsevier.com/retrieve/pii/S2405456918302256.

98. Payne KS, Mazur DJ, Hotaling JM, Pastuszak AW. Cannabis and male fertility: a systematic review. J Urol [Internet]. 2019 [cited 2019 Aug 13];101097JU0000000000000248. Available from: http://www.ncbi.nlm.nih.gov/pubmed/30916627.
99. Nassan FL, Arvizu M, Mínguez-Alarcón L, Williams PL, Attaman J, Petrozza J, et al. Marijuana smoking and markers of testicular function among men from a fertility centre. Hum Reprod [Internet]. 2019 [cited 2019 Aug 13];1–9. Available from: https://academic.oup.com/DocumentLibrary/humrep/PR_Papers/dez002.pdf.
100. Brents LK. Marijuana, the endocannabinoid system and the female reproductive system. Yale J Biol Med [Internet]. 2016 [cited 2019 Aug 13];89(2):175–91. Available from: http://www.ncbi.nlm.nih.gov/pubmed/27354844.
101. Jukic AMZ, Weinberg CR, Baird DD, Wilcox AJ. Lifestyle and reproductive factors associated with follicular phase length. J Womens Health (Larchmt) [Internet]. 2007 [cited 2019 Aug 13];16(9):1340–7. Available from: http://www.ncbi.nlm.nih.gov/pubmed/18001191.
102. Ilnitsky S, Van Uum S. Marijuana and fertility. CMAJ [Internet]. 2019 [cited 2019 Aug 13];191(23):E638. Available from: http://www.ncbi.nlm.nih.gov/pubmed/31182459.
103. Richter L, Pugh BS, Ball SA. Assessing the risk of marijuana use disorder among adolescents and adults who use marijuana. Am J Drug Alcohol Abuse [Internet]. 2017 [cited 2019 Aug 7];43(3):247–60. Available from: https://www.tandfonline.com/doi/full/10.3109/0095299 0.2016.1164711.
104. WHO. The health and social effects of nonmedical cannabis use. WHO [Internet]. 2016 [cited 2019 Aug 7]; Available from: https://www.who.int/substance_abuse/publications/cannabis_report/en/index5.html.
105. Hasin DS. US Epidemiology of cannabis use and associated problems. Neuropsychopharmacology [Internet]. 2018 [cited 2019 Aug 7];43(1):195–212. Available from: http://www.nature.com/articles/npp2017198.
106. Hasin DS, Shmulewitz D, Sarvet AL. Time trends in US cannabis use and cannabis use disorders overall and by sociodemographic subgroups: a narrative review and new findings. Am J Drug Alcohol Abuse [Internet]. 2019 [cited 2019 Aug 7];1–21. Available from: http://www.ncbi.nlm.nih.gov/pubmed/30870044.
107. Compton WM, Han B, Jones CM, Blanco C, Hughes A. Marijuana use and use disorders in adults in the USA, 2002–14: analysis of annual cross-sectional surveys. The Lancet Psychiatry [Internet]. 2016 [cited 2019 Jun 28];3(10):954–64. Available from: https://linkinghub.elsevier.com/retrieve/pii/S2215036616302085.
108. Davenport S. Falling rates of marijuana dependence among heavy users. Drug Alcohol Depend [Internet]. 2018 [cited 2019 Jun 28];191:52–5. Available from: http://www.ncbi.nlm.nih.gov/pubmed/30077891
109. Manthey J. Cannabis use in Europe: current trends and public health concerns. Int J Drug Policy [Internet]. 2019 [cited 2019 Jul 22];68:93–6. Available from: http://www.ncbi.nlm.nih.gov/pubmed/31030057.
110. Montanari L, Guarita B, Mounteney J, Zipfel N, Simon R. Cannabis use among people entering drug treatment in Europe: a growing phenomenon? Eur Addict Res [Internet]. 2017 [cited 2018 May 11];23:113–21. Available from: https://www.karger.com/Article/PDF/475810.
111. Curran HV, Freeman TP, Mokrysz C, Lewis DA, Morgan CJA, Parsons LH. Keep off the grass? Cannabis, cognition and addiction. Nat Rev Neurosci [Internet]. 2016 [cited 2019 Jul 24];17(5):293–306. Available from: http://www.nature.com/articles/nrn.2016.28.
112. Bonnet U, Preuss UW. The cannabis withdrawal syndrome: current insights. Subst Abuse Rehabil [Internet]. 2017 [cited 2019 Aug 13];8:9–37. Available from: http://www.ncbi.nlm.nih.gov/pubmed/28490916.
113. Patel J, Marwaha R. Cannabis use disorder [Internet]. StatPearls. StatPearls Publishing; 2019 [cited 2019 Aug 7]. Available from: http://www.ncbi.nlm.nih.gov/pubmed/30844158.
114. Livne O, Shmulewitz D, Lev-Ran S, Hasin DS. DSM-5 cannabis withdrawal syndrome: demographic and clinical correlates in U.S. adults. Drug Alcohol Depend [Internet]. 2019

[cited 2019 Feb 27];195:170–7. Available from: https://www.sciencedirect.com/science/article/pii/S0376871618307142.

115. Volkow ND, Swanson JM, Evins AE, DeLisi LE, Meier MH, Gonzalez R, et al. Effects of cannabis use on human behavior, including cognition, motivation, and psychosis: a review. JAMA Psychiatry [Internet]. 2016;73(3):292. Available from: http://archpsyc.jamanetwork.com/article.aspx?doi=10.1001/jamapsychiatry.2015.3278.

116. Lawn W, Freeman T, Pope R, Joye A, Harvey L, Hindocha C. Acute and chronic effects of cannabinoids on effort-related decision-making and reward learning: an evaluation of the cannabis 'amotivational' hypotheses. Psychopharmacol. 233(19–20):3537–52.

117. Duperrouzel JC, Granja K, Pacheco-Colón I, Gonzalez R. Adverse Effects of cannabis use on neurocognitive functioning: a systematic review of meta- analytic studies. J Dual Diagn [Internet]. 2019 Jun 22 [cited 2019 Jun 26];1–15. Available from: http://www.ncbi.nlm.nih.gov/pubmed/31e232216.

118. Gonzalez R, Pacheco-Colón I, Duperrouzel JC, Hawes SW. Does cannabis use cause declines in neuropsychological functioning? A review of longitudinal studies. J Int Neuropsychol Soc [Internet]. 2017 [cited 2019 Jul 25];23(9–10):893–902. Available from: https://www.cambridge.org/core/product/identifier/S1355617717000789/type/journal_article.

119. Silins E, Fergusson DM, Patton GC, Horwood LJ, Olsson CA, Hutchinson DM, et al. Adolescent substance use and educational attainment: an integrative data analysis comparing cannabis and alcohol from three Australasian cohorts. Drug Alcohol Depend. 2015;156:90–6.

120. Thompson K, Leadbeater B, Ames M, Merrin GJ. Associations between marijuana use trajectories and educational and occupational success in young adulthood. Prev Sci [Internet]. 2019 [cited 2019 May 28];20(2):257–69. Available from: http://link.springer.com/10.1007/s11121-018-0904-7.

121. Wright AC, Krieg JM. Getting into the weeds: does legal marijuana access blunt academic performance in college? Econ Inq [Internet]. 2018 [cited 2019 Feb 11]; Available from: http://doi.wiley.com/10.1111/ecin.12743.

122. Suerken CK, Reboussin BA, Egan KL, Sutfin EL, Wagoner KG, Spangler J, et al. Marijuana use trajectories and academic outcomes among college students. Drug Alcohol Depend [Internet]. 2016 [cited 2019 Jan 24];162:137–45. Available from: https://www.sciencedirect.com/science/article/pii/S037687161600140X.

123. Beverly HK, Castro Y, Opara I. Age of first marijuana use and its impact on education attainment and employment status. J Drug Issues [Internet]. 2019 [cited 2019 Aug 23];49(2):228–37. Available from: http://www.ncbi.nlm.nih.gov/pubmed/31341332.

124. Radoman M, Hoeppner SS, Schuster RM, Evins AE, Gilman JM. Marijuana use and major depressive disorder are additively associated with reduced verbal learning and altered cortical thickness. Cogn Affect Behav Neurosci [Internet]. 2019 [cited 2019 Mar 28]; Available from: http://www.ncbi.nlm.nih.gov/pubmed/30809764.

125. Marie O, Zölitz U. 'High' achievers? Cannabis access and academic performance. Rev Econ Stud [Internet]. 2017 [cited 2019 Aug 14]; Available from: https://academic.oup.com/restud/article-lookup/doi/10.1093/restud/rdx020.

126. Scott JC, Slomiak ST, Jones JD, Rosen AFG, Moore TM, Gur RC. Association of cannabis with cognitive functioning in adolescents and young adults: a systematic review and meta-analysis. JAMA Psychiatry [Internet]. [cited 2018 Apr 19]; Available from: https://jamanetwork.com/journals/jamapsychiatry/article-abstract/2678214.

127. Meier MH, Caspi A, Ambler A, Harrington H, Houts R, Keefe RSE, et al. Persistent cannabis users show neuropsychological decline from childhood to midlife. Proc Natl Acad Sci [Internet]. 2012;109(40):E2657–64.. Available from: http://www.pnas.org/cgi/doi/10.1073/pnas.1206820109.

128. Jackson NJ, Isen JD, Khoddam R, Irons D, Tuvblad C, Iacono WG, et al. Impact of adolescent marijuana use on intelligence: results from two longitudinal twin studies. Proc Natl Acad Sci U S A [Internet]. 2016 [cited 2019 Jul 25];113(5):E500–8. Available from: http://www.ncbi.nlm.nih.gov/pubmed/26787878.

129. Mokrysz C, Landy R, Gage S, Munafò M, Roiser J, Curran H. Are IQ and educational outcomes in teenagers related to their cannabis use? A prospective cohort study. J Psychopharmacol [Internet]. 2016 [cited 2019 Jul 25];30(2):159–68. Available from: http://journals.sagepub.com/doi/10.1177/0269881115622241.
130. Chye Y, Christensen E, Yücel M. Cannabis use in adolescence: a review of neuroimaging findings. J Dual Diagn [Internet]. 2019 Jul 16 [cited 2019 Jul 25];1–23. Available from: https://www.tandfonline.com/doi/full/10.1080/15504263.2019.1636171.
131. Lorenzetti V, Solowij N, Fornito A, Lubman DI, Yucel M. The association between regular cannabis exposure and alterations of human brain morphology: an updated review of the literature. Curr Pharm Des [Internet]. 2014 [cited 2019 Jul 25];20(13):2138–67. Available from: http://www.ncbi.nlm.nih.gov/pubmed/23829361.
132. Moore TH, Zammit S, Lingford-Hughes A, Barnes TR, Jones PB, Burke M, et al. Cannabis use and risk of psychotic or affective mental health outcomes: a systematic review. Lancet [Internet]. 2007 [cited 2019 Aug 13];370(9584):319–28. Available from: http://www.ncbi.nlm.nih.gov/pubmed/17662880.
133. Hall W, Degenhardt L. Cannabis use and the risk of developing a psychotic disorder. World Psychiatry [Internet]. 2008 [cited 2019 Jul 26];7(2):68–71. Available from: http://www.ncbi.nlm.nih.gov/pubmed/18560513.
134. Mustonen A, Niemelä S, Nordström T, Murray GK, Mäki P, Jääskeläinen E, et al. Adolescent cannabis use, baseline prodromal symptoms and the risk of psychosis. Br J Psychiatry [Internet]. 2018 [cited 2018 Mar 23];212(04):227–33. Available from: http://www.ncbi.nlm.nih.gov/pubmed/29557758.
135. Nesvåg R, Reichborn-Kjennerud T, Gillespie NA, Knudsen GP, Bramness JG, Kendler KS, et al. Genetic and environmental contributions to the association between cannabis use and psychotic-like experiences in young adult twins. Schizophr Bull [Internet]. 2016 [cited 2019 Jul 26];43(3):sbw101. Available from: https://academic.oup.com/schizophreniabulletin/article-lookup/doi/10.1093/schbul/sbw101.
136. Di Forti M, Morgan C, Dazzan P, Pariante C, Mondelli V, Marques TR, et al. High-potency cannabis and the risk of psychosis. Br J Psychiatry [Internet]. 2009 [cited 2019 Jul 25];195(6):488–91. Available from: https://www.cambridge.org/core/product/identifier/S0007125000251192/type/journal_article.
137. D'Souza DC, Perry E, MacDougall L, Ammerman Y, Cooper T, Wu Y, et al. The psychotomimetic effects of intravenous delta-9-tetrahydrocannabinol in healthy individuals: implications for psychosis. Neuropsychopharmacology [Internet]. 2004 [cited 2019 Aug 8];29(8):1558–72. Available from: http://www.nature.com/articles/1300496.
138. Morrison PD, Zois V, McKeown DA, Lee TD, Holt DW, Powell JF, et al. The acute effects of synthetic intravenous Δ9-tetrahydrocannabinol on psychosis, mood and cognitive functioning. Psychol Med [Internet]. 2009 [cited 2019 Jul 26];39(10):1607. Available from: http://www.journals.cambridge.org/abstract_S0033291709005522.
139. Di Forti M, Quattrone D, Freeman TP, Tripoli G, Gayer-Anderson C, Quigley H, et al. The contribution of cannabis use to variation in the incidence of psychotic disorder across Europe (EU-GEI): a multicentre case-control study. The lancet Psychiatry [Internet]. 2019 [cited 2019 Jul 25];6(5):427–36. Available from: http://www.ncbi.nlm.nih.gov/pubmed/30902669.
140. Witton J, Arseneault L, Cannon M, Murray R. Cannabis as a causal factor for psychosis – a review of the evidence. In: Search for the causes of schizophrenia [Internet]. Heidelberg: Steinkopff; 2004 [cited 2019 Jul 26]. p. 133–49. Available from: http://www.springerlink.com/index/10.1007/978-3-7985-1953-4_9.
141. Kuepper R, Morrison PD, van Os J, Murray RM, Kenis G, Henquet C. Does dopamine mediate the psychosis-inducing effects of cannabis? A review and integration of findings across disciplines. Schizophr Res [Internet]. 2010 [cited 2019 Jul 26];121(1–3):107–17. Available from: https://www.sciencedirect.com/science/article/abs/pii/S0920996410013526.

142. D'Souza DC, Radhakrishnan R, Sherif M, Cortes-Briones J, Cahill J, Gupta S, et al. Cannabinoids and psychosis. [cited 2019 Jul 26]; Available from: https://www.ingentaconnect.com/contentone/ben/cpd/2016/00000022/00000042/art00005.
143. Schoeler T, Theobald D, Pingault J-B, Farrington DP, Jennings WG, Piquero AR, et al. Continuity of cannabis use and violent offending over the life course. Psychol Med [Internet]. 2016 [cited 2019 Jul 22];46(8):1663–77. Available from: https://www.cambridge.org/core/product/identifier/S0033291715003001/type/journal_article.
144. Setién-Suero E, Neergaard K, Ortiz-García de la Foz V, Suárez-Pinilla P, Martínez-García O, Crespo-Facorro B, et al. Stopping cannabis use benefits outcome in psychosis: findings from 10-year follow-up study in the PAFIP -cohort. Acta Psychiatr Scand [Internet]. 2019 [cited 2019 Aug 8];acps.13081. Available from: http://www.ncbi.nlm.nih.gov/pubmed/31381129.
145. Colizzi M, Burnett N, Costa R, De Agostini M, Griffin J, Bhattacharyya S. Longitudinal assessment of the effect of cannabis use on hospital readmission rates in early psychosis: a 6-year follow-up in an inpatient cohort. Psychiatry Res [Internet]. 2018 [cited 2018 Sep 12];268:381–7. Available from: https://www.sciencedirect.com/science/article/pii/S0165178118302889.
146. Giordano GN, Ohlsson H, Sundquist K, Sundquist J, Kendler KS. The association between cannabis abuse and subsequent schizophrenia: a Swedish national co-relative control study. Psychol Med [Internet]. 2015 [cited 2018 Aug 22];45(2):407–14. Available from: http://www.journals.cambridge.org/abstract_S0033291714001524.
147. Starzer MSK, Nordentoft M, Hjorthøj C. Rates and predictors of conversion to schizophrenia or bipolar disorder following substance-induced psychosis. Am J Psychiatry [Internet]. 2017 [cited 2017 Dec 18];appi.ajp.2017.1. Available from: http://ajp.psychiatryonline.org/doi/10.1176/appi.ajp.2017.17020223.
148. Kendler KS, Ohlsson H, Sundquist J, Sundquist K. Prediction of onset of substance-induced psychotic disorder and its progression to schizophrenia in a Swedish national sample. Am J Psychiatry [Internet]. 2019 May 6 [cited 2019 Jul 22];appi.ajp.2019.1. Available from: http://ajp.psychiatryonline.org/doi/10.1176/appi.ajp.2019.18101217.
149. Niemi-Pynttäri JA, Sund R, Putkonen H, Vorma H, Wahlbeck K, Pirkola SP. Substance-induced psychoses converting into schizophrenia. J Clin Psychiatry [Internet]. 2013 [cited 2018 May 7];74(01):e94–9. Available from: http://www.ncbi.nlm.nih.gov/pubmed/23419236.
150. Gobbi G, Atkin T, Zytynski T, Wang S, Askari S, Boruff J, et al. Association of cannabis use in adolescence and risk of depression, anxiety, and suicidality in young adulthood. JAMA Psychiatry [Internet]. 2019 [cited 2019 May 16];76(4):426. Available from: http://archpsyc.jamanetwork.com/article.aspx?doi=10.1001/jamapsychiatry.2018.4500.
151. Sellers CM, Diaz-Valdes Iriarte A, Wyman Battalen A, O'Brien KHM. Alcohol and marijuana use as daily predictors of suicide ideation and attempts among adolescents prior to psychiatric hospitalization. Psychiatry Res [Internet]. 2019 [cited 2019 Aug 9];273:672–7. Available from: https://www.sciencedirect.com/science/article/abs/pii/S0165178118323321.
152. Silins E, Horwood LJ, Patton GC, Fergusson DM, Olsson CA, Hutchinson DM, et al. Young adult sequelae of adolescent cannabis use: an integrative analysis. Lancet Psychiatry [Internet]. 2014 [cited 2019 Jul 26];1(4):286–93. Available from: https://linkinghub.elsevier.com/retrieve/pii/S2215036614703074.
153. Carvalho AF, Stubbs B, Vancampfort D, Kloiber S, Maes M, Firth J, et al. Cannabis use and suicide attempts among 86,254 adolescents aged 12-15 years from 21 low- and middle-income countries. Eur Psychiatry [Internet]. 2019 [cited 2019 Aug 8];56:8–13. Available from: https://linkinghub.elsevier.com/retrieve/pii/S0924933818301913.
154. Adkisson K, Cunningham KC, Dedert EA, Dennis MF, Calhoun PS, Elbogen EB, et al. Cannabis use disorder and post-deployment suicide attempts in Iraq/Afghanistan-Era veterans. Arch Suicide Res [Internet]. 2018 [cited 2019 Aug 9];1–10. Available from: https://www.tandfonline.com/doi/full/10.1080/13811118.2018.1488638.

155. Center for Behavioral Health Statistics S. Results from the 2013 national survey on drug use and health: summary of national findings [Internet]. [cited 2019 Aug 15]. Available from: http://store.samhsa.gov/home.

156. Chadi N, Schroeder R, Jensen JW, Levy S. Association between electronic cigarette use and marijuana use among adolescents and young adults. JAMA Pediatr [Internet]. 2019 [cited 2019 Aug 13];e192574. Available from: https://jamanetwork.com/journals/jamapediatrics/fullarticle/2748383.

157. Audrain-Mcgovern J, Stone MD, Barrington-Trimis J, Unger JB, Leventhal AM. Adolescent E-cigarette, hookah, and conventional cigarette use and subsequent marijuana use. Pediatrics [Internet]. 2018 [cited 2018 Aug 16];142(3):20173616. Available from: www.aappublications.org/news.

158. Banks DE, Rowe AT, Mpofu P, Zapolski TCB. Trends in typologies of concurrent alcohol, marijuana, and cigarette use among US adolescents: an ecological examination by sex and race/ethnicity. Drug Alcohol Depend [Internet]. 2017 [cited 2019 Aug 15];179:71–7. Available from: http://www.ncbi.nlm.nih.gov/pubmed/28756102.

159. Schauer GL, Berg CJ, Kegler MC, Donovan DM, Windle M. Assessing the overlap between tobacco and marijuana: trends in patterns of co-use of tobacco and marijuana in adults from 2003–2012. Addict Behav [Internet]. 2015 [cited 2019 Aug 15];49:26–32. Available from: https://www.sciencedirect.com/science/article/abs/pii/S0306460315001768.

160. Schauer G, King B, Bunnell R, Promoff G, McAfee T. Toking, vaping, and eating for health or fun: marijuana use patterns in adults, U.S. Am J Prev Med. 2014;50(1):1–8.

161. Kandel D. Stages in adolescent involvement in drug use. Science (80-) [Internet]. 1975 [cited 2019 Aug 16];190(4217):912–4. Available from: http://www.ncbi.nlm.nih.gov/pubmed/1188374.

162. Keyes KM, Rutherford C, Miech R. Historical trends in the grade of onset and sequence of cigarette, alcohol, and marijuana use among adolescents from 1976–2016: implications for "Gateway" patterns in adolescence. Drug Alcohol Depend [Internet]. 2019 [cited 2019 May 16];194:51–8. Available from: https://www.sciencedirect.com/science/article/pii/S0376871618307555.

163. Patton GC, Coffey C, Carlin JB, Sawyer SM, Lynskey M. Reverse gateways? Frequent cannabis use as a predictor of tobacco initiation and nicotine dependence. Addiction [Internet]. 2005 [cited 2019 Aug 16];100(10):1518–25. Available from: http://www.ncbi.nlm.nih.gov/pubmed/16185213.

164. Schauer GL, Rosenberry ZR, Peters EN. Marijuana and tobacco co-administration in blunts, spliffs, and mulled cigarettes: a systematic literature review. Addict Behav [Internet]. 2017 [cited 2019 Jan 9];64:200–11. Available from: https://linkinghub.elsevier.com/retrieve/pii/S0306460316303306.

165. Fix BV, Smith D, O'Connor R, Heckman BW, Willemsen MC, Cummings M, et al. Cannabis use among a nationally representative cross-sectional sample of smokers and non-smokers in the Netherlands: results from the 2015 ITC Netherlands Gold Magic Survey. BMJ Open [Internet]. 2019 [cited 2019 Aug 16];9(3):E024497. Available from: http://www.ncbi.nlm.nih.gov/pubmed/30833306.

166. Akbar SA, Tomko RL, Salazar CA, Squeglia LM, McClure EA. Tobacco and cannabis co-use and interrelatedness among adults. Addict Behav [Internet]. 2019 [cited 2019 Feb 28];90:354–61. Available from: https://www.sciencedirect.com/science/article/abs/pii/S0306460318305082?via%3Dihub.

167. Goodwin RD, Pacek LR, Copeland J, Moeller SJ, Dierker L, Weinberger A, et al. Trends in Daily Cannabis Use Among Cigarette Smokers: United States, 2002-2014. Am J Public Health [Internet]. 2018 [cited 2017 Dec 18];108(1):137–42. Available from: http://ajph.aphapublications.org/doi/10.2105/AJPH.2017.304050.

168. Pacek LR, Copeland J, Dierker L, Cunningham CO, Martins SS, Goodwin RD. Among whom is cigarette smoking declining in the United States? The impact of cannabis use status, 2002–2015. Drug Alcohol Depend [Internet]. 2018 [cited 2018 Jun 5];0(0). Available from: http://linkinghub.elsevier.com/retrieve/pii/S0376871618301728.

169. Weinberger AH, Delnevo CD, Wyka K, Gbedemah M, Lee J, Copeland J, et al. Cannabis use is associated with increased risk of cigarette smoking initiation, persistence, and relapse among adults in the United States. Nicotine Tob Res [Internet]. 2019 [cited 2019 Aug 23]; Available from: http://www.ncbi.nlm.nih.gov/pubmed/31112595.
170. Caulkins JP (Jonathan P, Kilmer B, Kleiman M. Marijuana legalization: what everyone needs to know [Internet]. [cited 2019 Aug 12]. 284 p. Available from: https://books.google.no/books/about/Marijuana_Legalization.html?id=3UYnDAAAQBAJ&source=kp_cover&redir_esc=y.
171. Tucker JS, Pedersen ER, Seelam R, Dunbar MS, Shih RA, D'Amico EJ. Types of cannabis and tobacco/nicotine co-use and associated outcomes in young adulthood. Psychol Addict Behav [Internet]. 2019 [cited 2019 Apr 30]; Available from: http://www.ncbi.nlm.nih.gov/pubmed/30985164.
172. Subbaraman MS. Substitution and complementarity of alcohol and cannabis: a review of the literature. Subst Use Misuse [Internet]. 2016 [cited 2018 Nov 16];51(11):1399–414. Available from: http://www.ncbi.nlm.nih.gov/pubmed/27249324.
173. Ozgo D. Impact of retail marijuana legalization on alcohol sales in Colorado, Washington state and Oregon David Ozgo SVP, Strategic Analysis and Economic Affairs Distilled Spirits Council [Internet]. 2019 [cited 2019 Mar 5]. Available from: https://www.distilledspirits.org/wp-content/uploads/2019/01/Recreational-Marijuana-Impact-Study.pdf.
174. Subbaraman MS, Kerr WC. Simultaneous versus concurrent use of alcohol and cannabis in the National Alcohol Survey. Alcohol Clin Exp Res [Internet]. 2015 [cited 2019 Jan 7];39(5):872–9. Available from.: http://www.ncbi.nlm.nih.gov/pubmed/25872596.
175. Pape H, Rossow I, Storvoll EE. Under double influence: assessment of simultaneous alcohol and cannabis use in general youth populations. Drug Alcohol Depend [Internet]. 2009 [cited 2018 Nov 16];101(1–2):69–73. Available from: http://www.ncbi.nlm.nih.gov/pubmed/19095380.
176. Egan KL, Cox MJ, Suerken CK, Reboussin BA, Song EY, Wagoner KG, et al. More drugs, more problems? Simultaneous use of alcohol and marijuana at parties among youth and young adults. Drug Alcohol Depend [Internet]. 2019 [cited 2019 Aug 15];202:69–75. Available from: https://www.sciencedirect.com/science/article/abs/pii/S0376871619302121.
177. Terry-McElrath YM, O'Malley PM, Johnston LD. Alcohol and marijuana use patterns associated with unsafe driving among U.S. high school seniors: high use frequency, concurrent use, and simultaneous use. J Stud Alcohol Drugs [Internet]. 2014 [cited 2019 Aug 15];75(3):378–89. Available from: http://www.ncbi.nlm.nih.gov/pubmed/24766749.
178. Linden-Carmichael AN, Stamates AL, Lau-Barraco C. Simultaneous use of alcohol and marijuana: patterns and individual differences. Subst Use Misuse [Internet]. 2019 [cited 2019 Aug 14];1–11. Available from: https://www.tandfonline.com/doi/full/10.1080/10826084.2019.1638407.
179. Yurasek AM, Aston ER, Metrik J. Co-use of alcohol and cannabis: a review. Curr Addict Reports [Internet]. 2017 [cited 2019 Jan 7];4(2):184–93. Available from: http://link.springer.com/10.1007/s40429-017-0149-8.
180. Blanco C, Hasin DS, Wall MM, Flórez-Salamanca L, Hoertel N, Wang S, et al. Cannabis use and risk of psychiatric disorders. JAMA Psychiatry [Internet]. 2016 [cited 2019 Mar 27];73(4):388. Available from: http://archpsyc.jamanetwork.com/article.aspx?doi=10.1001/jamapsychiatry.2015.3229.
181. Green KM, Reboussin BA, Pacek LR, Storr CL, Mojtabai R, Cullen BA, et al. The effects of marijuana use on transitions through stages of alcohol involvement for men and women in the NESARC I and II. Subst Use Misuse [Internet]. 2019 [cited 2019 Aug 14];1–10. Available from: https://www.tandfonline.com/doi/full/10.1080/10826084.2019.1638408.
182. Cohn AM, Johnson AL, Rose SW, Pearson JL, Villanti AC, Stanton C. Population-level patterns and mental health and substance use correlates of alcohol, marijuana, and tobacco use and co-use in US young adults and adults: results from the population assessment for tobacco and health. Am J Addict [Internet]. 2018 [cited 2019 Aug 15];27(6):491–500. Available from: http://doi.wiley.com/10.1111/ajad.12766.

183. McPartland JM. A review of cannabis diseases. J Int Hemp Assoc [Internet]. 1996 [cited 2019 Aug 20];3(1):19–23. Available from: https://www.cabdirect.org/cabdirect/abstract/19971004184.

184. Thompson GR, Tuscano JM, Dennis M, Singapuri A, Libertini S, Gaudino R, et al. A microbiome assessment of medical marijuana. Clin Microbiol Infect [Internet]. 2017 [cited 2019 Aug 20];23(4):269–70. Available from: http://www.ncbi.nlm.nih.gov/pubmed/27956269.

185. Ruchlemer R, Amit-Kohn M, Raveh D, Hanuš L. Inhaled medicinal cannabis and the immunocompromised patient. [cited 2019 Aug 20]; Available from: https://www.mascc.org/assets/Pain_Center/2015_March/march2015-11.pdf.

186. McPartland JM, Pruitt PL. Medical marijuana and its use by the immunocompromised. Altern Ther Health Med [Internet]. 1997 [cited 2019 Aug 20];3(3):39–45. Available from: http://www.ncbi.nlm.nih.gov/pubmed/9141290.

187. Cescon DW, Page A V, Richardson S, Moore MJ, Boerner S, Gold WL. Invasive pulmonary aspergillosis associated with marijuana use in a man with colorectal cancer. J Clin Oncol [Internet]. 2008 [cited 2019 Aug 20];26(13):2214–5. Available from: http://ascopubs.org/doi/10.1200/JCO.2007.15.2777.

188. Chatkin JM, Zani-Silva L, Ferreira I, Zamel N. Cannabis-associated asthma and allergies. Clin Rev Allergy Immunol [Internet]. 2019 [cited 2019 Aug 20];56(2):196–206. Available from: http://www.ncbi.nlm.nih.gov/pubmed/28921405.

189. McPartland JM, McKernan KJ. Contaminants of concern in cannabis: microbes, heavy metals and pesticides. In: Cannabis sativa L – botany and biotechnology [Internet]. Cham: Springer International Publishing; 2017 [cited 2019 Aug 20]. p. 457–74. Available from: http://link.springer.com/10.1007/978-3-319-54564-6_22.

190. Martyny JW, Serrano KA, Schaeffer JW, Van Dyke M V. Potential exposures associated with indoor marijuana growing operations. J Occup Environ Hyg [Internet]. 2013 [cited 2019 Aug 20];10(11):622–39. Available from: http://www.ncbi.nlm.nih.gov/pubmed/24116667.

191. Cuypers E, Vanhove W, Gotink J, Bonneure A, Van Damme P, Tytgat J. The use of pesticides in Belgian illicit indoor cannabis plantations. Forensic Sci Int [Internet]. 2017 [cited 2019 Aug 20];277:59–65. Available from: http://www.ncbi.nlm.nih.gov/pubmed/28609661.

192. Busse F, Omidi L, Leichtle A, Windgassen M, Kluge E, Stumvoll M. Lead poisoning due to adulterated marijuana. N Engl J Med [Internet]. 2008 [cited 2019 Aug 20];358(15):1641–2. Available from: http://www.nejm.org/doi/abs/10.1056/NEJMc0707784.

193. Bloor RN, Wang TS, Španěl P, Smith D. Ammonia release from heated 'street' cannabis leaf and its potential toxic effects on cannabis users. Addiction [Internet]. 2008 [cited 2019 Aug 20];103(10):1671–7. Available from: http://www.ncbi.nlm.nih.gov/pubmed/18705690.

194. Gilbert CR, Baram M, Cavarocchi NC. "Smoking wet": respiratory failure related to smoking tainted marijuana cigarettes. Texas Hear Inst J [Internet]. 2013 [cited 2019 Aug 20];40(1):64–7. Available from: http://www.ncbi.nlm.nih.gov/pubmed/23466531.

195. Davidson M, Reed S, Oosthuizen J, O'Donnell G, Gaur P, Cross M, et al. Occupational health and safety in cannabis production: an Australian perspective. Int J Occup Environ Health [Internet]. 2018 [cited 2019 Aug 20];24(3–4):75–85. Available from: http://www.ncbi.nlm.nih.gov/pubmed/30281413.

196. Victory KR, Couch J, Lowe B, Green BJ. *Notes from the field:* occupational hazards associated with harvesting and processing cannabis – Washington, 2015–2016. MMWR Morb Mortal Wkly Rep [Internet]. 2018 [cited 2019 Aug 20];67(8):259–60. Available from: http://www.cdc.gov/mmwr/volumes/67/wr/mm6708a7.htm?s_cid=mm6708a7_w.

197. Secretary of State – Audits Division O. Oregon's framework for regulating marijuana should be strengthened to better mitigate diversion risk and improve laboratory testing. Oregon Liquor Control Commission, Oregon Health Authority. Oregon's framework for regulating marijuana should be strengthened to better mitigate diversion risk and improve laboratory testing report highlights [Internet]. 2019 [cited 2019 Sep 17]. Available from: https://sos.oregon.gov/audits/Documents/2019-04.pdf.

198. Daley DC. Family and social aspects of substance use disorders and treatment. J Food Drug Anal [Internet]. 2013 [cited 2019 Aug 7];21(4):S73–6. Available from: http://www.ncbi.nlm.nih.gov/pubmed/25214748.

199. Lander L, Howsare J, Byrne M. The impact of substance use disorders on families and children: from theory to practice. Soc Work Public Health [Internet]. 2013 [cited 2019 Aug 7];28(3–4):194–205. Available from: http://www.ncbi.nlm.nih.gov/pubmed/23731414.

200. Ólafsdóttir J, Hrafnsdóttir S, Orjasniemi T. Depression, anxiety, and stress from substance-use disorder among family members in Iceland. Nord Stud Alcohol Drugs [Internet]. 2018 [cited 2019 Aug 7];35(3):165–78. Available from: http://journals.sagepub.com/doi/10.1177/1455072518766129.

201. Wang X, Derakhshandeh R, Liu J, Narayan S, Nabavizadeh P, Le S, et al. One minute of marijuana secondhand smoke exposure substantially impairs vascular endothelial function. J Am Heart Assoc [Internet]. 2016 [cited 2018 Dec 19];5(8). Available from: http://www.ncbi.nlm.nih.gov/pubmed/27464788.

202. Wilson KM, Torok MR, Wei B, Wang L, Lowary M, Blount BC. Marijuana and tobacco coexposure in hospitalized children. Pediatrics [Internet]. 2018 [cited 2019 Jul 23];142(6):e20180820. Available from: http://www.ncbi.nlm.nih.gov/pubmed/30455340.

203. Posis A, Bellettiere J, Liles S, Alcaraz J, Nguyen B, Berardi V, et al. Indoor cannabis smoke and children's health. Prev Med Reports [Internet]. 2019 [cited 2019 May 14];14:100853. Available from: https://www.sciencedirect.com/science/article/pii/S2211335519300385#!.

204. Correlation between secondhand marijuana and tobacco smoke exposure and children ED visits: new research examines the impact of second hand smoke from tobacco to understand marijuana's impact on children – ScienceDaily [Internet]. [cited 2018 May 8]. Available from: https://www.sciencedaily.com/releases/2018/05/180505091833.htm.

205. Glantz SA, Halpern-Felsher B, Springer ML. Marijuana, secondhand smoke, and social acceptability. JAMA Intern Med [Internet]. 2018 [cited 2019 Feb 11];178(1):13. Available from: http://archinte.jamanetwork.com/article.aspx?doi=10.1001/jamainternmed.2017.5301.

206. Young-Wolff KC, Sarovar V, Tucker L-Y, Conway A, Alexeeff S, Weisner C, et al. Self-reported daily, weekly, and monthly cannabis use among women before and during pregnancy. JAMA Netw Open [Internet]. 2019 [cited 2019 Aug 9];2(7):e196471. Available from: https://jamanetwork.com/journals/jamanetworkopen/fullarticle/2738343.

207. Young-Wolff KC, Tucker L-Y, Alexeeff S, Armstrong MA, Conway A, Weisner C, et al. Trends in self-reported and biochemically tested marijuana use among pregnant females in California from 2009-2016. JAMA [Internet]. 2017 [cited 2018 May 7];318(24):2490. Available from: http://jama.jamanetwork.com/article.aspx?doi=10.1001/jama.2017.17225.

208. Young-Wolff KC, Sarovar V, Tucker L-Y, Avalos LA, Alexeeff S, Conway A, et al. Trends in marijuana use among pregnant women with and without nausea and vomiting in pregnancy, 2009–2016. Drug Alcohol Depend [Internet]. 2019 [cited 2019 Jul 22];196:66–70. Available from: http://www.ncbi.nlm.nih.gov/pubmed/30711893.

209. Volkow ND, Han B, Compton WM, McCance-Katz EF. Self-reported medical and non-medical cannabis use among pregnant women in the United States. JAMA [Internet]. 2019 [cited 2019 Jun 25]; Available from: http://jama.jamanetwork.com/article.aspx?doi=10.1001/jama.2019.7982.

210. Campo J. Washington State Office of Financial Management maternal and newborn inpatient stays with a substance use or use-related diagnosis [Internet]. 2016 [cited 2019 Jul 22]. Available from: https://www.ofm.wa.gov/sites/default/files/public/legacy/researchbriefs/2016/brief075.pdf.

211. Brown QL, Sarvet AL, Shmulewitz D, Martins SS, Wall MM, Hasin DS. Trends in marijuana use among pregnant and nonpregnant reproductive-aged women, 2002-2014. JAMA [Internet]. 2017 [cited 2019 Jan 16];317(2):207. Available from: http://jama.jamanetwork.com/article.aspx?doi=10.1001/jama.2016.17383.

212. Ko JY, Farr SL, Tong VT, Creanga AA, Callaghan WM. Prevalence and patterns of marijuana use among pregnant and nonpregnant women of reproductive age. Am J Obstet Gynecol

[Internet]. 2015 [cited 2019 Jul 22];213(2):201.e1–201.e10. Available from: http://www. ncbi.nlm.nih.gov/pubmed/25772211.

213. Petrangelo A, Czuzoj-Shulman N, Balayla J, Abenhaim HA. Cannabis abuse or dependence during pregnancy: a population-based cohort study on 12 million births. J Obstet Gynaecol Canada [Internet]. 2019 [cited 2019 Jul 22];41(5):623–30. Available from: https://linkinghub. elsevier.com/retrieve/pii/S1701216318307059.

214. Jansson LM, Jordan CJ, Velez ML. Perinatal marijuana use and the developing child. JAMA [Internet]. 2018 Aug 14 [cited 2018 Sep 5];320(6):545. Available from: http://jama.jamanet-work.com/article.aspx?doi=10.1001/jama.2018.8401

215. Corsi DJ, Walsh L, Weiss D, Hsu H, El-Chaar D, Hawken S, et al. Association between self-reported prenatal cannabis use and maternal, perinatal, and neonatal outcomes. JAMA [Internet]. 2019 [cited 2019 Jul 23];322(2):145. Available from: http://jama.jamanetwork. com/article.aspx?doi=10.1001/jama.2019.8734.

216. Gunn JKL, Rosales CB, Center KE, Nuñez A, Gibson SJ, Christ C, et al. Prenatal exposure to cannabis and maternal and child health outcomes: a systematic review and meta-analysis. BMJ Open [Internet]. 2016 [cited 2019 Aug 21];6(4):e009986. Available from: http://bmjo-pen.bmj.com/lookup/doi/10.1136/bmjopen-2015-009986.

217. Breit KR, Zamudio B, Thomas JD. The effects of alcohol and cannabinoid exposure during the brain growth spurt on behavioral development in rats. Birth Defects Res [Internet]. 2019 [cited 2019 Jul 24];111(12):760–74. Available from: https://onlinelibrary.wiley.com/ doi/abs/10.1002/bdr2.1487.

218. Boa-Amponsem O, Zhang C, Mukhopadhyay S, Ardrey I, Cole GJ. Ethanol and cannabinoids interact to alter behavior in a zebrafish fetal alcohol spectrum disorder model. Birth Defects Res [Internet]. 2019 [cited 2019 Jul 24];111(12):775–88. Available from: https:// onlinelibrary.wiley.com/doi/abs/10.1002/bdr2.1458.

219. Wright HR, Warrick CR, Kuyat JR, Rodriguez JW, Lugo, JM, McLaughlin RJ. Maternal cannabis vapor exposure dose-dependently impairs behavioral flexibility [Internet]. [cited 2019 Jul 22]. Available from: https://www.documentcloud.org/documents/5046724-WSU-Rats.html.

220. Bertrand KA, Hanan NJ, Honerkamp-Smith G, Best BM, Chambers CD. Marijuana use by breastfeeding mothers and cannabinoid concentrations in breast milk. Pediatrics [Internet]. 2018 [cited 2019 Jan 9];142(3):e20181076. Available from: http://www.ncbi.nlm.nih.gov/ pubmed/30150212.

221. Mourh J, Rowe H. Marijuana and breastfeeding: applicability of the current literature to clinical practice. Breastfeed Med [Internet]. 2017 [cited 2019 Jan 11];12(10):582–96. Available from: http://www.liebertpub.com/doi/10.1089/bfm.2017.0020.

222. Jarlenski M, Koma JW, Zank J, Bodnar LM, Bogen DL, Chang JC. Trends in perception of risk of regular marijuana use among US pregnant and nonpregnant reproductive-aged women. Am J Obstet Gynecol [Internet]. 2017 [cited 2019 Aug 7];217(6):705–7. Available from: http://www.ncbi.nlm.nih.gov/pubmed/28843740.

223. Bayrampour H, Zahradnik M, Lisonkova S, Janssen P. Women's perspectives about cannabis use during pregnancy and the postpartum period: an integrative review. Prev Med (Baltim) [Internet]. 2019 [cited 2019 Jan 24];119:17–23. Available from: https://www.sciencedirect. com/science/article/pii/S0091743518303773.

224. Dickson B, Mansfield C, Guiahi M, Allshouse AA, Borgelt LM, Sheeder J, et al. Recommendations from cannabis dispensaries about first-trimester cannabis use. Obstet Gynecol [Internet]. 2018 [cited 2018 May 11];1. Available from: http://insights.ovid.com/cro ssref?an=00006250-900000000-98083.

225. Blohm E, Sell P, Neavyn M. Cannabinoid toxicity in pediatrics. Curr Opin Pediatr [Internet]. 2019 [cited 2019 May 22];31(2):256–61. Available from: http://www.ncbi.nlm.nih.gov/ pubmed/30694824.

226. Leubitz A, Spiller HA, Jolliff H, Casavant M. Prevalence and clinical characteristics of unintentional ingestion of marijuana in children younger than 6 years in states with and with-

out legalized marijuana laws. Pediatr Emerg Care [Internet]. 2019 [cited 2019 Aug 12];1. Available from: http://insights.ovid.com/crossref?an=00006565-900000000-98140.

227. Claudet I, Mouvier S, Labadie M, Manin C, Michard-Lenoir A-P, Eyer D, et al. Unintentional cannabis intoxication in toddlers. Pediatrics [Internet]. 2017 Sep 1 [cited 2019 Jul 23];140(3):e20170017. Available from: https://pediatrics.aappublications.org/content/140/3/e20170017.

228. Brooks-Russell A, Hall K, Peterson A, Graves J, Van Dyke M. Cannabis in homes with children: use and storage practices in a legalised state. Inj Prev [Internet]. 2019 [cited 2019 Aug 6];injuryprev-2019-043318. Available from: http://www.ncbi.nlm.nih.gov/pubmed/31371385.

229. Wang GS, Le Lait M-C, Deakyne SJ, Bronstein AC, Bajaj L, Roosevelt G. Unintentional pediatric exposures to marijuana in Colorado, 2009-2015. JAMA Pediatr [Internet]. 2016 [cited 2019 Jul 23];170(9):e160971. Available from: http://www.ncbi.nlm.nih.gov/pubmed/27454910.

230. Onders B, Casavant MJ, Spiller HA, Chounthirath T, Smith GA. Marijuana exposure among children younger than six years in the United States. Clin Pediatr (Phila) [Internet]. 2016 [cited 2019 Jul 23];55(5):428–36. Available from: http://journals.sagepub.com/doi/10.1177/0009922815589912.

231. Whitehill JM, Harrington C, Lang CJ, Chary M, Bhutta WA, Burns MM. Incidence of pediatric cannabis exposure among children and teenagers aged 0 to 19 years before and after medical marijuana legalization in Massachusetts. JAMA Netw Open [Internet]. 2019 [cited 2019 Aug 22];2(8):e199456. Available from: https://jamanetwork.com/journals/jamanetworkopen/fullarticle/2748051.

232. Erkelens JL, Hazekamp A. That which we call Indica, by any other name would smell as sweet an essay on the history of the term Indica and the taxonomical conflict between the monotypic and polytypic views of Cannabis What's in a name? [Internet]. Vol. 9, Cannabinoids. 2014 [cited 2019 Aug 20]. Available from: www.cannabis-med.org.

233. INCB. The therapeutic use of cannabis. Available from: https://www.incb.org/documents/News/Alerts/Alert_on_Control_of_Narcotic_Drugs_June_2017.pdf.

234. Emcdda. Questions and answers for policymaking Medical use of cannabis and cannabinoids [Internet]. 2018 [cited 2019 Sep 12]. Available from: http://www.emcdda.europa.eu/system/files/publications/10171/20185584_TD0618186ENN_PDF.pdf.

235. Marijuana and cannabinoids. NCCIH [Internet]. [cited 2019 Aug 12]. Available from: https://nccih.nih.gov/health/marijuana.

236. Stockings E, Campbell G, Hall WD, Nielsen S, Zagic D, Rahman R, et al. Cannabis and cannabinoids for the treatment of people with chronic noncancer pain conditions: a systematic review and meta-analysis of controlled and observational studies. Pain [Internet]. 2018 [cited 2019 May 3];159(10):1932–54. Available from: http://www.ncbi.nlm.nih.gov/pubmed/29847469.

237. Häuser W, Welsch P, Klose P, Radbruch L, Fitzcharles M-A. Efficacy, tolerability and safety of cannabis-based medicines for cancer pain. Der Schmerz [Internet]. 2019 [cited 2019 Sep 23]; Available from: http://www.ncbi.nlm.nih.gov/pubmed/31073761.

238. Hill KP. Medical use of cannabis in 2019. JAMA [Internet]. 2019 Aug 9 [cited 2019 Sep 2]; Available from: https://jamanetwork.com/journals/jama/fullarticle/2748398.

239. Marijuana as medicine [Internet]. [cited 2019 Aug 20]. Available from: https://d14rmgtrw-zf5a.cloudfront.net/sites/default/files/marijuanamedicinedrugfacts_july2019_.pdf.

240. Fitzcharles M-A, Niaki OZ, Hauser W, Hazlewood G. Position statement: a pragmatic approach for medical cannabis and patients with rheumatic diseases. J Rheumatol [Internet]. 2019 [cited 2019 May 3];46(5):532–8. Available from: http://www.jrheum.org/lookup/doi/10.3899/jrheum.181120.

241. Klumpers LE, Thacker DL. A brief background on cannabis: from plant to medical indications. J AOAC Int [Internet]. 2019 Mar 1 [cited 2019 Aug 20];102(2):412–20. Available from: http://www.ncbi.nlm.nih.gov/pubmed/30139415.

242. Thomas BF, Pollard GT. Preparation and distribution of cannabis and cannabis-derived dosage formulations for investigational and therapeutic use in the United States. Front Pharmacol [Internet]. 2016 [cited 2019 Aug 21];7:285. Available from: http://www.ncbi.nlm.nih.gov/pubmed/27630566.

243. Bachhuber MA, Saloner B, Cunningham CO, Barry CL. Medical cannabis laws and opioid analgesic overdose mortality in the United States, 1999-2010. JAMA Intern Med [Internet]. 2014 [cited 2019 Sep 5];174(10):1668. Available from: http://archinte.jamanetwork.com/article.aspx?doi=10.1001/jamainternmed.2014.4005.

244. Chan NW, Burkhardt J, Flyr M. The effects of recreational marijuana legalization and dispensing on opioid mortality. Econ Inq [Internet]. 2019 [cited 2019 Aug 14];ecin.12819. Available from: https://onlinelibrary.wiley.com/doi/abs/10.1111/ecin.12819.

245. Lucas P, Walsh Z, Crosby K, Callaway R, Belle-Isle L, Kay R, et al. Substituting cannabis for prescription drugs, alcohol and other substances among medical cannabis patients: the impact of contextual factors. Drug Alcohol Rev. 2016;35(3):326–33.

246. Boehnke KF, Litinas E, Clauw DJ. Medical cannabis use is associated with decreased opiate medication use in a retrospective cross-sectional survey of patients with chronic pain. J Pain [Internet]. 2016 [cited 2019 Sep 5];17(6):739–44. Available from: https://linkinghub.elsevier.com/retrieve/pii/S1526590016005678.

247. Boehnke KF, Scott JR, Litinas E, Sisley S, Williams DA, Clauw DJ. Pills to pot: observational analyses of cannabis substitution among medical cannabis users with chronic pain. J Pain [Internet]. 2019 [cited 2019 May 15]; Available from: https://linkinghub.elsevier.com/retrieve/pii/S1526590018307351.

248. Shi Y, Liang D, Bao Y, An R, Wallace MS, Grant I. Recreational marijuana legalization and prescription opioids received by Medicaid enrollees. Drug Alcohol Depend [Internet]. 2019 [cited 2019 Jan 3];194:13–9. Available from: https://www.sciencedirect.com/science/article/pii/S0376871618307567.

249. Shover CL, Davis CS, Gordon SC, Humphreys K. Association between medical cannabis laws and opioid overdose mortality has reversed over time. Proc Natl Acad Sci [Internet]. 2019 [cited 2019 Jun 26];116(26):12624–6. Available from: https://www.pnas.org/content/116/26/12624.

250. Segura LE, Mauro CM, Levy NS, Khauli N, Philbin MM, Mauro PM, et al. Association of US medical marijuana laws with nonmedical prescription opioid use and prescription opioid use disorder. JAMA Netw Open [Internet]. 2019 [cited 2019 Aug 16];2(7):e197216. Available from: http://www.ncbi.nlm.nih.gov/pubmed/31314118.

251. Bhashyam AR, Heng M, Harris MB, Vrahas MS, Weaver MJ. Self-reported marijuana use is associated with increased use of prescription opioids following traumatic musculoskeletal injury. J Bone Jt Surg [Internet]. 2018 [cited 2019 Apr 24];100(24):2095–102. Available from: http://insights.ovid.com/crossref?an=00004623-201812190-00001.

252. Bauer F, Donahoo WT, Hollis HW, Tsai AG, Pottorf BJ, Johnson JM, et al. Marijuana's influence on pain scores, initial weight loss, and other bariatric surgical outcomes. Perm J [Internet]. 2018 [cited 2019 Apr 24];22:18–002. Available from: http://www.ncbi.nlm.nih.gov/pubmed/30010532.

253. Caputi TL, Humphreys K. Medical marijuana users are more likely to use prescription drugs medically and nonmedically. J Addict Med [Internet]. 2018 [cited 2018 Aug 24];12(4):295–9. Available from: https://www.ncbi.nlm.nih.gov/pubmed/29664895.

254. Campbell G, Hall WD, Peacock A, Lintzeris N, Bruno R, Larance B, et al. Effect of cannabis use in people with chronic non-cancer pain prescribed opioids: findings from a 4-year prospective cohort study. Lancet Public Heal [Internet]. 2018 [cited 2019 Aug 14];3(7):e341–50. Available from: http://www.ncbi.nlm.nih.gov/pubmed/29976328.

255. Rogers AH, Bakhshaie J, Buckner JD, Orr MF, Paulus DJ, Ditre JW, et al. Opioid and cannabis co-use among adults with chronic pain. J Addict Med [Internet]. 2018 [cited 2019 Apr 24];1. Available from: http://www.ncbi.nlm.nih.gov/pubmed/30557213.

256. Hefner K, Sofuoglu M, Rosenheck R. Concomitant cannabis abuse/dependence in patients treated with opioids for non-cancer pain. Am J Addict. 2015;24(6):538–45.
257. Regulating commercially legalized marijuana as a public health priority [Internet]. [cited 2019 Aug 26]. Available from: https://www.apha.org/policies-and-advocacy/public-health-policy-statements/policy-database/2015/01/23/10/17/regulating-commercially-legalized-marijuana-as-a-public-health-priority.
258. Aguilar S, Gutiérrez V, Sánchez L, Nougier M. Medicinal cannabis policies and practices around the world [Internet]. [cited 2019 Sep 17]. Available from: http://fileserver.idpc.net/library/Medicinal cannabis briefing_ENG_FINAL.PDF.
259. Bramness JG, Dom G, Gual A, Mann K, Wurst FM. A Survey On The Medical Use Of Cannabis In Europe: a position paper. Eur Addict Res [Internet]. 2018 [cited 2019 Sep 17];24(4):201–5. Available from: http://www.ncbi.nlm.nih.gov/pubmed/30134238.
260. 62% of Americans favor legalizing marijuana. Pew Research Center [Internet]. [cited 2019 Aug 26]. Available from: https://www.pewresearch.org/fact-tank/2018/10/08/americans-support-marijuana-legalization/.
261. Hammond D. Communicating THC levels and 'dose' to consumers: implications for product labelling and packaging of cannabis products in regulated markets. Int J Drug Policy [Internet]. 2019 [cited 2019 Aug 6]; Available from: https://www.sciencedirect.com/science/article/abs/pii/S0955395919301823?via%3Dihub.
262. McCambridge J, Mialon M, Hawkins B. Alcohol industry involvement in policymaking: a systematic review. Addiction [Internet]. 2018 [cited 2018 Aug 15];113(9):1571–84. Available from:.
263. Smith SW, Atkin CK, Roznowski J. Are "drink responsibly" alcohol campaigns strategically ambiguous? Health Commun [Internet]. 2006 [cited 2019 Mar 28];20(1):1–11. Available from: http://www.ncbi.nlm.nih.gov/pubmed/16813484.
264. Smith KC, Cukier S, Jernigan DH. Defining strategies for promoting product through 'drink responsibly' messages in magazine ads for beer, spirits and alcopops. Drug Alcohol Depend [Internet]. 2014 [cited 2019 Mar 28];142:168–73. Available from: http://www.ncbi.nlm.nih.gov/pubmed/24999061.
265. Maani Hessari N, Petticrew M. What does the alcohol industry mean by 'Responsible drinking'? A comparative analysis. J Public Health (Bangkok) [Internet]. 2018 [cited 2019 Mar 28];40(1):90–7. Available from: https://academic.oup.com/jpubhealth/article/40/1/90/3111234.
266. Duncan DF, Nicholson T, Clifford P, Hawkins W, Petosa R. Harm reduction: an emerging new paradigm for drug education. J Drug Educ [Internet]. 1994 [cited 2019 Aug 21];24(4):281–90. Available from: http://www.ncbi.nlm.nih.gov/pubmed/7869220.
267. Marijuana laws in Colorado. CDPHE [Internet]. [cited 2019 Aug 12]. Available from: https://responsibilitygrowshere.com/.

Chapter 19
Cannabis-Impaired Driving: Evidence and the Role of Toxicology Testing

Edward C. Wood and Robert L. Dupont

Experimental Evidence

Three types of experimental evidence have been used to determine the impairing effects of THC:

- *Laboratory experiments* are comparatively easy and inexpensive to perform. They are the most rigorous method of proving impairment. Laboratory assessment tools are used to measure impairment domains such as reaction time, memory, and motor control in study subjects after they have consumed cannabis. Study subjects may either be matched with comparable controls or the subjects may act as their own controls by being tested before and after dosing. Study subjects can be demographically pre-determined and can be stratified by cannabis use history. To control input variables, most studies rely upon a single source of cannabis, a defined THC concentration and a single mode of cannabis administration (e.g., smoking). These choices provide scientific rigor but cannot fully represent the many cannabis strains, THC concentrations, or modes of administration that are used in the real world.
- *On-road driving studies* are more expensive and more dangerous to perform than either laboratory or simulator studies, so there are few such studies. Studies may be conducted on closed courses or in real-world traffic. For safety considerations, doses of cannabis and other drugs have been relatively low in this type of study.

E. C. Wood (✉)
DUID Victim Voices, Morrison, CO, USA

R. L. Dupont (✉)
Institute for Behavior and Health, Inc., Rockville, MD, USA
e-mail: contactus@ibhinc.org

© Springer Nature Switzerland AG 2020
K. Finn (ed.), *Cannabis in Medicine*,
https://doi.org/10.1007/978-3-030-45968-0_19

• *Driving simulator studies* use devices that mimic driving conditions in a controlled environment. Use of the most sophisticated simulators is more difficult and expensive than performing laboratory experiments. Expense and logistic considerations require simulator studies to rely upon a small number of homogeneous study subjects. Simulator studies measure fewer dimensions of impairment than are possible with laboratory studies. To date, the most sensitive dimension is standard deviation of lane position (SDLP), which is a measurement of weaving in the lane.

Laboratory Experimental Evidence

Decades of research studies conducted around the world have concluded that THC causes measurable impairment in carefully controlled laboratory settings. Laboratory assays include evaluation of free recall, time and distance perception, reaction time, equilibrium, Wisconsin Card Sorting Task, Tower of London, virtual maze, critical tracking task, divided attention, and many other variants. Sewell's 2009 review of cognitive studies of the effects of cannabis [1] noted impairment of attentiveness, vigilance, perception of time and speed, and executive function. Impairment is prominently found in tasks requiring divided attention. When used together with alcohol, the impairing effects of the two drugs are at least additive and possibly multiplicative, which may depend upon the impairment dimension that is assessed.

The National Safety Council's 2017 research document [2] concluded that acute cannabis intoxication produces dose-related impairment in cognitive and psychomotor functions as well as risk-taking behavior. Cannabis also altered reaction time, short-term memory and attention, motor skills and tracking, all of which can impair driving skills.

The most helpful recent report on this topic is the systematic review published in 2016 by Solowij of 105 recent experimental studies of the effect of cannabis on cognition [3]. Results were summarized by primary cognitive domain in order of evidential strength for both acute and chronic exposure. Where data were available, the persistence of impairment of chronic users after abstinence was reported.

Solowij [3] found strong and largely consistent evidence that cannabis impaired focused, divided, and sustained attention for both chronic and occasional users regardless of gender. After an acute impairment episode, residual impairment in chronic users gradually subsided over a period of several weeks of abstinence. There was also strong and largely consistent evidence that cannabis impaired psychomotor function acutely, but the evidence was weaker for similar impairment of chronic users of cannabis. Impairment likely persists during abstinence after chronic use, but the data are mixed. Executive function impairment studies produced mixed results with a tendency to see greater impairment in older subjects with a long history of chronic cannabis use, indicating a perturbed development of the frontal lobes.

Although studies of cannabis-related cognitive impairment consistently report impairment across several cognitive domains, there are wide variations from one subject to the next that are usually attributed to biological variability, drug use history, polydrug use, and dosing variations. There is also some evidence that the cannabinoid cannabidiol (CBD) may attenuate some THC-caused deficits, especially verbal learning and memory [4].

Driving Experimental Evidence

Safety concerns have limited the number and extent of rigorous on-road driving experiments to determine the impact of cannabis consumption on safe driving. Huestis [5] reviewed three Dutch studies, all on young occasional cannabis users. Two of the studies demonstrated a strong dose-response effect of THC consumption on SDLP. The third study used low 100 μgm/Kg dose THC (approximately 7 mg, or one-third of a joint made with 5% THC cannabis) and found no effect on outcome measures. Other than journalistic publicity stunts, there have been no other published recent on-road driving experiments.

Sewell [1] pointed out that driving studies, whether they be on-road or simulator, suffer from the fact that the study subjects are fully aware of being observed. It is therefore likely that the outcome measures do not reflect driving behaviors of cannabis users on the road, but rather the driving behaviors they are capable of by compensating for their self-recognized impairment.

Simulator and Driving Experimental Evidence

While there is little disagreement that cannabis can cause measurable cognitive impairment, laboratory experiments such as those described above cannot determine the impact of the measured impairment on driving safety. Simulator studies have been developed to address that question.

Sewell [1] observed, based on early simulator and on-road experiments, that THC could impair some driving skills at low doses (about 7 mg THC) but that users were fairly self-aware and tended to compensate effectively for their impairment by driving more slowly and allowing more space between cars. Subjects were, however, much less able to compensate for their impairment when unexpected events occurred. Low dose THC combined with low dose alcohol was far more impairing than either substance separately, indicating a possible synergistic effect. Chronic cannabis users were generally less impaired than occasional users.

Huestis noted [5] that simulators permit measurement of driving performance aspects that cannot be achieved with actual road-driving experiments. Her research team reviewed nine simulator studies, two of which studied the effects of cannabis and alcohol. None evaluated chronic cannabis users. Study designs varied, with reaction time, tracking, speed and speed variation being the most commonly measured of the ten domains reported in the review. There were inconsistent results in half of the domains tested but eight of the nine studies reported impairment in at least one domain. Standard Deviation of Lane Position (SDLP) was the most sensitive road-tracking measure with two of four studies showing a THC-associated impairment.

After reviewing prior work, the Huestis team studied the impact of THC concentrations with and without alcohol using a highly instrumented simulator on 18 occasional cannabis users using vaporized cannabis [6]. That study found that 8.2 ng/ml of THC in whole blood provided a similar SDLP to an alcohol level of 0.05 gm/dl. Huestis cautioned that interpolated THC concentrations at the time of impairment measurement were not representative of forensically-determined THC levels due to the rapid redistribution of THC from the blood immediately post-dosing. The study found that the effects of THC and alcohol on SDLP were additive, rather than synergistic.

Epidemiological Evidence

Whereas experiments must be limited to a small number of study subjects, epidemiological studies consider large populations. Epidemiological studies of cannabis-impaired driving generally fall into the following categories:

- *Observational studies.* Most reports based on the Fatality Analysis Reporting System (FARS) sponsored by the National Highway Traffic Safety Administration (NHTSA) fall into this category. Outcomes of these studies are typically trend graphs and comparative ratio reports.
- *Case control studies* compare drivers in crash cases with similar drivers who were not involved in crashes. It is essential to establish a valid control group for these studies to have high value. Outcomes of these studies are typically Odds Ratios (ORs).
- *Culpability studies* examine drug presence in fatal and/or crash cases, comparing data from culpable drivers and non-culpable drivers. Outcomes of these studies are typically Odds Ratios (ORs).

Observational Studies

Perhaps the most widely reported observational studies are those published by states based upon fatal crash information collected for submission to NHTSA FARS reports. Data for these reports historically come primarily from coroners although excellent progress is being made in collecting toxicology data from surviving drivers as well. We will examine reports from two states that have legalized recreational cannabis, Colorado and Washington.

Rocky Mountain High Intensity Trafficking Area (RMHIDTA) has published The Legalization of Marijuana: *The Impact* annually since 2014, with periodic

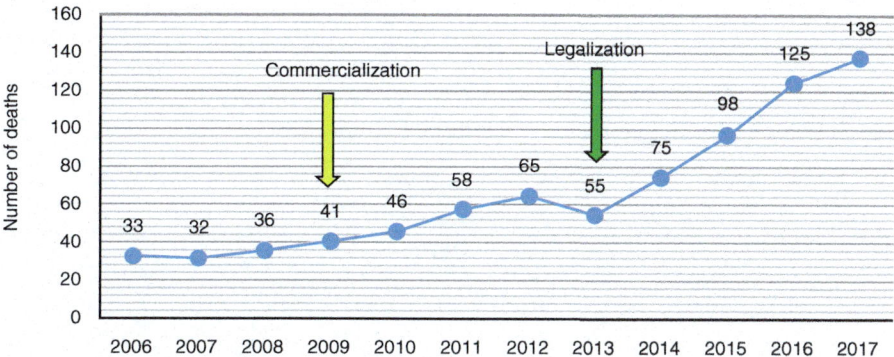

Fig. 19.1 Traffic deaths related to marijuana when a *driver* tested positive for Marijuana

updates. The reports contain valuable trend data (Fig. 19.1) along with bullet-point observations. The Volume 5 update of September 2018 [7] contains the following observations:

1. Since recreational marijuana was legalized, marijuana-related traffic deaths increased 151% while all Colorado traffic deaths increased 35%.
2. Since recreational marijuana was legalized, traffic deaths involving drivers who tested positive for marijuana more than doubled from 55 in 2013 to 138 people killed in 2017.
3. The percentage of all Colorado traffic deaths that were marijuana related increased from 11.43% in 2013 to 21.3% in 2017.

RMHIDTA was careful to define "marijuana-related" as a case where cannabis shows up in the toxicology report and includes both cannabis *only* cases and polydrug cases with cannabis. The term is not intended to mean "marijuana-impaired" since coroners provided much of the data and none of the coroners' subjects were ever charged with or convicted of impaired driving. Toxicology samples positive for THC, carboxy-THC, or both were considered cannabis-positive. Since 2016 the state has reported THC cases separately from cases with carboxy-THC *only*.

RMHIDTA's observations could be explained by an increase in impaired driving or an increasingly widespread use of cannabis brought about by legalization, even if cannabis caused no impairment whatsoever. A combination of both could also explain the observations.

NHTSA sponsored a series of roadside surveys in the state of Washington just prior to its legalization of recreational cannabis, 6 months after legalization, and 1 year after legalization [8]. Significant increases were found in the number of drivers testing positive for cannabinoids in the largest counties (13.3%, 20.9%, and 30.7%, respectively, for the three time periods), but no significant increases were seen in smaller counties. Due to the wide variations in cannabinoid-positive drivers between and within sites, the overall change was not significant.

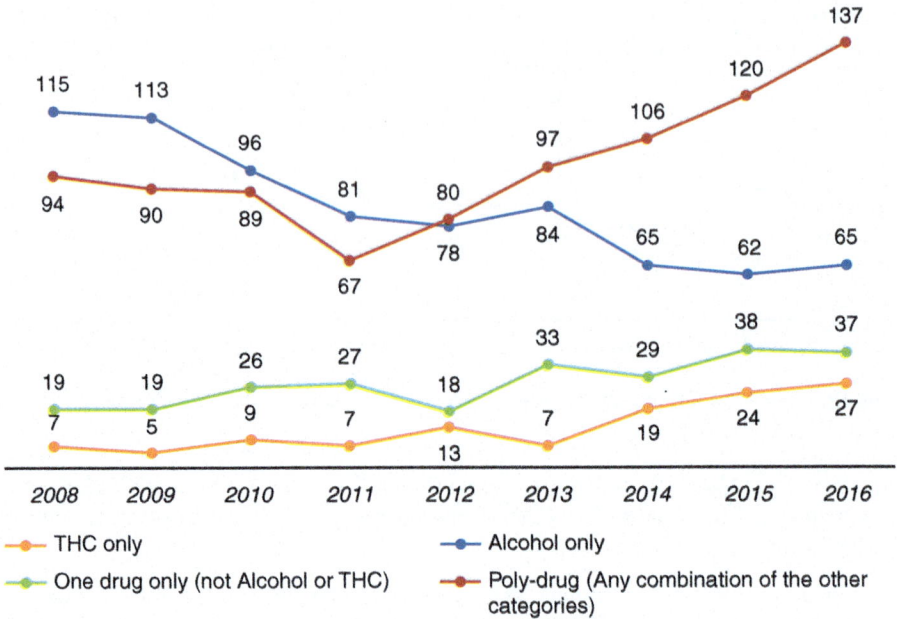

Fig. 19.2 Rising frequency of polydrug drivers in fatal crashes

Washington opened its first retail cannabis sales store in July 2014. The state has had a fairly stable 60% testing rate for both drugs and alcohol of drivers in fatal crashes from 2008 to 2016. Although toxicology tests indicated an increase in THC-positive drivers similar to the cannabinoid-positive drivers from the Colorado report, the more significant concern in Washington was polydrug-positive drivers (Fig. 19.2), most of which were cannabinoid and alcohol positive [9].

Washington has consistently reported THC separately from carboxy-THC, but like the Colorado data, THC trends could result from an increased impaired driving, an increase cannabis consumption in the driving population with no increases in impairment, or a combination of both.

Case-Control Epidemiological Evidence

Case-control epidemiological studies compare study subjects, typically those involved in fatal crashes, with control subjects who were not involved in crashes. Selection of comparable control subjects is critical for these studies to achieve validity. There have been literally thousands of reports of such studies, although only a few dozen qualify as highly-referenced original research. The best way to understand these studies is by understanding three recent meta-analyses, followed by the studies published since the last meta-analysis.

All three recent meta-analyses discussed below selected what the authors believed were high quality published research using different criteria, but generally considering issues such as:

1. Sufficiently large sample size
2. Appropriate controls selected to match the study subjects
3. Appropriate adjustments as needed to eliminate bias from study/control mismatching
4. Valid means of measuring drug presence with a preference for laboratory assays
5. Correct analytes studied: THC, not just cannabinoids, identification of poly-drug cases
6. Data presented to enable pooling with other studies

Li's 2011 meta-analysis [10] selected 9 studies out of a total surveyed population of 2960 published reports. This meta-analysis totaled 4236 cases and 88,993 controls and focused on cannabis use rather than THC presence. The most common source of exposure data were self-reports or urine tests, followed by blood tests. All but one study reported a significant risk to driving safety with cannabis use. The estimated summary OR was 2.66 (2.07, 3.41) of a fatal crash from cannabis use.

The meta-analysis from Asbridge's team published a few months later [11] also selected 9 studies out of a total surveyed population of 2975 published reports. There was some overlap of selected studies, but Asbridge included culpability studies, whereas Li did not. The most common source of exposure data was blood or serum assays rather than self-reports or urine analysis. Asbridge reported an estimated summary OR of 1.92 (1.35, 2.73) of a crash due to cannabis use and found that risks were higher in case control studies than culpability studies, and higher in fatal crashes than in non-fatal crashes.

These two studies led to a commonly accepted view that the OR of a fatal crash from cannabis use was about 2 [12]. Then 5 years later Rogeberg [13] critiqued and re-evaluated both the Li and Asbridge meta-analyses, restating their estimates to be 1.55 and 1.25, respectively. Rogeberg then performed a new meta-analysis of 28 studies and reported two OR estimates, one using a random-effects model, the other using meta-regression. The estimates were 1.36 (1.15–1.61) and 1.22 (1.1–1.36), respectively. Like Asbridge, Rogeberg found ORs to be higher in case-control studies than in culpability studies.

Li subsequently published two further OR studies, both based upon data from the FARS database. His 2013 report [14] found an OR for cannabis-related crashes to be 1.83 compared with 3.03 for narcotics, 3.57 for stimulants and 4.83 for depressants. His 2017 report [15] found an OR for cannabis-related crashes to be 1.54 compared with 16.33 for alcohol and 25.09 for the combination of cannabis and alcohol.

The wide variation in results from one researcher to another and even within a research team speaks to the difficulty of determining the quantitative effects of cannabis on driving safety. The best evidence to date is that it certainly isn't safe to drive while impaired by cannabis, that the OR is likely somewhat below 2, well below that of alcohol, and that the combination of THC and alcohol is synergistic.

Some of the difficulty in recent analyses comes from relying upon the FARS database, which is frequently used to assess safety of cannabis and driving despite caution from NHTSA [16]. Romano [17] and Li [14] published similar studies for the same time period, both using the FARS database for cases and the National Roadside Survey for controls. Yet the two studies found contrary ORs for the risk of cannabis on fatal crashes (0.86 from Romano and 1.83 from Li). Romano subsequently reconciled the two studies [18], resulting in a change to his OR estimate to 1.27 (0.88, 1.83). More importantly, Romano concluded that based in part on the limitations previously reported by NHTSA [16], the "FARS database should neither be used to examine trends in drug use or to obtain precise risk estimates."

Nevertheless, two recent reports [19, 20] based upon FARS data have been adopted by some in the commercial cannabis industry to downplay the effects of cannabis on road safety [21, 22]. Both referenced reports used a state's total traffic fatalities as a marker of the effect on road safety of legalized medical or recreational cannabis. Since at the time of their publication, cannabis-using drivers constituted a small minority of all drivers, it can be argued that total number of traffic fatalities is a blunt instrument with which to measure the impact of cannabis legalization. It should be noted that the Aydelotte study [20] reported 77 "excess traffic fatalities" due to cannabis legalization in Colorado and Washington. Aydelotte opined that "we do not view that as a clinically significant effect, but others might disagree." Presumably the "excess traffic fatalities" would disagree had they survived.

A case-control study sponsored by NHTSA and published in 2016 [23, 24] has been misreported [25, 26] as showing cannabis was not linked to car crashes. In fact, the study failed to find a link, which is far different than finding that a link does not exist. The study also failed to find links between crash risk and the use of any drug including cocaine, methamphetamine, opioids, or any combinations of those drugs, all of which have been shown to be more impairing than cannabis [14]. There are several reasons why the study failed to find these links. First, the sample size of the study was far too small to find a statistically significant link for many of the drugs. Second, unlike other epidemiological studies, the NHTSA study only included cases who volunteered to be assessed. It is unclear why a driver who knew he or she was impaired would volunteer to be assessed, but the report disclosed that many subjects chose not be assessed. Third, the study included principally property damage crashes, whereas prior studies [11] have demonstrated that ORs are higher for fatality crashes than for minor crashes. There were only 15 fatal crashes in the NHTSA study. Fourth, there were 3095 cases assessed in the 2682 crashes, indicating that at least 413 non-crash-initiators who might be expected to have drug-use levels similar to controls were included in the pool of study subjects. Their inclusion in a study of alcohol with its higher expected OR likely would not matter, but it likely does matter in a study of cannabis with an expected OR somewhat below 2. And finally, the study was conducted in Virginia Beach, Virginia, an atypical study site. Controls in Virginia Beach showed a 14.4% prevalence of drugs, compared with a 19–22% prevalence in the 2014 NHTSA National Roadside Survey, depending upon assay and time of day. The NHTSA study should certainly be included in the library of respected literature especially for its careful selection of controls, but its results do not deserve to overrule the body of high-quality contrary evidence available.

Culpability Epidemiological Evidence

Culpability studies of large populations have not unequivocally answered the question of the role of cannabis in traffic crashes, in part due to the wide variations in study design. Below we discuss only studies using blood testing and with two exceptions, those that distinguished THC from its inactive metabolite carboxy-THC. All studies found an effect of cannabis on crash risk, but one study (Longo) found no effect if the blood THC level was below 2 ng/ml.

Longo's 2000 study [27] involved 2500 injured and deceased drivers tested for alcohol, THC, benzodiazepines, and stimulants. Drivers were determined to be either culpable or non-culpable. The 6.2% who were determined to be contributory, rather than fully culpable were not included in the study. Drug- and alcohol-free drivers were culpable in 52.5% of the cases; THC-positive drivers were culpable 47.5% of the cases indicating no significant cannabis involvement. However, there were only 44 drivers found with THC *only* and those with a THC level at or above 2 ng/ml were culpable 66.7% of the time, indicating significant cannabis involvement. The time interval between crash and taking of a blood sample was not reported. Data were adjusted for risk factors, recognizing that cannabis users tend to be risk takers.

Drummer's 2004 study [28] involved 3398 fatal crashes, including 59 who tested positive for THC *only*. Like Longo, Drummer excluded drivers from his study whose culpability was only contributory. He found an odds ratio (OR) of 2.7 for being involved in a fatal crash if the driver was positive for THC, and 6.6 if the driver had a blood THC level above 5 ng/ml. In comparison, the OR for alcohol-positive drivers was 6.0 and 17.4 if both alcohol and THC were present.

Laumon's 2005 study [29] involved drivers in 10,748 fatal crashes, including 681 who were positive for THC *only*. The time between a crash and taking of a blood sample was not reported, but Beicheler [30] reported that a similar cohort had an average 4-hour delay between the two events. This would have a material effect on the validity of the THC laboratory findings as discussed below. After adjustment for risk factors, Laumon found an OR for involvement in a fatal crash to be 3.32 for THC-positive drivers.

Bédard's 2007 study [31] involved 32,543 drivers in the FARS database from 1993 to 2003 who were tested for both cannabinoids and alcohol and found negative for alcohol. A total of 1647 were cannabinoid-positive, including those positive for carboxy-THC only. Most tested samples were blood, with some urine. Culpability was determined by FARS-identified driver-related factors. Authors reported a 1.39 OR for involvement in a fatal crash, 1.29 after adjusting for risk factors. Inclusion of drivers positive for non-impairing carboxy-THC is the study group would tend to lower the OR for involvement in fatal crashes.

Beicheler's 2008 study [30] is similar to Laumon's, involving drivers in 9998 fatal crashes tested for both alcohol and THC. There were 391 drivers who tested positive for THC *only*. Most drivers were urine tested, and then blood tested if the urine tests were positive. Only blood test results were used in the study. The authors reported an average 3-hour delay between crash and taking a blood sample if no urine testing was required and a 4.5-hour delay if urine testing was performed first.

Drug- and alcohol-free drivers were culpable in 54.4% of the cases, THC *only* positive drivers were culpable 70.0% of the cases, indicating significant cannabis involvement.

Li's 2017 study [32] involved 14,742 culpable and 14,742 non-culpable drivers in the same fatal two-vehicle crashes between 1993 and 2014 that were reported in the FARS database: 2409 tested positive for cannabinoids, including carboxy-THC. The OR for initiating a fatal crash was 1.82 for cannabinoid-positive drivers, 1.64 after adjusting for risk factors. Adjusted risk ORs for alcohol $\geq$ .08 blood alcohol concentration (BAC) was 9.41 with no cannabinoids present and 10.57 if cannabinoids were present.

These culpability epidemiological studies show, albeit inconsistently, that drivers positive for THC were more likely to cause fatal crashes than drivers without THC. The increased risk to the driving public caused by cannabis-using drivers is measurable, but less than the risk caused by drunk drivers. However, when the two substances are combined, the risk is greater than the risk caused by either drug alone. In studies that evaluated drivers' use of alcohol and cannabis, more drivers were found using both drugs than were found using cannabis alone.

Tolerance

Some heavy users of cannabis claim they can drive safely after using the drug because they have built up a tolerance to its effects. Tolerance is measured primarily by how high a dose of a drug is required to achieve a desired effect. To some extent, this is based on individual susceptibility, body size, and body mass index. But even for a single individual, regular use of a drug creates a tolerance such that, with increasing use, a greater amount is needed to achieve a desired effect.

THC tolerance has been demonstrated by comparing counterclockwise hysteresis curves of frequent and occasional users. Frequent users can have a baseline THC blood level above zero, a much higher THC blood level after dosing, but don't feel as high as an occasional user [33, 34].

Because of THC's estimated 4.1-day terminal half-life in chronic users [35], THC is continuously released into the blood from the body's fat stores between doses, resulting in a chronic low blood THC level between doses. After dosing, chronic users have a much higher blood THC level than occasional users, yet do not feel as "high" as an occasional user after dosing [34]. These are all characteristics of a chronic user building up tolerance to THC.

Numerous studies have suggested that frequent cannabis users can develop a tolerance to some, but not all, impairing effects of THC [36–39]. More recent work by Ramaekers [40] found that chronic users, like occasional users, become acutely impaired after dosing with cannabis. However, because chronic users maintain a low level of chronic impairment, the acute increase in their level of impairment was less than that of an occasional user who was completely unimpaired prior to dosing. Ramaekers opined that prior work, including his own, did not detect this fact due to use of self-controls and the use of inadequate sample sizes. After a review of 10 recent studies of cannabis tolerance in chronic users, Solowij concluded that "tolerance generally manifests as a blunted effect rather than an absence of observable effects" [41].

Impairment Assessment

Although validated for scientific use, impairment measurement methods described in the first Laboratory Experimental Evidence paragraph above are time-consuming and impractical for use by police at the roadside. Furthermore, legal impairment not only can differ from scientific impairment, it can differ from state to state. Most states have statutes that define what driving under the influence means. Definitions range from "impairment to the slightest degree" to "incapable of driving safely." Colorado has both, the first offense defining Driving While Ability Impaired (DWAI) and the second defining Driving Under the Influence (DUI).

Forensically determining impairment is akin to diagnosing an illness. A physician studies both symptoms and laboratory tests in making a diagnosis and determining a treatment plan. Police also rely upon symptoms and chemical tests to determine impairment and to prove impairment in court. Just as some disease diagnoses are straightforward and others are more challenging, effectiveness of impairment assessments vary depending upon the impairing substance(s) and dose, symptoms, and of course, the diagnostician.

Symptoms of alcohol impairment are overt and the chemical assays are fairly definitive. Odor, bloodshot eyes, speech, behavior and balance are readily detected by even untrained observers. Horizontal Gaze Nystagmus is a validated [42] tool used by officers trained in Standardized Field Sobriety Tests to confirm alcohol impairment above 0.08 BAC. There is a very high correlation between BAC and levels of impairment [43]. For cannabis, symptoms are much more subtle and chemical assays play more of a supporting role than a definitive role.

Symptomatic Assessments

Aside from observed impaired driving behaviors which must be distinguished from simply bad driving, officers have several tools at their disposal to determine if a driver is impaired. These tools are relied upon to convict impaired drivers when laboratory assays are not available. There are three common levels of impairment detection training provided to law enforcement officers: SFST (Standardized Field Sobriety Test), ARIDE (Advanced Roadside Impaired Driving Enforcement), and DRE (Drug Recognition Expert), in increasing order of complexity and training time commitment. Colorado reported 5674 active SFST operators in 2018 compared with 1427 active ARIDE certificate holders and 228 DREs [44]. Criteria for all three classes of training were developed by NHTSA and the International Association of Chiefs of Police (IACP).

SFSTs consist of three tools – Horizontal Gaze Nystagmus (HGN), One Leg Stand (OLS), and Walk and Turn (WAT). The battery of tests has proven to be highly accurate identifying drivers above a BAC .10 [45] and BAC .08 [46, 47] with 93%, 95%, and 94% correct arrest decisions, respectively, in the three field studies. The battery of tests typically takes about 5 minutes to conduct in the field. To retain SFST certification, officers are required to complete a training update every 2 years.

SFSTs are only moderately successful identifying drug impairment, especially THC impairment [48, 49]. Papafotiou reported 65.8% and 76.3% correct identification of THC-impaired drivers with SFSTs, depending on the THC concentration of cannabis used [50]. Papafotiou used a driving simulator to determine THC impairment in his subjects. Cannabis rarely causes HGN, whereas HGN is the most sensitive of the SFST tools for detection of alcohol impairment [47, 48]. SFSTs are somewhat more successful identifying impairment by central nervous system (CNS) depressants, CNS stimulants, and narcotic analgesics [48].

Additional assessment tools may eventually be added to the SFST battery to enable more robust detection of drug impairment. The addition of finger-to-nose (FTN) and Modified Rombeg Balance (MRB) tests to OLS and WAT can provide a 96.7% reliability in detecting impairment confirmed by DRE assessments and laboratory confirmation [51]. Pupillary rebound dilation, lack of eye convergence, and peripheral vision have also been studied as useful tools to detect THC impairment [52]. Little has been done to determine these tests' ability to detect impairment by other drugs.

SFST-certified practitioners may take ARIDE training focused on drug impairment symptoms which requires an additional 16 hours of training beyond that required for SFST certification. Training on tools such as MRB is provided. There is no ARIDE periodic update or refresher course either required or available.

ARIDE-trained officers may continue their training with a 72-hour DRE training course requiring a field certification and a final examination. Updated training is required every 2 years to maintain DRE certification. DRE officers use a 12-step protocol to determine not only if a driver is impaired, but which class or classes of drugs are likely to be causing the observed impairment. The protocol is defined in the Drug Evaluation and Classification Program (DECP) administered by the IACP.

The DRE protocol has been validated in the laboratory [52] and in two field studies [53, 54]. The validation studies found that trained officers correctly identified the drug classes causing impairment observations 80–90% of the time and rarely claimed that a study subject was impaired by a drug when no drug was found by laboratory assessment. In a Los Angeles field study [53] only one of the 173 cases did an officer identify a subject as impaired when no drug or alcohol could be confirmed in the laboratory. The DRE protocol includes a laboratory assessment as step number 12 to prevent false positives from proceeding to conviction.

The three DECP validation studies were performed before the program's parameters were formalized and subjected to oversight by the IACP. Some validation studies used urine rather than blood for confirmation, all drug classes were not studied in all validation studies, and neither field validation study performed laboratory tests on subjects considered by officers to be unimpaired, which is necessary to identify false negatives. For these and other reasons, the validation studies themselves have been called into question [53]. Nevertheless, the DECP program has been accepted by law enforcement in all 50 states, several other countries, and results have been determined to be admissible as valid scientific evidence in court hearings.

DECP divided attention tests of walk and turn, one leg stand, modified Romberg balance, finger to nose, as well as the eye tests for lack of convergence, and rebound pupillary dilation are particularly sensitive to identify the presence of THC [51, 54, 55].

Few symptomatic impairment assays can be performed on a driver injured in a drugged driving crash. A driver strapped onto a backboard awaiting transport to a hospital is unable to be assessed by any of the SFSTs or most of the DRE protocol steps. In those cases, law enforcement officials must rely principally upon an examination of driving behavior that caused the crash.

Chemical Assays

In order of increasing invasiveness, chemical assays may be performed on breath, oral fluid, urine, or blood to confirm the presence of intoxicants after a driver's impairment symptoms have been observed and documented. Breath and blood tests are the preferred methods to detect and measure alcohol. Breath tests can be done at the roadside, whereas blood test results are not available for days or even weeks after an arrest.

Blood is the preferred matrix to detect and measure drugs other than alcohol. Oral fluid testing is gaining interest in the law enforcement community [56] because detection (not measurement) results can be available for many drugs at the roadside, and oral fluid samples may easily be taken at the roadside without the long sample delays common with blood sampling. Roadside oral fluid testing is being used routinely in some countries (e.g., Australia, Norway, Canada) but is still under evaluation in the United States. Urine tests are no longer recommended to support charges of drugged driving largely because urine reveals drug metabolites rather than the native drug. That is especially problematic for THC.

Chemical tests are useful but not infallible. NHTSA reported [57] that in 2011, 24% of those arrested for DUI refused to be tested, with a range between 4% and 82% among the states. Cases without chemical assays relied upon symptomatic assessments for prosecution and conviction.

The correlation between BAC and levels of impairment was documented by Borkenstein in 1964 and has since been replicated worldwide with similar results. The correlation isn't the same for each individual and there are even wide differences between ages and gender. For example, young males have a much higher risk of crashes after alcohol consumption than the general population [43]. Consequently, a high BAC cannot scientifically prove impairment, nor can a low BAC prove lack of impairment. Nevertheless, the correlation is so high that Department of Transportation Appropriations Act of 2001 required all states to adopt a BAC .08 limit as a DUI *per se* level. Delaware was the last state to adopt that standard in 2004 and Utah lowered its standard to BAC .05 in 2018, consistent with many European countries.

The reliance on BAC levels to convict of DUI *per se* and to support conviction of DUI has led to a popular belief that blood tests for alcohol prove DUI-alcohol and therefore should be used to prove DUI-cannabis as well [58]. Although roadside eye tests or other tools to measure impairment rather than drug presence may eventually provide a roadside equivalent for drugs to the alcohol preliminary breath testing devices, there will never be a BAC equivalent THC or any other drug. No roadside (or other) device to measure THC in blood will ever provide the simplified answer the public seeks to this complex problem.

Like alcohol impairment, THC impairment is a dose-related phenomenon. But due to the pharmacokinetic properties of THC, the dose of THC remaining in a driver at the time or arrest cannot be determined by forensic measurements of that driver's blood THC levels. Since THC is fat-soluble, circulating THC in blood is quickly absorbed by the brain and other highly-perfused fatty tissues, rapidly clearing it from the blood. On average, the maximum blood THC level can drop 73% (3.3%–89.5%) within the first 25 minutes after beginning to smoke a joint [59]. Since blood is typically drawn an hour after a routine traffic stop [60] and 2 hours after a crash [61], forensically-determined THC levels cannot represent THC levels at the time of the event leading to the blood draw. In contrast, water-soluble alcohol is cleared from blood via metabolism, rather than via redistribution. Alcohol's linear metabolic rate enables reasonably reliable retrograde extrapolation to infer alcohol blood levels at a time prior to a blood draw. That cannot be done with THC.

Sewell [1] demonstrated that, unlike alcohol, blood THC levels do not track subjective "high" ratings of users (Fig. 19.3). It is likely safe to presume that the same is true for other measures of driving impairment as well. Within the first 30 minutes after cannabis consumption, the serum THC levels decline at the same time the subjective effects of THC rise. Subjective effects remain elevated long after blood THC levels subside to levels that in some cases cannot even be detected.

The conclusions drawn from Sewell's chart should not be surprising when considering that blood is never impaired by THC, alcohol, or other drugs; the brain is impaired by these substances. Alcohol quickly establishes a fairly uniform concentration gradient across highly perfused tissues in the body, so blood testing provides an excellent indication of brain levels of alcohol. This is not so for fat-soluble THC. Mura [62] found that 100% of the 12 cadavers in his study had higher THC concentration in the brain than in the blood, sometimes even presenting with high levels of THC in the brain when none could be detected in blood.

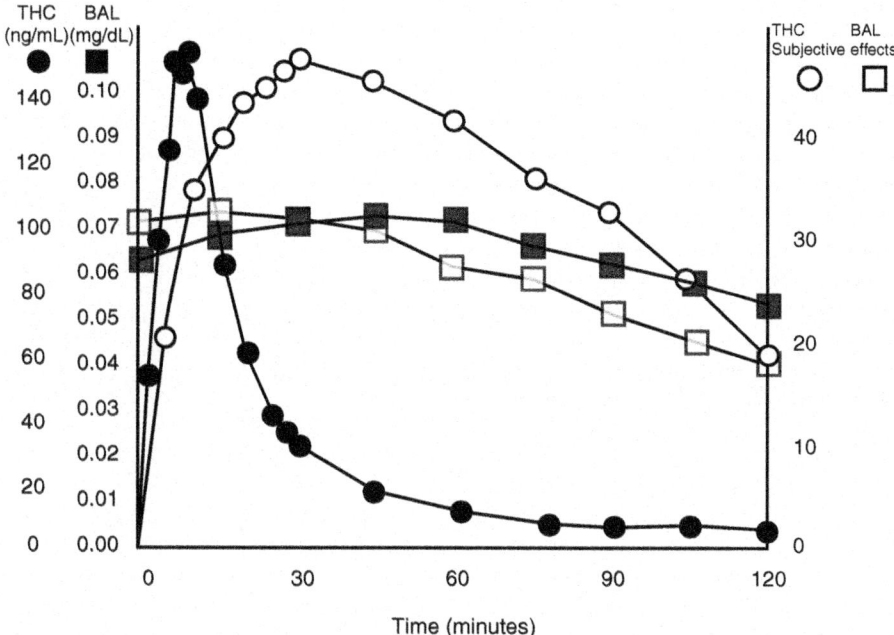

Fig. 19.3 Subjective effects vs. blood levels of alcohol and THC

Several states have established a legal THC *per se* level or permissible inference level of 5 ng/ml of THC in whole blood. Although states may choose whatever *per se* level they wish in the interests of highway safety, there is no scientific basis for a 5 mg/ml or any other *per se* level. The European Driving Under the Influence of Drugs (DRUID) culpability study of 7455 subjects found that the crash involvement OR of drivers with a THC level above 5 ng/ml was lower than the OR of drivers with a THC level of 3–5 ng/ml [65]. Three other studies of drivers arrested for DUI found no difference in impairment assessments for drivers above and below 5 ng/ml THC [55, 64, 65].

A further reason to avoid a 5 ng/ml THC legal limit is that blood THC levels differ depending upon the mode of consumption. The blood THC level of drivers impaired by a standard 10 mg dose of THC edible products rise no higher than 1 ng/ml and no higher than 3 ng/ml after consumption of five times the standard dose [66].

Chemical assays must play a different role in drugged driving forensic cases compared to drunk driving forensic cases. For alcohol, chemical assays are of primary importance. They can prove guilt of DUI *per se* and provide evidence that the observed impairment was likely dangerous. For drugged driving, symptomatic assessments are of primary importance and chemical assays are of secondary importance. Chemical assays merely provide evidence of which drug or drugs caused the observed impairment. However, chemical assays are of primary importance in jurisdictions that have established zero tolerance or legally-defined *per se* levels for selected drugs in impaired driving cases.

Public Safety

Fortunately, highways are generally very safe and have been getting safer, at least until the last few years. FARS data show that while annual vehicle crash deaths have hovered around the 40,000 mark for at least four decades, normalized deaths have steadily dropped from over 3 per 100 million miles driven to 1.18 in 2016. Fatal crashes are so rare than a driver who averages 20,000 miles per year may need 85 lifetimes before being involved in fatal crash. Normalized rates have been rising recently, which breaks a 40-year trend of improvement [67].

While we celebrate an improving highway safety record, the rarity of fatal crashes can make changing attitudes toward impaired driving more difficult. Drunk driving as a percentage of total fatalities was 48.2% in 1982. The "Friends don't let friends drive drunk" campaign was launched the following year. The percentage dropped to 30% by the late-1990s when the campaign was cancelled. Since that time, the drunk driving death rate has remained in the range of 30% [68].

As difficult as it is to change drunk driving attitudes when the relative risk for involvement in a fatal crash exceeds 10 for a young male with a BAC above 0.05, it is even more difficult to affect stoned-driving attitudes when the risk may be less than 20% of that for driving under the influence of alcohol.

One out of every five cannabis users in Colorado report driving within 2–3 hours after consumption of cannabis, the period when THC impairment has been shown to be the most serious [69]. That percentage has remained stable since cannabis for recreational use was legalized in that state, while the number of cannabis users continues to increase.

The educational challenge to change driving behaviors is daunting. A survey of people who drive under the influence of alcohol and cannabis revealed that 52% of them used cannabis to sober up after drinking too much to drive safely, even though cannabis actually increases the risk of a fatal crash [70].

An accurate understanding the public safety impact of cannabis-impaired driving has been crippled by the large proportion of cannabis users who are polydrug users and by a lack of good data. In 2018 Colorado, which has a 5 ng/ml THC permissible inference level, released the first report on causes of drugged driving created by linking the databases of forensic toxicology laboratories with judicial data [44]. By studying cases of drivers arrested for impaired driving, this enabled a better understanding of the *causes of drugged driving*, rather than the *presence of drugs in crashes* which is the foundation of most other reports. The report's power was limited by the fact that only 8.7% of the 27,244 DUI cases in 2016 had forensic toxicology tests for both alcohol and drugs, and even then, drug screening tests were inconsistent between the two primary forensic toxicology laboratories, and inconsistent among the various law enforcement agencies.

Nevertheless, several important lessons emerged from the report, including:

1. 52.5% of cannabinoid-positive drivers had a blood THC level below 5 ng/ml.
2. 54% of non-alcohol positive drug tests were for THC. The remainder were for other drugs, led by methamphetamine, alprazolam, and cocaine.

3. Among drivers tested for both alcohol and drugs, 89% of THC-positive drivers were polydrug users.
4. Although 82.8% of THC-positive were convicted of DUI, that was led by poly-drug impaired drivers.
5. For drivers impaired by THC *only* for whom blood THC levels were $\geq$5 ng/ml, 99.7% were convicted of impaired driving (DWAI) but only 59.8% were convicted of driving under the influence (DUI).
6. For drivers impaired by THC *only* for whom blood THC levels were <5 ng/ml, 91.4% were convicted of impaired driving (DWAI) but only 14.1% were convicted of driving under the influence (DUI).
7. Half of the 20 DUI vehicular homicide cases were due to alcohol – at least that was the only drug reported in those cases. The other half were due to non-alcohol drugs or polydrugs. Neither of the DUI vehicular homicide cases where THC was the only drug reported were convicted of DUI. Both were below 5 ng/ml THC. In contrast 80% of the alcohol and 71% of the polydrug cases were convicted of DUI.

The primary challenges for public safety remain changing attitudes toward the acceptance of drugged driving and ensuring justice for victims affected by drugged driving. In addition, it is important that effective actions be taken today to make roads and highways safer by reducing drugged driving. While more research is useful, it must not be the condition for more effective public education about the risks of drugged driving or for more active enforcement actions. There are many good policy solutions available today to reduce this serious public safety problem based on the substantial body of research reviewed in this chapter [71–73].

Conclusions

Laboratory experiments prove that cannabis adversely affects psychomotor skills and cognitive functions required for safe driving in both occasional and chronic cannabis users. Whereas laboratory evidence is strong and consistent, epidemiological evidence is far less so.

Epidemiological studies have demonstrated that alcohol increases driving crash risk far more than THC does. The large database created by the National Highway Traffic Safety Administration (NHTSA) through its Fatality Analysis Reporting System (FARS) has enabled determination of the odds ratio (OR) of being involved in a fatal crash across a variety of demographic characteristics [43]. There is a high correlation between alcohol blood levels and crash risk. Whereas the OR of a fatal crash for a driver using alcohol can range from 2 to 20 or higher depending upon the blood alcohol level, the OR of a fatal crash is typically around 2 for a driver using cannabis, regardless of the forensically-determined blood THC level [63]. Epidemiological results vary widely with some showing very little or no effect of cannabis use on driving fatalities [13]. These findings support the claim that driving under the influence of cannabis is safer than driving under the influence of alcohol, but more dangerous than sober driving.

The combination of alcohol and cannabis is more impairing than the effects of either substance separately. Impairing effects of the two substances (polydrug use) are either additive or synergistic, depending on the impairing domain being measured [15, 29, 32]. Polydrug impairment is not only more dangerous than impairment by THC alone, it is also more common. Most (64.1%) of THC-impaired drivers arrested for driving under the influence (DUI) in Colorado in 2016 tested positive for both alcohol and THC [44].

Although chronic users can develop a tolerance to some of cannabis's impairing effects, they can also maintain a chronic low level of impairment between dosing sessions. After dosing they become acutely impaired similar to occasional users.

Distracted driving further complicates understanding the impact of impaired driving. Some distractions such as traffic and road signs are beyond a driver's control, but others such as mobile phone use, monitoring a GPS, or talking with passengers are choices made by a driver. Regardless of the source of distractions, their impact on driving safety becomes magnified if the driver is suffering from a divided attention deficit, such as that induced by a driver's choice to use cannabis prior to driving. In the real world, we must frequently deal with cases where alcohol, drugs, and distractions are all contributing causes of a traffic crash, each one compounding the effects of the other.

There is no direct correlation between the degree of driving impairment and THC levels in blood. Forensic laboratory tests of drivers suspected of drugged driving are of secondary importance, playing a supportive role to that of collecting symptomatic evidence of impaired driving.

References

1. Sewell RA, Poling J, Sofuoglu M. The effects of cannabis compared with alcohol on driving. Am J Addict. 2009;18(3):185–93.
2. Marijuana and Driving. National Safety Council Research Document. Sept 2017.
3. Broyd SJ, van Hell HH, Beale C, Yücel M, Solowij N. Acute and chronic effects of cannabinoids on human cognition - a systematic review. Biol Psychiatry. 2016;79:557–67.
4. Solowij N, Broyd SJ, Beale C, Prick J-A, Greenwood L-m, van Hell H, Suo C, Galettis P, Pai N, Fu S, Croft RJ, Martin JH, Yücel M. Therapeutic effects of prolonged cannabidiol treatment on psychological symptoms and cognitive function in regular cannabis users: a pragmatic open-label clinical trial. Cannabis Cannabinoid Res. 2018;3(1):21–34.
5. Hartman RL, Huestis MA. Cannabis effects on driving skills. Clin Chem. 2013;59(3):478–92.
6. Hartman RL, Brown TL, Milavetz G, Spurgin A, Pierce RS, Gorelick DA, Gaffney G, Huestis MA. Cannabis effects on driving lateral control with and without alcohol. Drug Alcohol Depend. 2015;154:25–37.
7. Gorman T. The legalization of marijuana in Colorado: the impact. Vol 5. Sept 2018. Rocky Mountain High Intensity Drug Trafficking Area.
8. Ramirez A, Berning A, Carr K, Scherer M, Lacey JH, Kelley-Baker T, Fisher DA. Marijuana, other drugs, and alcohol use by drivers in Washington State (Report No. DOT HS 812 299). Washington, D.C.: National Highway Traffic Safety Administration; 2016, July.

9. Grondel D, Hoff S, Doane D. Marijuana use, alcohol use, and driving in Washington State. Washington Traffic Safety Commission. April 2018.
10. Li M-C, Brady JE, DiMaggio CJ, Lusardi AR, Tzong KY, Li G. Marijuana use and motor vehicle crashes. Epidemiol Rev. 2012;34(1):65–72.
11. Asbridge M, Hayden JA, Cartwright JL. Acute cannabis consumption and motor vehicle collision risk: systematic review of observational studies and meta-analysis. Br Med J. 2012;344:e536.
12. https://www.acmt.net/_Library/2015_Forensic_Course/Huestis_-_BW_-ACMTEffectsCanna bisDrivingWithWoutAlc12-9-15.pdf. Accessed 1 Mar 2019.
13. Rogeberg O, Elvik R. The effects of cannabis intoxication on motor vehicle collision revisited and revised. Addiction. 2016;111:1348–59.
14. Li G, Brady J, Chen Q. Drug use and fatal motor vehicle crashes: a case-control study. Accid Anal Prev. 2013;60:205–10.
15. Chihuri S, Li G, Chen Q. Interaction of marijuana and alcohol on fatal motor vehicle crash risk: a case-control study. Inj Epidemiol. 2017;4:8.
16. Berning A, Smither DD. Understanding the limitations of drug test information, reporting and testing practices in fatal crashes. NHTSA Traffic Safety Facts Research Note DOT HS 812 072 November 2014.
17. Romano E, Torres-Saavedra P, Voas RB, Lacey JH. Drugs and alcohol: their relative crash risk. J Stud Alcohol Drugs. 2014;75:56–64.
18. Romano E, Torres-Saavedra P, Voas RB, Lacey JH. Marijuana and the risk of fatal car crashes: what can we learn from FARS and NRS data? J Prim Prev. 2017;38:315–28.
19. Santaella-Tenorio J, Mauro CM, Wall MM, Kim JH, Cerdá M, Keyes KM, Hasin DS, Galea S, Martins SS. US traffic fatalities, 1985-2014, and their relationship to medical marijuana laws. Am J Public Health. 2017;107:336–42.
20. Aydelotte JD, Brown LH, Luftman KM, Mardock AL, Teixeira PGR, Coopwood B, Brown CVR. Crash fatality rates after recreational marijuana legalization in Washington and Colorado. Am J Public Health. 2017;107(8):1329–31.
21. Liszewski M, Angell T. State cannabis laws: a progress report. National Cannabis Industry Organization. May 2018.
22. Armentano P. The influence of cannabis on psychomotor performance and accident risk. NORML 2018 National Conference, Washington DC, 23 July 2018.
23. Lacey JH, Kelley-Baker T, Berning A, Romano E, Ramirez A, Yao J, Moore C, Brainard K, Carr K, Pell K, Compton R. Drug and alcohol crash risk: a case-control study. Dec 2016. DOT HS 812 355 NHTSA.
24. Compton RP, Berning A. Drug and alcohol crash risk. NHTSA Traffic Safety Facts Research Note DOT HS 812 117.
25. https://www.usatoday.com/story/college/2015/02/17/new-study-shows-no-link-between-mar ijuana-use-and-car-accidents/37400707/. Accessed 1 Mar 2019.
26. https://www.factcheck.org/2017/12/sessions-wrong-drugged-driving/. Accessed 1 Mar 2019.
27. Longo MC, Hunter CE, Lokan RJ, White JM, White MA. The prevalence of alcohol, cannabinoids, benzodiazepines and stimulants amongst injured drivers and their role in driver culpability. Accid Anal Prev. 2000;32:623–32.
28. Drummer OH, Gerostamoulos J, Batziris H, Chu M, Caplehorn J, Robertson MD, Swann P. The involvement of drugs in drivers of motor vehicles killed in Australian road traffic crashes. Accid Anal Prev. 2004;36:239–48.
29. Laumon B, Gadegbeku B, Martin J-L, Biecheler M-B. Cannabis intoxication and fatal road crashes in France: population based case-control study. BMJ. 2005;331:1371.
30. Biecheler M, Peytavin J, Facy F, Martineau H. SAM survey on drugs and fatal accidents: search of substances consumed and comparison between drivers involved under the influence of alcohol or cannabis. Traffic Inj Prev. 2008;9:11–21.
31. Bédard M, Dubois S, Weaver B. The impact of cannabis on driving. Can J Public Health. 2007;98(1):6–11.

32. Li G, Chihuri S, Brady J. Role of alcohol and marijuana use in the initiation of fatal two-vehicle crashes. Ann Epidemiol. 2017;27:342–7.
33. Schwope DM, Bosker WM, Ramaekers JG, Gorelick DA, Huestis MA. Psychomotor performance, subjective physiological effects and whole blood Δ9 tetrahydrocannabinol concentrations in heavy, chronic cannabis smokers following acute smoked cannabis. J Anal Toxicol. 2012;36(6):405–12.
34. https://www.acmt.net/_Library/2015_Forensic_Course/2_Huestis_-_BW_-_Acute_Chronic_Frequent_Cannibis.pdf. Accessed 1 Mar 2019.
35. Huestis MA. Human cannabinoid pharmacokinetics. Chem Biodivers. 2007;4(8):1770–804.
36. Desrosiers NA, Ramaekers JG, Chaucchard E. Smoked cannabis' psychomotor and neurocognitive effects in occasional and frequent smokers. J Anal Toxicol. 2015;39:251–61.
37. Ramaekers JG, Kauert G, Theunissen EL, Toennes SW, Moeller MR. Neurocognitive performance during acute THC intoxication in heavy and occasional cannabis users. J Psychopharmacol. 2009;23(3):266–77.
38. Grotenhermen F, Müller-Vahl K. The therapeutic potential of cannabis and cannabinoids. Dtsch Arztebl Int. 2012;109(29–30):495–501.
39. Hart CL, van Gorp W, Haney M. Effects of acute smoked marijuana on complex cognitive performance. Neuropsychopharmacology. 2001;25(5):757–65.
40. Ramaekers JG, van Wel JH, Spronk DB. Cannabis and tolerance: acute drug impairment as a function of cannabis use history. Sci Rep. 2016;6:26843.
41. Solowij N. Peering through the haze of smoked vs vaporized cannabis - to vape or not to vape? JAMA Netw Open. 2018;1(7):e1848838.
42. Burns M. The robustness of the horizontal gaze nystagmus test. Sept 2007. US DOT NHTSA DTNH22-98-D-55079.
43. Zador PL, Krawchuck SA, Voas RB. Relative risk of fatal and crash involvement by BAC, age and gender. NHTSA DOT HS 809 050. April 2000.
44. Bui B, Reed J. Driving under the influence of alcohol and drugs. A report pursuant to HB 17-1315. July 2018. Colorado Division of Criminal Justice.
45. Burns M, Anderson E. A colorado validation study of the standardized field sobriety test (SFST) battery. Colorado DOT 95-408-17-05. 1995.
46. Burns M. Dioquino T. A Florida validation study of the standardized field sobriety test (SFST) battery. Floriday DOT AL-97-05-14-01. 1997.
47. Stuster JW, Burns M. Validation of the standardized field sobriety test battery at BACs below 0.10 percent. NHTSA DOT HS 808 839. 1998.
48. Porath-Waller AJ, Beirness DJ. An examination of the validity of the SFST in detecting drug impairment using data from the DEC Program. Traffic Inj Prev. 2014;15(2):125–31.
49. Bosker WM, Theunissen EL, Conen S, Kuypers KPC, Jeffery WK, Walls HC, Kauert GF, Toennes SW, Moeller MR, Ramaekers JG. A placebo-controlled study to assess Standardized Field Sobriety Tests performance during alcohol and cannabis intoxication in heavy cannabis users and accuracy of point of collection testing devices for detecting THC in oral fluid. Psychopharmacology (Berl). 2011;223(4):439–46.
50. Papafotiou K, Carter JD, Stough C. The relationship between performance on the standardized field sobriety tests, driving performance and the level of Δ9-tetrahydrocannabinol (THC) in blood. Forensic Sci Int. 2005;155:172–8.
51. Hartman RL, Richman JE, Hayes CE. Drug Recognition Expert (DRE) examination characteristics of cannabis impairment. Accid Anal Prev. 2016;92:219–29.
52. Bigelow GE, Bickel WE, Roache JD, Liebson IA, Nowowieski P. Identifying types of drug intoxication: laboratory evaluation of a subject-examination procedure. NHTSA DOT HS 806-753 (1985).
53. Compton RP. Field evaluation of the Los Angeles Police Department drug detection program. NHTSA DOT HS 801 012. 1986.
54. Adler EV, Burns M. Drug recognition expert validation study. Arizona Department of Public Safety. 4 June 1994.

55. Hayes C. DU-high: taking a closer look at marijuana impaired driving. IACP webinar. 18 Dec 2018.
56. Flannigan J, Talpins S, Moore C. Oral fluid testing for impaired driving enforcement. The Police Chief. Jan 2017.
57. Namuswe ES, Coleman HL, Berning A. Breath test refusal rates in the United States - 2011 Update. NHTSA DOT HS 811 881. 2014.
58. Bichell RE. Scientists still seek a reliable DUI test for marijuana. NPR. 30 July 2017.
59. Hartman RL, Brown TL, Milavetz G, Spurgin A, Gorelick DA, Gaffney GR, Huestis MA. Effect of blood collection time on measured Δ9-tetrahydrocannabinol concentrations: implications for driving interpretation and drug policy. Clin Chem. 2016;62(2):367–77.
60. Urfer S, Morton J, Beall V, Feldmann J, Gunesch J. Analysis of Δ9-tetrahydrocannabinol driving under the influene of drugs cases in Colorado from January 2011 to February 2014. J Anal Toxicol. 2014;38:575–81.
61. Wood E, Brooks-Russell A, Drum P. Delays in DUI blood testing: impact on cannabis DUI assessments. Traffic Inj Prev. 2016;17(2):105–8.
62. Mura P, Kintz P, Dumestre V, Raui S, Hauet T. THC can be detected in brain while absent in blood. J Anal Toxicol. 2005;29:842–3.
63. Huestis MA. Effects of cannabis with and without alcohol on driving. ACMT Seminars in Forensic Toxicology. Denver, CO, 9 Dec 2015.
64. Logan BK, Kacinko SL, Beirness DJ. An evaluation of data from drivers arrested for DUI in relation to per se limits for cannabis (May 2016) AAA Foundation for Traffic Safety.
65. Declues K, Perez S, Figueroa A. A 2-year study of Δ9-tetrahydrocannbinol concentrations in drivers: examining driving and field sobriety test performance. J Forensic Sci. 2016;64:6.
66. Vandry R, Herrmann ES, Mitchell JM. Pharmacokinetic profile of oral cannabis in humans: blood and oral fluid disposition and relation to pharmacodynamic outcomes. J Anal Toxicol. 2017;41:83–99.
67. http://www.iihs.org/iihs/topics/t/general-statistics/fatalityfacts/overview-of-fatality-facts. Accessed 1 Mar 2019.
68. http://www.alcoholstats.com/wp-content/uploads/2017/12/Drunk-Driving-Trends-full-deck-2017-12-05.pdf. Accessed 1 Mar 2019.
69. Reed J. Impacts of Marijuana Legalization in Colorado. Colorado Department of Public Safety, Division of Criminal Justice. Oct 2018.
70. Dahl D. No, smoking pot will not sober you after drinking- but some drivers think it will. Bellingham Herald Dec 17, (2018); Shelley Baldwin, personal communication. 18 Dec 2018.
71. https://www.heritage.org/public-health/report/the-need-treat-driving-under-the-influence-drugs-seriously-driving-under-the. Accessed 1 Mar 2019.
72. DuPont RL, Holmes EA, Talpins SK, Walsh JM. Marijuana-impaired driving: a path through the controversies. In: Sabet KA, Winters KC, editors. Contemporary health issues on marijuana. New York: Oxford University Press; 2018. p. 183–218.
73. Talpins SK, DuPont RL, Voas RB, Holmes E, Sabet KA, Shea CL. License revocation as a tool for combating drugged driving. Impaired Driving Update. 2014;18(2):29–33.

Chapter 20
The Legal Aspects of Marijuana as Medicine

David G. Evans

This chapter discusses the legal liabilities of those in the medical profession who recommend or distribute marijuana to be used as a medicine. This is commonly known as "medical" marijuana and refers to marijuana that is used for medical purposes under some state laws but has not been approved by the FDA as a medicine.

The "marijuana industry" referred to here are those who illegally, negligently, or fraudulently produce, market, or distribute marijuana. "Illegally" includes being against federal law. The marijuana industry also includes front groups and pro-marijuana lobbying organizations and periodicals, and those seemingly independent third parties, who spread false and deceptive statements about the risks and benefits marijuana. It includes medical care providers and "dispensaries" and caregivers who recommend or distribute marijuana. See U.S. v. Philip Morris USA, Inc., 449 F.Supp.2d 1 (DDC 2006), aff'd in part, vacated in part, 566 F.3d 1095 (DCC 2009)

We use the term "medical care provider" because a physician can recommend marijuana or under some state laws a physician's assistant, nurse, or other professional may be licensed to "recommend" and not prescribe marijuana.

The problem for medical care providers is that most are woefully uninformed or misinformed about marijuana. In 2019, the JAMA online network published an article by Nathanial P. Morris, MD, titled "Educating Physicians About Marijuana." It showed the lack of knowledge among current medical providers about the risks associated with marijuana use. The article demonstrated that just 9% of medical schools had documented content on medical marijuana. A study of 51 resident physicians found that 76% did not know which category marijuana belonged to under

D. G. Evans (✉)
Cannabis Industry Victims Educating Litigators (CIVEL), Flemington, NJ, USA
e-mail: seniorcounsel@civel.org

© Springer Nature Switzerland AG 2020
K. Finn (ed.), *Cannabis in Medicine*,
https://doi.org/10.1007/978-3-030-45968-0_20

515

the Controlled Substances Act. It is a Schedule I drug, signifying a high potential for abuse and no accepted medical uses.[1]

Botanical Marijuana Poses Many Problems for Medical Care Providers

Botanical marijuana products are sold in "dispensaries" under state law. As used herein, the term "botanical marijuana" describes the illicit Schedule I drug that is derived from the leaves and flowering tops of the cannabis plant and is consumed in a variety of ways. The dried plant material is most often rolled in paper and smoked as a cigarette, called a "joint." It is often placed in smoking devices called "bongs," smoked in pipes, or smoked in "blunts," which are cigars from which the tobacco has been removed and replaced with marijuana. Sometimes it is baked in cookies or brownies and eaten, or brewed in tea and drunk. Concentrates such as oils can be derived from botanical marijuana that can also be consumed in many ways such as vaping. Other methods for consuming the drug are constantly being developed by the drug culture.

Botanical marijuana products pose many challenges for medical care providers to include:[2]

1. They are not homogeneous and are not a single or consistent substance.
2. THC content can vary widely depending on the strain, growing techniques, storage, and harvesting and other production practices.
3. The many methods of consumption do not guarantee that a patient will receive an identifiable, standardized, reproducible dose. As a result, patients cannot have certainty they will experience consistent "benefits" or side effects. They may also unwittingly ingest an excessive dose that causes very unpleasant effects.
4. Many sources document that marijuana products often have chemical contamination, pesticides, heavy metals, mold, fungus, and false claims, even in "regulated" marijuana states. Many CBD products have been demonstrated by the FDA to not be pure or safe and many CBD companies have made false medical claims and have misled medical care providers.[3]

---

[1] https://jamanetwork.com/journals/jamainternalmedicine/article-abstract/2734632

Denial of Petition to Initiate Proceedings to Reschedule Marijuana, by the Drug Enforcement Administration (DEA), Department of Justice. 81 FR 53767-01, 2016 WL 4240243 (August 12, 2016)

[2] "Medical Marijuana: Clinical Considerations and Concerns," Richard G. Soper, MD, AZ Medicine, Summer 2011

[3] "Medical Marijuana: Clinical Considerations and Concerns," Ibid

Marcel O. Bonn-Miller, PhD, et al. "Labeling Accuracy of Cannabidiol Extracts Sold Online," Research Letter November 7, 2017. JAMA. 2017;318(17):1708–1709.

§1:20 discussing marijuana contamination. 1 Drug Testing Law Tech. & Prac. Available on Westlaw.

Food and Drug Administration warning letters from 2015 to 2019. 2016 Test Results for Cannabidiol-Related Products, Food and Drug Administration, www.FDA.gov

5. The botanical marijuana distribution system does not equate to the system created by the FDA. Warnings are absent or inadequate, and unqualified non-medical dispensary staff routinely offer medical advice.

6. Medical care providers are in a conflict when it comes to marijuana used a medicine. On one hand, the state laws make them the gatekeepers of a patient's access to botanical marijuana, yet there is not enough reliable scientific information for medical care providers to provide effective advice and monitoring. The states normally do not provide a vehicle for data collection on the safety or efficacy of marijuana or to report adverse events such as required with FDA-approved medicines. As a result, medical care providers do not know if medical conditions are improved by use of marijuana or if there are contraindications or interactions with other drugs the patient is using. A medical care provider should not recommend marijuana when the provider does not have adequate information on the marijuana's composition, dosage, side effects, or what patients are appropriate. This is especially a concern due to the rise in potency of marijuana that heightens the risk of addiction and other side effects such as suicide.

7. People who use high-potency marijuana get intoxicated and that may mask symptoms that prevent the medical care provider and the patient from identifying the progression of their condition and may hinder patients from obtaining more appropriate treatment. Some marijuana products are now 99% THC.[4]

Many production variables influence the strength, quality, and purity of botanical marijuana. THC concentration and other cannabinoids in marijuana can vary greatly depending on growing conditions and the parts of the plant collected (flowers, leaves, stems, etc.), genetics of the plants, and processing. This lack of consistency of concentration of delta 9-THC in botanical marijuana from diverse sources makes the interpretation of clinical data very difficult.[5]

---

[4] Information on a 99% THC product available at: https://www.cannabis-mag.com/2017/03/07/hash-THC-a-crystallin/

Information on marijuana is available at: https://www.drugabuse.gov/publications/drugfacts/marijuana

§1:17.20. Marijuana use on the rise among adults and children and is causing severe damage; §1:17.40 discussing the rise in THC levels in marijuana; § 1:17.62 discussing effects of concentrates on users; § 1:17.80 discussing marijuana overdoses; §1:18 discussing effects of marijuana use, pharmacological, psychological, mental, physiological, and side effects; §1:18.30 discussing marijuana and employer concerns about driving, job performance, and safety; §1:18.60 discussing marijuana and other drug interactions; §1:18.70 discussing workplace and other violence and marijuana; §1:20 discussing marijuana contamination and employees' health; § 1:79 discussing safety and side effects; §1:91 Discussing Glaucoma; §1:87 discussing damage caused by medical marijuana.1 Drug Testing Law Tech. & Prac. Available on Westlaw

[5] The Potential Medical Liability for Physicians Recommending Marijuana as a Medicine, July 2003. Educating Voices, POB 6084, Naperville, IL 60567, www.educatingvoices.org

Vaping and Other Devices for Ingesting or Inhaling Marijuana

Drug paraphernalia such as vaporizers can be used to ingest, inhale, or otherwise introduce "medical" marijuana into the human body. When a medical care provider or dispensary sells or recommends a vaping device for "medical" marijuana, there are FDA issues to consider. This now makes the drug paraphernalia into "medical devices" for the delivery of a medical drug. Medical devices are strictly regulated by the FDA.[6]

The term "device" means an instrument, apparatus, implement, machine, contrivance, implant, in vitro reagent, or other similar or related article, including any component, part, or accessory, which is "intended for use in the diagnosis of disease or other conditions, or in the cure, mitigation, treatment, or prevention of disease, in man or other animals" 21 U.S.C.A. § 321(h)

In order for a vaporizer or other such device to be used, it will have to be approved as a medical device by the FDA. It will also have to be properly labeled under federal law and will have to have adequate directions for use such as mean directions under which the layman can use a device safely and for the purposes for which it is intended. Directions and labeling and approval for use can include:

1. The persons for whose use the device is represented or intended;
2. The conditions of use for the device, including conditions of use prescribed, recommended, or suggested in the labeling or advertising of the device, and other intended conditions of use;
3. The probable benefit to health from the use of the device weighed against any probable injury or illness from such use; and
4. The reliability of the device. 21 C.F.R. § 860.7

Directions for use may be inadequate because, among other reasons, of omission, in whole or in part, or incorrect specification of:

(a) Statements of all conditions, purposes, or uses for which such device is intended, including conditions, purposes, or uses for which it is prescribed, recommended, or suggested in its oral, written, printed, or graphic advertising, and conditions, purposes, or uses for which the device is commonly used; except that such statements shall not refer to conditions, uses, or purposes for which the device can be safely used only under the supervision of a practitioner licensed by law and for which it is advertised solely to such practitioner.

---

[6]21 U.S.C.A. § 321; 21 C.F.R. § 801.4; 21 C.F.R. § 801.5; 21 C.F.R. § 803.3; 21 C.F.R. § 808.3 (definitions and medical device reporting); 21 C.F.R. § 807.93 (Premarket Notification Procedures); 21 C.F.R. § 860.7 (Determination of safety and effectiveness)

For a news story on a vaping death see:

https://www.msn.com/en-us/news/us/oregon-vape-death-patient-used-thc-device-from-dispensary/ar-AAGO1pw

(b) Quantity of dose, including usual quantities for each of the uses for which it is intended and usual quantities for persons of different ages and different physical conditions.
(c) Frequency of administration or application.
(d) Duration of administration or application.
(e) Time of administration or application, in relation to time of meals, time of onset of symptoms, or other time factors.
(f) Route or method of administration or application.
(g) Preparation for use, i.e., adjustment of temperature, or other manipulation or process. See 21 Code of Federal Regulations 801.5.

Since vaping has also caused some deaths and illness, vaping promoted by a marijuana seller or medical care provider could lead to liability or licensing actions or action by the FDA.

Federal Scheduling of Marijuana

"Medical" botanical marijuana that is not approved by the FDA is classified under federal law as a Schedule I drug because: (1) the drug has a high potential for abuse; (2) the drug has no currently accepted medical use in treatment in the United States; and (3) there is a lack of accepted safety for use of the drug under medical supervision. 21 U.S.C. §§ 811, 812(b). Gonzales v. Raich, 545 U.S. 1, 15 (2005).

The DEA and FDA recently decided to keep "medical" marijuana as a Schedule I drug. Elansari v. United States, 2016 WL 4415012 (MD PA 2016); US v. Pickford, 100 F.Supp.3d 981, 1007–1009 (D CA 2015).[7]

Federal Standard of Care

A medical care provider can be liable to a patient, or a third party, for the damaging consequences of violating a standard of care. A medical care provider who recommends marijuana in violation of federal law may face a malpractice claim for recommending a drug for which there is no standard of care or approval under federal

---

[7] "Summary of the Medical Application of Marijuana: a Review of Published Clinical Studies," U.S. FDA Center for Drug Evaluation and Research, 81 FR 53767-01, 2016 WL 4240243 (August 12, 2016); Denial of Petition to Initiate Proceedings to Reschedule Marijuana, by the Drug Enforcement Administration (DEA), Department of Justice. 81 FR 53767-01, 2016 WL 4240243 (August 12, 2016)

law. One court held that "the presence of FDA marketing approval obviously is powerful evidence that a drug has currently accepted medical use and accepted safety for use under medical supervision." John Doe, Inc., v. Drug Enforcement Administration, 484 F.3d 561, 571 (CA DC 2007).

Marijuana products not approved by the FDA may be neither safe nor effective and put patients at risk. 21 U.S.C. § 321 (g)(1) and (p). The FDA has only approved one botanical marijuana product as a medicine, so all of the other medical claims for botanical marijuana should be considered to be false claims under the Food, Drug and Cosmetic Act (FDCA). 21 U.S.C. 321(g)(1) and (p); 21 U.S.C. 331 and 355 (b) (1) (drug must be safe and effective in use).

The federal Controlled Substances Act (CSA) provides that "except as authorized by this subchapter, it shall be unlawful for any person knowingly or intentionally . . . to manufacture, distribute, or dispense, or possess with intent to manufacture, distribute, or dispense, a controlled substance." United States v. Oakland Cannabis Buyers' Cooperative, 532 U.S. 483, 489 (2001) (citing 21 U.S.C. § 841(a)(i)). "Medical" marijuana is a Schedule I controlled substance that cannot be distributed outside of approved research projects and it is illegal for any purpose under federal law even though a number of states have legalized it for medical reasons and several states have decriminalized it for personal use. See also United States v. Dinh, 194 F. Supp. 3d 353, 356–57 (WD PA 2016) ("Despite the Commonwealth of Pennsylvania's enactment of its medical marijuana law, the distribution of marijuana remains illegal under federal law."). Arguments challenging the enforcement of federal marijuana laws have been repeatedly raised and summarily rejected by the courts.

The one botanical cannabinoid approved by the FDA as a medicine is Epidiolex, a pure CBD product. All other botanical marijuana/cannabis products (including CBD) dispensed under state law are illegal under federal law. The FDA has also approved synthetic prescription THC cannabinoids such as Marinol and Syndros for treatment of anorexia associated with weight loss in AIDS patients and chemotherapy-associated nausea.[8]

FDA approval of a medicine is not the only way to decide accepted medical use. A medicine must meet a five-part test:

1. The drug's chemistry must be known and reproducible.
2. There must be adequate studies showing it is safe to use.
3. There should be adequate and well-controlled studies showing proof of efficacy.
4. The use of the drug must be accepted by qualified experts.
5. The scientific evidence for the above must be widely available. Alliance for Cannabis Therapeutics v. DEA, 15 F.3d 1131,1135 (CA DC 1994).

---

[8] Highlights of Prescribing Information, Epidiolex®, www.FDA.gov
http://www.marinol.com

The FDA and the DEA have held that "medical" marijuana has not met these tests. The quality of the studies cited by the marijuana industry for "medical" marijuana does satisfy FDA standards for safety and effectiveness.[9]

Recently, the Commissioner of the FDA stated that:

> Cannabis and cannabis-derived products claiming in their marketing and promotional materials that they're intended for use in the diagnosis, cure, mitigation, treatment, or prevention of diseases (such as cancer, Alzheimer's disease, psychiatric disorders and diabetes) are considered new drugs or new animal drugs and must go through the FDA drug approval process for human or animal use before they are marketed in the U.S. Selling unapproved products with unsubstantiated therapeutic claims is not only a violation of the law, but also can put patients at risk, as these products have not been proven to be safe or effective. This deceptive marketing of unproven treatments raises significant public health concerns, as it may keep some patients from accessing appropriate, recognized therapies to treat serious and even fatal diseases.[10]

Can "Medical" Marijuana Be Prescribed?

Because "medical" marijuana is not approved as a medicine by the FDA, it cannot be prescribed because medical care providers have to follow federal law in writing prescriptions. 21 CFR § 1306.04; Wilcox v. Louisiana State Bd. of Medical Examiners, 446 So.2d 502 (Ct. App. La. 1984). "Medical" marijuana can be "recommended" under the state law, but in practice a prescription and a recommendation are the same. This is fraught with liability

States' Rights

"Medical" marijuana is not a "states' rights" issue. The US Supreme Court has twice upheld as constitutional the application of federal law to the intrastate growth and possession of marijuana for personal medicinal purposes as recommended by a doctor. The Supremacy Clause of the US Constitution unambiguously provides that if there is any conflict between federal and state law, federal law prevails. Gonzales v. Raich, 545 U.S. 1 (2005). See United States v. Oakland Cannabis Buyers' Cooperative, 532 U.S. 483, 490 (2001) (Holding that there is no medical-necessity

---

[9] Denial of Petition to Initiate Proceedings to Reschedule Marijuana, by the Drug Enforcement Administration (DEA), Department of Justice. 81 FR 53767-01, 2016 WL 4240243 (August 12, 2016)

"Summary of the Medical Application of Marijuana: A Review of Published Clinical Studies," U.S. FDA Center for Drug Evaluation and Research, 81 FR 53767-01, 2016 WL 4240243 (August 12, 2016);

[10] Statement from FDA Commissioner Scott Gottlieb, M.D., on signing of the Agriculture Improvement Act and the agency's regulation of products containing cannabis and cannabis-derived compounds. www.fda.gov

exception to federal law prohibitions on manufacturing and distributing marijuana); United States v. Wilde, 74 F.Supp.3d 1092, 1098 (NDCA 2014) (Federal courts have repeatedly rejected constitutional challenges to the classification of marijuana under federal law when applying traditional rational basis review); Kuromiya v. U.S., 37 F. Supp. 2d 717, 725 (EDPA. 1999). (There is no constitutional provision creating a fundamental right to possess, use, grow, or sell marijuana.)

It is indisputable that state "medical" marijuana laws cannot supersede federal laws that criminalize the possession of marijuana. US v. Hicks, 722 F.Supp.2d 829 (ED MI 2010).

Aiding and Abetting

Under some state "medical" marijuana laws, physicians provide written instructions for a registered qualifying patient or his care giver to present to a dispensary concerning the total amount of usable marijuana that a patient may be dispensed. This is far more than just a physician discussing with a patient the use of medical marijuana that may be protected by the First Amendment of the Constitution. This is taking an action to facilitate the use of marijuana. These actions by a physician violate federal law by aiding and abetting by acting with specific intent to provide the patient with the means to acquire marijuana knowing that the patient intends to acquire marijuana. Conant v. Walters, 309 F.3d 629 (CA 9 2002); cert denied Walters v. Conant, 540 U.S. 946 (U.S. Oct 14, 2003)

Legal Claims Against Medical Care Providers

The claims in lawsuits against the tobacco, opiate, and prescription drug industries can be used against the marijuana industry. Examples of the many claims that can be brought are found in Strayhorn v. Wyeth Pharmaceuticals, Inc., 882 F. Supp. 2d 1020 (WD TN 2012).

Malpractice and Negligence

Generally, in order to prevail on a medical malpractice claim, a Plaintiff must prove the following by a preponderance of the evidence:

1. That the Defendants were negligent under the law
2. That such negligence was the legal cause of damage to the Plaintiff[11]

---

[11] Adapted from: Eleventh Circuit, Pattern Jury Instructions, (Civil Cases), 2005; 1.3 Negligence Medical Malpractice Claim Against Hospital and Physician Statute of Limitations Defense; Page 468 http://federalevidence.com/pdf/JuryInst/11th_Civ_2005.pdf

Negligence Basics

Negligence is the failure by the Defendant to use reasonable care. Reasonable care is the degree of care a reasonably careful person would use under similar circumstances. Negligence is either taking an action that a reasonably careful person would not do under similar circumstances, or it is failing to take an action that a reasonably careful person would do under similar circumstances.

In the case of a medical care provider, it is the duty to apply to the diagnosis and treatment of a patient the ordinary skills, means, and methods that are recognized as necessary, and that are customarily followed in the diagnosis and treatment of similar cases, according to the prevailing professional standard of care of reasonably prudent medical care providers who are qualified by training and experience to practice in the same field or specialty in the community or a similar community. In general, medical care providers do not receive any or very little training on "medical" marijuana. There is no standard of care that is generally recognized.

It Can Be Malpractice to Recommend Treatments Not Approved by the FDA[12]

A medical care provider may be civilly liable to his patient, or a third party, for the damaging consequences of recommending marijuana. A physician who assists a patient to obtain marijuana may face a professional negligence claim for recommending a drug for which no standard of care has been adopted and which has an unknown likelihood of future harm.

Medical care providers who recommend "medical" marijuana that is not approved by the FDA should find it very difficult to demonstrate that they have provided good quality care or met the standards of care within accepted medical practice. The problem for these medical care providers is that the necessary medical research on marijuana as a medicine and its effectiveness, risks, benefits, dosages, interactions with other drugs, and impact on pre-existing conditions is not available. The science shows that marijuana is not safe or effective, or studies have not been done, or if studies have been done, marijuana's effect is minimal and the studies are not up to FDA standards. In addition, there may be poor or no quality controls in the manufacturing process for marijuana products many of which are full of contaminants.

Normally medical care providers have relied on the FDA process for approving medicines to protect them from liability should a drug turn out to be unsafe. However, when it comes to marijuana, the burden of proof of safety and

---

[12]The Potential Medical Liability for Physicians Recommending Marijuana as a Medicine, July 2003. Educating Voices, POB 6084, Naperville, IL 60567, www.educatingvoices.org

effectiveness has not been met and the FDA has not approved marijuana. For medical care providers recommending a non-FDA approved medicine drug requires an unsubstantiated guess that "medical" marijuana that is not approved by the FDA will turn out to be safe and effective and not cause "future harm" to the patient.

Informed Consent

A medical care provider must obtain the patient's informed consent before the medical care provider may treat the patient. The medical care provider has a duty to explain, in terms understandable to the patient, what the medical care provider intends to do before subjecting the patient to a course of treatment. The purpose of this legal requirement is to protect each person's right to self-determination in matters of medical treatment. There is also a duty to warn the patient of the risk of marijuana use.

Informed consent consists of:

1. A duty to evaluate the relevant information and disclose all courses of treatment that are medically reasonable under the circumstances. The medical care provider must tell the patient not only about the alternatives that the medical care provider recommends, but also about all medically reasonable alternatives that the medical care provider does not recommend. The medical care provider must discuss all medically reasonable courses of treatment, including non-treatment, and the probable risks and outcomes of each alternative. This is to ensure the patient's right to make an informed choice and effectively makes the choice for the patient.
2. A duty to explain, in words the patient can understand, all material medical information and risks. Medical information or a risk of a medical procedure is material when a reasonable patient in the plaintiff's position would be likely to attach significance to it in deciding whether or not to submit to the treatment.
3. The medical care provider is not required to disclose to the patient all the details of a proposed treatment or all the possible risks, no matter how small or remote. The medical care provider is not required to communicate those dangers known to the average person or those dangers the patient has already discovered. Taking into account what the medical care provider knows or should know to be the patient's need for information, the medical care provider must disclose the medical information and risks which a reasonably prudent patient would consider material or significant in making the decision about what course of treatment, if any, to accept. Such information would generally include a description of the patient's physical condition, the purposes and advantages of the proposed treatment, the material risks of the proposed treatment, and the material risks if such treatment is not provided, as well as the available options or alternatives that are medically reasonable under the circumstances and the advantages and risks of each alternative.[13]

---

[13] NJ-JICIV 5.50C, NJ J.I. CIV 5.50C, New Jersey Model Civil Jury Charges Chapter 5 – Negligence Charges Medical Negligence, 5.50C INFORMED CONSENT (Competent Adult and No Emergency)1,2 Approved 10/2000; revised 3/2002

The problem for medical care providers, hospitals, and marijuana dispensaries is that there is very little good quality scientific information on "medical" marijuana to provide to patients. They are flying blind.

Duty to Warn

A. Inadequate warnings about nonobvious risks that the medical care provider knew or should have known may render a product "defective or unreasonably dangerous." Plaintiffs may have a claim that the marijuana industry fails to warn people about the many acute effects of THC. Medical care providers have a duty to warn the patient about the risks of marijuana use. There are several types of risks from marijuana use that could require warnings:[14]

1. The possibility of a harmful interaction between marijuana and a food, beverage, dietary supplement (including vitamins and herbals), or another drug. Combinations of any of these products could increase the chance that there may be interactions.
2. The chance that marijuana may not work as expected.
3. The possibility that marijuana may cause additional problems such as side effects.
4. The improper use of marijuana edibles.
5. Product dangers such as misrepresenting marijuana as safer than alternatives such as opiates.
6. Adverse incidents such as overdoses, death, mental illness, suicide, etc.
7. Addiction risks and withdrawal from marijuana.
8. The harmful nature of marijuana or its side effects that the medical care provider purposefully or negligently failed to keep informed.
9. There may be health risks associated with the consumption of marijuana.
10. The product is intended for use only by patients of a certain age under state law.
11. The product is unlawful outside the state.
12. There may be additional health risks associated with the consumption of marijuana for women who are pregnant, breast-feeding, or planning on becoming pregnant.
13. The risk of driving or operating heavy machinery while using marijuana.
14. Marijuana and its potency.

---

[14] "Medical Marijuana: Clinical Considerations and Concerns," Richard G. Soper, MD, AZ Medicine, Summer 2011

"Human Performance Drug Fact Sheet, Marijuana," National Highway Traffic Safety Administration

Restatement (Third) of Torts: Prod. Liab. § 2 (1998) (10/2017 update) § 2 Categories of Product Defect

15. The product was produced without regulatory oversight for health, safety, or efficacy.
16. The intoxicating effects of this product may be delayed.

B. State or federal adverse events, warning letters, citations for violations
   If there is evidence of any adverse event reports (AERs) such as citations by a state agency for contamination problems, such evidence could be used to show that the defendants did not take certain steps to ensure their products were safe for consumers. In such cases if they also took no steps to warn, they could have failure-to-warn and design defect claims filed against them. For example, the state of Colorado publishes contamination reports and the FDA issues warning letters.[15]

C. Marijuana use is associated with many health problems, and medical care providers have a duty to warn patients of these risks.

Cancer The California Environmental Protection Agency concluded that marijuana smoking is statistically significantly associated with cancer of the lung, head, and neck, bladder, brain, and testis. Parental marijuana smoking before or during gestation has been statistically significantly associated with childhood cancer.[16]

Heart disease and stroke There is a causal link between marijuana use and strokes and heart attacks. [17]

Hepatocellular (liver) injury CBD can cause liver injury.[18]

---

[15] https://www.colorado.gov/pacific/revenue/search-results?search_api_views_fulltext=MARIJUANA%20PUBLIC%20HEALTH%20AND%20SAFETY%20ADVISORY&f%5B0%5D=og_group_ref%3A98751

   FDA CBD Warning letters

   Available at: https://www.fda.gov/NewsEvents/PublicHealthFocus/ucm484109.htm

[16] Evidence on the Carcinogenicity of Marijuana Smoke, August 2009, California Environmental Protection Agency.

[17] Pot Smoking Linked to Higher Stroke, Heart Risks: Study,16 Mar 2018 09:55 AM

   https://www.newsmax.com/health/health-news/pot-smoking-higher-stroke/2018/03/15/id/848861

   DeFilippis, E. M. et al. "Cocaine and Marijuana Use among Young Adults Presenting with Myocardial Infarction: The Partners YOUNG-MI Registry." J Am Coll Cardiol. 2018. https://doi.org/10.1016/j.jacc.2018.02.047.

   Desai, R. et al. "Recreational Marijuana Use and Acute Myocardial Infarction: Insights from Nationwide Inpatient Sample in the United States." Cureus. 2017;9:e1816. https://doi.org/10.7759/cureus.1816.

   Hackam DG. "Cannabis and Stroke: Systematic Appraisal of Case Reports." Stroke. 2015 Mar;46(3):852–856. https://doi.org/10.1161/STROKEAHA.115.008680.

   Desbois A, Cacoub P. "Cannabis-Associated Arterial Disease." Ann Vasc Surg. 2013 Oct;27(7):996–1005. https://doi.org/10.1016/j.avsg.2013.01.002. Epub 2013 Jul 10.

[18] Highlights of Prescribing Information, Epidiolex®, www.FDA.gov

Chronic vomiting   Studies show that chronic use of marijuana can lead to recurrent bouts of severe nausea, vomiting, and dehydration that can result in kidney failure and/or death.[19]

Addiction   The marijuana industry may claim that marijuana is not addictive but that is not accurate.[20]

Mental Illness and Violence   The use of marijuana can lead to mental illness, acts of suicide, and violence.[21] Marijuana is the number one substance found in suicides of young people in Colorado who are 15–19 years old.[22]

Glaucoma   The use of marijuana products can worsen glaucoma.[23]

Damage to Human Reproduction   Marijuana has been linked to infertility.[24] Low birth weight caused by maternal marijuana use sets the stage for infections and time

---

[19] Galli JA, Sawaya RA, Friedenberg FK. "Cannabinoid Hyperemesis Syndrome." Curr Drug Abuse Rev. 2011;4(4):241–249.

Sorensen CJ, DeSanto K, Borgelt L, Phillips KT, Monte AA. "Cannabinoid Hyperemesis Syndrome: Diagnosis, Pathophysiology, and Treatment-A Systematic Review." J Med Toxicol. 2017;13(1):71–87.

[20] 1:17.30. Marijuana is addictive, 1 Drug Testing Law Tech. & Prac (available on Westlaw)

"Health Effects of Cannabis and Cannabinoids: Current State of Evidence and Recommendations for Research" National Academies of Science

"What is marijuana?" (subchapter "Is marijuana addictive?), National Institute on Drug Abuse, Revised July 2019

Diagnostic and Statistical Manual of Mental Disorders -5, American Psychiatric Association. Cannabis use can create a strong desire and craving to use more and a need to use more to create the same effect. Page 509. There can be withdrawal just like the withdrawal from other addictive drugs. Page 517.

[21] American Psychiatric Association, 2013 "Position Statement on Marijuana as Medicine"

Health Effects of Cannabis and Cannabinoids: Current State of Evidence and Recommendations for Research. National Academies of Science

Berenson, Alex, Tell Your Children: The Truth About Marijuana, Mental Illness, and Violence

U.S. Surgeon General's Advisory: Marijuana Use and the Developing Brain https://www.hhs.gov/surgeongeneral/reports-and-publications/addiction-and-substance-misuse/advisory-on-marijuana-use-and-developing-brain/index.html

[22] Suicides in Colorado: Counts

Colorado Violent Death Reporting Systems https://cohealthviz.dphe.state.co.us/t/HSEBPublic/views/CoVDRS_12_1_17/Story1?:embed=y&:showAppBanner=false&:showShareOptions=true&:display_count=no&:showVizHome=no#4)

[23] Shelton, Beatrice, CBD Oil May Worsen Glaucoma, February 5, 2019, American Academy of Ophthalmology 2019

Marijuana for Glaucoma: Patients Beware! Found at: https://www.glaucomafoundation.org/news_detail.php?id=161

[24] "Marijuana Firmly Linked to Infertility," Scientific American, December 22, 2000

spent in neonatal intensive care.[25] Marijuana use can cause impaired neurodevelopment and other damage from paternal and maternal and fetal exposure to marijuana.[26]

D. The "learned intermediary doctrine"

The "learned intermediary doctrine" applies where manufacturers of unavoidably unsafe products who have a duty to give warnings may reasonably rely on intermediaries such as medical care providers to transmit their warnings and instructions. A medical care provider is a "learned intermediary" only if the medical care provider receives adequate warnings from the manufacturer; thus, the learned intermediary doctrine does not shield a drug manufacturer from liability for inadequate warnings to the physician. A drug manufacturer's duty to give adequate warnings is judged by the effect the warning has on the medical care provider and not the patient. Motus v. Pfizer, Inc., 127 F. Supp. 2d 1085 (C.D. Cal. 2000)

The problem here is that there is not the science on marijuana to be able to provide proper information.

E. Manufacturers' Warnings

Marijuana manufacturer's instructions and warnings can be used to establish a standard of care. For example, the Marinol warnings put medical care providers on notice that it has the potential for harm and must be used only in a controlled manner with dosages regulated and patients subject to monitoring.[27]

Failure to Provide Proper Documentation

A medical care provider must document all aspect of treatment to include:

1. The location and date when the "medical" marijuana was administered
2. All diagnoses that led to the recommendation to use marijuana
3. Detection and treatment of side effects of "medical" marijuana

---

[25] "Study shows prenatal cannabis use associated with low birth weights," Colorado School of Public Health, April 23, 2018

https://www.cuanschutztoday.org/study-shows-prenatal-cannabis-use-associated-with-low-birth-weights/

[26] Volkow ND, Compton WM, Wargo EM. "The Risks of Marijuana Use During Pregnancy." JAMA. 2017;317(2):129–130.

"Marijuana Use During Pregnancy and Lactation," American College of Obstetricians and Gynecologists. https://www.acog.org/Clinical-Guidance-and-Publications/Committee-Opinions/Committee-on-Obstetric-Practice/Marijuana-Use-During-Pregnancy-and-Lactation

U.S. Surgeon General's Advisory: Marijuana Use and the Developing Brain. https://www.hhs.gov/surgeongeneral/reports-and-publications/addiction-and-substance-misuse/advisory-on-marijuana-use-and-developing-brain/index.html

[27] Rheingold, Paul D. "Drug Products Liability and Malpractice Cases," 17 Am. Jur. Trials 1 August 2019 Update

http://www.marinol.com

See also: Highlights of Prescribing Information, Epidiolex®, www.FDA.gov

4. Prior use of marijuana
5. The amount or dose of "medical" marijuana and refills
6. All warnings given[28]

Labeling of Marijuana Used as a Medicine

Some states require some form of labeling, but it does not come close to FDA labeling requirements. At a minimum, information of marijuana should include:

1. Indications and usage
2. Dosage and administration
3. Dosage forms and strengths
4. Contraindications
5. Warnings and precautions
6. Adverse reactions
7. Drug interactions
8. Use in specific populations
9. Drug abuse and dependence
10. Overdosage
11. Description
12. Clinical pharmacology
13. Nonclinical toxicology
14. Clinical studies
15. References
16. How supplied, stored, and handled
17. Patient counseling information[29]

The problem is that this information does not exist for the forms of "medical" marijuana that are sold on the state level.

---

[28] The Potential Medical Liability for Physicians Recommending Marijuana as a Medicine, July 2003. Educating Voices, POB 6084, Naperville, IL 60567, www.educatingvoices.org

[29] Vandrey, R. G., et al. "Cannabinoid Dose and Label Accuracy in Edible Medical Cannabis Products." JAMA. 2015;313(24):2491–2493.

Freedman DA, Patel AD. "Inadequate Regulation Contributes to Mislabeled Online Cannabidiol Products." Pediatr Neurol Briefs. 2018;32:3. Published online 2018 Jun 18. https://doi.org/10.15844/pedneurbriefs-32-3.

FDA "Guidance for Industry, Labelling for Human Prescription Drug and Biological Products - Implementing the PLR Content and Format Requirements

U.S. v. Lane Labs-USA, Inc., 324 F. Supp. 2d 547 (D.N.J. 2004)

Strayhorn v. Wyeth Pharmaceuticals, Inc., 882 F. Supp. 2d 1020 (WD TN 2012).

Apparent Authority

If a hospital or marijuana dispensary uses a medical care provider, the defendant hospital or marijuana dispensary or dispensary may be liable for the medical care provider's negligence under a theory of "apparent authority." Apparent authority arises where a hospital or marijuana dispensary, through its actions, holds out a particular medical care provider as its agent and/or employee in a manner that leads a patient to reasonably believe that the medical care provider is rendering treatment on behalf of the hospital or marijuana dispensary. Thus, liability is determined based on the hospital or marijuana dispensary's actions rather than merely the existence of a contractual relationship. Many marijuana dispensaries are storefronts with a "doctor" inside who gives out recommendations for questionable reasons.[30]

Failure to Conduct a Proper Examination

The state laws permitting marijuana as a medicine often require medical care provider to recommend marijuana for a wide variety of medical conditions often without any documentation or a through medical examination. A medical care provider cannot exercise a competent medical judgment because the medical research does not show that marijuana is safe and effective or what are the proper dosages, interactions with other drugs, or the impact on pre-existing conditions. In addition, if there are already safe and effective drugs that have been approved by the FDA, the use of marijuana is very suspect.[31]

Third-Party Endangerment

A medical care provider can have a duty to protect unidentifiable, unknown third parties, who are endangered by a patient's treatment. Medical care providers can be liable if they fail to warn patients about the possible side effects of marijuana and the patient injures someone in a traffic accident because use of marijuana diminishes physical and mental abilities. Marijuana significantly impairs driving including time and distance estimation and reaction times and motor coordination.[32]

---

[30] NJ-JICIV 5.50, NJ J.I. CIV 5.50, New Jersey Model Civil Jury Charges Chapter 5 - Negligence Charges Medical Negligence, 5.50 Apparent Authority Charge (Approved 6/10)

[31] The Potential Medical Liability for Physicians Recommending Marijuana as a Medicine, July 2003. Educating Voices, POB 6084, Naperville, IL 60567, www.educatingvoices.org

[32] Ibid.

Loss of a Chance Doctrine

The "loss of a chance" doctrine applies when a medical care provider fails to diagnose an illness and the delay in treatment reduces the plaintiff's chances of survival. Use of marijuana instead of conventional treatment could also cause a loss of a chance to get well when a patient tells a medical care provider an anecdotal story of relief and cure provided by use of marijuana and requests treatment by marijuana. This all too frequent situation puts medical care providers in the position of accepting the self-diagnosis of the patient, thus missing the correct diagnosis and delaying proper treatment and possibly putting the medical care provider at risk of future lawsuits by patients or their families.[33]

Aggravation (Exacerbation) of a Pre-existing Condition

In the case of marijuana, its toxic and other negative effects can possibly cause an aggravation of a pre-existing condition. Examples are AIDS, glaucoma, and seizures. The aggravation of a pre-existing ailment or medical condition can be a separate element of compensable damages.[34]

Future Harm

Medical care providers can also be liable for causing future harm to a patient. Use of marijuana, particularly high potency marijuana, can cause a variety of harms.[35]

It is clear that use of marijuana can cause future harm or injury and cause fear for a plaintiff that such an injury may materialize in the future. Science shows that marijuana affects the reproductive process, damages unborn children, has more carcinogens than tobacco, is addictive, and is often a precursor drug to the use of other substances and many other harms. The use of marijuana and the later development of serious illnesses have many "future harm" implications as is the case with the use of tobacco.[36]

---

[33] Ibid.
[34] Ibid.
[35] Ibid.
[36] Ibid.

Emotional Distress: Intentional and Unintentional

Depending on state law, there may be emotional distress claims. These can be claimed in some cases even if there is no physical injury such as emotional distress based on a reasonable fear of an enhanced risk of disease if that fear was proximately caused by the negligent conduct of the medical care provider.

Respondeat Superior/Vicarious Liability

A hospital can be held liable under the theories of respondeat superior for the negligence of its pharmacy, marijuana dispensary, hospital medical care providers, nurses, and other staff. This may not apply to medical personnel who are not on the hospital staff. Hospitals may be liable if they use marijuana under any of these circumstances without federal approval:

1. Allowing a federally controlled substance such as marijuana to be used in violation of federal law.
2. Failing to educate medical care providers on marijuana and its dangers and side effects and proper use and dosage under state law. There is no proper use and dosage under federal law.
3. A failure to stop a medical care provider who is giving a wrong dose of marijuana or causing addiction.
4. Failure to consult with experts in a particular area of treatment.
5. If the hospital supplied marijuana, they could be sued for breach of warranty for any injuries because the hospital is a supplier of marijuana.
6. Lack of informed consent to use marijuana which is an unapproved medicine.
7. Medical experimentation with marijuana.[37]

Other Claims

There are a number of other possible malpractice claims medical care providers should be aware of:

1. Failing to detect or treat marijuana's side effects
2. Failing to keep up on the science on marijuana
3. Failing to be aware of contraindications to marijuana use
4. Failing to have a bona fide physician-patient relationship

---

[37] Rheingold, Paul D. "Drug Products Liability and Malpractice Cases," 17 Am. Jur. Trials 1 August 2019 Update

5. Allowing the patient to become addicted to marijuana
6. Failing to use alternative safer FDA-approved medical treatments
7. Failing to properly monitor the patient who is using marijuana
8. Failing to properly to dose marijuana. Deriving a standardized botanical dose poses major difficulties – especially with marijuana when there are widely varying strains and large numbers of marijuana components about which little is yet known

Loss of Malpractice Insurance

Medical care providers should check to see if their malpractice insurance covers them when recommending or being involved in dispensing "medical" marijuana.[38]

Conclusion

The use of "medical" marijuana as a medicine that has not been approved by the FDA is fraught with liability for medical care providers, especially when there are FDA approved medications that should be tried first. Lawsuits and loss of licenses could be the result.

Disclaimer of Legal Advice   This chapter should not be considered legal advice. This is for informational purposes only. Use of and access to these materials does not in itself create an attorney–client relationship between David G. Evans and CIVEL and the user or reader. Mr. Evans or CIVEL cannot vouch for any study cited herein since they did not do the study. The readers should consult the study and make their own interpretation as to its accuracy. Please also be advised that case law and statutory and regulatory laws cited herein may have been amended or changed by the time you read this. In addition, each state has laws that differ from other states. What may be true in one state may not be true in another. Federal law may also differ from state law. Please consult an attorney licensed in your state for legal advice.

David G. Evans, Esq., is Senior Counsel for the Cannabis Industry Victims Educating Litigators (CIVEL) who educate lawyers on how to make the marijuana industry accountable to their many victims. Mr. Evans was a plaintiffs' litigator in personal injury and employment law cases. Attorneys who desire more information can contact Mr. Evans at seniorcounsel@civel.org. The CIVEL website is: www.civel.org

---

[38] The Potential Medical Liability for Physicians Recommending Marijuana as a Medicine, July 2003. Educating Voices, POB 6084, Naperville, IL 60567, www.educatingvoices.org

Epilogue: The Medical Cannabis Landscape

Thida Thant and Paula Riggs

Clinical Implications of Expanding Cannabis Legalization

As of October 2019, more than 4/5 of states in the United States have legalized medical marijuana and more than 2/3 of these have legalized recreational use [1]. In the ever-expanding legalized cannabis environment, medical clinicians are struggling to better understand the clinical implications and health effects of cannabis in a growing number of patients. It is important to highlight that legalization of medical cannabis preceded the movement toward recreational cannabis legalization. It is also important to highlight that in medically legalized states, the approved indications or medical conditions for which cannabis could be legally used were not sanctioned by the medical community, because the safety and efficacy of cannabis for these conditions had not been established by the scientifically rigorous standards required for FDA approval. As a result, most medical clinicians in traditional practice settings lack training, education, and scientific knowledge about cannabis or its potential medicinal uses. This volume seeks to address these gaps. Given the growing number of individuals using cannabis for medical and recreational purposes, it is now essential for clinicians to be aware of current research on the health effects of cannabis and continue to track ongoing research advances in our scientific understanding of the risks potential benefit of cannabinoids.

The expanding cannabis legalization landscape is historically unprecedented, in that the federal government has granted individual states the authority to

T. Thant
Department of Psychiatry, The University of Colorado School of Medicine, Aurora, CO, USA
e-mail: Thida.thant@cuanschutz.edu

P. Riggs
Faculty Affairs, Division of Substance Dependence, Department of Psychiatry, University of Colorado School of Medicine, Aurora, CO, USA
e-mail: Paula.riggs@cuanschutz.edu

© Springer Nature Switzerland AG 2020   535
K. Finn (ed.), *Cannabis in Medicine*,
https://doi.org/10.1007/978-3-030-45968-0

legislatively legalize the medical use of a substance (cannabis) classified as Schedule 1 by the Food and Drug Administration (FDA). Schedule 1 drugs are defined as substances with no accepted medical use in the United States, a lack of accepted safety for use under medical supervision and a high potential for abuse.

In states that have legalized medical cannabis, state legislatures can approve the use of cannabis for specific medical conditions without the rigorous scientific support for medication safety and efficacy, dosage, or purity standards required for FDA-approved medications. Moreover, specific medical conditions that are approved as indications for medical cannabis vary state by state and are often based in part on anecdotal testimonies and endorsements by individual users and industry advocates at public hearings without the endorsement or approval of professional medical societies or regulatory boards. For example, at least three states have approved post-traumatic stress disorder (PTSD) as an approved condition or indication for medical cannabis without supporting evidence from even a single randomized controlled trial.

This chapter first provides a brief historical overview of cannabis legalization in the United States. This is followed by relevant highlights from current and emerging research in this volume and public health data from bell-weather states that were among the first to legalize medical and recreational cannabis. Taken together, this provides a scientifically grounded early signal and snapshot of the potential public health impact of ongoing national expansion cannabis legalization in the United States and begins to address what clinicians need to know about the health risks and potential benefits of cannabinoids.

Medical Cannabis: Recent History in the United States

The first medical cannabis program in the United States started in California in 1996. Since then, an increasing number of medical cannabis programs have opened with great variation in requirements and regulations [2, 3] with at least 33 states and DC participating in medical cannabis as of July 2019 [4]. In Colorado alone, medical cannabis sales went from $32.5 million in the first month after legalization in 2014 to almost $417 million in 2017 [5]. As of July 2019, it is estimated that there are more than three million medical cannabis users in the United States [4, 6].

Despite the proliferation of medical cannabis programs, little research exists to guide or inform policies and practice structure, and there is broad variability in regulatory requirements and medical cannabis licensing procedures [7, 8]. Programs range from utilizing dispensary-affiliated physicians certifying patients simply based on outside clinic records and patient self-report to a handful requiring their physicians to undergo state-based licensing or training prior to participating in medical cannabis clinics.

Medically oriented programs (those requiring bona fide physician-patient relationships, time-limited refills, links to state prescription monitoring programs, physician certification/training) are more likely to have been passed by state legislatures rather than by voter initiatives (90% vs 28.6%) and are more likely to have been passed in recent years [2].

Many states list similar qualifying conditions for medical cannabis the most common of which include cancer, HIV/AIDS, glaucoma, Hep C, chronic pain, muscle spasms, and spinal cord injuries (Table 1). While there is some scientific evidence supporting the use of medical cannabis for these conditions, the weight of evidence falls far short of the rigorous research and safety requirements required for FDA approval of conventional pharmaceuticals. Additionally, most legalized states allow the state health department to add conditions and some, including D.C. allow medical marijuana to be used for "any condition for which treatment with medical cannabis would be beneficial, as determined by the patient's physician" or as recently added in Colorado "any conditions for which a physician could prescribe an opioid."

Medical Cannabis Users: Who, Why, and How?

In most states, individuals must be evaluated and approved by a licensed physician to use medical cannabis for a specific indicated condition, after which similarities to traditional medical models of treatment and patient care disappear. First, most cannabis products do not meet standards for what can be classified as a "medication": impure with multiple contaminants; cannabinoids and other ingredients about which little is known; unstandardized dosages. Second, physician prescriptions are not required or applicable: physicians cannot write a prescription: refills, doses, and amount dispensed are usually not regulated or tracked through mechanisms such as prescription drug monitoring databases. In fact, physicians can only "recommend" medical marijuana in most states and are not required to undergo specific training or to provide evidence for their recommendations. Medical cannabis patients generally receive information about various cannabis product variants: dose, route of administration (edibles, vaping, smoked), and usage indications from nonmedically or pharmaceutically trained medical cannabis dispensary employees without any standardized training or certification requirements. The amount of medical cannabis used in terms of dose and frequency is entirely unregulated and unmonitored as are potential adverse effects, interactions with other medications, and contraindicated medical conditions.

Little is known about patterns of cannabis use in chronic medical illness other than reported indications. Gross et al. studied 136 epilepsy patients in a tertiary care epilepsy center and found that 21% of subjects had used cannabis in the past year [9]. Furler et al. studied 104 HIV patients and found that 43% reported any cannabis use, 29% reported medical use, and that 80% of medical users also reported recreational cannabis use [10]. Clark et al. found that in a small group of 34 multiple sclerosis medical cannabis users – almost 12% reported daily use, 23% reported use more than once per day, and 20% used once weekly [11]. They also found that medical cannabis use was associated with male gender, tobacco use, and recreational cannabis use.

Table 1 Summary of current approved conditions for adults by state with evidence stratification

Indications for medical cannabis enrollment stratified by clinical evidence level			
State	Moderate to strong	Mixed/limited	Little to none
Alaska	Severe pain related to cancer, spasticity related to MS	Severe nausea (HIV/AIDS), cachexia, seizures	Glaucoma, "any chronic or debilitating disease or treatment for such diseases, which produces conditions that may be alleviated by the medical use of marijuana"
Arizona	Severe pain related to cancer, spasticity related to MS and ALS	Severe nausea (HIV/AIDS), cachexia, seizures	Alzheimer's disease, HCV, glaucoma, ALS, Crohn's disease, PTSD
Arkansas	Cancer, severe and persistent muscle spasms	HIV/AIDS, a chronic or debilitating disease or medical condition or its treatment that produces one or more: cachexia/ wasting syndrome, peripheral neuropathy, intractable pain, severe nausea, seizures including without limitation of those characteristic of epilepsy	Glaucoma, HCV, ALS, Tourette's syndrome, Crohn's disease, ulcerative colitis, Alzheimer's disease, PTSD, severe arthritis, fibromyalgia
California	Severe pain related to cancer, spasticity related to MS	Severe nausea (AIDS), cachexia, anorexia, seizures	Glaucoma, arthritis, migraine, "other chronic or persistent medical symptoms"
Colorado	Severe pain related to cancer, spasticity related to MS	Severe nausea (HIV/AIDS), cachexia, anorexia	Glaucoma, seizures, PTSD, autism spectrum disorder, any condition for which opioids could be prescribed to treat

Connecticut	Severe pain related to cancer, spasticity related to MS, spinal cord injury with objective evidence, uncontrolled intractable seizure disorder	HIV/AIDS, cachexia, seizures	Glaucoma, Parkinson's disease, PTSD, Crohn's disease, PTSD, sickle cell disease, post-laminectomy syndrome with chronic radiculopathy, severe psoriasis, psoriatic arthritis, ALS, ulcerative colitis, complex regional pain syndrome, cerebral palsy, cystic fibrosis, neuropathic pain associated with fibromyalgia, severe rheumatoid arthritis, postherpetic neuralgia, hydrocephalus with intractable headache, intractable headache syndromes, neuropathic facial pain, muscular dystrophy, osteogenesis imperfecta, chronic neuropathic pain associated with degenerative spinal disorders, terminal illness requiring end-of-life care
Delaware	Severe pain related to cancer, spasticity related to MS, intractable epilepsy	Severe nausea (HIV/AIDS), cachexia, seizures	Alzheimer's disease, ALS, HCV, decompensated cirrhosis, PTSD, autism with aggressive behavior, glaucoma, chronic debilitating migraine, terminal illness
Florida	Severe pain related to cancer, spasticity related to MS	HIV/AIDS	Epilepsy, glaucoma, PTSD, ALS, Crohn's disease, Parkinson's disease, chronic nonmalignant pain, a terminal condition
Hawaii	Severe pain related to cancer, spasticity related to MS	Severe nausea (HIV/AIDS), cachexia, seizures	Glaucoma, Crohn's disease, ALS, glaucoma, lupus, epilepsy, rheumatoid arthritis, PTSD
Illinois	Severe pain related to cancer, spasticity related to MS, myoclonus, spinocerebellar ataxia, dystonia, muscular dystrophy, and spinal cord injury or disease	HIV/AIDS, cachexia, Tourette syndrome	Glaucoma, ALS, Alzheimer's disease, HCV, Parkinson's disease, Tarlov cysts, hydromyelia/syringomyelia, fibrous dysplasia, TBI and postconcussion syndrome, Arnold-Chiari malformation and syringomyelia, neurofibromatosis, Sjoren's syndrome, lupus, interstitial cystitis, hydrocephalus, myasthenia gravis, nail-patella syndrome, chronic inflammatory demyelinating polyneuropathy, Crohn's disease, complex regional pain syndrome, dystonia, PTSD, reflex sympathetic dystrophy. Alternative to opiate treatment, terminal illness with life expectancy of less than 6 months, neuropathic pain, severe pain (including severe fibromyalgia and rheumatoid arthritis)

(continued)

Table 1 (continued)

Indications for medical cannabis enrollment stratified by clinical evidence level			
State	Moderate to strong	Mixed/limited	Little to none
Louisiana	Cancer, spasticity related to MS	HIV/AIDS, cachexia/wasting syndrome, seizure disorders	Crohn's disease, muscular dystrophy, glaucoma, Parkinson's disease, intractable pain, PTSD, four conditions associated with autism spectrum disorder
Maine	Cancer, spasticity related to MS	Severe nausea (AIDS), HIV/AIDS, cachexia/wasting syndrome, seizures	Glaucoma, hepatitis C, ALS, Crohn's disease, Alzheimer's, nail-patella syndrome, chronic intractable pain
Maryland	Severe pain, spasticity related to MS	Severe nausea (HIV/AIDS), cachexia/wasting syndrome, anorexia, seizures	Chronic pain, glaucoma, PTSD, "or another chronic medical condition which is severe and for which other treatments have been ineffective"
Massachusetts	Cancer, spasticity related to MS	HIV/AIDS	Glaucoma, ALS, HCV, Parkinson's disease, Crohn's disease, "other conditions as determined in writing by a qualifying patient's physician"
Michigan	Severe pain related to cancer, spasticity related to MS	Severe nausea (HIV/AIDS), cachexia, seizures	Glaucoma, HCV, Crohn's disease, Alzheimer's disease, PTSD, nail-patella syndrome, arthritis, autism, chronic pain, colitis, IBD, OCD, Parkinson's, rheumatoid arthritis, spinal cord injury, Tourette's syndrome, ulcerative colitis
Minnesota	Severe pain related to cancer, spasticity related to MS	HIV/AIDS, Tourette syndrome, cachexia/severe wasting, severe nausea, seizures	Glaucoma, ALS, Crohn's disease, terminal illness with a life expectancy of <12 months, chronic pain, PTSD, intractable pain, autism spectrum disorders, OSA, terminal illness with a life expectancy of under 1 year

Missouri	Severe pain related to cancer, spasticity related to MS	HIV/AIDS, cachexia/wasting syndrome, seizures	Glaucoma, intractable migraines, Parkinson's disease, Tourette's syndrome, PTSD, chronic medical condition normally treated with a prescription medication that could lead to physical or psychological dependence, any other condition in the professional judgment of a physician such as HCV, ALS, IBD, Crohn's, Huntington's, autism, neuropathies, sickle cell anemia, Alzheimer's, terminal illness
Montana	Severe pain related to cancer, spasticity related to MS	Severe nausea (HIV/AIDS), cachexia/wasting syndrome, seizures	Glaucoma, Crohn's disease, painful peripheral neuropathy, PTSD, admittance to hospice care
Nevada	Severe pain related to cancer, spasticity related to MS	Severe nausea (HIV/AIDS), cachexia, seizures	Glaucoma, PTSD, severe pain, PTSD
New Hampshire	Severe pain related to cancer, spasticity related to MS, muscular dystrophy, spinal cord injury or disease	Severe nausea (HIV/AIDS), cachexia, anorexia, seizures	Glaucoma and elevated intraocular pressure, ALS, HCV, Crohn's disease, Alzheimer's disease, TBI, chronic pancreatitis, one or more injuries that significantly interferes with daily activities as documented by the patient's provider, PTSD, severe chronic pain
New Jersey	Severe pain related to cancer, spasticity related to MS, muscular dystrophy	Severe nausea (HIV/AIDS), cachexia, seizures	Glaucoma, ALS, IBD, terminal illness (physician-determined prognosis of <12 months of life), anxiety, chronic pain, dysmenorrhea, muscular dystrophy, opioid use disorder, PTSD, terminal illness with prognosis of less than 12 months to live, Tourette's syndrome
New Mexico	Severe pain related to cancer, spasticity related to MS, cervical dystonia, spinal cord injury, neuropathic pain	Severe nausea (HIV/AIDS), cachexia, anorexia, seizures	Glaucoma, ALS, HCV currently receiving antiviral treatment, Parkinson's disease, PTSD, Huntington's disease, inflammatory autoimmune-mediated arthritis, hospice care, inclusion body myositis, painful peripheral neuropathy, Parkinson's disease, PTSD, severe chronic pain, spasmodic torticollis, ulcerative colitis
New York	Severe pain related to cancer, spasticity related to MS, spinal cord injury, neuropathic pain	HIV/AIDS, cachexia/wasting syndrome, intractable nausea, seizures	ALS, Parkinson's disease, IBD, HCV, Huntington's disease, PTSD, "pain that degrades health and functional capability where the use... is an alternative to opioid use" and substance use disorder treatment

(continued)

Table 1 (continued)

Indications for medical cannabis enrollment stratified by clinical evidence level			
State	Moderate to strong	Mixed/limited	Little to none
North Dakota	Severe pain related to cancer, intractable spasticity	HIV/AIDS, seizures	HCV, ALS, PTSD, Alzheimer's disease, dementia, Crohn's disease, fibromyalgia, spinal stenosis or chronic back pain, glaucoma, severe debilitating pain that has not responded to previously prescribed medication or surgical measures for more than 3 months or for which other treatment options produced serious side effects
Ohio	Severe pain related to cancer	AIDS/HIV, seizures	Alzheimer's disease, ALS, chronic traumatic encephalopathy, Crohn's disease, fibromyalgia, glaucoma, HCV, IBD, chronic pain, Parkinson's disease, PTSD, sickle cell anemia, spinal cord injury, Tourette's syndrome, traumatic brain injury, ulcerative colitis
Oklahoma			"A medical marijuana license must be recommended to the accepted standards a reasonable and prudent physician would follow when recommending or approving any medication"
Oregon	Severe pain related to cancer, spasticity related to MS	Severe nausea (HIV/AIDS), cachexia, seizures	Glaucoma, degenerative or pervasive neurological condition, PTSD
Pennsylvania	Intractable spasticity	HIV/AIDS, intractable seizures, seizures	ALS, anxiety disorders, autism, Crohn's disease, dyskinetic and spastic movement disorders, glaucoma, Huntington's disease, IBD, neurodegenerative diseases, neuropthies, opioid use disorder for which conventional therapeutic interventions are contraindicated or ineffective, Parkinson's disease, PTSD, chronic or intractable neuropathic pain, sickle cell anemia, terminal illness, Tourette syndrome
Rhode Island	Severe pain related to cancer, spasticity related to MS	Severe nausea (HIV/AIDS), cachexia, seizures	Glaucoma, HCV, Crohn's disease, Alzheimer's disease

Utah	Severe pain related to cancer, spasticity related to MS	HIV/AIDS, cachexia, seizures	Alzheimer's disease, ALS, persistent nausea, Crohn's disease, ulcerative colitis, autism, terminal illness with life expectancy of 6 months or less, hospice care, rare condition or disease that affects fewer than 200,000 individuals in the United States, pain
Vermont	Severe pain related to cancer, spasticity related to MS	Severe nausea (HIV/AIDS), cachexia/wasting syndrome, seizures	Glaucoma, chronic pain, Parkinson's disease, Crohn's disease, PTSD
Washington	Severe pain related to cancer (unrelieved by standard treatment), spasticity related to MS	Severe nausea (HIV/AIDS), cachexia, anorexia, seizures	Glaucoma, HCV, Crohn's disease, chronic renal failure requiring hemodialysis, intractable pain, PTSD, traumatic brain injury
Washington D.C.	Severe pain related to cancer, spasticity related to MS	Severe nausea (HIV/AIDS), seizures	Glaucoma, patients undergoing chemotherapy or radiotherapy, using azidothymidine or protease inhibitors, decompensated cirrhosis, ALS, Alzheimer's disease
West Virginia	Spasticity	Cachexia/wasting syndrome, anorexia, severe nausea, seizures	Hospice or receiving palliative care, severe or chronic pain, refractory generalized anxiety disorder, PTSD

aUpdated through October 2019
Refs. [2, 4, 18–20]

Who Are Medical Cannabis Patients?

In Colorado, medical cannabis patients tend to be men (61% vs 38% women) in their early 40s [12]. A study of 9 Californian medical cannabis assessment clinics also found a predominance of men (almost 80% vs 27%) with most ages spanning 25–54 years old [13].

Young adult medical cannabis patients in Los Angeles, California, reported greater mean days of cannabis use (76.4%) compared to young adult non-medical cannabis patient users with approximately one quarter of both medical and non-medical cannabis users reporting diversion of dispensary cannabis [14].

A Michigan medical cannabis clinic found frequent reports of lifetime cannabis use in all participants (96% of 331 patients) with 61% reporting daily or almost daily use (76% for patients renewing their medical cannabis card vs 51% for first-time card registrants) [15]. Additionally, returning medical cannabis patients reported a higher prevalence of lifetime illicit substance use, primarily cocaine, amphetamine, inhalant, and hallucinogens. Many states continue to explore how to track people using medical marijuana – Washington state, despite creation of a medical marijuana program in 1998, only passed legislation creating a voluntary patient database in 2015 [16].

Literature on patterns of use in chronic medical illness patients is even sparser. Based on available data, most patients present for pain [12, 13, 15, 17]. Other studies find patients also tend to use medical cannabis for sleep, stress, mood, muscle spasm, appetite stimulation, and weight gain [10, 11].

Despite the minimal clinical evidence for numerous medical cannabis indications such as glaucoma, PTSD, depression, inflammation/chronic infection, autism (Table 1), studies report anywhere from 1% to 15% of patients reporting medical cannabis use for these indications [12, 13, 15].

While we have a better sense of who uses cannabis (and even why) and the twisted path the industry took to arrive in its current form, a frightening number of gaps in our understanding of cannabis remain. We highlight these gaps in our book, not to emulate the "Reefer Madness" claims of the past but to remind the medical community and the public that when it comes to cannabis the cart was most certainly placed before the horse. It is not too late to improve the knowledge of ourselves and our patients, and clinicians should receive more education about cannabis and its use, potencies, strains, risks, and benefits. The confusion among ourselves is clear, and if you review Table 1 it becomes apparent that different US states are also struggling with how to manage the medical cannabis era. Some stick with the classic indications of pain (yet another indication for which evidence is lacking with dispensary cannabis), seizures, glaucoma, and GI symptoms, while others have thrown the gates wide open to any and all comers regardless of current evidence (or lack thereof). In such times, we hope volumes such as this can act as a compass and provide guidance to all of us navigating this new landscape. As Dr. Murray pointed out in his prologue, the nationwide experiment with cannabis is underway and leading us toward a future of unanticipated (and already seeded) consequences.

References

1. DISA. Map of Marijuana Legality by State [Internet]. [cited 2019 Nov]. Available from: https://disa.com/map-of-marijuana-legality-by-state.
2. Compton MT. Marijuana and mental health. Arlington: American Psychiatric Association Publishing; 2016.
3. Pacula RL, Sevigny EL. Marijuana liberalization policies: why we cant learn much from policy still in motion. J Policy Anal Manage. 2013;33(1):212–21.
4. Should Marijuana be a medical option? [Internet]. Should marijuana be a medical option? [cited 2019 Jul]. Available from: https://medicalmarijuana.procon.org/.
5. Marijuana Sales Reports. Colorado Department of Revenue, Office of Research and Analysis. 2019.
6. Project MP. Marijuana policy project: we change laws [Internet]. MPP. [cited 2019Jul]. Available from: https://www.mpp.org/.
7. Sevigny EL, Pacula RL, Heaton P. The effects of medical marijuana laws on potency. Int J Drug Policy. 2014;25(2):308–19.
8. Wilkinson ST, D'Souza DC. Problems with the medicalization of marijuana. JAMA. 2014;311(23):2377–8.
9. Gross DW, Hamm J, Ashworth NL, Quigley D. Marijuana use and epilepsy: Prevalence in patients of a tertiary care epilepsy center. Neurology. 2004;62(11):2095–7.
10. Furler MD, Einarson TR, Millson M, Walmsley S, Bendayan R. Medicinal and recreational marijuana use by patients infected with HIV. AIDS Patient Care STDs. 2004;18(4):215–28.
11. Clark AJ, Ware MA, Yazer E, Murray TJ, Lynch ME. Patterns of cannabis use among patients with multiple sclerosis. Neurology. 2004;62(11):2098–100.
12. Medical Marijuana Registry Program Statistics October 2019.
13. Reinarman C, Nunberg H, Lanthier F, Heddleston T. Who are medical marijuana patients? Population characteristics from nine California assessment clinics. J Psychoactive Drugs. 2011;43(2):128–35.
14. Lankenau SE, Fedorova EV, Reed M, Schrager SM, Iverson E, Wong CF. Marijuana practices and patterns of use among young adult medical marijuana patients and non-patient marijuana users. Drug Alcohol Depend. 2017;170:181–8.
15. Ilgen MA, Bohnert K, Kleinberg F, Jannausch M, Bohnert AS, Walton M, et al. Characteristics of adults seeking medical marijuana certification. Drug Alcohol Depend. 2013;132(3):654–9.
16. History of Washington State Marijuana Laws [Internet]. History of Washington State Marijuana Laws. National Conference of State Legislatures; Available from: http://www.ncsl.org/documents/summit/summit2015/onlineresources/wa_mj_law_history.pdf.
17. Medical Marijuana Registry Program Statistics June 2019.
18. Whiting PF, Wolff RF, Deshpande S, Nisio MD, Duffy S, Hernandez AV, et al. Cannabinoids for medical use. JAMA. 2015;313(24):2456–73.
19. Hill KP. Medical marijuana for treatment of chronic pain and other medical and psychiatric problems. JAMA. 2015;313(24):2474–83.
20. The health effects of cannabis and cannabinoids: the current state of evidence and recommendations for research. Washington, DC: the National Academies Press; 2017.

Index

© Springer Nature Switzerland AG 2020
K. Finn (ed.), *Cannabis in Medicine*,
https://doi.org/10.1007/978-3-030-45968-0

The manufacturer's authorised representative in the EU is Springer
Nature Customer Service Centre GmbH, Europaplatz 3, 69115 Heidelberg,
Germany. If you have any concerns regarding our products, please
contact ProductSafety@springernature.com

Printed and bound by CPI Group (UK) Ltd, Croydon, CR0 4YY
24/04/2026
02096309-0003